CALCIUM ENTRY AND
ACTION AT THE PRESYNAPTIC
NERVE TERMINAL

ANNALS OF THE NEW YORK ACADEMY OF SCIENCES
Volume 635

CALCIUM ENTRY AND ACTION AT THE PRESYNAPTIC NERVE TERMINAL

Edited by Elis F. Stanley, Martha C. Nowycky, and David J. Triggle

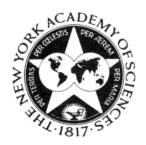

The New York Academy of Sciences
New York, New York
1991

Library of Congress Cataloging-in-Publication Data

Calcium entry and action at the presynaptic nerve terminal / edited by
    Elis F. Stanley, Martha C. Nowycky, and David J. Triggle.
      p.   cm. — (Annals of the New York Academy of Sciences, ISSN
0077-8923; v. 635)
    Result of a conference held in Baltimore, Md., on Oct. 15–17,
1990, by the New York Academy of Sciences.
    Includes bibliographical references and index.
    ISBN 0-89766-685-2 (cloth: alk. paper). — ISBN 0-89766-686-0
(paper: alk. paper)
    1. Synapses—Congresses.   2. Calcium channels—Congresses.
3. Calcium—Physiological effect—Congresses.   4. Neurotransmitters—
    Secretion—Congresses.   I. Stanley, Elis F.   II. Nowycky, Martha
C.   III. Triggle, D. J.   IV. New York Academy of Sciences.
V. Series.
    [DNLM: 1. Calcium—pharmacology—congresses.   2. Calcium Channels—
physiology—congresses.   3. Nerve Endings—physiology—congresses.
4. Receptors, Synaptic—physiology—congresses.   W1 An626YL   v. 635
/ WL 102.9 C144 1990]
Q11.N5   vol. 635
[QP364]
500 s—dc20
[591.1′88]
DNLM/DLC
for Library of Congress   91-36658
                                                   CIP

SP
Printed in the United States of America
ISBN 0-89766-685-2 (cloth)
ISBN 0-89766-686-0 (paper)
ISSN 0077-8923

ANNALS OF THE NEW YORK ACADEMY OF SCIENCES

Volume 635
October 14, 1991

CALCIUM ENTRY AND ACTION AT THE PRESYNAPTIC NERVE TERMINAL[a]

Editors and Conference Organizers
ELIS F. STANLEY, MARTHA C. NOWYCKY, AND DAVID J. TRIGGLE

CONTENTS

[a]This volume is the result of a conference entitled **Calcium Entry and Action at the Presynaptic Nerve Terminal,** held in Baltimore, Maryland on October 15–17, 1990, by the New York Academy of Sciences.

Financial assistance was received from:

Supporters
- HOFFMANN-LA ROCHE INC.
- NATIONAL INSTITUTE OF MENTAL HEALTH
- NATIONAL SCIENCE FOUNDATION
- U. S. ARMY MEDICAL RESEARCH AND DEVELOPMENT COMMAND, DAMD 17-90-Z0029

Contributors
- AMERICAN CYANAMID COMPANY
- BRISTOL-MYERS COMPANY
- BURROUGHS WELLCOME COMPANY
- GENENTECH, INC.
- HOECHST-ROUSSEL PHARMACEUTICALS INC.
- ICI PHARMACEUTICALS GROUP
- LILLY RESEARCH LABORATORIES
- MERCK SHARP & DOHME RESEARCH LABORATORIES
- MERRELL DOW RESEARCH INSTITUTE
- MILES INC.
- PARKE-DAVIS
- PFIZER CENTRAL RESEARCH
- SCHERING-PLOUGH RESEARCH
- SMITHKLINE BEECHAM
- THE SQUIBB INSTITUTE FOR MEDICAL RESEARCH
- STERLING DRUG INC.

Introduction

ELIS F. STANLEY

Laboratory of Biophysics
National Institute of Neurological Disorders and Stroke
Building 9, Room 1E124
National Institutes of Health
Bethesda, Maryland 20892

The mechanism by which impulses in nerve terminals are translated into the release of chemical neurotransmitters is one of the most basic issues in neurobiology that remains unexplained. This question has eluded researchers, despite much effort and the passage of a substantial period of time since the elements of the process were identified. Thus, the release of transmitters in quanta was noted in 1952,[1] the existence of secretory vesicles was first reported in 1954,[2,3] the importance of calcium ions in the indirect excitation of muscle was described in 1894,[4] and evidence identifying this ion as a link between the action potential and transmitter release was elegantly demonstrated in 1967.[5]

Although a full understanding of neurotransmitter release remains elusive, the study of the role of calcium ions has resulted in two particularly important clues: First, transmitter release is a steep function of calcium entry[6,7]; second, the interval between calcium entry and transmitter release can be very short, in the order of 0.1 millisecond. These observations, together with the high selectivity of the activation site for calcium over the ubiquitous divalent cation, magnesium, strongly suggest that secretion involves the specific binding of calcium ions to a protein.

The one aspect of presynaptic nerve terminal function that is yielding to research is the means by which calcium ions enter the nerve terminal. The entry of calcium ions, first demonstrated in the squid giant synapse by calcium-sensitive dyes[8] and later by voltage clamp,[9] can now also be detected in vertebrate models (see Stanley and Cox, and Lindgren Moore, this volume) and even by direct voltage clamp.[10] This development will allow the examination of some of the more subtle aspects of the extracellular regulation of transmitter release—questions that have important implications to the control of neural networks in the brain.

The other end of the process, the fusion and discharge of synaptic vesicle contents, has only been examined to a limited extent directly on presynaptic nerve terminals. Important clues to this process have been obtained, however, by studies on cell-free systems, such as lipid vesicles and bilayers (see Meers *et al.* and Niles and Cohen, this volume), and in studies on the beige-mouse mast cells with their large, individually identifiable, secretory granules (see Almers *et al.* and Zimmerberg *et al.*, this volume). Although these are fascinating models of exocytosis, it is not yet clear that these results are directly relevant to secretion from nerve terminals. In many regards the biological demands on a secreting mast cell and on a secreting presynaptic nerve terminal are diametrically opposite. The mast cell is capable of secreting substantial quantities of product from large 1 μm diameter vesicles (see Chandler, this volume), with minimum time constraints, in the seconds or minutes range, and by a process that may not be critically dependent on calcium. By contrast, the presynaptic nerve terminal secretes much smaller quantities from 200 times smaller vesicles, within a time frame of less than 1 ms, and this process is highly calcium-dependent.

Furthermore, the initial fusion of the mast cell granule to the cell membrane is by way of an intervening membrane tube, in contrast to the synaptic vesicle that appears to fuse directly at the release site. Although it is attractive to hypothesize that the same mechanism of fusion is operative in all cases of secretory vesicle discharge, it would not, perhaps, be surprising if this notion proves to be incorrect.

Previous meetings have addressed various themes that are highly relevant to presynaptic nerve terminal function, such as calcium channels or exocytosis, but no recent meeting has provided an overview of the basic mechanism of transmitter release at synapses. We have attempted to cover the critical aspects of this process by following the passage of the calcium ion through the various steps that ultimately lead to synaptic vesicle discharge. Thus, we begin this meeting with a discussion of presynaptic calcium channels and end with the role of calcium in gating neurosecretion.

A reader new to this field might note that studies on presynaptic nerve terminals are often indirect and use experimental techniques with rather limited time resolution. This limitation can usually be attributed to the technical difficulty of experimentation on structures that are typically minute and inaccessible. Studies on nerve terminal function that require real time resolution have relied, in general, on electrophysiological recordings of postsynaptic potentials as a mirror on the presynaptic nerve terminal. Although this may be a reasonable approach for some questions, the detailed understanding of nerve terminal function will probably require techniques that can analyze these processes directly in the nerve terminal. The isolated neurosecretosome model (see articles by Nowycky and Bookman, this volume) is progressing in this direction. In this hormone-secreting nerve terminal, it is possible to obtain information on calcium channels, by recording calcium currents, and also on secretion, by recording capacitance changes. Perhaps studies on this and similar experimental models will allow us to finally identify the crucial intermediate events in the evoked discharge of synaptic vesicles.

REFERENCES

1. FATT, P. & B. KATZ. 1952. J. Physiol. **117:** 109.
2. DE ROBERTIS, E. & S.H. BENNETT. 1954. Fed. Proc. Fed. Am. Soc. Exp. Biol. **13:** 38.
3. PALADE, G. E. & S. L. PALAY. 1954. Anat. Rec. **118:** 335.
4. LOCKE, F. S. 1894. Zentralbl. Physiol. **8:** 166.
5. KATZ, B. & R. MILEDI. 1967. J. Physiol. **189:** 535.
6. DODGE, F. A. & R. RAHAMIMOFF. 1967. J. Physiol. **193:** 419.
7. JENKINSON, D.H. 1957. J. Physiol. **138:** 434.
8. LLINÁS, R. R., J. R. BLINKS & C. NICHOLSON. 1972. Science **176:** 1127.
9. LLINÁS, R. R., I. Z. STEINBERG & K. WALTON. 1981. Biophys. J. **33:** 289.
10. STANLEY, E. F. 1989. Brain Res. **505:** 341.

Depolarization Release Coupling:
An Overview

RODOLFO R. LLINÁS

Department of Physiology and Biophysics
New York University Medical Center
550 First Avenue
New York, New York 10016

It is now well-established that in many chemical junctions transmitter release is regulated by intracellular calcium concentration changes brought about by presynaptic depolarization.[1] The biophysical properties of this voltage-dependent calcium inflow is best studied under presynaptic voltage clamp conditions as may be implemented, for instance, in the squid giant synapse.[2] Under such conditions and following pharmacological block of sodium and potassium currents, a depolarizing voltage step will result in the activation of an inward transmembrane calcium current, which demonstrates little inactivation, and, at pulse brake, in a fast inward tail current carried by the same ion.[3-6] This presynaptic calcium current was shown to be accompanied, after a short delay, by the generation of a postsynaptic response.[3,4,7,8] In addition it was demonstrated that the calcium conductance change is accompanied by a discernible increase in intracellular calcium concentration changes[9,10] (cf. ref. 11) and that the actual injection of calcium into the preterminal[12-15] is sufficient to produce transmitter release.

VOLTAGE CLAMP STUDIES

The correspondence between the amplitude of the presynaptic voltage clamp depolarization and the amplitude of the inward calcium current (I_{Ca}) has been shown in several preparations[3] (cf. ref. 16). Following the onset of a sustained presynaptic depolarization, the membrane permeability to calcium was shown to increase slowly and to reach a peak whose amplitude varies with the level of depolarization. At low levels of depolarization (-40 mV from a holding potential of -70 mV) (FIG. 1A), a small inward current (middle record) was observed with a slow onset. At the end of the pulse, a fast tail current was observed. The postsynaptic response (PSP) associated with this current is illustrated in the top trace of FIGURE 1A. Note that the postsynaptic response during the pulse also has, as I_{Ca}, a close-to-linear rate of rise and that the PSP that followed the break of the voltage clamp pulse ("off" response) was generated by the inward tail current. With increasing levels of depolarization, I_{Ca} increases in amplitude, reaching a maximum at -10 mV. At this level, the sigmoidal character of the current onset becomes evident (FIG. 1B, middle trace, for a pulse to -18 mV). In accordance with the view that calcium entry is the parameter of interest in transmitter release, this peak amplitude in I_{Ca} is accompanied by a peaking in both amplitude and rate of rise in the postsynaptic response.[7]

As the presynaptic voltage step is increased beyond -10 mV, the steady-state presynaptic current decreases in amplitude, while the tail current increases to reach a maximum near $+30$ mV. At the same time, the rate of rise and amplitude of the "on" excitatory postsynaptic potential (EPSP) decreases, while the off response

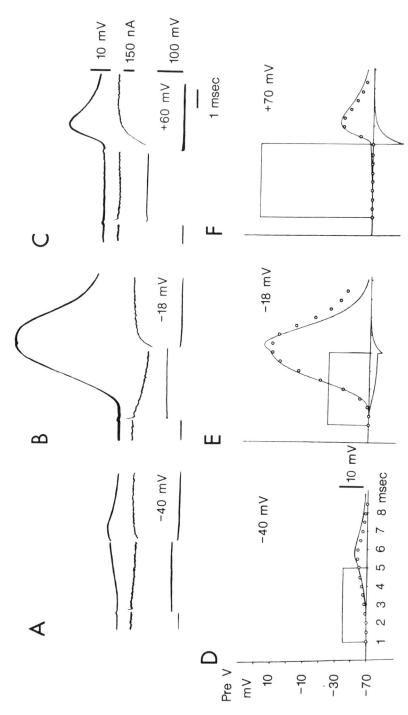

FIGURE 1. Synaptic transmission during voltage clamp of presynaptic terminal. **A–C:** Experimental data. Top trace, postsynaptic response; middle trace, calcium current; lower trace, presynaptic voltage. The S shape of the current onset can be seen at 60 mV depolarization from a holding potential of −70 mV. Note the fast tail current and the "on" and "off" excitatory postsynaptic potential (EPSP). **D–F:** Numerical solution to mathematical model. Top trace, vesicle depletion; other traces as in A–C. (Modified from Llinás, Steinberg, and Walton.[3,7])

increases. The steady-state current continues to decrease beyond $+40$ mV, until the suppression potential[17] is reached at close to $+60$ mV depolarization (FIG. 1C, middle trace). At this voltage level, no current is seen during the voltage pulse, but a large tail current is observed following the pulse break. Similarly, no synaptic transmission is observed for the duration of the pulse, and a sharp, short-latency off postsynaptic response is generated by the tail current. A clear correlation can thus be seen between the characteristics of presynaptic I_{Ca} and the postsynaptic response, the on EPSP being related to the I_{Ca} during the pulse and the off EPSP to the tail I_{Ca}. A comparison of the experimental results 1A, B, and C with the numerical solution from our synaptic transmissions model[7] is illustrated in D, E, and F for similar voltage-clamp steps. Open circles represent the postsynaptic voltages illustrated in A, B, and C, whereas the continuous lines are the numerical solutions to the model.

Presynaptic Voltage and I_{Ca}

The relation between the amplitude of the presynaptic voltage clamp depolarization and the amplitude of the inward steady-state I_{Ca} and of the tail current is shown in FIGURE 2A. As seen in that figure, I_{Ca} follows a bell-shaped curve with a rather rapid rise, reaching a peak near -10 mV. By contrast, the tail current increases sharply for increasing levels of depolarization up to about $+10$ mV, at which point it begins to saturate, reaching a maximum near $+30$ mV.[7]

Calcium Current and Postsynaptic Potentials

The relation between presynaptic voltage and I_{Ca} and that of I_{Ca} to the amplitude of the postsynaptic response were found to be quite similar (FIGURE 2 A and B). Moreover, a comparison between presynaptic voltage and the amplitude of the on (filled circles) and off (crosses) EPSP with the numerical solution for the mathematical model described below (continuous line) agrees quite well, suggesting a low stoichiometry for the I_{Ca}-EPSP relation. Therefore, a close-to-linear relationship between these two variables was suggested.[7,18] Indeed when I_{Ca} was plotted against the on EPSP amplitude using double-logarithmic coordinates, a mean slope of 1.36 was obtained.[7] A mean slope of 1.11 was also obtained when tail-current amplitude and off EPSP amplitudes were plotted using double-logarithmic coordinates[7] or when calcium was related to transmitter release with a short pulse.[7,18] These findings indicate that the bell-shaped curve relating presynaptic depolarization to postsynaptic response[9,17,19] reflects chiefly the nonlinear dependence of g_{Ca} on voltage and that transmitter release demonstrates a first- to second-order dependence on I_{Ca}, at least at the levels studied. This close-to-linear relationship was questioned by other investigators who view this relation as steeper.[8,20] More recently, however, a linear relation was reported, in agreement with our original findings, for short presynaptic pulses.[21] A higher stoichiometry was proposed for longer pulses in the same publication. We continue to read our results as demonstrating a close to linear relation for both short and long pulses; so this important point continues to be one of some controversy.

SYNAPTIC DELAY

Another important parameter in attempting to understand the nature of synaptic transmissions is that provided by the synaptic delay under presynaptic voltage

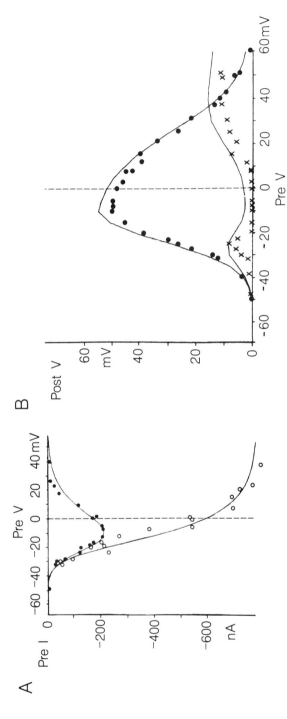

FIGURE 2. Dependence of calcium current (A) and EPSP (B) on presynaptic depolarization. **A:** (●) Steady state I_{Ca}; (○) tail current. **B:** (●) On EPSP; (x) off EPSP. The continuous line in panels A and B shows that the solution of mathematical model $[Ca^{2+}]_o$ equals 10 mM. In the Pre-V axis, 0 corresponds to a holding potential of −70 mV. (Modified from Llinás, Steinberg, and Walton.[3,7])

control. The temporal relationship between depolarization and transmitter release may be divided into two parts, a and b.[22] The first component (a) is related to the time required for opening of the calcium channels, whereas the second (b) relates to the time between calcium entry and the onset of the postsynaptic potential. Examples of how these two components affect synaptic delay can be obtained by comparing the delay for the on and off release as shown in FIGURE 3 A and B. Here, in record A, a presynaptic voltage-clamp step (to -10 mV) demonstrates a characteristic 1-ms delay for the on response (composed of components a and b). The record in FIGURE 3B was taken at the suppression potential and illustrates the tail calcium current and the latency (about 200 μs, comprising the b component alone) for the off synaptic potential generated by this short current injection. The actual synaptic delay may, in fact, be slightly shorter inasmuch as the falling phase of the pulse is not instantaneous. These two components were measured directly[22] by comparing the onset time of the voltage-clamp pulse to the time of onset for the inward calcium current (giving a value for the a component) and then discerning the delay between the current onset and the initiation of the postsynaptic potential (giving a value for b). A plot for the on and off synaptic delays for synapses are shown in FIGURE 3E.[7] Note that the values for these two levels of voltage steps are similar to those predicted by our model (FIG. 3 C and D).

A MATHEMATICAL MODEL FOR SYNAPTIC TRANSMISSION

A kinetic model based on the above findings was developed that related numerically presynaptic depolarization to calcium current and calcium current to transmitter release.[2,3,7,18] The model for the calcium current that best fits these results assumed a fourth- to fifth-order Michaelis-Menten kinetics, which further assumed that four to five noncooperative conformational changes occur prior to channel opening. These conformational changes are voltage- and time-dependent and are thought to be regulated by way of forward and backward rate constants between the active and inactive states of the subunits in the channels. According to the model, each Ca channel is composed of n subunits, each of which exists in either of two active states: S and S*. The modulation between these states is governed by the rate constants, k_1 and k_2. Thus,

$$S \overset{k_1}{\underset{k_2}{\rightleftharpoons}} S^*$$

where a gate or channel is open when all n subunits are in the S* state. The number of "open" channels [G] is proportional to $(S^*)^n$, and the Ca current is given by [G] times the current flow per gate per unit time (j). Thus,

$$I_{Ca} = [G] \cdot j$$

$$[G] = [G]_0 \left(\frac{k_1}{k_1 + k_2} [1 - \exp\{-(k_1 + k_2)|t|\}] \right)^n$$

$$j = \frac{\beta_1 K[c_o \exp(-80V_n) - c_i]}{1 + K_{c_o} \exp(-80V_n)}$$

where $[G]_0$ is the total number of channels, open and closed; k_1 and k_2 are the rate constants for the opening and closing, respectively, of a channel subunit; t is the time; V is membrane voltage relative to absolute zero; c_i is $[Ca^{2+}]_i$; c_o is $[Ca^{2+}]_o$; K is the

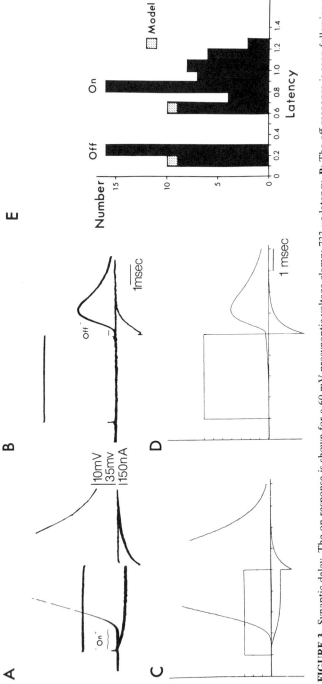

FIGURE 3. Synaptic delay. The on response is shown for a 60 mV presynaptic voltage clamp. **B:** The off response is seen following a voltage clamp to the suppression potential (140 mV); 200 μs latency. **C** and **D:** EPSPs generated by the mathematical model for a 60 mV clamp (on response latency, 675 μs), and a 140 mV clamp (off response latency, 150 μs). **E:** Histogram showing the variation in latency observed for the on response (mean 0.894 ± 0.168, n = 51), and the off response (mean 0.192 ± 0.27, n = 25). (Modified from Llinás, Steinberg and Walton.[3,7])

equilibrium constant for the transfer of calcium from outside the cell to the calcium site in the channel, at zero membrane potential; β_1 is a proportionality factor; and 80 is the solution to $2e/kT$, where e is the elementary electric charge, k is the Boltzmann constant, and T is the absolute temperature ($291°K = 18°C$). In FIGURE 1 D, E, and F the solution for I_{Ca} from this equation for presynaptic clamp voltages of -40, -18, and $+70$ from a holding potential of -70 mV is illustrated (continuous lines).

By simplifying the equation to eliminate the time-dependent component, an expression for the steady-state I_{Ca} is furnished. When modeling the remaining steps in synaptic transmission several factors must be taken into account: (1) The high specificity of calcium ions in promoting vesicle fusion and transmitter release (cf. ref. 1) strongly supports the notion that a specific binding entity for calcium in addition to the calcium-binding protein[23,24] may be involved in the process. Such a factor is included in this model and was referred to as the fusion-promoting factor (fpf).[3] (2) As fusion is initiated we assume that vesicles are depleted from the immediate vicinity of the plasma membrane (the immediately available store) and that this may affect the transmission process. (3) The time required for the diffusion of the transmitter across the synaptic gap is expected to be very short (less than 1 µs for a gap width of 200 Å and a diffusion coefficient of 10^{-5} cm^2 sec^{-1}) and thus is not a significant consideration. (4) The opening and closing time constants for the gating of the postsynaptic receptor transmitter complex have been assumed to be proportional to the rate of transmitter release, and it is also assumed that the postsynaptic receptors are far from saturation. (5) The electrical constants of the postsynaptic terminal membrane are included.

A three-compartment scheme to model transmitter release and postsynaptic current was thus proposed in which each compartment has forward and backward first-order rate constants.[7] The first compartment consists of a calcium protein reaction involving fpf. The behavior of fpf is assumed to be as follows: If a pulse of calcium ions enters the presynaptic digit, fpf binds these ions, forming a complex fpf · Ca^{2+} directly determined by the amplitude of I_{Ca} and the time of exposure to the calcium ions. This complex then becomes activated by first-order kinetics into a species fpf* · Ca^{2+} that facilitates fusion of vesicles with the plasma membrane at a rate proportional to its amount. The species fpf* · Ca^{2+} can then revert to an inactive form, again by first-order kinetics. Similarly, the complex fpf · Ca^{2+} can be inactivated directly without being converted into fpf · Ca^{2+}. The concatenation may be summarized as shown below.

$$\text{fpf} \cdot Ca^{2+} \xrightarrow{k_a} \text{fpf} * \cdot Ca^{2+} \xrightarrow{k_i} \text{inactive form}$$

$$\downarrow k_b$$

$$\text{inactive form}$$

In the above reactions, k_a is the rate constant for activation, and k_b and k_i are the rate constants for the inactivation of fpf · Ca^{2+} and fpf* · Ca^{2+}, respectively.

The second compartment relates to a membrane fusion factor—synaptic vesicle reaction leading to transmitter release (TR). Thus,

$$TR = k_f (\text{fpfCa}^{2+})Q$$

where k_f is the rate constant for vesicle fusion, and Q is the fractional number of vesicles still available from the immediate store. (The rate constants k_a, k_b, k_i, and k_f are voltage-dependent.) The third component involves synaptic transmitter triggering, the postsynaptic conductance generating the EPSP.

The computation of EPSP amplitude and time course for three levels of presynaptic voltage clamp are illustrated in FIGURE 1 D–F. Values obtained experimentally are given by open circles: those calculated using the model for the peak postsynaptic on and off EPSP are given by the continuous lines.

In short then, this very simple model for presynaptic calcium current, transmitter release, and postsynaptic response does correspond quite well to the experimental voltage-clamp data (FIGURES 1 and 2) and was further shown to predict accurately transmissions by simulated action potentials.[18,21]

SYNAPSIN I AND THE ISSUE OF VESICULAR AVAILABILITY

From the above model it seems clear that synaptic transmission must comprise more than a single compartment for the effect of calcium on transmitter release. Simultaneous with these studies, a then-unrelated study of the biochemistry of the presynaptic terminal had been developed by Greengard and collaborators, and a protein now known as Synapsin I had been isolated.[25] Although the actual role of this protein in synaptic transmissions was not known at that time, the possibility was clearly evident that it could be involved in at least one aspect of the multicompartment mechanism that regulates transmitter release. In fact several findings had suggested a prominent role for the protein Synapsin I in synaptic transmission, as this protein had been found in most presynaptic terminals and in contact with the cytoplasmic surface of synaptic vesicles.[26] Following these two leads experiments in the squid giant synapse indeed showed that intracellular injection of dephospho-Synapsin I could block synaptic transmission, and that CaM kinase II had a facilitory effect.[27–29]

Based on these and other findings, we hypothesized that the dephosphorylated form of Synapsin I could serve to immobilize synaptic vesicles by binding them to cytoskeletal elements, and that phosphorylation of Synapsin I by CaM kinase II liberated vesicles from these attachments.[26–28,30] The size of the postsynaptic response would then depend on both the size of the inward calcium current and the number of vesicles available for release.

Recent research on this topic[29] has shown that, as indicated in our original findings, dephospho-Synapsin I has a blocking effect on transmitter release. This may be seen in FIGURE 3 where the injection of dephospho-Synapsin I at the proximal region of the preterminal was directly monitored using fluorescent dephospho-Synapsin I. The results directly demonstrate that this protein markedly reduces transmitter release (FIG. 4, upper trace) without modifying inward calcium current (FIG. 4B). Moreover, the reduction was clearly related (FIG. 5) to the degree of penetration of Synapsin I into the preterminal digit as indicated by the time marks after initial injection (immediately to the left in minutes) and by the plot of postsynaptic reduction against time (FIG. 4B). This demonstrated that the effect on the release process is truly local in the sense that the effect required local increase in dephospho-Synapsin I. Finally, the results also demonstrate that the phosphorylated form of Synapsin I (phospho-Synapsin I) has no obvious effect as transmitter release (FIG. 4B). As in the previous experiments the mobilization of this protein was monitored directly, using fluorescence imaging.[29]

Effect of Dephosphorylated Synapsin I on Synaptic Noise

Although miniature-potential recording is possible in the squid giant synapse[31,32] a technique more suited for the study of spontaneous transmitter release and its

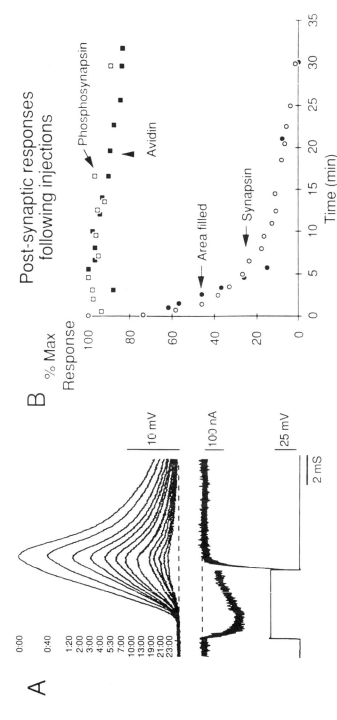

FIGURE 4. Postsynaptic voltage, above; presynaptic I_{Ca} below, following preinjection of Synapsin I. **A:** Constant 50 mV prevoltage steps lasting 5 ms were delivered at regular intervals. The postsynaptic responses were recorded at regular intervals given to the left (in minutes). **B:** Time course of the reduction of the EPSP following synaptic injection at the proximal end of the terminal digit. Ordinates, a percent of EPSP amplitudes (open circles). Closed circles are the inverse of the filled area by Synapsin I injection as visualized with Texas Red (dark-filled circles). Open squares and black squares are similar to injections of phospho-Synapsin I, and avidin produced no reduction of EPSP amplitude. (Modified from Llinás, Gruner, Sugimori, McGuinness, and Greengard.[29])

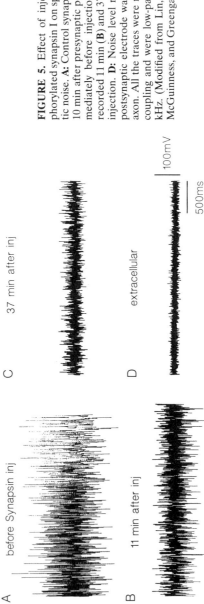

FIGURE 5. Effect of injection of dephosphorylated synapsin I on spontaneous synaptic noise. **A:** Control synaptic noise recorded 10 min after presynaptic penetration but immediately before injection. Synaptic noise recorded 11 min (**B**) and 37 min (**C**) after the injection. **D:** Noise level recorded after the postsynaptic electrode was withdrawn from axon. All the traces were recorded under ac coupling and were low-pass filtered at 1.25 kHz. (Modified from Lin, Sugimori, Llinás, McGuinness, and Greengard.[33])

regulation by Synapsin I was implemented.[33] The voltage noise recorded in the postsynaptic axon at rest was shown to be similar to that rendered for the spontaneous transmitter release in the neuromuscular junction.[34] The injection of dephospho-Synapsin I has been shown to produce a rapid and robust decline of synaptic noise.[33] An example of this effect is illustrated in FIGURE 5 where traces obtained at different times after the protein injection are shown. The thickness of the traces reflects the level of spontaneous release (A to C). The extracellular noise trace is displayed in panel D to illustrate the resolution of the recording system. Measurement of noise level over time, following dephospho-Synapsin I injection demonstrated a reduction in the average noise level to 21% of the control after 20 minutes, whereas following phospho-Synapsin I or vehicle injection, the noise level showed only a small drop (70% to 90%) to control over time.[33] Similar results were also found when evoked release was monitored following the injection of dephospho-Synapsin I.

The results obtained using this approach were very similar to that measured from the amplitude of the postsynaptic potentials after dephospho-Synapsin I injection and, as previously stated, reflect the time course of dephospho-Synapsin I diffusion into the terminal.

CaM KINASE II

As a second approach to test the hypothesis that Synapsin I regulates transmitter release, the effect of presynaptic injection of CaM kinase II (an enzyme known to phophorylate Synapsin I[28]) was undertaken. This enzyme should in fact dissociate vesicles from their attachments by phosphorylating an endogenous Synapsin I–like molecule.[35] Thus, increasing the endogenous CaM kinase II normally present in the terminal should increase transmitter release as was originally reported in our initial publication.[27]

Further studies demonstrated that facilitation of transmitter release by the CaM kinase II injection occurred at a mean percent of 409 ± 157%. The maximum facilitation usually occurred between 10 and 20 minutes after injection with no modification of presynaptic I_{Ca}.[29]

A double voltage clamp experiment showing facilitation of synaptic transmission following CaM kinase II injection demonstrates the time course and amplitude of I_{post} at three different times after the injection (FIG. 6A).[29] The postsynaptic current increased to the point of saturation, as evidenced by the flattened top of the response. Similar results were observed in eight experiments, three of which are plotted in FIGURE 6B.

Effect of CaM Kinase II on Synaptic Noise

In contrast to the effect of Synapsin I on postsynaptic noise, little effect was seen on spontaneous release following CaM kinase injection. Evoked release, however, increased gradually following such CaM kinase II injection (FIG. 6C). The increase in evoked release was indicated by an elevation of noise that occurred during a small presynaptic depolarizing clamp pulse (a 2 s, 15 mV pulse from a holding potential of -70 mV). This is illustrated in FIGURE 6C where the same presynaptic depolarization produced a larger noise after CaM kinase II injection. The insensitivity of spontaneous release to CaM kinase II injection suggests that the resting level of intracellular calcium was not high enough to substantially activate this enzyme.

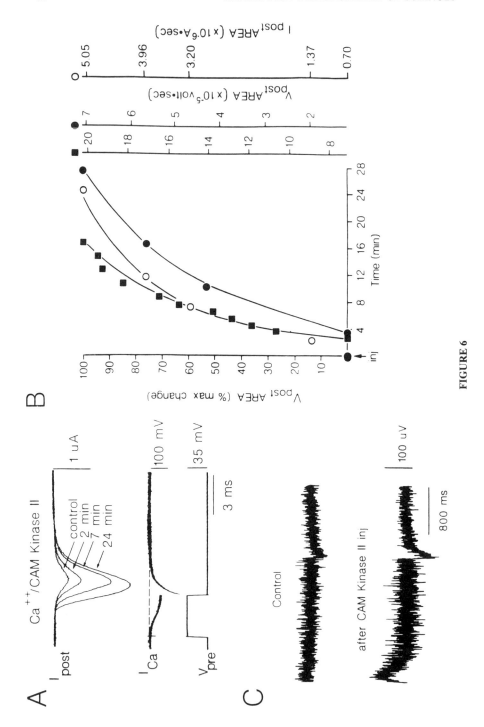

FIGURE 6

DISCUSSION

Depolarization Release Coupling

Investigation of the question of depolarization release coupling at chemical junctions seems to have advanced quite steadily over the last two or three decades. Close to universally agreement has been reached regarding several issues, although others still remain controversial. Among those that may be regarded as settled are the following. (1) Presynaptic depolarization is the most common triggering signal for release, and it works by activating an influx of calcium into the preterminal. Whereas some believe that potential itself may modify release sufficiently fast to regulate spike-evoked transmission,[36,37] this view is not universally held.[35] (2) The intracellular calcium concentration microprofiles that follow calcium channel activation[38-41] are complex enough that a single compartment model relating I_{Ca} to release are far too simplistic to be of use. Equally simplistic is the view that the stoichiometry of I_{Ca} versus release addresses questions such as the number of calcium ions required to release a single vesicle. (3) From the above it also follows that the residual calcium hypothesis for synaptic facilitation must be replaced by a more tenable explanation where calcium concentration microdomains, intracellular biochemical processes, and ultrastructural cell biology are considered as interrelated parts of the release mechanism.

Modulation of Transmitter Release by Synapsin I and CaM Kinase II

The major findings concerning transmitter modulation by these proteins may be summarized as follows. (1) Dephospho-Synapsin I: (a) This protein reversibly inhibits transmitter release and reduces evoked and spontaneous synaptic noise. (b) The inhibition is related to the extent of its diffusion into the presynaptic terminal. (c) Phospho-Synapsin I injection does not affect release.[27-29] These results are supported by recent data on the Mauthner cell synapse[42] and the crayfish neuromuscular junction.[43] All these data suggest that Synapsin I modifies release by acting locally at the active zones. (2) CaM kinase II: (a) This protein facilitates synaptic release by several fold without affecting presynaptic I_{Ca}. (b) It does not facilitate spontaneous synaptic noise, but does increase evoked noise. (c) Facilitation is related to the extent of its diffusion into the presynaptic terminal digit. The changes in postsynaptic amplitude seen after these injections have recently been confirmed in mammalian brain synaptosomes.[44] These changes are most likely due to change in the availability of synaptic vesicles[27-29] and supported by *in vitro* studies. (cf. ref. 28) This interpretation agrees with the view that dephosphorylated Synapsin I cross-links

FIGURE 6. Presynaptic injection of CaM kinase II. **A:** Increase in postsynaptic current produced by injection of CaM kinase II presynaptically as recorded at three different times after injection (2, 7, and 24 min). Midtrace and lower trace, respectively: calcium current and presynaptic voltage step. Note the lack of change in presynaptic calcium current following CaM kinase injection. **B:** Example of percentage increase of the postsynaptic response following CaM kinase injection for three different synapses. The postsynaptic response as an area is plotted against time after Synapsin I injection. **C:** Effect of CaM kinase II on synaptic noise in control and after CaM kinase I during a small depolarizing step. (Modified from Llinás, Gruner, Sugimori, McGuinness, and Greengard.[29])

synaptic vesicles to elements such as actin[45] and that these vesicles need to be dissociated (or decaged) from such structures before they can move to release sites.

We concluded that these proteins do not alter channel kinetics or the dynamics of vesicular exocytosis. Rather, by dephosphorylating Synapsin I, CaM kinase II modifies the availability of synaptic vesicles in the immediate vicinity of the active zones, thus regulating transmitter release.

REFERENCES

1. KATZ, B. 1969. The Release of Neural Transmitter Substances. The Sherrington Lectures X. Charles C. Thomas. Springfield, IL.
2. LLINÁS, R., I. Z. STEINBERG & K. WALTON. 1976. Proc. Natl. Acad. Sci. USA **73:** 2913–2922.
3. LLINÁS, R., I. Z. STEINBERG & K. WALTON. 1981. Biophys. J. **33:** 289–321.
4. AUGUSTINE, G. J., M. P. CHARLTON & S. J. SMITH. 1985. J Physiol. (Lond.) **367:** 143–62.
5. STANLEY, E. F. 1989. Brain Res. **505:** 341–345.
6. FUCHS, P. A., M. G. EVANS & B. W. MURROW. 1990. J. Physiol. (London) **429:** 553–568.
7. LLINÁS, R., I. Z. STEINBERG & K. WALTON. 1981. Biophys. J. **33:** 323–352.
8. AUGUSTINE, G. J., M. P. CHARLTON & S. J. SMITH. 1985. J. Physiol. (London) **367:** 163–81.
9. LLINÁS, R. & C. NICHOLSON. 1975. Proc. Natl. Acad. Sci. USA **72:** 187–90.
10. LLINÁS, R. R. 1984. *In* The Squid Axon, Curent Topics in Membrane and Transport. P. F. Baker, Ed.: **22:** 519–546. Academic Press. New York.
11. SMITH, S. J. & G. J. AUGUSTINE. 1988. Trends Neurosci. **11:** 458–464.
12. MILEDI, R. 1973. Proc. R. Soc. Lond. B Biol. Sci. **183:** 421–5.
13. CHARLTON, M. P., S. J. SMITH & R. S. ZUCKER. 1982. J. Physiol. (London) **323:** 173–193.
14. LLINÁS, R., M. SUGIMORI & K. WALTON. 1987. Adv. Exp. Med. Biol. **221:** 1–17.
15. DELANEY, K.-R. & R.-S. ZUCKER. 1990. J. Physiol. (London) **426:** 473–498.
16. AUGUSTINE, G. J., M. P. CHARLTON & S. J. SMITH. 1988. *In* Calcium and Ion Channel Modulation. A. D. Grinnell, D. Armstrong & M. B. Jackson, Eds.: 157–168. Plenum Press. New York.
17. KATZ, B. & R. MILEDI. 1967. J. Physiol. (London) **192:** 407–436.
18. LLINÁS, R., M. SUGIMORI & S. M. SIMON. 1982. Proc. Natl. Acad. Sci. USA **79:** 2415–2419.
19. KUSANO, K., D. R. LIVENGOOD & R. WERMAN. 1967. J. Gen. Physiol. **50:** 2579–2601.
20. AUGUSTINE, G. J. & M. P. CHARLTON. 1986. J. Physiol. (London) **381:** 619–640.
21. AUGUSTINE, G. J. 1990. J. Physiol. (London) **431:** 343–364.
22. LLINÁS, R. R. 1977. *In* Approaches to the Cell Biology of Neurons. W. M. Cowan & J. A. Ferendelli, Eds.: 139–160. Society for Neuroscience. Bethesda, MD.
23. BAKER, P. F. & W. W. SCHAEPFER. 1978. J. Physiol. (London) **270:** 103–125.
24. KRINKS, M. H., C. B. KLEE, H. C. PANT & H. GAINER. 1988. J. Neurosci. **8:** 2172–2182.
25. DECAMILLI, P., R. CAMERON & P. GREENGARD. 1983. J. Cell Biol. **96:** 1337–1354.
26. DECAMILLI, P. & P. GREENGARD. 1986. Biochem. Pharmacol. **35:** 4348–4355.
27. LLINÁS, R., T. MCGUINNESS, C. S. LEONARD, M. SUGIMORI & P. GREENGARD. 1985. Proc. Natl. Acad. Sci. USA **82:** 3035–3039.
28. GREENGARD, P., M. D. BROWNING, T. L. MCGUINNESS & R. LLINÁS. 1987. Adv. Exp. Med. Biol. **221:** 135–153.
29. LLINÁS, R., J. GRUNER, M. SUGIMORI, T. L. MCGUINNESS & P. GREENGARD. 1991. J. Physiol. (London) **436:** 251–282.
30. MCGUINNESS, T. L., S. T. BRADY, J. A. GRUNER, M. SUGIMORI, R. LLINÁS & P. GREENGARD. 1989. J. Neurosci. **9:** 4138–4149.
31. MILEDI, R. 1966. Nature **212:** 1240–1242.
32. MANN, D. W. & R. W. JOYNER. 1978. J. Neurobiol. **9:** 329–35.
33. LIN, J.-W., M. SUGIMORI, R. LLINÁS, T. MCGUINNESS & P. GREENGARD. 1990. Proc. Natl. Acad. Sci. USA **87:** 8257–8261.
34. FATT, P. J. & B. KATZ. 1952. J. Physiol. (London) **117:** 108–128.
35. HUTTNER, W. B., W. SCHEIBLER, P. GREENGARD & P. DECAMILLI. 1983. J. Cell. Biol. **96:** 1374–1388.

36. DUDEL, J., I. PARNAS & H. PARNAS. 1983. Pfluegers Arch. **399:** 1–10.
37. PARNAS, H., J. DUDEL & I. PARNAS. 1986. Pfluegers Arch. **406:** 121–130.
38. CHAD, J. E. & R. ECKERT. 1984. Biophys. J. **45:** 993–999.
39. SIMON, S. M., M. SUGIMORI & R. LLINÁS. 1984. Biophy. J. **45:** 264a.
40. SIMON, S. M. & R. R. LLINÁS. 1985. Biophys. J. **48:** 485–498.
41. FOGELSON, A. L. & R. S. ZUCKER. 1985. Biophys. J. **48:** 1003–1017.
42. HACKETT, J. T., S. L. COCHRAN, L. J. GREENFIELD, D. C. BROSIUS & T. UEDA. 1990. J. Neurophysiol. **63:** 701–706.
43. DELANEY, K. R., Y. YAMAGATA, D. TANK, P. GREENGARD & R. LLINÁS. 1990. Biol. Bull. (Woods Hole) **179:** 229.
44. NICHOLS, R. A., W. C. WU, J. W. HAYCOCK & P. GREENGARD. 1989. J. Neurochem. **52:** 521–529.
45. BAHLER, M. & P. GREENGARD. 1987. Nature **326:** 704–707.

Ion Permeation through Calcium Channels

A One-Site Model[a]

CLAY M. ARMSTRONG[b] AND JACQUES NEYTON[c]

[b]Department of Physiology
University of Pennsylvania
Philadelphia, Pennsylvania 19104-6085

[c]Laboratoire de Neurobiologie
Ecole Normale Supérieure
46, rue d'Ulm
Paris, France

INTRODUCTION

Several interesting permeation phenomena have led previous investigators to conclude that calcium channels are large in diameter compared to the crystal radius of a calcium ion[1] and that they have two ion binding sites, one at either end of the channel.[2-4] An ion passing from outside to inside occupies first the outer site, then the inner, and finally passes into the cytoplasm. The model proposes that both sites have a high affinity for Ca, but that the presence of a Ca ion in the other site lowers the affinity for both through mutual repulsion. The model assumes that an ion can only move into a site that is vacant. For example, an external Ca ion (call it Ca_1) can occupy the outer site, provided it is empty. It cannot move to the inner site if that site is Ca-occupied (by Ca_2), but its presence destabilizes Ca_2 and makes it more likely to move into the cytoplasm. If Ca_2 does move inward, leaving the inner site vacant, Ca_1 can easily move through the channel to occupy the inner site.

The two-site model provides an explanation for several well-known properties of Ca channels, for example, monovalent conduction through the channels in the absence of divalent cations; the ability of very low divalent concentrations to inhibit monovalent conduction; saturation of the current as a function of [Ca]; and the ability of low Ca concentrations to inhibit Ba conduction through the channels.

We show here that these phenomena can also be explained by a one-site model. The model we present grew out of fierce discussions between the authors regarding ion permeation mechanisms in general. We were encouraged to explore the one-site model by Chow's[5] excellent analysis of Cd block of Ca channels.

THE MODEL

We postulate that the Ca channel has a single ion binding site, which has a net charge of -2 e. The site has physical plausibility if thought of as two carboxyl oxygens, each with a radius of 1.32 Å. For convenience, we draw the site as a single sphere with charge of -2 e and radius 1.32 Å.

---

[a]This work was supported by NIH Grant No. NS12547.

The electrostatic energy of a divalent cation interacting with this site is taken to be

$$\text{Energy} = 100 \, kT/\text{center to center distance}$$
$$= 100 \, kT/(1.32 \, \text{Å} + \text{cation radius}).$$

For present purposes, the site can be anywhere in the channel, but we have drawn it near the channel's outer end, in conformity with Chow's analysis.[5]

In this paper we use Pauling radii for the cations and for oxygen. We were heavily influenced in our modeling by the numerous excellent papers of Levitt,[6] and Jordan and coworkers,[7] which examined theoretical interactions of ions with gramicidin A channels. Our analysis takes into account only ion-ion interactions and ignores the energy changes arising from the Born self-charging energy, mainly because nothing is known about this factor in Ca channels. A more complete treatment would include a term for Born energy.

RESULTS

Conduction by Knock-On (or Ion Exchange)

The two-site model assumes that an intruding ion can only enter a vacant site. This assumption, though reasonable for a neutral site, is incorrect for a charged site. For one thing, it is highly improbable that a charged site is vacant. As an example, withdrawing a calcium ion from a membrane site with a charge of -2 e would cost approximately $43 \, kT$ of energy. This means that a vacant site is roughly 10^{18} times less probable than an occupied site!

Thus, for a charged site, conduction cannot occur by a vacancy mechanism, because there is never a vacancy. Instead, a replacement ion must be present at the site before the occupying ion can withdraw. There is no energy barrier (due to ion-ion interaction) in bringing a second divalent cation to a two-carboxyl site that is occupied: the second cation is approaching a complex (site plus occupying ion) that is electrically neutral; or, stated another way, the repulsion from the occupying cation is balanced by the attraction to the negative charges of the site (FIG. 1). The conclusion is that conduction can occur with a charged site, and the mechanism requires ion exchange, or knock-on: the appearance of a second ion at the site makes its possible for the occupying ion to leave.

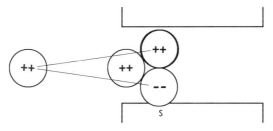

FIGURE 1. The approach and arrival of a second divalent cation (light circle) to a doubly charged site that is already occupied by a divalent cation (heavy circle). For the entering cation, repulsion from the occupying cation is balanced by attraction to the negative site. As a result, there is no energy increase due to ion-ion interaction.

Monovalent Cation Conduction

It has been found that calcium channels conduct monovalent cations in the absence of divalents. Monovalent cations through a one-site channel would occur as diagrammed in FIGURE 2. In Step I the site is occupied by two monovalent cations. The complex has a net charge of zero, and a third monovalent can easily approach. The arrival (Step II) of a third cation makes it possible for the right cation to withdraw (Step III), for it is receding from a complex that has a net charge of zero. Thus, during monovalent conduction, the site changes back and forth from double to triple occupancy.

Calcium Inhibition of Monovalent Conduction

Addition of 1 μM Ca to the external medium largely prevents monovalent conduction through calcium channels. This phenomenon can be understood in terms of the one-site model by examining FIGURE 3, which shows that a divalent cation occupying the site cannot be replaced by a monovalent cation. Step I of the FIGURE shows the approach of a monovalent cation to a divalent occupied site, a step that requires no energy, because the monovalent cation is approaching a neutral complex. The divalent, however, cannot withdraw, for it would be leaving a site with a net negative charge. The energy barrier, in this case, for a charge of $+2$ e receding from a charge of -1 e would be approximately 19 kT, corresponding to a probability of roughly 10^{-8}. Thus, a low concentration of calcium would lead to almost exclusive occupation of the sites by calcium and very low monovalent conduction.

Could two monovalent cations replace a divalent? This is unlikely, for the following reason. The complex of one monovalent plus one divalent plus site has a net charge of $+1$ e and would repel a second monovalent cation attempting to approach the site. Thus replacement of a divalent cation by either one or two monovalent cations is improbable.

Saturation of Current Magnitude as a Function of [Ca] or [Ba]

It has been observed that Ca current saturates as a function of calcium concentration, with a K_D of about 14 mM (Hess, Lansman, and Tsien[8]; although Yue and Marban[9] have evidence that the relationship is more complex than a simple saturation function). The single-site model can explain a K_D of 14 mM with physically plausible assumptions concerning cation arrangement near the site.

FIGURE 4 shows a site occupied by one or two cations. Taking the energy of the singly occupied site as the reference level, the energy is actually below the reference level when a second cation is present in the position shown. The reason is that the attraction to the site ($-100\ kT/(1.32 + 0.99)$) is stronger than the mutual repulsion between cations ($100\ kT/(1.98 + 0.58)$) because of the gap between the cations. A gap of only 0.58 Å would lower the energy by 4.3 kT, sufficient to explain the K_D of 14 mM. Thus, at 14 mM Ca, single and double occupancy would be equally probable.

During conduction the site alternates between single and double occupancy, and the rate-limiting step would be the departure of a cation from the doubly occupied site: this step involves a positive energy change, whereas conversion of a singly occupied site to a doubly occupied site involves an energy decrease. The rate of conduction is thus proportional to the probability of double occupancy, and this

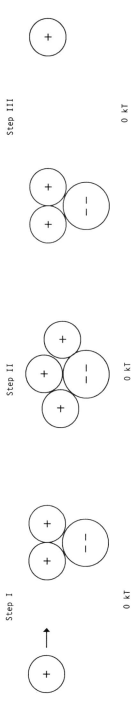

FIGURE 2. Monovalent cation conduction. If a site (-2 e) is occupied by two monovalent cations, the approach of a third cation to the site requires no energy, because the site, plus two occupying cations, is net neutral. The withdrawal of the third cation (step III) also requires no energy, because the cation is withdrawing from a neutral complex (site plus two occupying ions). The numbers under each step give the change in ion-ion energy, in kT.

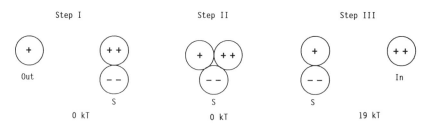

FIGURE 3. Inhibition of monovalent current by calcium. The illustration shows the steps required for the replacement of a divalent cation in the site by a monovalent. Step III would be very unlikely because the divalent cation withdraws from a complex that has a charge of -1 e, a step that would require 19 kT of energy. The numbers under each step give the change in ion-ion energy, in kT.

probability is a saturating function of [Ca], with K_D of 14 mM. For the Ba ion, similar arguments lead to the arrangement shown in the lower part of FIGURE 4. To explain the observed K_D of 28 mM,[8] the doubly occupied site must be 3.8 kT below the singly occupied site. This would require the approximate spacing shown in the FIGURE.

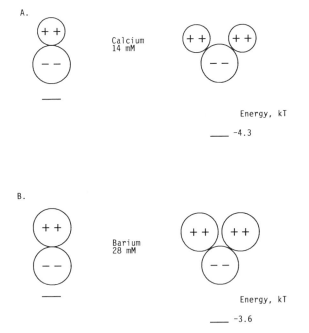

FIGURE 4. The ion-ion energy of a doubly occupied site is lower than for a singly occupied one. **A:** The illustration shows an arrangement of cations in a singly and a doubly occupied site. The approximate distances shown make the ion-ion energy of the doubly occupied site lower by 4.3 kT. **B:** With these approximate spacings, the ion-ion energy of the doubly occupied site is 3.6 kT lower. For calibration, the negatively charged sphere representing the site is 1.32 Å.

Channel Conductance in Ba and Ca

Ba carries current through Ca channels more effectively than does Ca, by a ratio of about two. This can be understood from inspecting the energy levels summarized in FIGURE 5. The reference (zero) level is taken as the energy of a singly Ba-occupied site. Based on the K_D of Ba conduction through the Ca channel, the doubly Ba-occupied site is $-3.6\,kT,$ as described in the preceding section.

Relative to the zero level, the energy of a singly Ca-occupied site is $-5.7\,kT,$ based on the crystal radii of barium, calcium, and oxygen (-2). Because Ca is smaller than Ba, it binds $5.7\,kT$ more tightly to the oxygen. The doubly Ca-occupied site is 4.3 kT lower in energy than the singly Ca-occupied site, as required to explain the K_D of 14 mM, making it $-10\,kT.$

Given these energies it is easy to understand the relative conductances for Ca and Ba. In pure Ba the site alternates from singly to doubly occupied, and the dominant

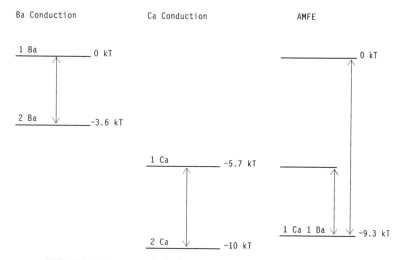

FIGURE 5. Energy levels for ions in various occupancy states. See text.

energy barrier is 3.6 kT (Ba). For Ca conduction, the energy jump from doubly to singly occupied is higher, 4.3 kT. Because of the higher barrier in Ca, conductance is lower by a factor of two, or

$$e(4.3 - 3.6)kT/kT.$$

The "Anomalous Mole Fraction Effect"

It has been observed in whole-cell recordings of current through Ca channels that conductance in mixtures of Ba and Ca is lower than in either of the pure solutions. Thus conductance is highest in pure Ba, lowest in a mixture of approximately 10% Ca and 90% Ba, and somewhat higher than the minimum value in 100% calcium. This effect has rather quaintly been called the "anomalous mole fraction effect"[2,4] following terminology of Eisenman. At the single channel level, conductance is about the same in 10% Ca and 90% Ba as in 100% Ca, and in a strict sense there is no anomalous mole fraction effect.[9] Nonetheless it seems clear that addition of a small amount of Ca profoundly inhibits Ba flux through the channels.

The one-site model considered here predicts inhibition of Ba current by Ca, and, with appropriate selection of energy levels, an anomalous mole-fraction effect. In mixtures of Ca and Ba, a fraction of the sites are occupied by 1 Ca, or 1 Ca and 1 barium. Because Ca has a higher affinity for the site, a relatively large fraction of the singly occupied sites contain Ca, even at low Ca concentration.

Now suppose that the external medium is 10% Ca and 90% Ba, and consider the substantial fraction of the channels that contain 1 calcium. Conduction requires that a second ion from the external medium enter the site, and the original Ca ion must pass on through the membrane. Because the concentration ratio outside is 9 to 1 in favor of Ba, the entering ion is most likely Ba. We must now ask, How likely is it that Ba can replace Ca in the site?

To answer, we must know the energy of a site occupied by 1 Ba and 1 Ca. In FIGURE 5 we have assumed that the energy of such a site is lower than a 1 Ca-occupied site by 3.6 kT. That is, Ba as a second ion lowers the energy by the same amount whether the first ion is Ba or Ca.

Considering still the sites that were originally occupied by 1 Ca, conduction requires jumping to the 1 Ba-occupied state (and passage of the Ca ion to the inside). The barrier for this event is 9.3 kT, compared to only 3.6 kT for a transition to the 1 Ca-occupied state. Thus, return of the Ba ion to external medium, with no resulting transport across the membrane, is the more likely event, by a factor of

$$e(9.3 - 3.6)kT/kT$$

or 299.

The net result is that the substantial fraction of the channels that are 1 Ca-occupied do not conduct effectively. Conductance thus is depressed by replacing a small fraction of the Ba ions in a pure Ba solution by Ca. Quantitative calculations confirm these qualitative predictions. The degree of the depression depends, of course, on the energy levels, and it is arguable that the selection of levels in FIGURE 5 is not the only reasonable possibility.

DISCUSSION

The one-site model that is presented here can reproduce all of the major selectivity phenomena that have been reported for Ca channels. An obvious question, for which as yet we have no clear answer, is whether the one-site model is preferable to the two-site model. In defense of the one-site model, it can be said that it gives a reasonable physical basis for selectivity, whereas the two-site model simply assigns energy levels on an arbitrary basis, as necessary to fit the data. Perhaps the strongest argument, however, is experimental: the one-site model is clearly compatible with Chow's detailed analysis of the interaction of the Cd ion with Ca channels. From his analysis Chow concluded that there is a single site very close to the outer end of the channel. Although he did not explicitly consider a two-site model, it seems somewhat unlikely to be compatible with his data. Clearly these questions need more study.

The one-site model provides a plausible physical explanation for all of the selectivity properties reported for Ca channels. It will be interesting to see whether it can meet future experimental tests. One such test is to provide an explanation for the slow increase of conductance with concentration that has been observed by Yue and Marban.[9] This phenomenon, they conclude, is not explained by the two-site model and is probably outside the scope of the model presented here.

REFERENCES

1. MCCLESKEY, E. W. & W. ALMERS. 1985. The Ca channel in skeletal muscle is a large pore. Proc. Natl. Acad. Sci. USA **82:** 7149–7153.
2. HESS, P. & R. W. TSIEN. 1984. Mechanism of ion permeation through calcium channels. Nature **309:** 453–456.
3. ALMERS, W., E. W. MCCLESKEY & P. T. PALADE. 1984a. A non-selective cation conductance in frog muscle membrane blocked by micromolar external calcium ions. J. Physiol. (London) **353:** 565–583.
4. ALMERS, W. & E. W. MCCLESKEY. 1984b. Non-selective conductance in calcium channels of frog muscle: calcium selectivity in a single-file pore. J. Physiol. **353:** 585–608.
5. CHOW, R. H. 1991. J. Gen. Physiol. In press.
6. LEVITT, D. G. 1978. Electrostatic calculations of an ion channel. Energy and potential profiles and interactions between ions. Biophys. J. **22:** 209–219.
7. JORDAN, P. C. 1984. The total electrostatic potential in a gramicidin channel. J. Membr. Biol. **78:** 91–102.
8. HESS, P., J. B. LANSMAN & R. W. TSIEN. 1986. J. Gen. Physiol. **88:** 293–319.
9. YUE, D. T. & E. MARBAN. 1990. Permeation in the dihydropyridine-sensitive calcium channel. Multi-ion occupancy but no anomalous mole-fraction effect between Ba^{2+} and Ca^{2+}. J. Gen. Physiol. **95:** 911.

Enzymatic Gating of Voltage-Activated Calcium Channels

D. L. ARMSTRONG,[a] M. F. ROSSIER,
A. D. SHCHERBATKO, AND R. E. WHITE

Laboratory of Cellular and Molecular Pharmacology
National Institute of Environmental Health Sciences
Research Triangle Park, North Carolina 27709

More than a decade has passed since electrophysiologists began to recognize that signaling in the nervous system involves more complicated metabolic pathways than activating ion channels directly through membrane depolarization or ligand binding.[1-3] During that time, substantial evidence has accumulated to support Paul Greengard's original proposal that protein kinases might mediate many of the effects of neurotransmitters on cell function by phosphorylating specific target proteins.[4] Phosphate esters can be attached enzymatically and removed many times per second with dramatic consequences on protein conformation.[5] Some of the earliest and most compelling evidence for ion channel modulation by second messengers through protein phosphorylation was obtained from cardiac muscle cells.[6-8] By activating adenylyl cyclase to produce cAMP, which in turn stimulates a cAMP-dependent protein kinase, noradrenaline rapidly increases the number of voltage-activated calcium channels that respond to membrane depolarization.[9,10]

DIHYDROPYRIDINE-SENSITIVE CALCIUM CHANNELS

The high affinity of dihydropyridine binding to these calcium channels has been exploited to purify the channel protein from skeletal muscle and determine its primary and subunit structure.[11] The α1 subunit that binds dihydropyridines is an essential component of the voltage-activated calcium channel in skeletal muscle and shows remarkable sequence homology to other voltage-activated channels.[12-14] As expected from the physiological studies on cardiac muscle, the dihydropyridine-binding protein from skeletal muscle is phosphorylated rapidly by several protein kinases,[15-17] but the physiological significance of phosphorylation in skeletal muscle, where many of the dihydropyridine receptors do not function as calcium channels,[18] remains to be determined.

In the brain, calcium influx through dihydropyridine-sensitive calcium channels in the plasma membrane stimulates neurite outgrowth, synaptic plasticity, and gene activation.[19-21] Whether calcium influx through dihydropyridine-sensitive calcium channels also contributes directly to neurotransmitter release from presynaptic terminals is discussed further in other chapters of this book. In the pituitary, however, secretion depends almost entirely on calcium entry through dihydropyridine-sensitive calcium channels,[22,23] even when secretion is stimulated by neuropeptides that mobilize intracellular calcium through activation of phospholipase C.[24] Despite

[a] Address for correspondence: LCMP (7-07) NIEHS, P.O. Box 12233, Research Triangle Park, NC 27709

a small conductance (~ 60 ions/ms at 0 mV) in standard physiological saline and the brevity of the average opening (≤ 1 ms), these channels are very efficient at raising intracellular calcium.[25] Consequently, small changes in the frequency or duration of channel openings could have profound effects on calcium signaling.

PROTEIN PHOSPHORYLATION ALTERS GATING

The introduction of patch-clamp techniques[26,27] for detecting transitions between functional conformations of individual channels in the absence of much of the cell's

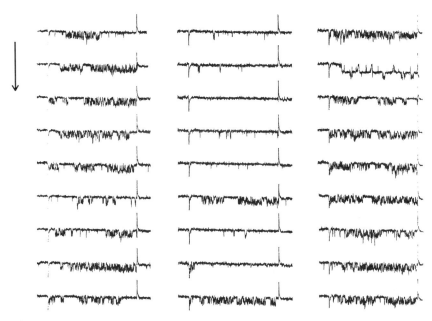

FIGURE 1. Dihydropyridine-sensitive calcium channels exhibit three modes of gating in cell-attached patches; leak-subtracted unitary currents recorded with 90 mM Ba^{2+}, 20 mM tetraethylammonium, and 1 μM tetrodotoxin in the pipette and 140 mM K^+, 10 mM Mg^{2+}, and 0.1 mM Ca^{2+} in the bath. Successive responses to identical 100 ms pulses from -40 to $+10$ mV delivered at 0.3 Hz are displayed from top to bottom, left to right. Mode 0, few or no openings; mode 1, many short bursts of very brief openings; mode 2 (second trace at upper right), continuous openings of much longer duration. Note how infrequently the channel shifts modes.

metabolic regulatory machinery has made it possible to examine the consequences of phosphorylation on ion channel gating at the molecular level.[28,29] With the collaboration of Paul Greengard, Angus Nairn, and Yvonne Lai in the Laboratory of Molecular and Cellular Neuroscience at the Rockefeller University, we have investigated how protein phosphorylation controls the response of dihydropyridine-sensitive calcium channels to membrane depolarization in clonal cell lines derived from a rat pituitary tumor.

In cell-attached patches on these mammalian endocrine cells, dihydropyridine-sensitive calcium channels exhibit three distinct modes of gating (FIG. 1): mode 0, few or no openings; mode 1, many short bursts of very brief openings; and mode 2 (second trace at upper right), continuous openings of much longer duration. These qualitatively different responses to membrane depolarization were first observed in cardiac muscle and dorsal root ganglion neurons.[30,31] Because the average activity within a mode is constant, and because transitions between modes occur on a time scale of seconds, Tsien *et al.* postulated that the modes reflect covalent modifications of the channel protein. Furthermore, the effects of neurotransmitters and dihydropyridines that modulate calcium channel gating appear to result from selectively stabilizing the channel in a particular mode of activity.[32,33] Our experiments on cell-free patches with purified protein kinases[34–36] have tentatively identified the enzymes that catalyze transitions between the modes of gating. FIGURE 2 summarizes those results.

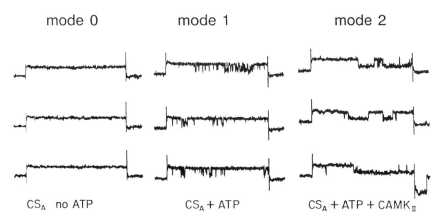

FIGURE 2. Protein phosphorylation determines the mode of channel gating. Examples of unitary barium current responses to voltage steps from −40 to 0 mV when affinity-purified protein kinases are applied to cell-free patches in the inside out configuration. In CsCl solutions containing 2 mM Mg^{2+}, 10 μM calmodulin, no added Ca^{2+}, no EGTA, and 1 μg/mL catalytic subunit of the cAMP-dependent protein kinase (CSA) purified from bovine heart produces no activity (mode 0) in the absence of ATP. Addition of ATP produces only mode 1 gating even in the presence of micromolar calcium and calmodulin. Subsequent addition of calcium- and calmodulin-dependent protein kinase type II subunits purified from rat forebrain produces mode 2–like activity.

Cyclic AMP–Dependent Protein Kinase

In the absence of ATP-Mg to support protein phosphorylation, dihydropyridine-sensitive channels in cell-free patches rapidly enter mode 0.[35] This loss of activity can be slowed substantially in dialyzed cells by buffering calcium on the cytoplasmic side of the membrane, by cooling, or by hyperpolarization of the membrane, but it is not prevented.[37–39] Although the primary amino acid sequences of voltage-activated calcium and sodium channels are highly conserved in the putative membrane spanning domains,[14] this behavior is very different from the behavior of voltage-activated sodium channels, which continue to respond to depolarization for hours in minimal physiological saline solutions. Therefore, it is likely that other regions of the molecule also determine the response to depolarization.

The dihydropyridine-binding protein (α_1) contains several consensus sequences for serine/threonine kinases,[15-17] most of which are located in the large cytoplasmic tail at the carboxy terminal where the amino acid sequence has diverged most from the sodium channel. The β subunit is also phosphorylated *in vitro*,[11] however, and voltage-activated channels have been reconstituted with the purified α_1 subunit in the absence of ATP.[12] Nevertheless, phosphorylation by the cAMP-dependent protein kinase (PKA) is necessary and sufficient to restore activity to these cell-free patches.[34,35] Therefore, we have postulated that dihydropyridine-sensitive calcium channels must be phosphorylated to respond to membrane depolarization. In addition, ATP-Mg alone often sustains activity in cell-free patches, but that effect is blocked by a protein inhibitor of PKA that was isolated originally from skeletal muscle by Walsh *et al.*[40] Therefore, we concluded that an endogenous PKA is often associated with the membrane in sufficient proximity to the channel to regulate its gating on a physiological time scale. Similar observations have now been reported on many cell types.[41-43] In all cases, however, the predominant effect of cAMP-dependent phosphorylation is to promote mode 1 activity.

Calcium/Calmodulin-Dependent Protein Kinase II

More recently we have discovered that mode 2 activity can be stimulated in the absence of any dihydropyridines by a calcium/calmodulin- and ATP-dependent process that can be reconstituted in cell-free patches with the multifunctional calcium and calmodulin-dependent protein kinase type II (CaMKII) purified from rat forebrain.[36] The involvement of a calcium-dependent process may explain why mode 2 activity in cell-attached patches has been difficult to detect.[44,45] In order to voltage-clamp cell-attached patches at fixed voltages, investigators routinely zero the cell's resting membrane potential by bathing the cell in 140 mM K^+. This has the unwelcome side effect of activating the voltage-dependent channels in the membrane outside the patch. To avoid calcium-dependent inactivation (see below) of the dihydropyridine-sensitive calcium channels in the patch, EGTA is added routinely to the bath solution. This reduces calcium entry through voltage-activated calcium channels, but it also depletes intracellular calcium. We have restored mode 2 gating to channels in cell-attached patches by using high Mg^{2+}/low Ca^{2+} solutions to limit calcium entry across the plasma membrane. Thus, mode 2 activity can also be observed at physiological voltages on intact cells in the complete absence of dihydropyridines or neurotransmitters.[46-48]

Protein Kinase C

Although the purified dihydropyridine binding protein from cardiac muscle can be phosphorylated by protein kinase C (PKC) as well as PKA and CaMKII,[16,17] we have found no evidence for direct effects of PKC on dihydropyridine-sensitive calcium channel gating in rat pituitary tumor cells. By contrast, there are many reports of the inhibitory effects of phorbol esters on calcium channel gating in mammalian neurons.[49] In many of those systems, however, the class of calcium channels that were modulated was not identified unambiguously. Furthermore, phorbol esters have been reported to have direct effects on calcium channels that are unrelated to PKC activation[50,51] and to stimulate phospholipase A2, which may alter calcium channel gating through lipoxygenase metabolites of arachidonic acid.[52,53] In summary, in cells where dihydropyridine-sensitive channels can be studied confidently in isolation, stimulation of PKC through receptor activation of phospholipase C has had no direct effects on channel gating.[54–56]

DEPHOSPHORYLATION INACTIVATES THE CHANNEL

If protein kinases stimulate activity, one may expect protein phosphatases to inhibit activity. As noted above, in the absence of ATP-Mg the channels remain in mode 0. In addition, purified protein phosphatases reverse the effects of protein phosphorylation and inhibit dihydropyridine-sensitive calcium channels.[57–59] One of these phosphatases, calcineurin, is activated by calcium/calmodulin and may be responsible for the calcium-dependent inactivation of macroscopic currents.[60,61]

Thus, intracellular calcium stimulates both activation and inactivation of the dihydropyridine-sensitive calcium channel through calmodulin-dependent enzymes. The net effect of intracellular calcium transients on channel activity will depend on the magnitude and distribution of the increase. Large increases near the membrane associated with calcium channel activity might plausibly activate calcineurin because it is associated with the membrane through the myristic acid moiety on its amino terminal glycine. By contrast, smaller sustained rises in intracellular calcium might preferentially activate the cytoplasmic CaMKII. Once activated, the two enzymes also turn off differently. Although calcineurin activity declines rapidly when calcium is reduced, CaMKII enzymes that have been autophosphorylated remain active.[62]

DIHYDROPYRIDINES MODULATE GATING

It has been suggested that dihydropyridines modulate calcium channel activity by stabilizing the less common modes of gating:[30,31] antagonists like nimodipine promote mode 0, and agonists like BAY K 8644 promote mode 2. Other dihydropyridines, like nitrendipine or nifedipine, produce both effects: increasing the frequency of null sweeps (mode 0) but shifting the channel from mode 1 to mode 2 in the active sweeps. Nevertheless, all these compounds appear to bind competitively to one site on the α_1 subunit.[63] Therefore, it is intriguing how one ligand produces two very different effects.

We began to study calcium channel modulation by dihydropyridines to address the questions raised by the successful reconstitution of calcium channel gating in lipid bilayers without ATP. Although the frequency of successful reconstitution was too low to rule out the possibility that the active channels were still phosphorylated,[64] we were interested in the fact that the best success was obtained when the channels were purified in the presence of BAY K 8644.[65] Therefore, we investigated the effect of BAY K 8644 on channel rundown in cell-free patches. When cells were exposed to 1 μM BAY K 8644 before the patch was excised, the channels remained active in the absence of ATP for 30 minutes or more in every case. By contrast, preexposing the cells to 100 nM vasoactive intestinal peptide to maximally activate G_S and adenylyl cyclase had no significant effect over controls. BAY K 8644 also slows calcium-dependent inactivation of the dihydropyridine-sensitive calcium channels.[66,67]

Thus, BAY K 8644 slows two processes that are reversed by cAMP-dependent phosphorylation, and we have postulated that BAY K 8644 produces its effects on channel gating by slowing dephosphorylation of the channel.[35] That would explain why calcium current stimulation by BAY K 8644 and β-adrenergic agonists is additive in cardiac muscle cells.[10] One reduces the rate of channel dephosphorylation, whereas the other stimulates the rate of channel phosphorylation. We do not believe this is a direct effect of BAY K 8644 on the phosphatase, although dihydropyridines do inhibit calmodulin at higher concentrations. Instead we believe that BAY K 8644 produces its effect allosterically. Whether the increase in open-channel lifetime that is associated with mode 2 activity is an independent allosteric effect or whether it results directly from inhibition of dephosphorylation (see below) remains to be determined.

These observations led us to speculate that dihydropyridine antagonists might produce their effects by slowing rephosphorylation of the channel.[34] In other words, what makes a dihydropyridine an agonist or an antagonist is its relative affinity for phosphorylated or dephosphorylated channels. In that context it is easy to explain the action of a drug like nitrendipine, which is expected to show relatively equal affinity for the phosphorylated and dephosphorylated site. We have recently tested this hypothesis by examining the effect of cAMP-dependent phosphorylation on the effectiveness of nimodipine block on single dihydropyridine-sensitive calcium channels in cell-attached and cell-free patches from rat pituitary tumor cells.[68] In both

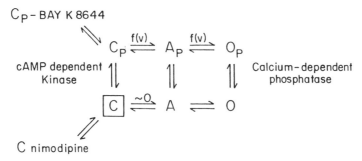

FIGURE 3. State diagram to explain modulation of dihydropyridine-sensitive channels by phosphorylation and dihydropyridines: two closed states, C and A, and one open state, O, each of which can be phosphorylated, as indicated by the subscript p, or dephosphorylated.

cases, cAMP-dependent phosphorylation reduces the effectiveness of block by nimodipine.

A MODEL FOR ENZYMATIC GATING

All the results that are summarized above can be explained by the state diagram illustrated in FIGURE 3. Although the model is very simple, it is not unique. Nevertheless, the model has the virtue of explaining the kinetic observations under very different metabolic conditions. Only three states are postulated: a resting closed state, C; an activated state, A, that is also closed; and an open state, O. Two closed states are postulated because two exponentials are required to fit the closed time distributions of single-channel records.[69] In addition, in our model each state can be phosphorylated by a cAMP-dependent kinase (denoted by the subscript p) and dephosphorylated by a Ca^{2+}-dependent phosphatase, both of which have been shown to act on the channel protein.[15] Forward transitions from C_p to A_p and from A_p to O_p are believed to be voltage-dependent, but the dephosphorylated channel exhibits a much slower, almost negligible, forward rate from C to A. Thus, in this model C is the inactivated state of the channel. The ratio of phosphorylated to dephosphorylated channels is determined by the relative activity of the kinase and the phosphatase. Thus, the microscopic kinetics of gating in the model are determined in part by the rate constants of enzymatic reactions. Gating can be modulated by altering those rate constants. For example, calcium produces inactivation by stimulating dephosphorylation of the "resting" state, C_p.

The state diagram also provides a convenient way of understanding the mechanism of dihydropyridine action. Nimodipine slows rephosphorylation of the channel by binding selectively to the dephosphorylated state. By contrast, BAY K 8644 binds selectively to the phosphorylated state and reduces the rate of channel dephosphorylation. For simplicity, dihydropyridines are only shown binding to the resting closed states. No transitions between phosphorylated and dephosphorylated channels are indicated for dihydropyridine-bound channels to emphasize the hypothesis that dihydropyridines produce their effects by slowing those transitions.

IMPLICATIONS

Finally, the model raises two interesting possibilities that remain to be considered. The first question is, Which open state corresponds to which mode of gating? If BAY K 8644 and CaMKII produce mode 2 activity by inhibiting dephosphorylation of the cAMP-dependent site, then mode 2 activity represents the opening of phosphorylated channels. In that case, however, mode 1 gating must reflect the activity of the dephosphorylated channels (state O). In other words, the channels are usually dephosphorylated before or shortly after they open, they oscillate back and forth between state A and state O, and then they must be rephosphorylated when the channel returns to the inactivated closed state, C. This could explain why hyperpolarization slows rundown,[39] why both activation and inactivation are slower in BAY K 8644,[67] and why both cAMP-dependent phosphorylation and large depolarizations increase the frequency of mode 2 openings.[32,46,47]

Second, the hypothesis that activated channels have a much higher probability of being dephosphorylated could also explain the voltage-dependent relief of nimodipine block in pituitary tumor cells that exhibit no steady-state inactivation at those voltages.[68] In pituitary tumor cells, the rate of phosphorylation is much greater than the rate of dephosphorylation under resting conditions because cAMP levels are high, as indicated by the high probability of finding channels in cell-attached patches in mode 1 when the membrane is depolarized (FIG. 1). Consequently, dephosphorylated channels are rapidly rephosphorylated in the absence of intracellular accumulation of calcium, so barium currents do not show any "voltage-dependent" inactivation.

By contrast, in unstimulated heart muscle cells the probability of channel opening is very low, and β-adrenergic stimulation increases activity dramatically.[10] Thus, one might infer that under resting conditions the rate of dephosphorylation is much greater than the rate of phosphorylation. In that case, channels that enter the activated state during weak depolarizations will be dephosphorylated rapidly and rephosphorylated slowly. In other words, the channels will accumulate in the inactivated state. This novel view of voltage-dependent inactivation of dihydropyridine-sensitive calcium channels is very similar to the current understanding of sodium-channel inactivation, which is believed to be voltage-dependent because inactivation proceeds from a closed state that is only occupied at more positive voltages.[70] In fact, the sodium channels' transition to the inactivated state shows no more intrinsic dependence on voltage than the inactivation of barium currents through dihydropyridine-sensitive calcium channels in GH_3 cells. This conclusion is also supported by the observation that voltage-dependent inactivation of both sodium and calcium channels can be removed altogether by mild trypsin treatment of the cytoplasmic side of the membrane[70,71] because it is assumed that the trypsin is unable to cleave portions of the channel protein that are buried in the membrane where they could feel the field.

SUMMARY

The model of calcium-channel gating described above, although almost certainly too simple, suggests a direct role for protein kinases and phosphatases in determining the kinetics of calcium channel gating on a subsecond time scale. In addition, it provides a unique perspective for understanding studies of calcium channel gating under widely different metabolic and pharmacological conditions. Although many of these effects may be specific to the dihydropyridine-sensitive or L-type calcium channel, they give an indication of the range of possibilities for integrating calcium-channel activity with cellular biochemistry.

REFERENCES

1. KEHOE, J. & A. MARTY. 1980. Annu. Rev. Biophys. Bioeng. **9:** 437–465.
2. HARTZELL, H. C. 1981. Nature **291:** 539–544.
3. KOSTYUK, P. G. 1984. Neurosci. **13:** 983–989.
4. GREENGARD, P. 1976. Nature **260:** 101–108.
5. SPRANG, S. R., K. R. ACHARYA, E. J. GOLDSMITH, D. I. STUART, K. VARVILL, R. J. FLETTERICK, N. B. MADSEN & L. N. JOHNSON. 1988. Nature **336:** 215–221.
6. TSIEN, R. W., W. GILES & P. GREENGARD. 1972. Nature New Biol. **240:** 181–183.
7. KAMEYAMA, M., F. HOFMANN & W. TRAUTWEIN. 1985. Pflugers Arch. **405:** 285–293.
8. KAMEYAMA, M., J. HESCHELER, F. HOFMANN & W. TRAUTWEIN. 1986. Pflugers Arch. **407:** 123–128.
9. REUTER, H. 1979. Annu. Rev. Physiol. **41:** 413–424.
10. TSIEN, R. W., B. P. BEAN, P. HESS, J. B. LANSMAN, B. NILIUS & M. C. NOWYCKY. 1986. J. Mol. Cell. Cardiol. **18:** 691–710.
11. CATTERALL, W. A., M. J. SEAGAR & M. TAKAHASHI. 1988. J. Biol. Chem. **263:** 3535–3538.
12. FLOCKERZI, V., H. OEKEN, F. HOFMANN, D. PELZER, A. CAVALIE & W. TRAUTWEIN. 1986. Nature **323:** 66–68.
13. TANABE, T., K. G. BEAM, J. A. POWELL & S. NUMA. 1988. Nature **336:** 134–138.
14. TANABE, T., H. TAKESHIMA, A. MIKAMI, V. FLOCKERZI, H. TAKAHASHI, K. KANGAWA, M. KOJIMA, H. MATSUO, T. HIROSE & S. NUMA. 1987. Nature **328:** 313–318.
15. HOSEY, M. M., M. BORSOTTO & M. LAZDUNSKI. 1986. Proc. Natl. Acad. Sci. USA **83:** 3733–3737.
16. O'CALLAHAN, C. M. & M. M. HOSEY. 1988. Biochemistry **27:** 6071–6077.
17. JAHN, H., W. NASTAINCZYK, A. ROHRKASTEN, T. SCHNEIDER & F. HOFMANN. 1988. Eur. J. Biochem. **178:** 535–542.
18. SCHWARTZ, L. M., E. W. MCCLESKY & W. ALMERS. 1985. Nature **314:** 747–751.
19. SILVER, R. A., A. G. LAMB & S. R. BOLSOVER. Nature **343:** 751–754.
20. HOCKBERGER, P. E., H. TSENG & J. A. CONNOR. 1989. J. Neurosci. **9:** 2272–2284.
21. MORGAN, J. I. & T. CURRAN. 1988. Cell Calcium **9:** 303–311.
22. KIDOKORO, Y. 1975. Nature **258:** 741–742.
23. ENYEART, J. J., T. AIZAWA & P. M. HINKLE. 1985. Am. J. Physiol. **248:** C510–C519.
24. BENHAM, C. D. 1989. J. Physiol. **415:** 143–158.
25. SCHLEGEL, W., B. P. WINIGER, P. MOLLARD, P. VACHER, F. WUARIN, G. R. ZAHND, C. B. WOLLHEIM & B. DUFY. 1987. Nature **329:** 719–721.

26. HORN, R. & J. B. PATLACK. 1980. Proc. Natl. Acad. Sci. USA **77:** 6930–6934.
27. HAMILL, O. P., A. MARTY, E. NEHER, B. SAKMANN & F. J. SIGWORTH. 1981. Pfluegers Arch. **391:** 85–100.
28. SHUSTER, M. J., J. S. CAMARDO, S. A. SIEGELBAUM & E. R. KANDEL. 1985. Nature **313:** 392–395.
29. EWALD, D. A., A. WILLIAMS & I. B. LEVITAN. 1985. Nature **315:** 503–506.
30. HESS, P., J. B. LANSMAN & R. W. TSIEN. 1984. Nature **311:** 538–544.
31. NOWYCKY, M. C., A. P. FOX & R. W. TSIEN. Proc. Natl. Acad. Sci. USA **82:** 2178–2182.
32. YUE, D. T., S. HERZIG & E. MARBAN. 1990. Proc. Natl. Acad. Sci. USA **87:** 753–757.
33. OCHI, R. & Y. KAWASHIMA. 1990. J. Physiol. **424:** 187–204.
34. ARMSTRONG, D. L. 1988. Biomed. Res. **9:** 11–15.
35. ARMSTRONG, D. L. & R. ECKERT. 1987. Proc. Natl. Acad. Sci. USA **84:** 2518–2522.
36. ARMSTRONG, D. L., C. ERXLEBEN, D. KALMAN, Y. LAI, A. NAIRN & P. GREENGARD. 1988. J. Gen. Physiol. **92:** 10a.
37. HAGIWARA, S. & S. NAKAJIMA. 1966. J. Gen. Physiol. **49:** 807–818.
38. FENWICK, E. M., A. MARTY & E. NEHER. 1982. J. Physiol. **331:** 599–635.
39. SCHOUTEN, V. J. A. & M. MORAD. 1989. Pfluegers Arch. **415:** 1–11.
40. WALSH, D. A., C. D. ASHBY, C. GONZALEZ, D. CALKINS, E. FISCHER & E. G. KREBS. 1971. J. Biol. Chem. **246:** 1977–1985.
41. NUNOKI, K., V. FLORIO & W. A. CATTERALL. 1989. Proc. Natl. Acad. Sci. USA **86:** 6816–6820.
42. OHYA, Y. & N. SPERELAKIS. 1989. Pfluegers Arch. **414:** 257–264.
43. ROMAINEN, C., P. GROSSWAGEN & H. SCHINDLER. 1989. Biophys. J. **55:** 299a.
44. CAVALIE, A., D. PELZER & W. TRAUTWEIN. 1986. Pfluegers Arch. **406:** 241–258.
45. LACERDA, A. E. & A. M. BROWN. 1989. J. Gen. Physiol. **93:** 1243–1273.
46. PIETROBON, D. & P. HESS. 1990. Nature **346:** 651–655.
47. MAZZANTI, M. & L. J. DEFELICE. 1990. Biophys. J. **58:** 1059–1065.
48. ARTALEJO, C. R., M. A. ARIANO, R. L. PERLMAN & A. P. FOX. 1990. Nature **348:** 239–242.
49. MILLER, R. J. 1990. FASEB J. **4:** 3291–3299.
50. HOCKBERGER, P., M. TOSELLI, D. SWANDULLA & H. D. LUX. 1989. Nature **338:** 340–342.
51. DOERNER, D., M. ABDEL-LATIF, T. B. ROGERS & B. E. ALGER. 1990. J. Neurosci. **10:** 1699–1706.
52. CARLSON, R. O. & I. B. LEVITAN. 1990. J. Membr. Biol. **116:** 249–260.
53. KEYSER, D. O. & B. E. ALGER. 1990. Neuron **5:** 545–553.
54. DUBINSKY, J. M. & G. S. OXFORD. 1985. Proc. Natl. Acad. Sci. USA **82:** 4282–4286.
55. WALSH, K. B. & R. S. KASS. 1988. Science **242:** 67–69.
56. APKON, M. & J. M. NERBONNE. 1988. Proc. Natl. Acad. Sci. USA **85:** 8756–8760.
57. CHAD, J. E. & R. ECKERT. 1986. J. Physiol. **378:** 31–51.
58. HESCHELER, J., M. KAMEYAMA, W. TRAUTWEIN, G. MIESKES & H. SOLING. 1987. Eur. J. Biochem. **165:** 261–266.
59. HESCHELER, J., G. MIESKES, J. C. RUEGG, A. TAKAI & W. TRAUTWEIN. 1988. Pfluegers Arch. **412:** 248–252.
60. KALMAN, D., P. H. O'LAGUE, C. ERXLEBEN & D. L. ARMSTRONG. 1988. J. Gen. Physiol. **92:** 531–548.
61. ARMSTRONG, D. L. 1989. Trends Neurosci. **12:** 117–122.
62. LAI, Y., A. C. NAIRN & P. GREENGARD. 1986. Proc. Natl. Acad. Sci. USA **83:** 4253–4257.
63. KWON, Y. W., G. FRANCKOWIAK, D. A. LANGE, M. HAWTHORN, A. JOSLYN & D. J. TRIGGLE. 1989. Naunyn-Schmiedeberg's Arch. Pharmakol. **339:** 19–30.
64. CURTIS, B. M. & W. A. CATTERALL. 1986. Biochemistry **25:** 3077–3083.
65. AFFOLTER, H. & R. CORONADO. 1985. Biophys. J. **48:** 341–347.
66. KALMAN, D. & D. L. ARMSTRONG. 1988. *In* The Calcium Channel: Structure, Function, and Implications. M. Morad, W. Naylor, S. Kazda & M. Schramm, Eds.: 103–114. Springer-Verlag. Berlin.
67. LORY, P., J. NARGEOT, S. RICHARD & F. TIAHO. 1989. J. Physiol. **418:** 25P.
68. ARMSTRONG, D. L. & D. KALMAN. 1990. Biophys. J. **57:** 516a.
69. HAGIWARA, S. & H. OHMORI. 1983. J. Physiol. **336:** 649–661.
70. GONOI, T. & B. HILLE. 1987. J. Gen. Physiol. **89:** 253–274.
71. HESCHELER, J. & W. TRAUTWEIN. 1988. J. Physiol. **404:** 259–274.

The Sea Urchin Cortical Reaction

A Model System for Studying the Final Steps of Calcium-Triggered Vesicle Fusion

STEVEN S. VOGEL,[a] KERRY DELANEY,[b] AND
JOSHUA ZIMMERBERG[a]

[a] Laboratory of Theoretical and Physical Biology
National Institute of Child Health and Human Development
National Institutes of Health
Bethesda, Maryland 20892

[b] New York University and
A.T. & T. Bell Labs
Murray Hill, New Jersey 07974

INTRODUCTION

Calcium-triggered vesicle fusion is a fundamental step of chemical-synaptic release. To fully understand complex synaptic functions, such as potentiation, facilitation, and presynaptic inhibition, we wish to first understand, on a molecular level, this basic step of neuronal communication. Certain aspects of the study of calcium-triggered vesicle fusion at synaptic terminals are difficult because of the small size of synaptic terminals, the functional fragility of these systems, and the inaccessibility of the terminal's interior to experimental control. Studies of calcium-mediated vesicle fusion in less limiting, nonneuronal systems have taught much, and although we cannot extrapolate directly to the synapse, these studies have been very useful for the development of hypotheses.[1–5]

To study the mechanism by which calcium leads to membrane fusion, one must devise methods to isolate the fusion reaction from others that either prime, maintain, or modulate fusion. In the context of the topic of this volume, we will first describe the sea urchin cortical reaction, compare calcium-triggered membrane fusion in the sea urchin egg to the synapse, and finally describe how we have used this system to dissect different steps of calcium-triggered vesicle fusion.

CORTICAL GRANULE EXOCYTOSIS IN THE EGG

When Echinoderm (and many other) eggs are fertilized there are two mechanisms that block multiple sperm from entering the egg: a fast change in membrane potential called the fast block to polyspermy,[6] and a slower block due to the raising and hardening of the fertilization envelope, called the cortical reaction.[7,8] The cortical reaction can be broken into three steps: 1) the sperm fertilizing the egg results in the release of calcium from intracellular stores; 2) the rise of intracellular free calcium triggers the fusion of cortical granules (exocytotic vesicles that line the inner leaflet of the egg plasma membrane) with the egg membrane; 3) granular contents (mostly enzymes and mucopolysaccharides) released into the perivitelline space result in the raising of the fertilization envelope. In the egg, three lines of evidence suggest that calcium triggers the cortical reaction. First, cortical granule fusion can be seen when calcium is injected into the egg.[9] Second, the cortical reaction can be triggered by calcium ionophores in a calcium-dependent manner.[10-12] Finally, the sperm-induced cortical reaction can be blocked by injection of calcium chelators into the egg.[13]

COMPARISON OF THE CORTICAL REACTION AND SYNAPTIC RELEASE

Calcium-triggered vesicle fusion observed in sea urchin eggs appears to be similar to the fusion of other biological membranes in that it results in vectorial, nonleaky transport of the secretory granule contents to the extracellular space by way of omega-shaped intermediates that demonstrate the coalescence of cortical granule membrane and plasma membranes.[14] The concentrations of calcium required to trigger the cortical reaction in permeabilized cells are similar to the concentrations capable of triggering vesicle fusion in other systems: micromolar free calcium.[1,12] TABLE 1 shows a comparison of synaptic release and the cortical reaction. Differences between the two systems might reflect the different physiological constraints on the systems. (1) Synapses need to communicate at speeds of 1 ms; the cortical reaction does not have to be as fast because of the fast electrical block to polyspermy.[6] (2) All cortical granules need to fuse during the cortical reaction to build a substantial fertilization barrier around the egg, whereas only a small percentage of synaptic vesicles need to fuse after an action potential in order to communicate with a postsynaptic element.[15] (3) Synaptic vesicles need to fuse near specialized regions of the presynaptic terminal membrane in order to release their contents onto specific postsynaptic elements; cortical granules must fuse in every region of the egg plasma membrane to construct a fertilization barrier all around the egg. Some of these mechanistic differences may result from the substantial differences between the calcium delivery systems in synaptic terminals and eggs. Calcium influx through voltage-dependent calcium channels in presynaptic terminals produces highly localized, transient (< 1 ms) increases in calcium concentration at release sites.[16,17] In the sea urchin, egg fertilization results in release of calcium from internal stores, which elevates bulk calcium for tens of seconds.[18]

Similarities may reflect elements common to calcium-mediated exocytosis: (1) Similar calcium concentrations are capable of triggering the reaction.[1] (2) The extent of fusion is a sigmoidal function of the calcium concentration when eggs and synaptosomes are permeabilized in the presence of calcium.[1] (3) The rate of fusion increases as a function of calcium concentration[19,20] (see FIG. 1). (4) The predominant mode of fusion in both systems is simple, as compared to compound, exocytosis. Although compound exocytosis has been occasionally observed in the intact sea

TABLE 1.

	Synapse	Sea Urchin Egg
Primary trigger	membrane depolarization	sperm
Final trigger	μM calcium	μM calcium
Shortest lag time observed (from calcium to fusion)	0.2 ms	10–35 ms
Extent of fusion vs. calcium	sigmoidal	sigmoidal
Rate of fusion vs. calcium	increases	increases
Main mode of exocytosis: simple or compound	simple	simple
Compound exocytosis observed	?	yes

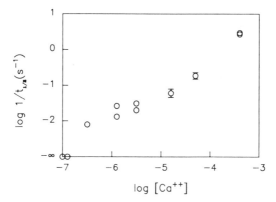

FIGURE 1. The half-time of the cortical reaction in isolated planar cortices was measured as the time between calcium perfusion and half-maximal light-scattering change at various calcium concentrations. (Zimmerberg *et al.*[25] With permission from the *Journal of Cell Biology.*)

urchin egg (Zimmerberg and Kachar, unpublished observation), and although purified granules are capable of fusing with each other,[21,22] the evidence for compound exocytosis in neuronal tissue is still not conclusive.[23,24]

The fact that vesicles are "predocked," (bound to the plasma membrane prior to activation) distinguishes these two systems from other examples of exocytosis. For example, in the mast cell and neutrophil, granules are separated from the plasma membrane by as much as 200 nm,[14] and only after activation does the plasma membrane contact the secretory vesicle. In the sea urchin egg, the attachment site is a specialized zone of adhesion, where the two opposing bilayers are connected by amorphous material at the resolution of the electron microscope.[25]

The observation that the extent of exocytosis is a sigmoidal function of calcium concentration in both sea urchin eggs, and synaptosomes (isolated nerve terminals),[1] we find especially interesting. Because vesicle fusion is an irreversible reaction, we would expect that if suprathreshold calcium was introduced into the fusion site, and the fusion reaction was allowed to proceed indefinitely, all docked vesicles should ultimately fuse. This is not observed, so this reaction does not follow simple kinetics. Rather, a percentage of vesicles fuse, and this percentage of fused vesicles is determined by the calcium concentration. This can be explained in two ways:[26] First, the vesicles may not be homogeneous in their ability to fuse in response to calcium. The second explanation suggests that some other kinetic process that interferes with vesicle fusion is also operating, perhaps with slower kinetics. This would produce a system that is sensitive to the rate of change of the calcium concentration, in addition to the concentration itself.[26] Regardless of which mechanism is responsible for this common behavior between most permeabilized exocytotic systems, the fact that both synaptosomes and the cortical reaction exhibit this unique kinetic behavior suggests that they may share a common mechanism. Clearly more experimentation is required to determine the basis for the kinetics of fusion in these systems.

EXOCYTOSIS IN THE ISOLATED PLANAR CORTEX

One of the great advantages of using the cortical reaction to study calcium-triggered fusion is easy access to the intracellular compartment. When eggs are placed on polycation-coated glass slides, they adhere to the treated surface.[27] When a jet of buffer is applied, the eggs break and the cytoplasmic contents are washed away leaving the plasma membrane attached to the glass with cortical granules still bound to the membrane.[28] When this open egg preparation (isolated planar cortex) is perfused with buffers containing sufficient concentrations of calcium, the bound cortical granules fuse with the egg membrane.[25,29] As in the egg, the extent of fusion is a sigmoidal function of calcium concentration. Reagents that perturb cytoskeletal elements do not inhibit fusion.[29] Fusion proceeds perfectly well in solutions devoid of significant electrolyte, and altering membrane permeability neither halts nor triggers fusion.[30] The surface potential of the calcium-binding site for fusion has been studied in this preparation.[31] Proteins probably mediate, at least in part, the cortical reaction because both trypsin and N-ethylmaleimide (NEM) are known inhibitors of the reaction.[32,33] It is not known, however, if these reagents affect granule/plasma membrane attachment, the fusion reaction itself, fusion pore widening, or content dispersal.

KINETICS

One approach for study of a reaction mechanism has been kinetic analysis. Using the sea urchin planar cortex, we have devised a light-scattering assay that measures granule fusion in well-buffered solutions of fixed-calcium concentration, independent of biosynthesis and calcium mobilization.[25] This *in vitro* preparation responds to calcium at micromolar concentrations and is ideal for kinetic analysis. After perfusion with a buffered-calcium solution, the time course of fusion in the isolated planar cortex of the sea urchin egg is complex (FIG. 2). As noted above, the reaction does not go to completion, and the time course is not simply described. The first step is to quantify the relationship between rate of membrane fusion and calcium concentration, to determine the orders of the reactions. One way of quantifying the rate of this complex cortical reaction is to plot the reciprocal of the half time of the total cortical reaction as a function of calcium concentration. In this way, this reaction is pseudo-first-order with respect to calcium (FIG. 1).

While perfusion experiments are useful for applying a step in known calcium, they are limited by fluid dynamics. The fluid change takes time, and then the rate of change of calcium at the release site is dependent upon diffusion of the calcium buffer system through the unstirred layer. Another experimental approach that shows promise is the use of "caged" compounds. Chelators are synthesized that release calcium upon exposure to ultraviolet light.[34] By equilibrating the cortex with a solution containing caged calcium, the calcium can now be stored only angstroms from the membrane surface. After photoactivation of the chelator, there is no appreciable diffusional delay. Preliminary experiments were performed with DM-nitrophen, a chelator whose affinity for calcium decreases after photon absorption.[34] In the cortex, the ability to release calcium directly at the fusion site allows us to measure the initial rate of the cortical reaction (FIG. 3). As the duration of the photolysis pulse increases, more calcium is released, and the initial reaction rate increases. Ongoing experiments are directed towards quantifying the relationship between calcium concentration and vesicle fusion using caged calcium compounds.

Caged calcium compounds can also be used to measure the delay times from calcium release to onset of fusion. Initial experiments with caged calcium compounds allow us to determine delay times for the cortical reaction on the order of 10 milliseconds. Faster photolysis will allow us to measure the delay more accurately. This speed is similar to the time domain of calcium-triggered muscle contraction. In

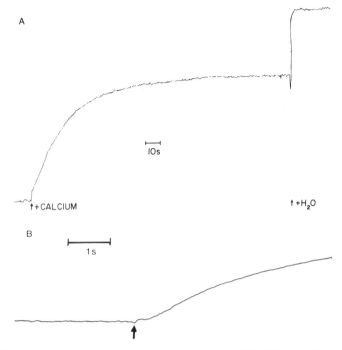

FIGURE 2. A. Sea urchin cortices were prepared in an isotonic 0.1 μM free-calcium buffer and placed in a perfusion chamber while fusion activity (light scattering) was monitored as previously described.[25] At the arrow marked +CALCIUM the cortices were perfused with a buffer containing 17 μM free calcium. The time of calcium addition was detected by a temperature transient recorded from a thermistor built into the perfusion chamber. At the arrow marked +H$_2$O, distilled water was perfused through the chamber to lyse any remaining granules. B. Cortices were treated as in A, but only the initial calcium response was recorded at a higher gain. (Zimmerberg *et al.*[25] With permission from the *Journal of Cell Biology*.)

the squid synapse, the synaptic delay is < 0.2 milliseconds.[35] Biologically, the lag times of both the cortical reaction and synaptic release fall into a time domain that is faster than the biosynthesis of most proteins, yet slower than the fastest of enzyme reactions.[36] From this data we cannot rule out the possibility that proteins, acting in a simple enzymatic manner, might mediate calcium-triggered vesicle fusion.

CORTICAL GRANULE/CORTICAL GRANULE FUSION

While the isolated planar cortex has been very useful as a model system for studying calcium-triggered vesicle fusion, as mentioned above, a serious limitation of the utility of the system has been the inability to differentiate between inhibitors of granule/plasma membrane attachment and inhibitors of the fusion reaction itself. Fortunately, recent developments in the field suggest a way to discriminate between these reaction steps. It has been shown that granules, removed from the egg cortex, and subsequently added back to the cytoplasmic surface of the planar cortex, will fuse with the plasma membrane upon the re-addition of calcium.[21,37] Thus the native,

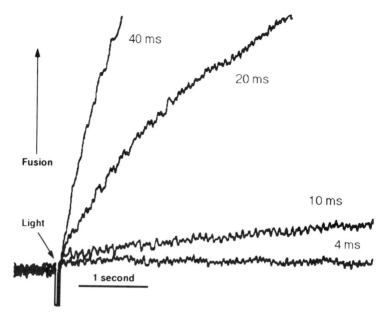

FIGURE 3. Sea urchin cortices were prepared, and fusion activity (light scattering) was monitored as described in FIG. 1, except that cortices were placed in a sealed microscope slide containing an isotonic buffer with the caged calcium compound DM-nitrophen (1 mM, 50% loaded with calcium; Calbiochem, La Jolla, CA). To trigger the release of calcium from the caged compound, the sample chamber was illuminated using a 100 W Hg arc lamp with single UV light pulses of various lengths (4–40 ms) through the epifluorescence port of an IM-35 Zeiss microscope. Control experiments where the DM-nitrophen was not loaded with calcium did not result in fusion.

contact site can be disrupted and reformed upon bringing the membranes back together.

We have further simplified the system by demonstrating that purified cortical granules can also fuse with each other in response to calcium (50% fusion at 32 μM free calcium.[22]). Using the cortical granule/cortical granule reconstituted fusion system, we can now readily control and distinguish certain aspects of binding, fusion, and content release. We believe that cortical granule/cortical granule fusion can be used to study the membrane fusion step of exocytosis in isolation from the adhesion step of exocytosis. We have been able to demonstrate that manipulations that force membranes to come into contact do not trigger fusion themselves, but rather allow membrane fusion in response to the physiological stimulus, calcium (FIG. 4A); and forcing membranes together after treatment with either trypsin or NEM, in the presence of 440 μM free calcium, does not result in membrane fusion (FIGURES 4B and 4C). Thus it is likely that these reagents are affecting steps in fusion that occur after membrane contact. We suggest that the fusion mechanism involved in calcium-triggered exocytosis contains trypsin and NEM-labile sites, presumably proteins, that reside on the surface of the exocytotic granules.

The ability to reconstitute calcium-triggered vesicle fusion between isolated cortical granules opens the door to several lines of research on vesicle fusion that are not currently possible using components from synaptic terminals. (1) It might be possible to isolate the fusion reaction from other reactions either temporally, by triggering this reaction rapidly with caged calcium compounds, or chemically, by introducing inhibitors of other known calcium-dependent reactions. (2) Because this is an open system, we can directly control the calcium concentration and the rate of change of the calcium concentration. In these ways we might be able to ascertain what mechanism is responsible for the sigmoidal extent of exocytosis observed in both synaptosomes and sea urchin eggs. (3) Because isolated granules can be labeled

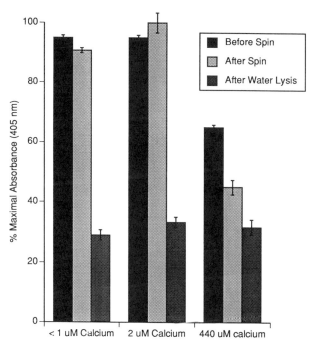

FIGURE 4A. Cortical granules were prepared from *Strongylocentrotus purpuratus* adults. Eggs were prepared as previously described.[25] Cortical granules were isolated as follows: Eggs were attached to the bottoms of tissue culture flasks. Unattached eggs were removed by washing with PKME (50 mM PIPES, pH 6.7; 425 mM KCl, 10 mM $MgCl_2$, 5 mM EGTA). Immobilized eggs were lysed in PKME by hitting the sides of the flask. After several washes in PKME, to remove free cytoplasm and loosely attached vesicles, the egg cortex remained. Cortical granules were removed from the attached cortex by incubation in KEA (450 mM KCl, 5 mM EGTA, 50 mM NH_4Cl, pH 9.1) and again hitting the sides of the flask. Cortical granules were pelleted at $1000 \times g$ for 10 min at 4°C (in a Beckman TJ-6 centrifuge using a TH-4 rotor) and resuspended in 1 mL KEA/flask of eggs (~ 0.2 mg/mL). Isolated cortical granules were kept on ice until ready for use. Prior to use the pH of the cortical granules was adjusted with 1M PIPES, pH 6.1, to pH 6.7. Suspensions of cortical granules (100 μL/well) were mixed with PKME solutions (100 μL) containing varying calcium concentrations. Final free-calcium concentrations were measured using a calcium electrode[38] calibrated with defined reference buffers.[39] The absorption at 405 nm was determined on a Titertek™ Multiscan microtiter plate reader. The suspended granules were then pelleted by centrifugation in a Beckman TH-4 rotor with microtiter plate adaptors $1000 \times g$ for 5 min), and the absorbance was measured again. All points are mean absorbance ± SE, n = 5. The remaining granules were then lysed by the addition of 100 μL water/well.

with fluorescent dyes that partition into membranes, it may be possible to follow the fusion of granules by following the redistribution of dye from one granule membrane to a granule membrane with which it fuses. (4) Finally, the ability of isolated cortical granules, without any soluble factors, save calcium, to undergo membrane fusion argues that the proteins that mediate this reaction must reside on the granules themselves. How can we identify these proteins? One approach would be to raise antibodies against cortical granule membrane proteins. Antibodies could easily be screened for their ability to inhibit granule/granule fusion using this system, thus facilitating the purification of proteins that we have shown are required for calcium-triggered vesicle fusion.

In summary, the cortical granule exocytosis of the sea urchin egg provides unique

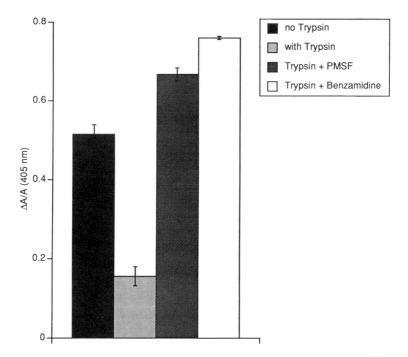

FIGURE 4B. Cortical granules were centrifuged to the bottom of 96-well titer dishes at a density that gave an initial A_{405nm} of ~ 0.215. Granules were then incubated for 1.5 h at room temperature with either 0 or 1 mg/mL trypsin in the presence or absence of either 1 mM PMSF or 10 mM benzamidine. Subsequently an equal volume of either PKME or PKME with 10.966 mM $CaCl_2$ (final free calcium was measured to be 440 μM) was added to each point. The samples were again centrifuged to maximize CG/CG contact. The A_{405nm} was then measured for each reaction point. Because there was a small decrease in absorbance in all the samples that were incubated with trypsin (regardless of the concentration used), we plot the results as the difference of absorption between samples that were incubated with PKME or with PKME + Ca^{2+}, normalized to the signal in the absence of calcium at each trypsin concentration. $\Delta A/A$ was calculated using this equation: $(A_{405nm}$ with PKME $- A_{405nm}$ with PKME + $Ca^{2+})/(A_{405nm}$ with PKME). All points represent the mean $\pm$ SE, n = 5. Presumably, the increase in $\Delta A/A$ over the control without added trypsin, seen for the samples coincubated with protease inhibitors, is due to the inactivation of a trypsin-like protease, contained inside cortical granules, that might be released from lysed granules in our preparation.

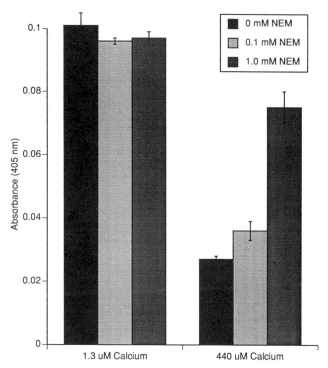

FIGURE 4C. Cortical granules were centrifuged to the bottom of 96-well titer dishes at a density that gave an initial A_{405nm} of ~0.113. Granules were then incubated for 30 min at room temperature in PKME containing 0, 0.1, and 1 mM NEM. The NEM solutions were prepared immediately prior to use. Subsequently the samples were recentrifuged, and half of the supernatant (100 µL) was removed from each well. An equal volume of either PKME or PKME with either 10.966 or 2.19 mM $CaCl_2$ (final free calcium was measured to be 440 and 1.3 µM) was then added to each point. The samples were again centrifuged to maximize CG/CG contact. The A_{405nm} was then measured for each reaction point. All points represent the mean ± SE, n = 3.

experimental opportunities for biophysical and biochemical studies of the final steps of calcium-triggered vesicle fusion, which cannot be studied in the synapse at this time. Questions of both composition and mechanism can now be attacked by eliminating biological components not required for the fusion reaction, and then adding back defined components to reconstruct fusion. We have eliminated one element, the plasma membrane; so we are one step closer to a minimal system for reconstitution of the fusion reaction from purified components. At the same time, we have new techniques for applying calcium directly to the fusion apparatus.

REFERENCES

1. KNIGHT, D. E. & M. C. SCRUTTON. 1986. Biochem. J. **234:** 497–506.
2. CHERNOMORDIK, L. V., G. B. MELIKYAN & Y. A. CHIZMADZHEV. 1987. Biochim. Biophys. Acta **906:** 309–352.

3. PLATTNER, H. 1989. Int. Rev. Cytol. **119:** 197–286.
4. STEGMANN, T., R. W. DOMS & A. HELENIUS. 1989. Annu. Rev. Biophys. Biophys. Chem. **18:** 187–211.
5. ZIMMERBERG, J. 1990. *In* Membrane Fusion. J. Wilschut & D. Hoekstra, Eds.: 183–193. Marcel Dekker, Inc. New York.
6. JAFFE, L. A. & N. L. CROSS. 1986. Annu. Rev. Physiol. **48:** 191–200.
7. MOSER, F. 1939. J. Exp. Zool. **80:** 423–445.
8. ANDERSON, E. 1968. J. Cell Biol. **37:** 514–539.
9. HAMAGUCHI, R. & Y. HIRAMOTO. 1981. Exp. Cell Res. **134:** 171–179.
10. STEINHARDT, R. A. & D. EPEL. 1974. Proc. Natl. Acad. Sci. USA **71:** 1915–1919.
11. STEINHARDT, R., R. ZUCKER & G. SCHATTEN. 1977. Dev. Biol. **58:** 185–195.
12. BAKER, P. F. & M. J. WHITAKER. 1978. Nature **276:** 513–515.
13. ZUCKER, R. S. & R. A. STEINHARDT. 1978. Biochim. Biophys. Acta. **541:** 459–466.
14. CHANDLER, D. E. & J. E. HEUSER. 1980. J. Cell Biol. **86:** 666–674.
15. HEUSER, J. E., T. S. REESE, M. J. DENNIS, Y. JAN, L. JAN & L. EVANS. 1979. J. Cell Biol. **81:** 275–300.
16. PARSEGIAN, V. A. 1977. *In* Neurosciences Research Program Bulletin, Volume 15. R. R. Llinas & J. E. Heuser, Eds.: 620–622. MIT Press. Boston.
17. SIMON, S. M. & R. R. LLINAS. 1985. Biophys. J. **48:** 485–495.
18. POENIE, M., J. ALDERTON, R. Y. TSIEN & R. A. STEINHARDT. 1985. Nature (London) **315:** 147–149.
19. ZUCKER, R. S. & P. G. HAYDEN. 1988. Nature (London) **335:** 360–362.
20. DELANEY, K. R. & R. S. ZUCKER. 1990. J. Physiol. (London) **426:** 473–498.
21. WHALLEY, T. & M. J. WHITAKER. 1988. Biosc. Rep. **8:** 335–343.
22. VOGEL, S. S. & J. ZIMMERBERG. 1991. Biophys. J. **59:** 131a.
23. PECOT-DECHAVASSINE, M. & R. COUTEAUX. 1975. C. R. Acad. Sci. D **280:** 1099–1101.
24. GRATZL, M., G. DAHL, J. T. RUSSEL & N. A. THORN. 1977. Biochim. Biophys. Acta **470:** 45–57.
25. ZIMMERBERG, J., C. SARDET & D. EPEL. 1985. J. Cell Biol. **101:** 2398–2410.
26. KNIGHT, D. E. & P. F. BAKER. 1982. J. Membr. Biol. **68:** 107–140.
27. MAZIA, D., G. SCATTEN & W. SALE. 1975. J. Cell Biol. **66:** 198–200.
28. VACQUIER, V. D. 1975. Dev. Biol. **43:** 62–74.
29. WHITAKER, M. J. & P. F. BAKER. 1983. Proc. R. Soc. London Ser. B. **218:** 397–413.
30. ZIMMERBERG, J. & J. LIU. 1988. J. Membr. Biol. **101:** 199–207.
31. MCLAUGHLIN, S. & M. WHITAKER. 1988. J. Physiol. **396:** 189–204.
32. HAGGERTY, J. G. & R. C. JACKSON. 1983. J. Biol. Chem. **258:** 1819–1825.
33. JACKSON, R. C., K. K. WARD & J. G. HAGGERTY. 1985. J. Cell. Biol. **101:** 6–11.
34. KAPLAN, J. H. & C. R. ELLIS-DAVIES. 1988. Proc. Nat. Acad. Sci. USA **85:** 6571–6575.
35. LLINAS, R., I. Z. STEINBERG & K. WALTON. 1981. Biophys. J. **33:** 323–351.
36. HILLE, B. 1984. *In* Ionic Channels of Excitable Membranes. Sinauer Associates, Inc. Sunderland, MA pp. 331–334.
37. CRABB, J. H. & R. C. JACKSON. 1985. J. Cell Biol. **101:** 2263–2273.
38. SIMON, W. & E. CARFOLI. 1979. Methods Enzymol. **56:** 439–448.
39. TSIEN, R. Y. & T. J. RINK. 1980. Biochim. Biophys. Acta **599:** 623–638.

Two High-Threshold Ca^{2+} Channels Contribute Ca^{2+} for Depolarization-Secretion Coupling in the Mammalian Neurohypophysis

MARTHA C. NOWYCKY

Department of Anatomy and Neurobiology
Medical College of Pennsylvania
Philadelphia, Pennsylvania 19129

INTRODUCTION

Voltage-gated Ca^{2+} channels play a pivotal role in the coupling of electrical activity to neurotransmitter release. At neuronal somata, several classes of Ca^{2+} channels have been described that differ in their time- and voltage-dependent properties as well as in their pharmacological profiles (for reviews see refs. 1 and 2). Obtaining detailed information about the kinetic properties of channels located at actual release sites has proven to be remarkably difficult. With the exception of certain giant presynaptic structures in invertebrates, most kinetic studies have been limited to the cell soma, because most vertebrate nerve terminals are very small or have shapes that do not lend themselves easily to electrical recordings. Large nerve terminals exist in the central nervous system, but usually these are difficult to separate from the neuropil.

The vertebrate neurohypophysis circumvents most of these difficulties. The use of the neurohypophysis as a model system for stimulus-secretion coupling dates back to W. W. Douglas, who demonstrated that Ca^{2+}-triggered release of "neurohumors" was a general phenomenon, with similar mechanisms operating in the neurohypophysis, neuromuscular junction, and chromaffin cells.[3,4] The neurohypophysis (also called posterior pituitary) consists of the terminal swellings or nerve endings of neuronal cell bodies in the hypothalamus (predominantly supraoptic and paraventricular nuclei). Individual neurons in either nucleus synthesize either the peptide hormone vasopressin or oxytocin. These are packaged along with associated specific neurophysins into large dense cored vesicles that are transported by way of the neurohypophysial stalk to the endings that abut on a vascular portal system. Several laboratories have taken advantage of the lack of neuronal soma or dendrites in the neurohypophysis to make preparations of isolated nerve endings. A critical breakthrough occurred in 1987 when Nordmann's laboratory developed an isolation procedure that yielded terminals that secreted the peptides in a Ca^{2+}-dependent manner.[5]

Physiologically, the peptide hormones are released into the blood stream in response to specific and characteristic bursts of action-potential activity. These bursts are 1–100 seconds in duration, separated by interburst intervals of several seconds to minutes (reviewed in ref. 6). Additional patterning is seen within bursts. The first action potentials are only ~1 ms in duration, whereas later ones broaden to ~3 milliseconds.[7,8] Bursts typical for vasopressin cells start at 10–30 Hz and decline to a mean value of ~3 Hz. Oxytocin cells often exhibit higher frequency activity of 70–80 Hz that is maintained for a few seconds.[9]

Isolated neurohypophysial nerve endings are large enough for the use of standard patch clamp techniques.[8,10-12] This article will review the properties of Ca^{2+} channels located in these nerve endings and investigate their probable contribution to stimulus-secretion coupling.[11,12]

METHODS

The neurohypophysis (NHP) of adult rats is dissected free of adhering pars intermedia. Nerve terminals are isolated from the NHP by very light homogenization without enzymatic treatment and plated on glass coverslips. Standard patch clamp techniques are used. Typical solutions are in mM (intracellular): 130 CsCl or CsGlutamate, 0.5 or 10 CsEGTA, 20 HEPES, 2 $MgCl_2$, 0.25 cAMP, and 2 Mg-ATP, pH 7.2; (extracellular): 145 NaCl, 5 KCl, 10 $CaCl_2$ or $BaCl_2$, 10 HEPES, and 10 glucose, pH 7.2. All recordings are performed at room temperature.

RESULTS

Properties of Two Types of Ca^{2+} Channels

Whole Cell Recordings

Macroscopic currents were recorded in solutions that minimize ion flow through Na^+ and K^+ channels. Two types of high-threshold Ca^{2+} channels are present in essentially all terminals.[11] When the terminal is depolarized from a negative steady-state potential (V_m), the two channel types contribute approximately equally to the peak currents. There is no evidence for low-threshold currents. One of the currents is identical to L-type channels found in many excitable cells. The other is a member of the broad N-type family of high-threshold Ca^{2+} currents. We will refer to it as N_t (terminal) to emphasize differences in kinetics from previously described N-type channels.[2]

FIGURE 1A illustrates the two currents. A terminal was held at a membrane potential of $V_m = -60$. Depolarization elicited a rapid inward Na^+ current followed by a maintained current (L-type Ca^{2+} current). On changing V_m to -90 mV, depolarization to the same potential elicits a larger Ca^{2+} current that now has a prominent decaying component and represents the sum of the two types of Ca^{2+} channels. Current through L-type channels inactivates little even during prolonged depolarization. Single exponential fits to traces of ~600 ms duration gave time constant values for τ_{decay} of many hundreds of ms, for example, >700 ms in FIGURE 2B. This number is probably a lower limit on the actual rate of decay. By contrast, the current elicited from the more negative V_m decays with a single exponential time constant of between 25–40 ms (FIGURES 2A and C). The inactivation rates of the two currents differ by a factor of at least 20-fold.

Both Ca^{2+} currents activate relatively rapidly, with a time constant that equals ~.8 ms whether Ca^{2+} or Ba^{2+} ions are the charge carriers (FIG. 1B), and reach peak values between 2–4 ms after depolarization. Both are also high-threshold currents. Because the two channels inactivate at such different rates, it is possible to isolate

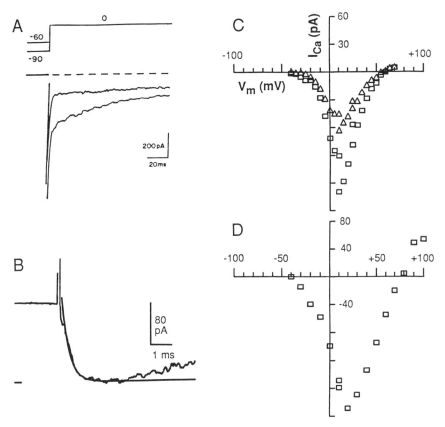

FIGURE 1. Activation properties of the two types of Ca^{2+} channels present in neurohypophy-sial terminals. **A:** Inward macroscopic currents with 10 mM Ca as the charge carrier; two superimposed traces from $V_h = -60$ and -90 mV to 0 mV. The early downward spike is a large sodium current that briefly saturates the patch clamp amplifier. The slow inward current elicited from $V_h = -60$ is essentially flat (noninactivating), whereas the current elicited from $V_h = -90$ mV has a pronounced inactivating component. (Lemos & Nowycky.[11] With permission from *Neuron.*) **B:** Depolarizing step from V_h -90 to $+10$ mV elicits combination of L- and N-type currents in a solution of 10 Ba with tetraethylammonium (TEA) substituting for Na^+. The activation time course is fit with a single exponential time constant with $\tau = 0.8$ ms. Sampling rate was 10 μs. **C** and **D:** The current-voltage relationships of the peak (squares: N- and L-type) and late currents (triangles: L-type only). C is from a terminal with Cl−, whereas D is a terminal with glutamate as the major anion.

L-type current by giving a depolarization approximately five times the average τ_{decay} of the N_t-type current. The current at the end of such a depolarization is almost exclusively L-type, which at this time has not yet undergone much inactivation. This can be subtracted from the current at the peak, and the remainder will largely reflect N_t-type current. With this strategy we determined the activation ranges of the two channels. These were essentially indistinguishable. Both had a threshold of ~ -30 mV and peaks at $+10$ mV in CsCl solution and $+30$ mV in CsGlutamate (FIGURES

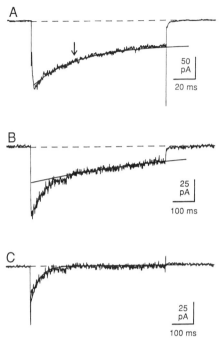

FIGURE 2. Inactivation of L- and N-type currents during a maintained depolarization. Ca^{2+} currents were elicited by a step to $+10$ mV from -90 mV in a 10 mM Ba^{2+}, 135 mM TEA extracellular solution. **A:** 140-ms duration pulse elicited an inward current that was fit with a single exponential with $\tau = 40$ ms (arrow), assuming that the latter part of the current was flat. **B:** 700-ms duration pulse. The latter portion of the current was fit with a single exponential with $\tau = 770$ ms, assuming that the baseline was at zero current level. The early, more rapidly decaying portion of the curve was ignored. **C:** Subtraction of the slow single exponential of **B** from the total current yields a rapidly decaying current that can be fit with a single exponential with $\tau = 38$ ms, comparable to the value obtained in **A.** Thus the inward current of neurosecretosomes is adequately described by the sum of two exponentials, corresponding to inactivation of the N_t- and L-type channels.

1C and D). The apparent reversal potentials were $+60$ and $+80$ mV in the two solutions. Cells recorded with CsGlutamate as the major intracellular anion more frequently exhibited contaminating outward currents, which tended to increase during the experiment.

The steady-state inactivation of the two types of currents were estimated with a similar strategy. For these experiments, the terminal was held at a given potential for 30 s and then depolarized to a constant test potential. For L-type channels, the midpoint of inactivation is ~ -60 mV (in CsCl), and channel inactivation range is very broad with full inactivation around -10 or 0 mV (FIG. 3). The midpoint of N_t-type channel inactivation with this protocol is -72 mV, and the range is narrower. In FIGURE 3, full inactivation occurs at -40 mV. Earlier, we had used the same protocol in the occasional terminal, which has predominantly N_t-type current. In one such terminal the midpoint was -75 mV, and the range was narrower, with full inactivation by -60 to -50 mV.

Single Channel Recordings

L- and N$_t$-type Ca^{2+} channels can also be distinguished with single-channel recordings. Recordings were performed in the cell-attached patch mode. The pipette contained 110 mM Ba^{2+} to maximize current through Ca^{2+} channels and to block current through Na$^+$ and K$^+$ channels.

The L-type channel is more readily seen because of its larger conductance. In terminals whose resting potential had been zeroed by the use of isotonic extracellular K$^+$, depolarizations to relatively negative test potentials (approximately −30 to 0 mV) elicited occasional large and brief openings of an inward channel (FIG. 4A). Addition of the dihydropyridine (DHP) Ca^{2+} channel agonist, BayK 8644, to the external solution rapidly and dramatically increased the frequency and duration of the channel openings (FIG. 4B).

In experiments with DHP-induced long openings, an accurate estimate of the slope conductance of the channel is obtained. This is linear with a value of 28 pS between the −30 and +20 mV, with 110 mM Ba^{2+} as the charge carrier.

Some patches contained inward currents that had two distinct amplitudes (FIG. 5A). The larger openings are easily distinguished and are due to L-type channels as identified by their single-channel conductance and their responsiveness to BayK 8644. The smaller openings are harder to measure but are approximately one half the amplitude. These were unresponsive to BayK 8644. The frequency of opening of both channels increased with stronger depolarizations (FIG. 5A, 0 through +30 mV). At the two most positive potentials there is a clear clustering of activity in the first

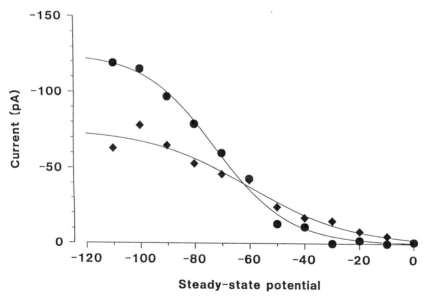

FIGURE 3. Steady-state inactivation of the L- and N$_t$-type channels. Inactivation of the late current (L-type, diamonds) was compared to inactivation of the peak current from which the late current had been subtracted (N$_t$-type, circles). Both are fit with the Boltzmann distribution with −110 mV used as full availability. V$_{1/2}$ = −60 and −72 for L- and N$_t$-type current; k = 18 and 13, respectively.

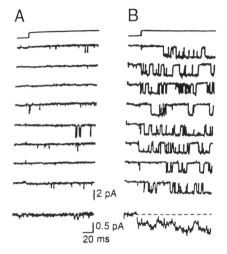

FIGURE 4. Terminal-attached recording of L-type channel. Patch was held at RP −30 mV and depolarized to RP +80 mV (RP estimated at −90 for this terminal). Sequential steps before (**A**) and after (**B**) addition of 1 μM Bay K8644 to the bath. Last trace in each column is average of a number of traces. (Lemos & Nowycky.[11] With permission from *Neuron.*)

half of the sweep, which can be seen more prominently in the averaged current at the bottom.

The identity of the second type of inward activity as underlying the N_t-type current is strengthened by data from a different patch (FIG. 5B). This patch contained a minimum of five channels, all with the same small amplitude as seen in FIGURE 5A at +30 mV. The activity of these channels is clearly clustered at the beginning of the sweeps. Averages of large number of traces at different potentials show the marked voltage-dependence of the activity. Single-exponential fits to these traces gave time constants for decay of 20–30 ms, remarkably similar to those obtained in whole-cell recordings. The channel opening probabilities were very sensitive to changes in holding potential: activity was completely eliminated at $V_m = -30$ mV and fully recovered by returning to the original $V_m = -80$ mV.

In summary, two types of Ca^{2+} channels coexist in both individual terminals and in small membrane patches. Their properties are summarized in TABLE 1. Our single-channel recordings to date do not indicate any marked clustering of either channel type within the terminal membrane. Estimates of channel density are difficult to provide because of the low opening probability, particularly of the L-type channel in control conditions and because of the different ionic conditions used for whole cell versus single-channel recordings (FIGURES 4A, 5A). Most patches, however, contained only a small number of channels (0–5).

Kinetics During a Burst of Activity

Neurohypophysial hormones are released most efficaciously by bursts of action potentials separated by relatively long interburst intervals (reviewed in ref. 13). Vasopressin release, elicited by physiological stimuli such as hemorrhage, dehydration, or plasma hypertonicity is mediated by a bursting activity of vasopressin-synthesizing cells of the hypothalamus. These bursts are 1–100 s in duration and are separated by similar long silent intervals. The intraburst frequency at the beginning of the burst is often just above 20 Hz and then decreases to about 3 to 5 Hz (reviewed in ref. 6). The only well-studied stimulus for oxytocin release, suckling in lactating females, causes a high-frequency discharge (~ 80 Hz) in oxytocin-synthesizing cells, which lasts for several seconds and then is followed by a completely silent interval of seconds to minutes.

Because the two types of channels have different kinetic properties, their relative contribution to Ca²⁺ influx would differ during a burst of activity. As discussed above, both channels are activated over the same voltage range and at approximately the

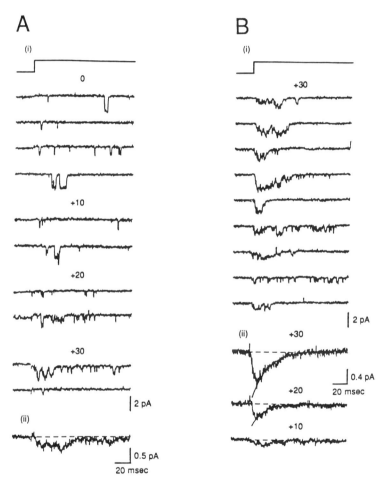

FIGURE 5. Smaller, inactivating channel activity. A: Terminal-attached recordings from patch with two-single channel amplitudes. (i) Steps from RP (estimated at −70 mV) to approximately 0, +10, +20, and +30 mV. Several representative traces shown at each potential. (ii) Average of 28 sweeps from +20 and +30 mV. B: Patch with >5 small amplitude channels and no large L-type channels. (i) Representative single traces. (ii) Averaged activity from a large number of sweeps at each of the indicated potentials. (Lemos & Nowycky.[11] With permission from *Neuron*.)

TABLE 1. Calcium Channels in Neurohypophysial Nerve Terminals

	L-type	N_t-type
Activation threshold	> -30 mV	> -20 mV
τ activation ($+10$ mV)	~ 0.8 ms	~ 0.8 ms
τ decay ($+10$ mV)	> 500 ms	25–40 ms
Steady state inactivation		
$\quad V_{1/2}$	-60 mV	-75 mV
$\quad$ k (slope factor)	> 15 mV	< 10 mV
DHP-sensitive	Yes	No
Single-channel conductance (110 Ba)	28 pS	10–15 pS

same rate. Thus, they will probably contribute equal amounts of Ca^{2+} influx at the beginning of a burst of activity. They differ, however, in inactivation properties: the N_t-type channel inactivates at least 20-fold more rapidly than the L-type, and removal of inactivation is quite slow, with a time constant near half a second.

The ultra-slow inactivation properties of L-type channels imply that these channels would almost certainly continue to open during even a prolonged burst of action potentials. Predictions of the behavior of N_t-type channels are less certain. We have shown above that N_t-type channels inactivate with an average time constant of ~ 30 ms during a maintained strong depolarization. During physiological activity, however, the channels would experience brief periods of depolarizations alternating with longer hyperpolarized intervals. Under these conditions, their behavior would reflect the various closed and open states available to the channel and transition rates between these.

The activity of the N_t-type channel during a series of brief depolarizations was tested by simulating action-potential activity as 2-ms duration depolarizing prepulses to either $+10$ or $+60$ mV separated by 10-ms duration returns to the holding potential (-90 mV). The availability of N_t-type channels was determined with a 20-ms duration test pulse to $+10$ mV. The current elicited by this depolarization was compared to an identical depolarization that had been preceded by a 10-s rest period. We find that as few as four prepulses produced a very small amount of inactivation (FIG. 6). Significant inactivation, however, was not seen until the test pulse was preceded by 32 to 64 prepulses of 2 ms duration. As many as 128 to 256 prepulses were needed to inactivate a majority of N_t-type channels. This suggests that N_t-type channels provide Ca^{2+} influx during a significant portion of a burst. The slower time course of inactivation elicited by prepulses when compared to a maintained depolarization is due to the interprepulse interval, during which Ca^{2+} channels could return to a closed state, or move to a more distant closed state. Of course, such simulated activity cannot accurately predict the behavior of the two channels during physiological bursts of activity. For example, we stimulated at near-maximal rates (final rate of 83.3 Hz) for oxytocin cells, and one would expect even less inactivation at average frequencies of 20 Hz or less. On the other hand, the N_t-type channel is also sensitive to steady-state inactivation. One common feature of bursts of activity in these and other cells is a gradually depolarizing resting, or return, potential. This was not simulated in these experiments but would decrease N_t-type channel availability.

The kinetic properties of the channels suggest that both types will be activated at the beginning of a burst of activity, with L-type activity continuing nearly undiminished, while the N_t-type channels become progressively unavailable but contributing to a significant portion of the burst.

Capacitance

There is a great deal of interest in the identification of the Ca^{2+} channels that trigger secretion. Because of difficulties in applying electrophysiological techniques to the majority of nerve terminals, most studies have exploited pharmacological differences between Ca^{2+} channel types. On the basis of such studies, several laboratories proposed that DHP-sensitive L-type channels are the dominant channel for regulating secretion of peptide transmitters packaged in large dense cored vesicles (100–400 nm diameter), whereas N-type channels more often regulate the release of small classical transmitters packaged in small (40–60 nm), clear synaptic vesicles.[14-21] The neurohypophysial peptide hormones, oxytocin and vasopressin, are packaged with their associated neurophysins in typical large dense cored vesicles. There are conflicting reports whether secretion of the peptides is DHP-sensitive: DHP-sensitivity is reported for endings from the rat[22] but not from the mouse.[23] According to both studies, secretion is blocked by ω-conotoxin (ω-CTX).

The feasibility of patch clamping isolated neurohypophysial nerve terminals allowed us to apply another technique for determining the participation of Ca^{2+} channels types in triggering secretion. Neher and Marty[24] demonstrated that by using sinusoidal stimulation during patch clamp recordings, it was possible to monitor

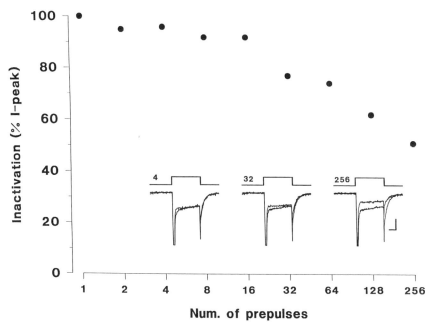

FIGURE 6. Inactivation of Ca^{2+} channels by simulated action potentials. Two-millisecond duration depolarizing prepulses to +10 mV were applied at 10-ms intervals followed by a 20-ms duration test pulse. The peak current amplitude of the test pulse was compared to identical control pulses given 10 seconds later. Data are plotted as a percentage of the control peak amplitude. The insets illustrate superimposed test and control currents from three representative sets of prepulses. The prominent tail currents are of unknown identity but do not represent the closure of Ca^{2+} channels. Scale bars: 5 ms and 100 pA.

exocytosis in real time by detecting small changes in the current flowing through the cell membrane capacitance. Inasmuch as all cellular membranes have the same specific capacitance (~ 1 $\mu F/cm^2$), the addition of vesicular membrane to the surface membrane increases its area and therefore its total capacitance. With appropriate choice of stimulus parameters the technique is extremely sensitive, capable of detecting single chromaffin granule fusions.[24] Since the original publication, there have been several modifications to the technique[25]; recently, its implementation was greatly simplified by using software-based phase-detection techniques instead of phase-lock amplifiers.[26,27]

By combining capacitance detection and voltage control of isolated nerve terminals, we can take advantage of the kinetic properties of L- and N_t-type channels to determine their contribution to the secretory response. Increases in capacitance, and thus in exocytosis, were compared for Ca^{2+} currents elicited from two steady-state

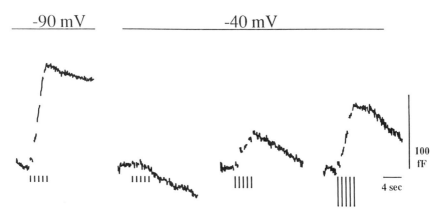

FIGURE 7. Capacitance measurements of exocytosis triggered by Ca currents through N_t- and L-type channels ($V_h = -90$ mV) or L-type only ($V_h = -40$ mV). Left panel: Five depolarizations to +30 mV of 46-ms duration. (Duration of depolarizations is graphically indicated by length of bars under capacitance trace.) Each capacitance point represents one calculation/100 ms. From a holding potential of -40 mV, 46-ms duration pulses did not elicit any capacitance increase. Increasing the duration to 98, however, and then 256 ms (panels on right) caused progressively greater increases in the capacitance trace.

holding potentials: a negative potential at which both types of channels were available and a more positive holding potential that completely inactivated the N_t-type channel. The panel on the left (FIG. 7) shows a capacitance trace during which five 46 ms-long depolarizations, administered at 1 s intervals, elicit a total of ~ 140 fF of release. This corresponds to the fusion of approximately 35–140 vesicles,[12] assuming a range of diameters of 180–400 nm[28] (also B. Salzberg, personal communication). The same duration depolarizations elicited from a positive steady-state potential ($V_m = -40$ mV) produces no change in capacitance. If, however, the pulse duration of the five depolarizations is broadened in this experiment to 98 and then to 256 ms (extreme right), progressively more secretion is observed. It appears that if there is sufficient Ca^{2+} entry, manipulated here by prolonging the duration of time L-type channels are open or depolarizing from a potential at which both L- and N_t-types are available, exocytosis will occur.

Quantification of the response is not possible at this time because the relationship between total $[Ca^{2+}]_i$ and amount of release is highly nonlinear and poorly understood (work in progress). To summarize, the amount of Ca^{2+} entry, irrespective of pathway or other stimulation details, is the relevant trigger for exocytosis in neurohypophysial endings.

Ca^{2+} influx through either channel produces all features of the neurohypophysial secretory response. In the extreme left- and right-most traces, we observe the following typical characteristics: facilitation, depression or fatigue, and poststimulus release. Facilitation refers to the observation that within a burst the response to the first depolarization is always smaller than to the second and/or third,[12] despite the fact that there is somewhat less Ca^{2+} entry during the later depolarizations because of N_t-type channel inactivation (this applies only to the traces from $V_m = -90$ mV). Fatigue or depression is seen as the smaller response to the fourth or fifth depolarization. We have previously shown that this phenomenon is not due to N_t-type channel inactivation, inasmuch as the secretory response takes longer to recover from depression than do the Ca^{2+} currents (> 20 seconds[12]). In this experiment, depression is seen for depolarizations that only elicit L-type current, which is unlikely to be significantly inactivated during these protocols. Finally, the capacitance traces elicited at both holding potentials increase, both with a rapid "jump," which reflects exocytosis during the depolarization, as well as with a slower upward drift after the second through fourth depolarization, presumably due to poststimulus or "residual" release as Ca^{2+} levels remain high.[29,30]

DISCUSSION

Two types of Ca^{2+} channels coexist in essentially all nerve endings prepared from the rat neurohypophysis. One of these corresponds to the DHP-sensitive L-type channel found in many excitable cells.[1,31] The other is a high-threshold, relatively rapidly inactivating, DHP-insensitive channel, and thus is classified as a member of the N-type family. It differs from most other N-type channels in kinetic details with a higher threshold and more rapid inactivation.[1,2,31–33] These properties are also more uniform across individual terminals than is usually the case for N-type channels described in neuronal somata. It is unclear if this is due to superior voltage control in the small, perfectly spherical isolated terminals or whether it reflects a greater homogeneity of properties and/or channel types in neurohypophysial endings.

A typical physiological burst of action potential (AP) activity, which is optimally effective in eliciting secretion of neurohypophysial peptides, consists of several hundred APs with a starting frequency of ~ 20 Hz, diminishing to ~ 5 Hz for vasopressin cells and a maintained frequency of ~ 70–80 Hz in oxytocin cells.[16,34] The kinetic properties of the two types of Ca^{2+} channels predict that both will be opened during the initial tens of APs, providing for a large amount of Ca^{2+} influx at the beginning of a burst. Then due to the inactivation of the N_t-type channel, less Ca^{2+} will enter during the second phase of the burst, when only the L-type channel will be available. One function of the relatively long silent periods between bursts may be to fully restore the availability of the N_t-type channel.

From the results obtained with capacitance measurements, it appears likely that exocytosis occurs in response to Ca^{2+} entry through either channel. These experiments support results of Dayanithi et al.,[22] who found that vasopressin secretion was sensitive to both ω-CTX and DHPs. Interestingly, the DHP nicardipine was a more potent inhibitor if secretion was stimulated with a high K^+ solution than with electrical stimulation mimicking physiological bursting activity. This suggests that in the neurohypophysis the method or pattern of stimulation will determine which type of Ca^{2+} channel is active. Further work is necessary to see to what extent this applies to other nerve terminals. At the neuromuscular junction, release of acetylcholine is very sensitive to ω-CTX in a number of species,[16,34] yet several groups have reported modulation by DHPs.[35,36] On the other hand, mammalian sympathetic neurons contain predominantly N-type channels, and these are likely to dominate the release process.[18,20] Depolarization-secretion coupling is a complex function of the physiological patterns of activity, kinetic properties of available Ca^{2+} channels, Ca^{2+} handling within the terminal, and finally, Ca^{2+}-sensing properties of the secretory machinery.

REFERENCES

1. TSIEN, R. W., A. P. FOX, L. D. HIRNING, D. V. MADISON, E. W. MCCLESKEY, R. J. MILLER & M. C. NOWYCKY. 1988. Multiple types of neuronal calcium channels. Symp. Neurosci. **6:** 1–10.
2. BEAN, B. P. 1989. Classes of calcium channels in vertebrate cells. Annu. Rev. Physiol. **51:** 367–384.
3. DOUGLAS, W. W. & A. M. POISNER. 1964a. Stimulus-secretion coupling in a neurosecretory organ: the role of calcium in the release of vasopressin from the neurohypophysis. J. Physiol. **172:** 1–18.
4. DOUGLAS, W. W. & A. M. POISNER. 1964b. Calcium movement in the neurohypophysis of the rat and its relation to the release of vasopressin. J. Physiol. **172:** 19–30.
5. CAZALIS, M., G. DAYANITHI & J. J. NORDMANN. 1987. Requirements for hormone release from permeabilized nerve endings isolated from the rat neurohypophysis. J. Physiol. **390:** 71–91.
6. POULAIN, D. A. & J. B. WAKERLEY. 1982. Electrophysiology of hypothalamic magnocellular neurones secreting oxytocin and vasopressin. Neuroscience **7:** 773–808.
7. BOURQUE, C. W. 1990. Intraterminal recordings from the rat neurohypophysis *in vitro.* J. Physiol. **421:** 247–262.
8. JACKSON, M. B., A. KONNERTH & G. J. AUGUSTINE. 1991. Action potential broadening and frequency-dependent facilitation of calcium signals in pituitary nerve terminals. Proc. Natl. Acad. Sci. USA. **88:** 380–384.
9. LINCOLN, D. W. & J. B. WAKERLEY. 1974. Electrophysiological evidence for the activation of supraoptic neurones during the release of oxytocin. J. Physiol. **242:** 533–554.
10. MASON, W. T. & R. E. J. DYBALL. 1986. Single ion channel activity in peptidergic nerve terminals of the isolated rat neurohyophysis related to stimulation of neural stalk axons. Brain Res. **283:** 279–286.
11. LEMOS, J. R. & M. C. NOWYCKY. 1989. Two types of calcium channels coexist in peptide-releasing vertebrate nerve terminals. Neuron **2:** 1419–1426.
12. LIM, N. F., M. C. NOWYCKY & R. J. BOOKMAN. 1990. Direct measurement of exocytosis and calcium currents in single vertebrate nerve terminals. Nature **344:** 449–451.
13. LENG, G., ED. 1988. Pulsatility in neuroendocrine systems. CRC. Boca Raton, FL.
14. MIDDLEMISS, D. N. & M. SPEDDING. 1985. A functional correlate for the dihydropyridine binding site in rat brain. Nature **314:** 94–96.
15. PERNEY, T. M., L. D. HIRNING, S. E. LEEMAN & R. J. MILLER. 1986. Multiple calcium channels mediate neurotransmitter release from peripheral neurons. Proc. Natl. Acad. Sci. USA **83:** 6656–6659.
16. YEAGER, R. E., D. YOSHIKAMI, J. RIVIER, L. J. CRUZ & G. P. MILJANICH. 1987. Transmitter release from presynaptic terminals of electric organ: inhibition by the calcium channel antagonist, omega Conus toxin. J. Neurosci. **7:** 2390–2396.
17. HOLZ, G. G., K. DUNLAP & R. M. KREAM. 1988. Characterization of the electrically evoked release of Substance P from dorsal root ganglion neurons: methods and dihydropyridine sensitivity. J. Neurosci. **8:** 463–471.
18. HIRNING, L. D., A. P. FOX, E. W. MCCLESKEY, B. M. OLIVERA, S. A. THAYER, R. J. MILLER & R. W. TSIEN. 1988. Dominant role of N-type Ca^{2+} channels in evoked release of norepinephrine from sympathetic neurons. Science **239:** 57–61.

19. NAVONE, F., G. DIGIOIA, R. JAHN, M. BROWNING, P. GREENGARD & P. DeCAMILLI. 1989. Microvesicles of the neurohypophysis are biochemically related to small synaptic vesicles of presynaptic nerve terminals. J. Cell Biol. **109:** 3425–3433.
20. LIPSCOMBE, D., S. KONGSAMUT & R. W. TSIEN. 1989. α-Adrenergic inhibition of sympathetic neurotransmitter release mediated by modulation of N-type calcium-channel gating. Nature **340:** 639–642.
21. GRAY, D. B., D. ZELAZNY, N. MANTHAY & G. PILAR. 1991. Endogenous modulation of ACh release by somatostatin and the differential roles of Ca⁺⁺ channels. J. Neurosci. In press.
22. DAYANITHI, G., N. MARTIN-MOUTOT, S. BARLIER, D. A. COLIN, M. KRETZ-ZAEPFEL, F. COURAUD & J. J. NORDMANN. 1988. The calcium channel antagonist, ω-Conotoxin, inhibits secretion from peptidergic nerve terminals. Biochem. Biophys. Res. Commun. **156:** 255–262.
23. SALZBERG, B. M. & A. L. OBAID. 1988. Optical studies of the secretory event at vertebrate nerve terminals. J. Exp. Biol. **139:** 195–231.
24. NEHER, E. & A. MARTY. 1982. Discrete changes of cell membrane capacitance observed under conditions of enhanced secretion in bovine adrenal chromaffin cells. Proc. Natl. Acad. Sci. USA **79:** 6712–6716.
25. LINDAU, M. & E. NEHER. 1988. Patch-clamp technique for time-resolved capacitance measurements in single cells. Pfluegers. Arch. Gesamte. Physiol. Menschen Tiere **411:** 137–146.
26. JOSHI, C. & J. M. FERNANDEZ. 1988. Capacitance measurements. An analysis of the phase detector technique used to study exocytosis and endocytosis. Biophys. J. **53:** 885–892.
27. FIDLER, N. H. & J. M. FERNANDEZ. 1989. Phase tracking: an improved phase detection technique for cell membrane capacitance measurements. Biophys. J. **56:** 1153–1162.
28. MORRIS, J. F. 1976. J. Endocrinol. **68:** 209–224.
29. THOMAS, P., A. SURPRENANT & W. ALMERS. 1990. Cytosolic Ca²⁺, exocytosis, and endocytosis in single melanotrophs of the rat pituitary. Neuron **5:** 723–733.
30. BOOKMAN, R. J. & T. SCHWEITZER. 1988. J. Gen. Physiol. **92:** 4a .
31. FOX, A. P., M. C. NOWYCKY & R. W. TSIEN. 1987a. Single-channel recordings of three types of calcium channels in chick sensory neurones. J. Physiol. **394:** 173–200.
32. FOX, A. P., M. C. NOWYCKY & R. W. TSIEN. 1987b. Kinetic and pharmacological properties distinguishing three types of calcium channels in chick sensory neurones. J. Physiol. **394:** 149–172.
33. NOWYCKY, M. C., A. P. FOX & R. W. TSIEN. 1985. Three types of neuronal calcium channel with different calcium agonist sensitivity. Nature **316:** 440–442.
34. YOSHIKAMI, D., Z. BAGABALDO & B. M. OLIVERA. 1989. The inhibitory effects of omega-conotoxins on Ca channels and synapses. Ann. N.Y. Acad. Sci. **560:** 230–248.
35. ATCHINSON, W. D. & S. M. O'LEARY. 1987. BAY K 8644 increases release of acetylcholine at the murine neuromuscular junction. Brain Res. **419:** 315–319.
36. LINDGREN, C. A. & J. W. MOORE. 1989. Identification of ionic currents at presynaptic endings of the lizard. J. Physiol. **414:** 201–222.

Calcium Current in Motor Nerve Endings of the Lizard

CLARK A. LINDGREN[a] AND JOHN W. MOORE[b]

[a]Department of Biology
Allegheny College
Meadville, Pennsylvania 16335

[b]Department of Neurobiology
Duke University
Durham, North Carolina

INTRODUCTION

For many years the neuromuscular junction has been the preparation of choice for studying synaptic transmission. This is because the neuromuscular junction is a highly accessible and robust synapse at which transmitter release can be monitored with extreme precision by measuring voltage changes in the muscle. Furthermore, release can be induced simply by stimulating the motor nerve bundle and allowing the nerve impulse to propagate down the axon to the presynaptic terminals. Because motor nerve terminals are small, however, presynaptic mechanisms, such as the activation of transmitter release by Ca^{2+} ions, have been difficult to study.

Recent work of Brigant and Mallart[1] has demonstrated that the small size of presynaptic motor terminals can be overcome in certain preparations by using extracellular electrodes. They showed that it is possible to measure highly localized currents from motor nerve endings and interpret the current patterns in terms of known ionic conductances in the presynaptic membrane.[1] The ceratomandibularis muscle in the lizard, *Anolis carolinensis,* is particularly well-suited for making measurements of currents in motor nerve terminals.[2] This muscle is extremely thin and flat, and the presynaptic nerve endings contain large boutons. These features allow the nerve endings to be visualized with exceptional clarity using differential interference contrast optics. The ability to see the nerve terminals clearly greatly simplifies the process of recording currents at precise locations over the nerve terminal.

One of the currents that can be recorded in the motor nerve endings with this technique is a calcium current.[2] Because the release of neurotransmitter is triggered by the influx of calcium into the nerve terminal, the ability to measure this influx directly could be exploited in various studies aimed at elucidating the role of calcium in activating neurotransmitter release. It is first necessary, however, to establish how closely the calcium current correlates with the release of neurotransmitter. Inasmuch as multiple types of calcium channels exist,[3] with more than one type coexisting in a single cell,[4-6] it is entirely possible that a calcium current measured at discrete locations over a nerve terminal is not associated directly with the release of the neurotransmitter.

One way to identify and isolate the components of calcium current in a cell is through the application of selective pharmacological modifiers of calcium channel function.[6] Because the release of neurotransmitter can be detected by measuring current in the muscle (*i.e.* end-plate currents (EPC)) and the calcium current can be measured independently in the motor nerve ending, the pharmacological approach was applied to the neuromuscular junction of the ceratomandibularis muscle. The presynaptic calcium current and the postsynaptic EPC were both measured before and after application of various calcium channel modifiers. Under all of the conditions studied, changes in EPC were paralleled by identical changes in presynaptic calcium current. This pharmacological similarity suggests that the calcium influx measured directly as calcium current in the motor nerve terminals with focal, extracellular electrodes is the same [or very similar to the] calcium influx associated with the release of neurotransmitter.

Thus, a calcium current can be measured directly in motor nerve endings of the ceratomandibularis muscle in the lizard, which has the same pharmacological profile as the release of neurotransmitter, measured as current in the underlying muscle. This preparation promises to be extremely useful for investigating the initiation and regulation of neurotransmitter release by the influx of calcium into the nerve terminal.

MATERIAL AND METHODS

Preparation

The motor nerve terminals on muscle fibers in the lizard are compact, extending only 25–50 μm.[7] The terminals are composed of several boutons or varicosities, approximately 5 μm in diameter, connected by short segments of unmyelinated axon. This is representative of the single en plaque innervation characteristic of the twitch muscle fiber type described in the scalenus[8] and intercostal muscles of the lizard.[7] There are also some fibers in the ceratomandibularis muscle that contain nerve endings consisting of smaller boutons (2–5 μm in diameter), connected by very fine segments of axon, 1 μm (or less) in diameter. This type is morphologically similar to the fast twitch fibers described in mammalian EDL fibers[9] as well as lizard intercostal muscle (John Walrond, personal communication). There was no obvious difference in the electrical properties of these two types of endings. Thus, we made no attempt to distinguish between them in our description of the nerve terminal currents.

Dissection and Solutions

Small (2–3 in.) lizards, *Anolis carolinensis,* were obtained from the Carolina Biological Supply Company (Burlington, NC). Prior to experiments they were cold anesthetized and then decerebrated immediately. The ceratomandibularis muscle and its motor nerve (a small branch of the hypoglossal nerve) were then dissected from the lower jaw and perfused with saline[8] of the following composition (mM): NaCl, 130; KCl, 3; NaHCO$_3$, 20; CaCl$_2$, 2; and glucose, 5. The saline was gassed with a mixture of oxygen (95%) and CO$_2$ (5%) and maintained between 15°C and 25°C (±0.1) with a thermoelectric cooling device.

Tetraethylammonium bromide (TEA), 3,4-diaminopyridine (DAP), and nifedipine were obtained from Sigma Chemical Company. Omega-conotoxin GVIA was purchased from two different sources, Peninsula Laboratories (Belmont, CA) and American International Chemicals (Natick, MA). The Bay K 8644 was kindly provided by Dr. Alexander Scriabine (Miles Laboratories).

Electrode Positioning and Current Measurement

The recording electrodes, filled with standard saline (see *Dissection and Solutions*), had resistances of about 1 megohm. Often the tip of the electrode became mechanically "stuck" to the underlying nerve terminal membrane and/or connective-tissue sheath, allowing for prolonged and stable recording. The resistance of the seal, however, was only about 100–200 Kohms—not in the range of *gigaohms* normally employed in patch-clamp recording.

Currents were measured and filtered by a conventional patch clamp amplifier (Axopatch made by Axon Instruments, Burlingame, CA). The signals were digitized by a 12-bit analog-to-digital converter (Data Translation 2818) and stored on disks in an IBM PC-AT computer for averaging, analysis, and plotting. To improve the signal-to-noise ratio, 25 to 100 current signals were averaged and, when necessary, further smoothed by passing the average signal through a 3- or 5-point "boxcar" filter.

Interpretation of Electrode Signals

Ordinarily there is no calibration, in terms of current density, for extracellular current measurements because neither the spatial resolution of the electrode nor the resistance to ground of the measurement point is known. In order to gain insight into the interpretation of the extracellularly recorded signals, an attempt was made to estimate the spatial resolution and densities of the recorded currents.

Spatial Resolution

The spatial resolution of the extracellular current recordings were examined by computer simulation. (This work was assisted by Dr. Michael Hines, Department of Neurobiology, Duke University.) The currents, which would be measured by a 5 μm × 5 μm electrode at various locations relative to a 5 μm × 5 μm current source residing in a nonconducting infinite plane, were calculated. The current source was designed to represent a synaptic bouton (diameter 5 μm) on the surface of a cylindrical muscle fiber (diameter 100 μm), which at distances less than one-tenth its diameter (*i.e.* 10 μm) can be approximated by an infinite plane. To simplify calculations, the dimensions of the electrode glass and the partial electrical seal at its tip were ignored. This, of course, is a simplification that gives the minimum or worst-case resolution.

The results of these calculations are summarized in FIGURE 1. The predicted lateral resolution of the recording electrode is shown at 10, 1, 0.1 and 0.01 μm from the surface of the plane. They show that the spatial resolution improves rapidly as the electrode approaches the plane (muscle) but saturates at a distance of about 0.1 μm. At this distance, the resolution curve has a half-width of about 7.5 micrometers. As the electrode is moved in closer than 0.1 μm from the bouton membrane, there is little appreciable improvement in either signal amplitude or resolution.

These observations, that the spatial resolution is not much larger than the measuring electrode, suggest that there is relatively little contribution to the measured signal from currents flowing through the membrane only 10 μm from the center of the electrode. Thus, currents measured at the different locations through-

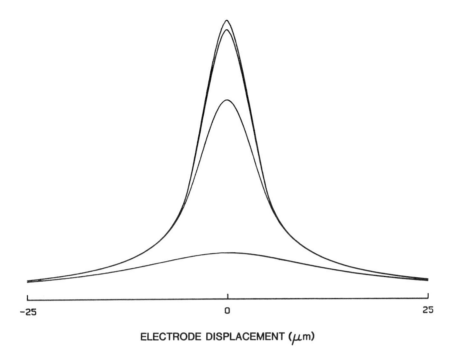

FIGURE 1. Predicted resolution of extracellular current recordings. Synaptic boutons were estimated as 5 μm × 5 μm current sources located in a nonconducting infinite plane. The current, which would be measured by a 5 μm × 5 μm electrode at various locations relative to such a synaptic bouton, was calculated. The four curves represent (from top to bottom) the predicted current measurements for an electrode located 0.01, 0.1, 1.0, and 10 μm from the surface of the plane and displaced ± 25 μm from the center of the bouton (current source).

out the 30–60 μm region of nerve terminal originate from localized patches of membrane approximately 10 μm in diameter.

Estimating Current Densities

Because the resistance of the electrode is approximately an order of magnitude greater than the seal resistance, it can measure only a small fraction of the total current traversing the 10 μm patch of membrane beneath its tip. From the above simulations of the electrode resolution the contribution of other nearby boutons to the measured signal can be measured. For an electrode placed less than 0.1 μm from the surface of a synaptic bouton of 5 μm diameter, two adjacent boutons of 5 μm diameter and centered at a distance of 7.5 μm away would contribute an additional 45% to the potential measured from the bouton directly under the electrode. Because the current patterns in adjacent boutons would very likely be quite similar, the net effect should be just a multiplication (×1.45) of the amplitude of that from the central bouton. Therefore, because the fraction of the current that actually flows through the electrode can be estimated, from the ratio of the seal-to-electrode

resistance, to be about 10%, the measured current should be about 15% (*i.e.*
1.45 * 10%) of the actual current density of the bouton on which the electrode is
centered. Therefore to obtain an approximation of the total current flowing through
the 5 μm patch of membrane beneath the tip of the electrode, the actual current
measurements should be multiplied by 6.9 (1/.15). Current density can then be
estimated by dividing this number by the area of the patch (5 μm diameter). Using
this conversion factor, current densities in motor nerve endings on the ceratomandibularis muscle of the lizard are estimated to range from 1.2 ma/cm^2 to 3.5 ma/cm^2.
The fact that this varies by almost a factor of three is interpreted as the variability in
centering the electrode over the boutons.

Elimination of Postsynaptic Current

Although postsynaptic current signals are useful as a measure of transmitter
release, they were eliminated in some of the measurements to avoid contamination
of the much smaller nerve terminal current signals. Surprisingly, postsynaptic
currents were only partially blocked by tubocurarine chloride at a concentration of
50 μM (see FIG. 2). For comparison, 20 μM tubocurarine was found to be sufficient
to block the ACh channels at the mouse neuromuscular junction completely.[1]
Although curare was only partially effective, complete blockade of the postsynaptic
current was obtained by bath application of the curariform drug, pancuronium
bromide, at a concentration of only 5 μM (FIG. 2). The high-affinity ACh receptor
antagonist, α-bungarotoxin (5 μg/mL), also blocked the postsynaptic response

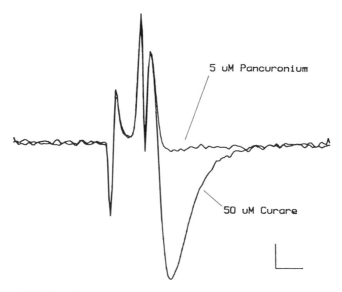

FIGURE 2. Inhibition of postsynaptic current. Current was measured over a motor nerve
ending on the ceratomandibularis muscle of the lizard, *Anolis carolinensis.* Each trace represents the average of 40 measurements made in the presence of either 50 μM tubocurarine
chloride (curare) or 5 μM pancuronium bromide. Stimulation rate, 0.5 Hz; calcium, 2 mM;
temperature, 21°C; calibration: 10 pA, 1 ms.

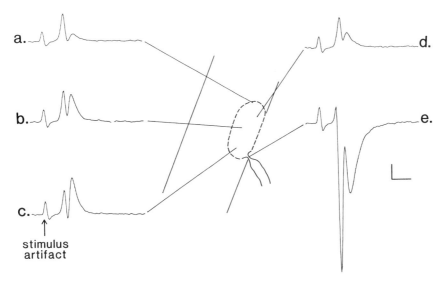

FIGURE 3. Current patterns at various locations in motor nerve endings of the lizard. Current was measured with an extracellular electrode at five positions (a–e) over a motor nerve ending on the ceratomandibularis muscle of the lizard, *Anolis carolinensis.* The approximate positions of the recording electrode are indicated on the drawing. Downward peaks correspond to inward current. Postsynaptic current was blocked completely with 10 μM pancuronium bromide; temperature, 20°C. Each pattern is the average of 100 traces obtained at a stimulation rate of 0.5 Hz. Calibration: 25 pA, 1 ms.

completely. Therefore all presynaptic current measurements were made in the presence of either pancuronium bromide or α-bungarotoxin.

RESULTS AND DISCUSSION

Spatial Distribution of Ionic Currents

Ionic currents resulting from the invasion of an action potential into the nerve terminal were recorded at different locations along the terminal, as shown in FIGURE 3, by carefully positioning the heat-polished tip (ca. 5 μm i.d.) of an extracellular electrode. These records are quite similar to those observed at motor nerve endings of the mouse by Brigant and Mallart.[1] The current flow is predominantly inward at the transition between the myelinated and nonmyelinated portions of the axon (e). This region is called a "heminode" because it is anatomically equivalent to one-half a node of Ranvier. Over the remainder of the terminal, the predominant net current flow is outward (a–d). Brigant and Mallart[1] explained their current patterns at motor nerve terminals of the mouse by arguing that Na current dominates in the heminode and that K current dominates in the terminal branches and boutons. The current patterns recorded in lizard motor nerve terminals can be explained by a similar segregation of Na and K channels.[2]

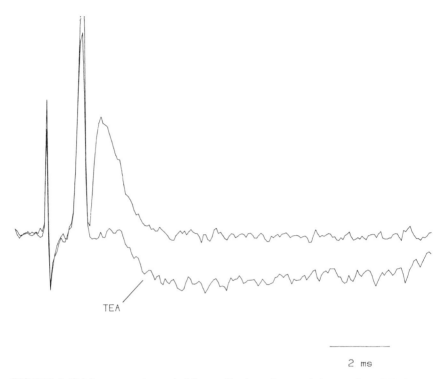

2 ms

FIGURE 4. Calcium current revealed by application of tetraethylammonium (TEA). An inward calcium current is revealed by blocking the K channels with TEA (10 mM). Each trace is the average of 25 measurements obtained at a stimulation rate of 0.5 Hz. Calcium, 2 mM; pancuronium, 10 μM; temperature, 18°C.

Measurement of Calcium Current in Presynaptic Nerve Terminals

Application of the potassium channel blocker, TEA, unmasked a small, but prolonged, inward current (see FIG. 4). In this preparation, blocking the K conductance with TEA increases the duration of the action potential severalfold.[10] Appropriate for the increase in duration of the action potential, the duration of this new current component was much longer than the original K current and is consistent with a calcium conductance located in the nerve terminal.

This inward current was identified as calcium current because it was abolished by substituting cobalt for calcium in the bath, and its amplitude and duration were decreased by reducing the calcium concentration in the bath.[2] During a normal brief action potential, this calcium current is obscured by the presence of the large K current flowing in the opposite direction (FIG. 4). The calcium current is revealed only when the K current is blocked and when the action potential is prolonged.

Inasmuch as several different types of calcium channel exist,[3] and multiple types even coexist in individual neurones,[4–6] the identity and function of this calcium current is not immediately obvious. Although it is likely that this current, or at least a portion of it, is associated with the influx of calcium responsible for the release of neurotransmitter, this is not necessarily true. It is possible that the calcium current measured at precise locations over the nerve ending with focal, extracellular electrodes is created by calcium channels that are relatively distant from that portion of the nerve ending involved in neurotransmitter release. The calcium channels responsible for the extracellularly recorded calcium current may not be directly involved in neurotransmitter release or may be involved only under unusual circumstances.[3]

Theoretical calculations have estimated that the influx of Ca^{2+} through calcium channels in the presynaptic membrane is highly localized.[11,12] The sphere of influence of the entering Ca^{2+} is thought to be limited to the immediate vicinity of the calcium channel. Thus, in the presynaptic motor nerve terminals of the lizard, neurotransmitter release may be activated by a highly restricted influx of Ca^{2+} through a small subpopulation of channels located exclusively at the sites of neurotransmitter release. Additional calcium channels, not involved directly in neurotransmitter release, may be located over the remainder of the terminal. Furthermore, the subpopulation of calcium channels associated with neurotransmitter release may be so small as to contribute only negligibly to the calcium current measured with extracellular electrodes.

Because many of the known calcium channel types can be distinguished on the basis of their sensitivity to pharmacological agonists and antagonists (*e.g.* the L, N, and T channels in sensory neurons from chick[6]), the sensitivity of the calcium current and neurotransmitter release to several calcium channel modifiers was determined. If the calcium current measured with extracellular electrodes is created by the same influx of Ca^{2+} that induces neurotransmitter release, then the calcium current and neurotransmitter release should be affected similarly. If, on the other hand, neurotransmitter release is induced by the influx of Ca^{2+} through a type of calcium channel different from the type creating the majority of calcium current in the nerve terminal, then neurotransmitter release and the calcium current may have different pharmacological sensitivities.

Pharmacological Sensitivity of Calcium Current

To determine the pharmacological properties of the calcium current, the calcium current was measured before and after applying the following inorganic and organic calcium channel blockers: cadmium, nickel, omega-conotoxin GVIA, and nifedipine. The results are summarized in TABLE 1. Cadmium blocked the calcium current

TABLE 1. Pharmacological Sensitivity of Calcium Current and End-Plate Current (EPC) at the Neuromuscular Junction in the Ceratomandibularis Muscle of the Lizard, *Anolis carolinensis*

	Calcium Current	EPC
Blockers		
Cadmium (50 μM)	100% inhibition (reversible)	100% inhibition (reversible)
Nickel (100 μM)	No effect	10% inhibition
ω-Conotoxin GVIA (5 μM)	100% inhibition (irreversible)	100% inhibition (irreversible)
Nifedipine (5–10 μM)	100% inhibition[a] (partial reversal)	85% inhibition[a] (partial reversal)
Activator		
Bay K 8644 (5 μM)	No effect	111% increase (reversible)

[a]The preparation was exposed to either TEA or TEA and 3,4-DAP.

rapidly and reversibly at only 50 μM; however, nickel was ineffective at concentrations up to 100 μM (much higher concentrations, *e.g.* 1 mM, were effective). Omega-conotoxin GVIA, a 27–amino acid peptide component of the venom of the marine snail *Conus geographus,*[13] blocked the calcium current irreversibly. This is consistent with reports of the irreversibility of conotoxin at the frog neuromuscular junction[14] and in sensory neurons.[15]

In initial experiments, the dihydropyridine calcium channel antagonist, nifedipine, produced variable effects on the calcium current. Previous work in cardiac muscle fibers[16,17] and neurons from dorsal root ganglia (DRG)[18,19] demonstrated that the effectiveness of dihydropyridines in blocking calcium channels is increased by depolarization. Unfortunately, measurement of calcium current in motor nerve endings on the ceratomandibularis muscle requires that the nerve impulse propagate into the presynaptic ending. Thus, it is not possible to depolarize the preparation and still measure calcium current in the motor nerve endings, such as was possible in the DRG neurons or cardiac muscle fibers, because this would inactivate the Na channels and render the motor nerve inexcitable. As an alternative to long-term depolarization, the nerve was stimulated repetitively, and the duration of each individual action potential was increased severalfold by applying TEA for at least one hour (5–10 minutes was the normal time of application). Under these conditions, nifedipine blocked the calcium current consistently and reversibly.

After the action potential duration had been increased to at least 20 ms, nifedipine was applied (5–10 μM), and the nerve was given 100 stimuli (at 0.5 Hz) every 5 minutes. Under these conditions, nifedipine progressively reduced the calcium current until the current was blocked completely (at least 25 minutes). Subsequent removal of the nifedipine gradually reversed its effects, even though the simulation protocol was continued. Although washing the preparation with control saline caused the current to return to its control amplitude, it was never completely restored to its initial duration.

The improvement in nifedipine's ability to block the calcium current under the above conditions presumably relates to the voltage dependance of its binding to the calcium channels. The combination of repetitive stimulation and prolonged action potentials appears to produce the same effect at the lizard neuromuscular junction as long-term depolarization produces in DRG neurons and cardiac muscle cells. This suggests that the dihydropyridine sensitivity of the calcium channels in lizard motor endings has a similar voltage and time dependence as the high-threshold calcium channels in DRG neurons and cardiac muscle cells.

The nifedipine analogue, Bay K 8644, which enhances dihydropyridine-sensitive calcium current in DRG neurons,[6,19] had an erratic effect on the calcium current in motor nerve endings of the lizard (increase, n = 2; decrease, n = 2; no effect, n = 2). This lack of effect was surprising given the effectiveness of the dihydropyridine antagonist, nifedipine. Failure to observe a consistent effect of the Bay K 8644 may have been the result of a small, chronic depolarization of the lizard motor endings associated with the application of TEA (which was required to reveal and measure the calcium current). In marked contrast to dihydropyridine antagonists, such as nifedipine, depolarization decreases the effectiveness of Bay K 8644 as a calcium channel agonist.[20] Depolarization may even cause the Bay K to function as an antagonist.[21] Application of TEA (10 mM) does lead to a slight (10–15 mV) depolarization of the lizard motor axon.[10] Thus, the erratic results with the Bay K may have been caused by the complex voltage dependence of its modulation of calcium channels.

Pharmacological Sensitivity of Neurotransmitter Release

To determine whether the influx of calcium responsible for neurotransmitter release is the same as the calcium influx detected in the motor ending by direct measurement of calcium current, the pharmacological sensitivity of neurotransmitter release was also tested. Changes in neurotransmitter release were monitored by measuring current in the underlying muscle (*i.e.* end-plate currents). EPC were measured under conditions of reduced calcium (0.25–0.5 mM) and elevated magnesium (2–8 mM). These conditions were chosen so that the amplitude of spontaneous miniature end-plate currents (MEPC) could be monitored. A change in postsynaptic sensitivity to ACh would be reflected as a change in the average amplitude of the MEPC. Inasmuch as none of the agents tested altered MEPC amplitude, the amplitude of EPC accurately reflected changes in transmitter release.

The effects of nickel, cadmium, and omega-conotoxin on the EPC are summarized in TABLE 1. In normal saline, the EPC is a large inward current peaking approximately 1 ms after the first appearance of current at the presynaptic ending (see FIG. 2). Nickel (100 μM) reduced the EPC only slightly. Cadmium (50 μM) and omega-conotoxin (5 μM) abolished it completely. Thus, these three calcium channel blockers have the same pattern of effects on transmitter release as they had on calcium current.

Nifedipine also inhibited transmitter release. In five out of seven experiments, nifedipine reduced transmitter release an average of 39 percent. As with the experiments on calcium current, nifedipine's efficacy was enhanced by treating the preparation with TEA or with a combination of TEA and 3,4-DAP to prolong the presynaptic action potential. Following pretreatment with either of these K channel blocking solutions, the effect of nifedipine on the EPC was enhanced significantly. Under these conditions, nifedipine (10 μM) reduced the amplitude of the EPC an average of 85 percent.

Because, in addition to its effect on presynaptic K channels, TEA also has a postsynaptic blocking effect, MEPC were reduced in amplitude below the noise level and could not be measured during this latter series of experiments. Thus it was not possible to monitor changes in postsynaptic sensitivity. It is possible, therefore, that some of the decrease in postsynaptic current observed in the presence of TEA was due to a decreased responsiveness of the muscle to ACh and not to a decrease in transmitter release *per se.* Because nifedipine, however, did not alter MEPC amplitude in the experiments performed without TEA, and because presynaptic calcium current was blocked so convincingly by nifedipine in the presence of TEA, it seems most likely that the entirety of nifedipine's effect on the EPC resulted from reduced presynaptic release of neurotransmitter.

Bay K 8644 increased the EPC in a highly reproducible manner. In seven experiments, Bay K 8644 increased the EPC an average of 111% with a range of 25 to 350 percent. The effect of the Bay K could be reversed in most cases (5 out of 7) by washing the preparation in control saline for at least 30 minutes. Bay K also increased the frequency of MEPC. This increase could not be reversed with washing. Application of Bay K for ten minutes was sufficient to initiate a continuous and rapid increase in the frequency of MEPC, sometimes to extremely high levels (> 100/ min.). Atchison and O'Leary[22] have also reported that Bay K 8644 increases the frequency of miniature end-plate potentials at the neuromuscular junction of the rat. Inasmuch as an increase in the frequency of spontaneous transmitter release usually indicates that the resting, background level of calcium has increased, this result suggests that Bay K may have multiple effects on calcium homeostasis at the vertebrate neuromuscular junction.

CONCLUSION

At the neuromuscular junction on the ceratomandibularis muscle of the lizard, the release of neurotransmitter, measured as current in the underlying muscle, can be related directly to the presynaptic currents that activate its release, measured from localized regions of the presynaptic nerve terminal. In particular, using extracellular electrodes, a calcium current can be measured in the presynaptic motor nerve terminals, which has a pharmacological sensitivity identical to the postsynaptic current recorded in the muscle. This suggests that the nerve-muscle synapse on the ceratomandibularis muscle in the lizard will be extremely useful for answering questions related to the initiation and regulation of neurotransmitter release by Ca^{2+} ions in a vertebrate nerve terminal.

REFERENCES

1. BRIGANT, J. L. & A. MALLART. 1982. Presynaptic currents in mouse motor endings. J. Physiol. **333:** 619–636.
2. LINDGREN, C. A. & J. W. MOORE. 1989. Identification of ionic currents at presynaptic nerve endings of the lizard. J. Physiol. **414:** 201–222.
3. MILLER, F. J. 1987. Multiple calcium channels and neuronal function. Science **235:** 46–52.
4. DUPONT, J. L., J. L. BOSSU & A. FELTZ. 1986. Effect of internal calcium concentration on calcium currents in rat sensory neurones. Pflugers Archives **406:** 433–435.
5. KOSTYUK, P. G., M. F. SHUBA & A. N. SAVCHENKO. 1987. Three types of calcium channels in the membrane of mouse sensory neurons. Biol. Membr. **4:** 366–373.
6. FOX, A. P., M. C. NOWYCKY & R. W. TSIEN. 1987. Kinetic and pharmacological properties distinguishing three types of calcium currents in chick sensory neurones. J. Physiol. **394:** 149–172.
7. WALROND, J. P. & T. S. REESE. 1985. Structure of axon terminals and active zones at synapses on lizard twitch and tonic muscle fibers. J. Neurosci. **5:** 1118–1131.
8. PROSKE, U. & P. VAUGHAN. 1968. Histological and electrophysiological investigation of lizard skeletal muscle. J. Physiol. **199:** 495–509.
9. ELLISMAN, M. H., J. E. RASH, L. A. STAEHELIN & K. R. PORTER. 1976. Studies of Excitable Membranes: II. A comparison of specializations at neuromuscular junctions and nonjunctional sarcolemmas of mammalian fast and slow twitch muscle fibers. J. Cell Biol. **68:** 752–774.
10. BARRETT, E. F., K. MORITA & K. A. SCAPPATICCI. 1988. Effects of tetraethylammonium on depolarizing afterpotential and passive properties of lizard myelinated axons. J. Physiol. **402:** 65–78.
11. STOCKBRIDGE, N. & J. W. MOORE. 1984. Dynamics of intracellular calcium and its possible relationship to phasic transmitter release and facilitation at the frog neuromuscular junction. J. Neurosci. **5:** 1118–1131.
12. SIMON, S. M. & R. LLINÁS. 1985. Compartmentalization of the submembrane calcium activity during calcium influx and its significance in transmitter release. Biophys. J. **48:** 485–498.
13. OLIVERA, B. M., W. R. GRAY, R. ZEIKUS, J. M. MCINTOSH, J. VARGA, J. RIVIER, B. DE SANTUS & L. CRUZ. 1985. Peptide neurotoxins from fish-hunting cone snails. Science **230:** 1338–1343.
14. KERR, L. M. & D. YOSHIKAMI. 1984. A venom peptide with a novel presynaptic blocking action. Nature **308:** 282–284.
15. MCCLESKEY, E. W., A. P. FOX, D. H. FELDMAN, L. J. CRUZ, B. M. OLIVERA, R. W. TSIEN & D. YOSHIKAMI. 1987. Omega-conotoxin: direct and persistent block of specific types of calcium channels in neurons but not muscle. Proc. Natl. Acad. Sci. USA **84:** 4327–4331.
16. SANGUINETTI, M. C. & R. S. KASS. 1984. Voltage-dependent block of calcium channel current in the calf cardiac Purkinje fiber by dihydropyridine calcium channel antagonists. Circ. Res. **55:** 336–348.

17. BEAN, B. P. 1984. Nitrendipine block of cardiac calcium channels: high-affinity binding to the inactivated state. Proc. Natl. Acad. Sci. USA **81:** 6388–6392.
18. RANE, S. G., G. G. HOLZ & K. DUNLAP. 1987. Dihydropyridine inhibition of neuronal calcium current and substance P release. Pfluegers Arch. **409:** 361–366.
19. HOLZ, G. G., K. DUNLAP & R. M. KREAM. 1988. Characterization of the electrically evoked release of substance P from dorsal root ganglion neurons: methods and dihydropyridine sensitivity. J. Neurosci. **8:** 463–471.
20. SANGUINETTI, M. C., D. S. KRAFTE & R. S. KASS. 1986. Voltage-dependent modulation of calcium channel current in heart cells by Bay K 8644. J. Gen. Physiol. **88:** 369–392.
21. CAZALIS, M., G. DAYANITHI & J. J. NORDMANN. 1987. Hormone release from isolated nerve endings of the rat neurohypophysis. J. Physiol. **390:** 55–70.
22. ATCHISON, W. D. & S. M. O'LEARY. 1987. Bay K 8644 increases release of acetylcholine at the murine neuromuscular junction. Brain Res. **419:** 315–319.

Calcium Channels in the Presynaptic Nerve Terminal of the Chick Ciliary Ganglion Giant Synapse

E. F. STANLEY AND C. COX

Laboratory of Biophysics
National Institute of Neurological Disorders and Stroke
Building 9, Room 1 E124
National Institutes of Health
Bethesda, Maryland 20892

INTRODUCTION

The detection of calcium ion movement directly into a presynaptic nerve terminal using the voltage clamp technique has proved possible only in invertebrate preparations, notably the squid giant synapse. In vertebrates, the study of presynaptic calcium channels has been limited by the small size and inaccessibility of these structures. Thus, the properties of these channels have been inferred primarily by the action of pharmacological agents on the secretion of neurotransmitters or the uptake of radiolabeled calcium ions into synaptosomes. These procedures are either too indirect, or too slow, for definitive channel characterization. Thus, it is not clear whether presynaptic calcium channels are N-type,[1] L-type,[2,3] a combination, or neither.[4,5] Furthermore, it has been suggested that synaptic strength can be regulated by the indirect modulation of presynaptic calcium channels. This is based on the observation that calcium channels in neuron cell bodies are modulated by neurotransmitters acting through second messengers.[6] It remains to be demonstrated, however, that these pharmacological agents can also modulate the calcium current recorded directly from a presynaptic nerve terminal.

We have used the chick embryo ciliary ganglion "calyx" synapse to develop a preparation in which it is possible to apply voltage clamp techniques directly to a presynaptic nerve terminal. In this synapse the axonal input does not form the usual bouton-type terminals on the postsynaptic cell, the ciliary neuron, but instead envelopes the neurons to form a calyx[7-10] (FIG. 1). These calyces can be very extensive, enclosing a large fraction of the neuron. Transmission across this synapse is initially chemical but gradually becomes mixed, chemical and electrical.[11,12] Gap junctions are inserted,[13] and the calyx/ciliary neuron synapse myelinates and eventually occupies an internodal region.[11] Thereafter, the calyx gradually breaks into multiple small bouton-like contacts.[11,14] It is likely that the purpose of calyx formation is to ensure the capture of each ciliary neuron by a single presynaptic axon. Without such a developmental stage the eventual transition to a one-to-one electrically transmitting synapse might not be possible.

Calyces can be readily visualized by the anterograde fill of the presynaptic axons by Lucifer yellow dye.[15-17] The teased ciliary neurons are observed under fluorescent illumination, and the calyces appear as thin crescents encircling the neurons (FIG. 2). Lucifer yellow is known to pass through gap junctions and is often used to demonstrate cytoplasmic continuity through gap junctions.[18] Thus, dye-coupling might be

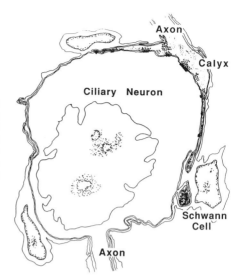

FIGURE 1. Schematic illustration of the structure of the chick ciliary ganglion calyx synapse. In this example, the calyx is shown to envelop only a small fraction of the ciliary neurons, but dye-filled calyces often totally surround the postsynaptic neuron. Note the Schwann cells that enclose the entire synapse.

expected in the calyx-ciliary neuron synapse, particularly at the later stages of development. Prominent transfer of the dye from the calyx to the ciliary neuron, however, as would be indicated by staining that did not distinguish the calyx from the postsynaptic neuron, was never observed. At embryonic day 14 (stage 40), when electrical coupling is known to be very weak,[19] Lucifer-filled calyces were clearly demarcated from the ciliary neurons. Similar results were obtained up to day 20 (stage 45–46) when electrical coupling is strong, and even at 1 to 3 days after hatching.[15] A faint staining of the ciliary neurons was detectable at all stages, but it was not clear if this was due to the over- and underlying calyx rather than dye transfer. Thus, some dye-coupling may be present but, if so, this is only through a small number of gap junctions. Perhaps the rate of diffusion of the dye out of the ciliary neuron by way of the axon was more rapid than the rate of influx from the calyx. Attempts to enhance dye-coupling by depolarizing the ganglion in high K^+ solutions were without effect, as were attempts to reduce the staining of the ciliary neurons by blocking agents used on other cell systems, such as octanol. Thus, electrical transmission develops during a period when there is no discernible increase in gap junctions, as assayed by dye transfer. These results support the hypothesis[11,12] that the increase in electrical coupling from day 14 to 20 is due, in most part, to the formation of the myelin sheath rather than the continued insertion of more gap junction proteins.

Presynaptic calyces have also been reported in the ciliary ganglion of reptiles including the turtle[9] and lizard.[20] Lucifer-filled lizard calyces were similar to those in the chick, also appearing as thin crescents that encircled the ciliary neuron (FIG. 2). In general, however, there seemed to be less staining over the ciliary neuron itself. It is not clear if the darker ciliary neurons were due to the absence of dye-transfer; there is no electrical coupling in the lizard.[20] To date we have attempted to dye-fill ciliary ganglion calyces from chick, lizard, turtle, and garter snake. Of these the chick calyx remains the most promising for patch-clamp studies, because it is the most extensive and has the greatest intermembrane thickness.

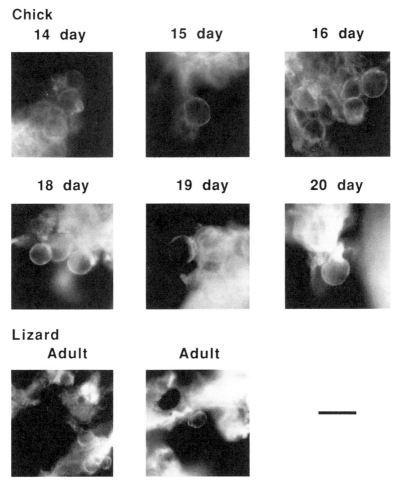

FIGURE 2. Anterograde Lucifer dye-fill of chick and lizard calyces. The presynaptic oculomotor nerve was drawn up into a pipette filled with Lucifer yellow dye, and the dye was allowed to perfuse into the nerve fibers for 2 to 3 hours. The ganglia were teased apart and were observed under fluorescent illumination. The dye-filled nerve endings can be seen as crescents surrounding a dark area that corresponds to the ciliary neuron. Note that staining was similar in ganglia stained from the 14th to 20th day *in ovo*. Calibration bar: 50 μm for chick and 100 μm for lizard.

PRESYNAPTIC CALCIUM CHANNELS

Ciliary neurons were dissociated with intact calyces by enzyme treatment and gentle trituration, as described in detail.[16,17] Under light microscopy the neurons appeared as round structures, generally without any processes. Many of the neurons had overlying calyces, but only in a few were the Schwann cells completely removed. In addition, some of the neurons were completely devoid of their neural capsules and were exposed to direct experimentation.

Standard patch-clamp techniques were used to record ion currents in calyces, whereas ciliary neurons that were dissociated free of their neural capsules served as controls. The type of structure contacted by the electrode was confirmed by including Lucifer yellow dye in the intracellular buffer solution in the pipette. The dye perfused the patched structure when the intervening membrane was ruptured. Calyces were similar in appearance to that observed by anterograde dye fill,[16,17] except that axons were generally lost during the dissociation procedure.[17]

Membrane currents were recorded in ciliary neurons and in calyces from a holding potential of -80 mV. In the neuron a large inward current was recorded that had two obvious components: a small current that decayed during the voltage pulse and a large sustained current. A similar voltage step in the calyces resulted in a qualitatively different inward current. This current activated rapidly and was sustained for the duration of the pulse. In no case was there evidence for a decaying component at this or any other pulse potential.[16,17] At the end of the pulse a prominent tail current was observed. The inward current in the calyx could be completely blocked by locally applied Cd.[17]

EFFECT OF A DEPOLARIZING PREPULSE ON CA CURRENTS

We tested the sensitivity of the calyx Ca currents to voltage-dependent inactivation by preceding a 50 ms test pulse with a 1 s depolarizing prepulse. In the ciliary neurons the decaying component of the high-voltage–activated Ca current was inactivated by the prepulse (FIG. 3), similar to reports in chick motoneurons,[21] leaving only the sustained current. Subtracting the prepulse-resistant current from the total current evoked without the prepulse revealed the decaying component. In the calyx, however, the prepulse had no discernible effect on the current trace, and subtraction of the current traces failed to reveal a voltage-inactivated current component (FIG. 3). Although the noise associated with the high gain precludes the conclusion that a ciliary neuron-like voltage-inactivated Ca current was totally absent in the calyx, it was clear that the bulk of the current was prepulse-insensitive.

EFFECT OF ω-CONOTOXIN ON CALCIUM CURRENTS

The calyx calcium current[17] and synaptic transmission[5] in the ciliary ganglion are blocked by locally applied ω-conotoxin GVIA (ω-CTX). We have examined the effect of low concentrations of this toxin on the calcium current of calyces and ciliary neurons.

Ciliary neurons were held at -80 mV, and calcium currents were activated by step depolarizations to $+30$ mV at 0.3 Hz. Synthetic ω-conotoxin was applied to the cells from the tip of a micropipette positioned within 50 μm of the cell. At a pipette toxin of 10 nM, calcium current block proceeded slowly and did not affect both components of the Ca current equally (FIG. 4). The toxin reduced the peak Ca current more rapidly than the current at the end of the pulse, indicating that the decaying component was more sensitive to the ω-CTX than the sustained component. This was confirmed by subtracting current traces averaged at different times after the onset of ω-CTX treatment. The decaying component of the Ca current was blocked very soon after toxin exposure (see also refs. 22 and 23). With a longer duration of toxin treatment there was also a decline in the sustained component.

The calyx Ca current was also blocked by ω-CTX at 10 nM (FIG. 4). In this case,

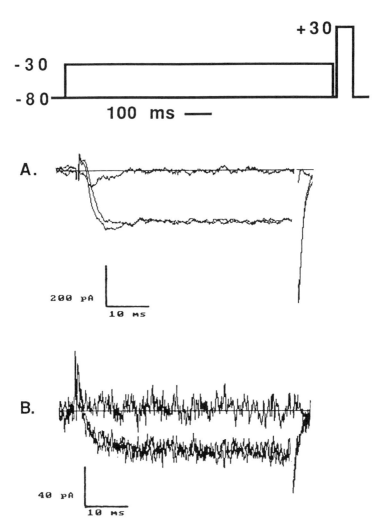

FIGURE 3. Effect of a sustained depolarizing prepulse on inward currents in the ciliary neuron and calyx. Top: Voltage clamp pulse. A 50 ms test pulse was preceded by a 1 s prepulse to −30 mV. This was compared to a test pulse alone. **A:** Ion currents recorded during the test pulse in a ciliary neuron. The lowest trace shows the control current, the middle trace shows the ciliary neuron current with the prepulse, and the top trace shows the difference. The prepulse eliminated a small fraction of the total current, leaving only a noninactivating component. **B:** Same as A but recorded in a calyx. The control and prepulse traces are superimposed, and no current is evident in the subtracted trace. Thus, the bulk of the ion current recorded in the calyx is not inactivated by prior depolarization.

however, the toxin did not affect an early component of the current trace. Subtraction of the current trace after toxin treatment from the pretreatment control did not reveal an inactivating inward current component.

Subtracting the post– from the pre–ω-CTX current trace is an effective method of revealing the calyx Ca current free from other minor contaminating current compo-

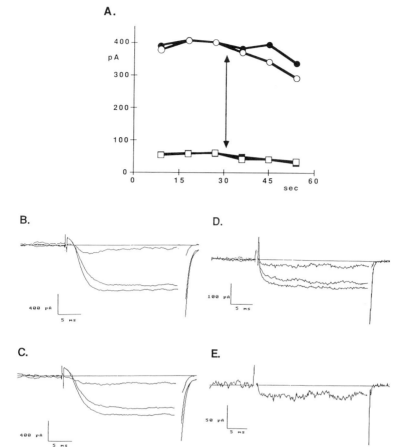

FIGURE 4. Effect of 10 nM ω-CTX on ion currents in the ciliary neuron and the calyx. **A:** Current amplitudes measured at the peak (open symbols) and end (filled symbols) of the inward current recorded in a ciliary neuron (circles) or at the same intervals in a calyx (squares) before and during exposure to 10 nM ω-CTX (double-headed arrow). Each point is the mean of three consecutive current recordings at a frequency of 0.3 Hz, stepping from a −80 mV holding potential to +30 mV. The time course of toxin action is variable, but note the more rapid reduction of the peak than the end current in the ciliary neuron. This was due to a faster action of the toxin on the inactivating than the sustained inward current (see **B** and **C**). No such difference was observed in the calyx. **B:** Bottom trace, averaged current traces prior to ω-CTX exposure in the ciliary neuron. Middle trace, average of four traces over the period of 3 to 15 s after the onset of toxin treatment. Top trace, the subtracted difference between bottom and middle current traces showing the fraction of calcium current blocked early after toxin exposure. Note the decay of the subtracted trace, indicating that the inactivating component of the total current was more sensitive to the toxin. **C:** Bottom trace (same as middle trace in **A**), current after a few seconds of toxin treatment. Middle trace, average of four traces from 18 to 30 s after toxin exposure. Top trace, difference between bottom and middle traces; fraction of calcium current blocked later after toxin exposure. Note the absence of any decay in the subtracted current trace, indicating that with longer exposure the sustained component of the current was also blocked by the toxin. **D:** Bottom trace, averaged traces prior to ω-CTX exposure. Middle trace, average of five traces from 3 to 18 s after onset of toxin exposure. Top trace, subtracted difference between bottom and middle traces. The Ca current in the calyx is also blocked by ω-CTX, but note the lack of decay in the subtracted trace. **E:** Subtracted trace in C at a higher gain to illustrate the ω-CTX–sensitive inward Ca current in the calyx. The subtraction eliminates non-Ca current elements of the membrane current, such as the early outward current.

nents. The ω-CTX–sensitive current activated rapidly (within 5 ms), was sustained for the duration of the pulse, and deactivated rapidly. The time constant of deactivation of the calyx calcium current has been reported to be about 0.5 ms at −80 mV.[17]

MODULATION OF THE PRESYNAPTIC CALCIUM CURRENT

We have begun to test the effect of agents that have been reported to modulate calcium channels in cultured neurons on the calcium current recorded from the calyx. The first agent we selected to test was somatostatin (SST), as this peptide is present in the ciliary ganglion,[24] is known to modulate calcium currents,[25] and depresses transmitter release in cat parasympathetic ganglion presynaptic nerve terminals.[26]

Somatostatin (1 μM) was applied to the calyx from a closely positioned, blunt-tipped pipette while evoking inward calcium currents with a train of voltage step to +30 mV. Peptide treatment resulted in a reduction of the sustained calcium current of about 30% (FIG. 5). We used extracellular recording from the intact ciliary ganglion[5,27] to test the effect of SST on synaptic transmission. The ciliary ganglion was isolated, and the oculomotor nerve leading into the ganglion was stimulated while recording compound nerve action potentials (CNAP) from the postsynaptic ciliary nerve. The amplitude of the CNAP is a direct measure of the number of ciliary neurons activated by synaptic transmission. SST (1 μM) failed to reduce the amplitude of the CNAP in standard extracellular buffer (FIG. 5). We reasoned that a significant effect of SST might be obscured by a large safety factor to synaptic transmission. The safety factor was essentially eliminated by reducing the extracellular calcium concentration from the standard level of 2 mM to 0.8 mM. With the low extracellular calcium, some of the ciliary neuron synapses failed to transmit, and the CNAP was reduced by over 50 percent. The CNAP was very sensitive to any further reduction in synaptic strength as the remaining synapses were transmitting marginally. Under these conditions 1 μM SST treatment resulted in a significant and reversible decline in the CNAP. These results indicate that SST can modulate presynaptic calcium currents and that this effect can be biologically significant but, at least in this case, only when synaptic transmission is already compromised.

DISCUSSION

The ciliary ganglion calyx is the first vertebrate presynaptic nerve terminal in which it has proved possible to record inward calcium currents directly.[16,20] The properties of the calyx may be of direct relevance to well-established, but less accessible experimental preparations [notably the neuromuscular junction], as this synapse is both fast-transmitting and cholinergic.

The calcium channels in the calyx have properties that are both consistent, and at odds, with predictions from previous studies. It is usually assumed that the dominant presynaptic calcium channel is of the N-type (see ref. 1). This conclusion was based on the insensitivity of synaptic transmission to the dihydropyridine (DHP) blockers, together with the block of transmitter release by ω-CTX, albeit with several exceptions.[28] We have demonstrated that the calyx calcium channels and synaptic transmission in the ciliary ganglion are, indeed, DHP-block resistant, even under conditions where this resistance cannot be attributed to voltage sensitivity of these agents.[5] In

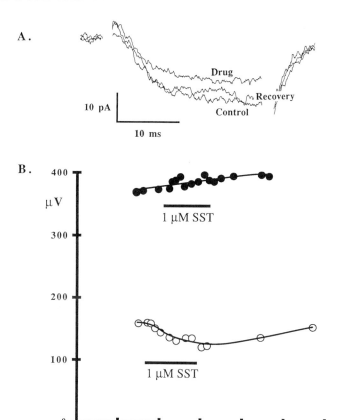

FIGURE 5. **A:** Effect of SST on the calcium current recorded from the calyx. Depolarizing pulses were given to +30 mV at a frequency of 0.3 Hz from a holding potential of −80 mV to evoke inward calcium currents. During the train the calyx was treated with SST (1 μM) from a closely positioned blunt-tipped pipette. Each trace is the mean of three to four current pulses prior (control), during (drug), or after (recovery) SST treatment. The inward calcium current was reduced by about 30%. **B:** Effect of SST on the amplitude of the CNAP recorded from the postsynaptic ciliary nerve in response to a stimulus to the presynaptic oculomotor nerve in the presence of 2 mM (filled circles) or 0.8 mM (empty circles) external calcium (see text).

addition, the calyx calcium channels and ciliary ganglion transmission are blocked by ω-CTX (see also refs. 16 and 17). Thus, in some respects these channels are typical of the N-type. N-type calcium channels, however, have also been reported to be sensitive to voltage-dependent inactivation[29,30] (but see refs. 23 and 31). The calyx calcium current is insensitive to voltage-dependent inactivation, at least as far as can be ascertained when the space clamp difficulties of this structure are considered.[16,17] Thus, this calcium current exhibits no decay during long depolarizing pulses[17] (up to several hundred milliseconds, unpublished observations) and relatively little inactivation with a depolarization of the holding potential to −40 mV from −80 mV.[17]

Furthermore, as shown here, a prolonged depolarizing prepulse does not inactivate the calcium current, in contrast to the small decaying component in the ciliary neurons. At present we prefer to designate these channels as N-like or N_{PT}-type (N-like, presynaptic nerve terminal) until the range, and possible subdivision, of this category of calcium channel is more clearly established.

The calyx calcium channels are capable of very rapid activation and deactivation.[17] These properties are essential for calcium channels involved in impulse secretion at fast-transmitting nerve terminals.[32] The duration of the action potential is typically of 1 ms or less and, hence, in order to contribute to transmitter release the calcium channels must be activated during this period. Calyx calcium currents exhibited activation time constants with a minimum of about 1.3 ms at +30 mV.[17] If this value is a good estimate of the actual activation rate it implies that only a fraction of the available calcium channels will be activated during an action potential. This relatively slow activation rate (compared, for example, with sodium channels) may have some advantages, however. If only 50 to 60% of the channels are activated during a typical action potential, there remains a large capacity for modulation of the calcium current, and hence, transmitter release. Thus, transmitter release could be up- or down-regulated by factors that change the number of available calcium channels, the channel activation rate, or simply the duration of the action potential.

The demonstration that the calyx calcium current and synaptic transmission can be down-regulated by SST confirms the suggestion in numerous previous studies that the modulation of calcium channels in presynaptic nerve terminals is a mechanism whereby external factors can control synaptic strength. There is direct evidence for such an effect, as SST can reduce transmitter release from preganglionic nerve terminals in the parasympathetic ganglia of the cat.[26] Presumably, SST acts by way of a second-messenger G protein, similar to the regulation of calcium channels in other cells.[33]

The calyx calcium channel has properties that are consistent with many studies on the biology of presynaptic nerve terminals at fast-transmitting synapses. This ion channel may, therefore, be representative of calcium channels at a number of vertebrate presynaptic nerve terminals.

REFERENCES

1. MILLER, R. 1987. Multiple calcium channels and neuronal function. Science 235: 46–52.
2. LINDGREN, C. A. & J. W. MOORE. 1989. Identification of ionic currents at presynaptic nerve endings of the lizard. J. Physiol. (London) 414: 201–22.
3. RANE, S. G., G. G. HOLZ IV & K. DUNLAP. 1987. Dihydropyridine inhibition of neuronal calcium current and substance P release. Pfluegers Arch. 409: 361–366.
4. SUSZKIW, J. B., M. M. MURAWSKY & M. SHI. 1989. Further characterization of phasic calcium influx in rat cerebrocortical synaptosomes: Inferences regarding calcium channel type(s) in nerve endings. J. Neurochem. 52: 1260–1269.
5. STANLEY, E. F. & A. H. ATRAKCHI. 1990. The calcium current in the presynaptic nerve terminal of the chick giant synapse is insensitive to the dihydropyridine nifedipine. Proc. Natl. Acad. Sci. USA 87: 9683–9687.
6. REUTER, H. 1983. Calcium channel modulation by neurotransmitters, enzymes and drugs. Nature 301: 569–574.
7. CARPENTER, R. W. 1911. The ciliary ganglion of birds. Folia Neuro. Biol. 5: 738–754.
8. TERZUOLO, C. 1951. Richerche sul ganglio ciliari degli Ucelli. Connessioni mutamenti in relazione all'eta e dopo recisione delle fibre pregangliari. Z. Zellforsch. Mikrosk. Anat. 36: 255–267.
9. SZENTAGOTHAI, J. 1964. The structure of the autonomic interneuronal synapse. Acta Neuroveg. 26: 338–359.

10. DE LORENZO, A. J. 1960. The fine structure of synapses in the chick ciliary ganglion. J. Biophys. Biochem. Cytol. **7:** 31–36.
11. HESS, A. 1965. Developmental changes in the structure of the synapse on the myelinated cell bodies of the chicken ciliary ganglion. J. Cell Biol. **25:** 1–19.
12. HESS, A., G. PILAR & J. N. WEAKLEY. 1969. Correlation between transmission and structure in avian ciliary ganglion synapses. J. Physiol. (London) **202:** 339–354.
13. CANTINO, D. & E. MUGNAINI. 1975. The structural basis for electronic coupling in the avian ciliary ganglion. J. Neurocytol. **4:** 505–536.
14. HAMORY, J. & L. N. DYACHKOVA. 1964. Electron microscope studies on developmental differentiation of ciliary ganglion synapses in the chick. Acta Biol. Acad. Sci. Hung. **15:** 213–230.
15. STANLEY, E. 1987. Light microscopic visualization of the presynaptic nerve terminal calyx in dissociated chick ciliary ganglion neurons. Brain Res. **421:** 367–369.
16. STANLEY, E. F. 1989. Calcium currents in a vertebrate presynaptic nerve terminal: the chick ciliary ganglion calyx. Brain Res. **505:** 341–343.
17. STANLEY, E. F. & G. GOPING. 1989. Characterization of a calcium current in a vertebrate cholinergic presynaptic nerve terminal. J. Neurosci. **11:** 985–993.
18. STEWART, W. W. 1981. Lucifer dyes—highly fluorescent dyes for biological tracing. Nature (London) **292:** 17–21.
19. LANDMESSER, L. & G. PILAR. 1972. The onset and development of transmission in the chick ciliary ganglion. J. Physiol. (London) **222:** 691–713.
20. MARTIN, A. R., V. PATEL, L. FAILLE & A. MALLART. 1989. Presynaptic calcium currents recorded from calyciform nerve terminals in the lizard ciliary ganglion. Neurosci. Lett. **105:** 14–18.
21. McCOBB, D. P., P. M. BEST & K. G. BEAM. 1989. Development alters the expression of calcium currents in chick limb motoneurons. Neuron **2:** 1633–1643.
22. KASAI, H., T. AOSAKI & J. FUKUDA. 1987. Presynaptic Ca-antagonist ω-conotoxin irreversibly blocks N-type Ca-channels in chick sensory neurons. Neurosci. Res. **4:** 228–235.
23. AOSAKI, T. & H. KASAI. 1989. Characterization of two kinds of high-voltage-activated Ca-channel currents in chick sensory neurons. Pfluegers Arch. **414:** 150–156.
24. EPSTEIN, M. L., J. P. DAVIS, L. E. GELLMAN, J. R. LAMB & J. L. DAHL. 1988. Cholinergic neurons of the chicken ciliary ganglion contain somatostatin. Neurosci. **3:** 1053–1060.
25. LUINI, A., D. LEWIS, S. GUILD, G. SCHOFIELD & F. WEIGHT. 1986. Somatostatin, an inhibitor of ACTH secretion, decreases cytostolic free calcium and voltage-dependent calcium current in a pituitary cell line. J. Neurosci. **6:** 3128–3132.
26. KATAYAMA, Y. & K. HIRAI. 1989. Somatostatin presynaptically inhibits transmitter release in feline parasympathetic ganglia. Brain Res. **487:** 62–68.
27. MARTIN, A. R. & G. PILAR. 1963. Transmission through the ciliary ganglion of the chick. J. Physiol. (London) **168:** 464–475.
28. YOSHIKAMI, D., Z. BAGABOLDO & B. M. OLIVERA. 1989. The inhibitory effects of omega-conotoxins on Ca channels and synapses. Ann. N.Y. Acad. Sci. **560:** 230–248.
29. NOWYCKY, M. C., A. P. FOX & R. W. TSIEN. 1985. Three types of neuronal calcium channel with different calcium agonist sensitivity. Nature (London) **316:** 440–443.
30. FOX, A. P., M. C. NOWYCKY & R. W. TSIEN. 1987. Kinetic and pharmacological properties distinguishing three types of calcium currents in chick sensory neurons. J. Physiol. **394:** 149–172.
31. PLUMMER, M. R., D. E. LOGOTHETIS & P. HESS. 1989. Elementary properties and pharmacological sensitivities of calcium channels in mammalian peripheral neurons. Neuron **2:** 1453–1463.
32. LLINÁS, R. R., M. SUGIMORI & S. M. SIMON. 1982. Transmission by presynaptic spike-like depolarization in the squid synapse. Proc. Natl. Acad. Sci. USA **79:** 2415–2419.
33. HESCHELER, J., W. ROSENTHAL, W. TRAUTWEIN & G. SCHULTZ. 1987. The GTP binding protein, Go, regulates neuronal calcium channels. Nature **325:** 445–447.

Properties of Calcium Channels Isolated with Spider Toxin, FTX

BRUCE D. CHERKSEY, MUTSUYUKI SUGIMORI, AND
RODOLFO R. LLINÁS

Department of Physiology and Biophysics
New York University Medical Center
New York, New York 10016

Our ability to define more precisely the molecular structures responsible for calcium inflow which triggers synaptic transmitter release has suffered from the lack of a selective blocking agent for the Ca^{2+} channels present in presynaptic terminals. Recently we discovered an agent that blocks presynaptic calcium currents in the squid stellate ganglions,[1] a junction where the calcium blockers, Ω-conotoxin and dihydroxypyridine, do not influence calcium currents.

The toxin in question was isolated from the venom of the American grass spiders, also known as funnel-web spiders, including *Agelenopsis aperta, Hololina curta,* and *Calilena.* Although this venom has proven to be a rich source of channel blockers, none of the previously defined components[2] was able to block Ca^{2+} currents in either guinea pig cerebellar Purkinje cells or in the squid giant synapse. Only the fraction which we have termed FTX proved to be an effective Ca^{2+} channel blocker in these systems. FTX is specific in that it does not block fast or slow sodium currents nor does it directly block potassium currents.[3,4] Thus, as our initial effort, we felt that it would be important to characterize further the structure of FTX.

STRUCTURE OF NATURAL FTX

In an earlier paper we reported that FTX was a low-molecular-weight compound.[5] Initially the molecular weight of FTX was estimated using gel-permeation chromatography on Sephadex G-10 and G-15. The fraction with the FTX activity (determined electrophysiologically) was in the 200–400 molecular-weight range. In addition, the FTX activity was found to be dialyzable through MW 1200 tubing, further suggesting a low molecular weight for the toxin. The apparent molecular weight of FTX was not altered by extensive boiling, by reduction with dithiothreitol, or by trypsin. In our early studies we used the low-molecular-weight fraction FTX, but the purity of this material was insufficient for structural characterization.

Early attempts to purify FTX using HPLC were not successful. The FTX activity would unreliably run through an ODS column or stick to it completely for reasons we have not yet determined. In view of our experience with Sephadex, we next turned our attention to the FPLC purification methods which yielded more satisfactory results (FIG. 1A). Size-exclusion chromatography on a Superose 6 column demonstrated a predictable separation with results similar to that of the Sephadex G-10, with the FTX activity in the low-molecular-weight region. Although the results were consistent from run to run, contamination of the sample with dipeptides and single amino acids could not be ruled out. Thus, an improved method of purification was desirable, and so ion-exchange chromatography was employed. Initially we used Mono-Q, a strong anion exchanger. The FTX activity was found to elute immediately from the column. Cation exchange on Mono-S yielded a preferable result in that the FTX activity eluted late in the run and was essentially free of contaminants. Currently, our preferred procedure for purification of FTX is to follow cation exchange with anion exchange to purify further the toxin and to strip off the residual salt.

With a purified, electrophysiologically active form of FTX it was possible to perform a variety of chemical analyses aimed at elucidating its structure. When UV spectroscopy was performed on FTX (as shown in FIG. 1B), the most significant finding was that the toxin did not absorb in the aromatic region of 260–290 nm and thus lacked tyrosine, phenylalanine, or tryptophan-like residues. For a natural product this was somewhat surprising. The compound, however, did absorb in the 200–220 nm range and exhibited a large acid-base shift in its absorption spectra, which suggested the presence of an amine or amines, and perhaps a guanidino moiety. Further studies using Fourier-Transform infrared spectroscopy (FT-IR, shown in FIG. 1C) revealed a particularly unremarkable structure. Noteworthy was the lack of a carbonyl group. The NMR spectra obtained were also unremarkable.

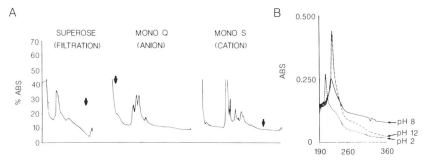

FIGURE 1. Chemical characterization of the natural FTX fraction from *A. aperta*. Panel **A:** FPLC of deproteinated spider venom. Arrows show fraction with electrophysiological activity against P channels. **B:** pH dependence of UV spectra of FTX; note absence of aromatic absorption and very pronounced shifts in wavelength between pH 2 and pH 8. **C:** FT-IR of FTX using repetitive scanning technique.

Elemental analysis suggested only the presence of carbon, nitrogen, and hydrogen in a ratio of 2:1:1, an extremely high nitrogen content. With this information, it was possible to speculate on a range of structures for FTX.

SYNTHETIC FTX

The analytical data we obtained suggested that FTX might be a nonaromatic polyamine.[5] Initially, we tested parent compounds including spermine, spermidine, and putrescine for channel-blocking activity. Neither spermine nor putresceine blocked the calcium currents in Purkinje cells or in squid giant synapse. Spermidine, however, exhibited weak effects as a blocker. Thus, model compounds were developed using spermidine as the synthetic base. From the physical characterization of FTX, a reasonable first step was to couple the amino acid arginine to spermidine. Although this would still contain the carbonyl group thought to be absent in FTX, it was synthetically much easier to prepare. When the arginine-spermidine adduct was tested electrophysiologically, it was found to be far more potent than spermidine

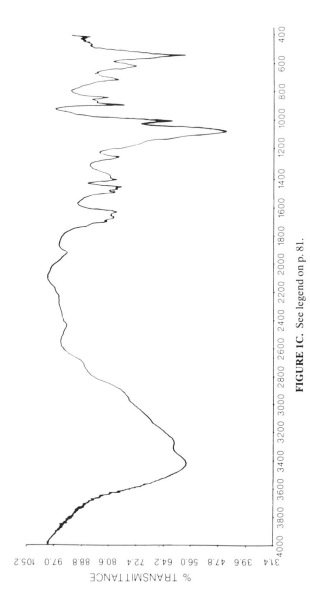

FIGURE 1C. See legend on p. 81.

itself, as a Ca^{2+} channel blocker. We then proceeded to prepare further analogues of synthetic FTX, initially to test if the free amine of the compound would insert itself into the channel. To do this we prepared a diarginyl adduct—that is, a compound with arginine at each end. This compound was found to be inactive.

A second type of model compound which we prepared replaced arginine with lysine. This minor biochemical modification abolished the activity of synthetic FTX. More recently we have substituted symmetric triamines for spermidine, which has resulted in a substantial enhancement of activity.

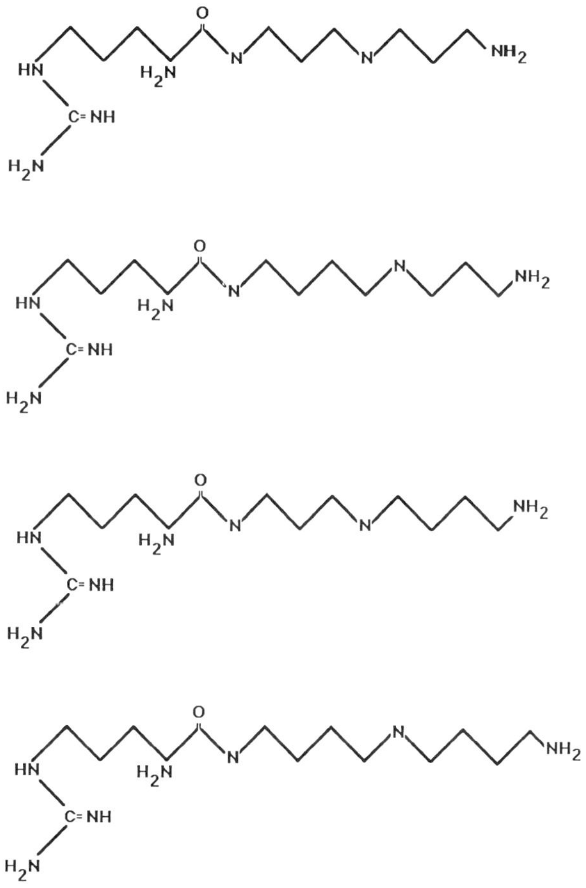

STRUCTURE 1.

These structures, which are shown above, include (a) FTX (3:3) symmetric polyamine in which each of the terminal nitrogens is separated from the central nitrogen by three methylene (CH_2) groups; (b) FTX (4:3), the resolved regioisomer of spermidine in which the 4-methylene-group-containing end is coupled to arginine; (c) FTX (3:4), the resolved regioisomer in which the 3-methylene-group-containing end of spermidine is coupled to the arginine; and (d) FTX (4:4), similar to (3:3) but with four methylene groups rather than three.

To understand further the structure-activity relationships for FTX channel block, we have synthesized a wide series of compounds. The most interesting findings to date are that the amino group alpha to the carbonyl group is necessary for Ca^{2+} channel block in our preparations. Removal of this nitrogen converts the compounds into sodium-channel blockers or nonselective blockers, depending on the length of the carbon chain between the guanidino group and the coupled polyamine. A further finding was that substitution of a diamine such as 1,10 diamino decane for spermidine yielded a compound that acts as a substantially selective potassium-channel blocker. Substitution of phenylalanine, tyrosine, tryptophan, or histidine produced compounds with no discernible activity in our systems.

FTX ACTIVITY ON PRESYNAPTIC CALCIUM CURRENTS AND TRANSMITTER RELEASE IN THE SQUID GIANT SYNAPSE

As was previously reported, both purified FTX[1-4] and synthetic FTX can block transmission in the squid giant synapse.[5,6] Pre- and postsynaptic recordings were made in squid giant synapse with presynaptic voltage-clamp techniques. In previous

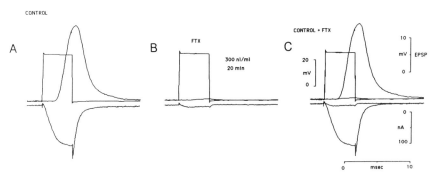

FIGURE 2. Voltage-clamp study in squid giant synapse. A: Presynaptic voltage step (upper trace) generates an inward calcium current (lower trace) and a powerful postsynaptic response (middle trace). B: After synthetic FTX is added to the bath, the calcium current and the postsynaptic response is markedly reduced. C: Comparison of A and B. Voltage current and time calibrations as indicated in the FIGURE.

studies it had been determined that synthetic FTX at a concentration of 30 μmole blocks calcium currents as well as the postsynaptic response and without modifying the postsynaptic responsiveness to glutamic acid applied directly into the bath and without affecting presynaptic action potential except for the small component of afterhyperpolarization. This later change is probably due to the reduction of calcium-dependent potassium conductance, which adds a small component to this afterhyperpolarization. The results shown in FIGURE 2 indicate that synthetic FTX (3:3) at a concentration of 300 nL/mL (30 μM) produced a total block of presynaptic calcium currents and of the associated transmitter release in 20 minutes of exposure. Once the transmission is blocked, the "washout time" for the toxin is very long indeed, and synaptic transmission never seems to recuperate fully.

BIOCHEMICAL STUDIES OF ISOLATED CA²⁺ CHANNELS

A limiting problem which we experienced in attempting to characterize the protein isolated using an FTX affinity gel was the small amount of toxin available, but this has been solved by the development of synthetic analogues. Affinity gels have been constructed using synthetic FTX. Arginine was first coupled to Sepharose CL 4B via a butane diglycidyl ether spacer group following reaction with spermidine. To obtain the large amounts of material required for the biochemical studies, we used cow cerebellum freshly obtained from a slaughterhouse. The material was processed as we have previously described.[4,7] The activity of the isolated protein was determined using the lipid-bilayer technique and was found to exhibit activity similar to that in proteins obtained from guinea pig cerebellum. The results we obtained in the lipid-bilayer studies are shown in FIGURE 3A–C, tracings of the channel behavior at potentials of −10 mV, −30 mV, and −50 mV, which illustrate the voltage dependence of the open probability of the isolated channel. FIGURE 3D shows the results obtained for the ensemble average of a large number (> 1000) of 15 mV and 25 mV voltage steps. With a 15 mV pulse, the channel shows little or no inactivation over the time scale of the experiment. With the larger pulse, a slight degree of inactivation is seen. These results have been compared with a mathematical model of the predicted channel behavior (FIG. 3D, smooth lines) with favorable results. Although the properties of this channel show some resemblance to those of the N-type channel, the isolated protein is not blocked by conotoxin. Also, when the ability of monovalent ions to permeate the channel in the absence of divalents was tested (FIG. 3E), a unique series unlike that for the N channel was found. For the P-type channel, Cs^+ was essentially impermeant, although Rb^+ was highly permeant.

Structural determination of the isolated protein was performed using both size-exclusion HPLC and SDS-polyacrylamide gel electrophoresis (SDS-PAGE). As shown in FIG. 4A, on HPLC the protein showed a molecular weight of approximately 120,000. Upon reduction (FIG. 4A, lower panel), at least two, and possibly three, subunits are in evidence. One subunit of MW 70,000 produces a sharp HPLC peak, although the second subunit peak is broad in the range of 20,000–30,000. This broad peak could be due to either two distinct subunits of similar molecular weight or one subunit in different states of glycosylation. SDS-PAGE of the nonreduced protein (FIG. 4B, second lane) showed a single sharp band at an apparent molecular weight of 90,000–100,000, similar to the result obtained by size-exclusion HPLC. The small difference in apparent molecular weights is probably due to trapped detergent in the HPLC measurement.

The isolated protein has been used to inoculate rabbits to form polyclonal antibodies. Western blot analysis of these antibodies (FIG. 4B, third lane) shows that they react with the isolated protein. In addition, when tested against whole cerebellar homogenate (FIG. 4B, fourth lane, membrane preparation, silver stained), the antibodies reacted only with the protein at a single band (FIG. 4B, fifth lane), which is consistent with the isolated channel protein.

CONCLUSIONS

The utilization of specific channel-blocking agents has become an important tool with respect to the characterization of the biophysics and biochemistry of ionic channels. Most of the categorization of these channels into particular groups is based on either pharmacological or biophysical properties. With regard to calcium chan-

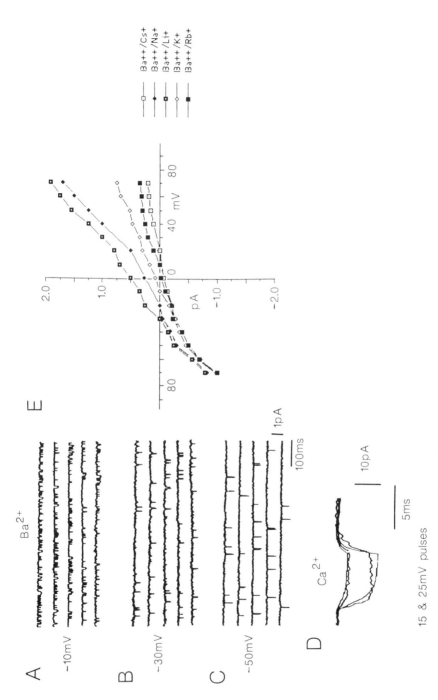

FIGURE 3. Behavior of synthetic FTX-purified CNS protein when reconstituted into lipid bilayer. **A**, **B**, and **C** show voltage dependence of single channels. **D**: Ensemble average of currents obtained with voltage-step stimulation. **E**: Monovalent ion selectivity obtained in absence of divalents on one side of the membrane; Ba^{2+} on the other side.

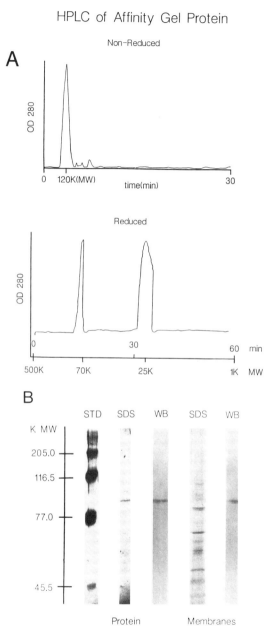

FIGURE 4. Biochemical characterization of synthetic FTX–purified CNS protein. **A:** Size-exclusion chromatography under nonreduced condition is reduced protein. **B:** SDS-PAGE and Western blot of purified protein and polyvalent antibody raised against this protein.

nels such operational definitions have generated a certain degree of confusion, which must be addressed if further understanding of these molecular entities is to follow. We have presented evidence that a polyamine, which can be extracted from the venom of American grass spiders, can block voltage-dependent calcium channels in the squid presynaptic terminal. This block is quite specific for the calcium channel and does not alter the postsynaptic potentials or sodium-generated action potentials. A similar specificity is found for similar calcium currents in other species. In particular, in *Xenopus* oocytes, it has been found that FTX can block one of the components of calcium current while the second component is blocked by omega conotoxin.[8]

Similar results were found in immature cultured granule cells[9] and in mammalian neurohypophysis.[10] Reports of calcium-channel blockage at very low synthetic-FTX concentrations were also reported for the pike retina.[11] In contrast to results recently published and discussed in this volume, we found that synthetic FTX could easily distinguish calcium P channel from those which are blocked by Ω-conotoxin (N channel). Furthermore, we found that in mammalian central neurons, *in vitro,* FTX as defined below failed to block the low-threshold or transient calcium conductances of the high-threshold (L-type) conductances without affecting sodium or potassium conductances.[12,13]

In our hands, then, the polyamines described are quite specific enough and have permitted the isolation of a protein that behaves in many ways like the P channel described in previous papers.[4,7,12,13]

Synthetic FTX

Results recently obtained used a variation of the polyamine structure where the carbon chain varied in the 4:3, 3:4, and 3:3 manner, indicating the most potent blocker to be the 3:3 compound. It must be emphasized that even when we tested elevated concentrations of either the very potent 3:3 or the 4:3 (into the high micromole and the millimole level), interference with sodium or potassium conductances was not seen. The 3:4 compound did not produce calcium block at concentrations ten times higher than those employed for FTX (3:3) or FTX (4:3).

From the above we conclude that polyamines having the structure given above are capable of specific blocking of calcium channels, and the calcium channels most likely affected belong to the category we call the P type. Of interest here is the fact that as research continues in polyamine-ionic channel pharmacology, it has been possible to refine further the pharmacological effects of these molecules. This is not surprising if they are used by the body as global channel modulators, as polyamines are manufactured by the body and found in the brain.

THE CALCIUM CHANNEL

Use of the synthetic FTX has allowed the development of an affinity gel that yielded a protein with a molecular weight of 90,000. On presentation to the lipid bilayer, it reproduces ionic conductances similar to the squid and the Purkinje cell. These results further support the view that this polyamine produces a specific blockade of the P-type channel and give us a glimpse at the structure of the P channel itself.

Additional experiments in this area are now being designed to analyze further the nature of this protein and to develop even more potent polyamine-type compounds for the biochemical and pharmacologic properties of a variety of CNS channel types.

REFERENCES

1. SUGIMORI, M., J.-W. LIN, B. CHERKSEY & R. LLINÁS. 1988. Biol. Bull. (Woods Hole) **175:** 308.
2. ADAMS, M. E., V. P. BINDOKAS, A. C. DOLPHIN, J. S. IMPERIAL, B. M. OLIVERA, R. H. SCOTT & V. J. VENEMA. 1989. Soc. Neurosci. (Abst.) **15:** 652.
3. SUGIMORI, M. & R. LLINÁS. 1987. Soc. Neurosci. (Abst.) **13:** 228.
4. LLINÁS, R., M. SUGIMORI, J.-W. LIN & B. CHERKSEY. 1989. Proc. Natl. Acad. Sci. USA **86:** 1689.
5. CHERKSEY, B., R. LLINÁS, M. SUGIMORI & J.-W. LIN. 1989. Biol. Bull. (Woods Hole) **177:** 321.
6. LLINÁS, R., M. SUGIMORI, J.-W. LIN & B. CHERKSEY. 1989. Biol. Bull. (Woods Hole) **177:** 324.
7. CHERKSEY, B. D., M. SUGIMORI, J.-W. LIN & R. LLINÁS. 1988. Biol. Bull. (Woods Hole) **175:** 304.
8. LIN, J.-W., B. RUDY & R. LLINÁS. 1990. Proc. Natl. Acad. Sci. USA **87:** 4538–4542.
9. BERTOLINO, M., S. VINCINI, R. LLINÁS & E. COSTA. 1990. Soc. Neurosci. (Abst.) **16:** 956.
10. OBAID, A. L. *et al.* 1990. Biol. Bull. (Woods Hole) **179:** 232.
11. SULLIVAN, J. M. & E. M. LASATER. 1990. Soc. Neurosci. (Abst.) **16:** 257.
12. CHERKSEY, B., J.-W. LIN, M. SUGIMORI & R. LLINÁS. 1989. Soc. Neurosci. (Abst.) **14:** 652.
13. LLINÁS, R. R., M. SUGIMORI & B. CHERKSEY. 1989. Ann. N.Y. Acad. Sci. **560:** 103–111.

Endoplasmic Reticulum as a Source of Ca^{2+} in Neurotransmitter Secretion

RENE ETCHEBERRIGARAY, JENNY L. FIEDLER,
HARVEY B. POLLARD, AND EDUARDO ROJAS

Laboratory of Cell Biology and Genetics
National Institute of Diabetes and Digestive and Kidney Diseases
National Institutes of Health
Bethesda, Maryland 20892

INTRODUCTION

Adenine nucleotides (ATP) are stored in presynaptic vesicles and are released together with specific neurotransmitters.[1,2] Although the physiological role of the secreted nucleotides is unknown, many observations suggest that they could act as neurotransmitters and neuromodulators in the nervous system.[3] Support for this idea has come from recent reports showing that adenine nucleotides inhibit electrical activity of some neurons.[4] Several results show that membrane depolarization causes the release of specific neurotransmitters and ATP from different types of synaptosomal preparations.[5,6]

We and others have shown that it is possible to measure on-line the time course of ATP secretion from adrenal medullary chromaffin cells[7] and rat brain synaptosomes[8,9] by including in the reaction medium the enzyme mixture luciferin-luciferase. We have employed this method to study the effects of extracellular calcium on both the extent and the kinetics of ATP release evoked by membrane depolarization.[10] We found and report here that, in addition to the classical $[Ca^{2+}]_0$-dependent secretion, membrane depolarization induced $[Ca^{2+}]_0$-independent secretion ($[Ca^{2+}]_0 < 1 \ \mu M$). It is widely accepted that Ca^{2+} is essential for exocytotic secretion. Therefore, the source of Ca^{2+} for the latter modality of ATP release described here must be the intracellular Ca^{2+} stores. In skeletal muscle from vertebrates,[11,12] the control of Ca^{2+}-release from the reticulum into the cytoplasm involves the activation of Ca^{2+}-channels gated by intracellular messengers such as inositol 1,2,4 trisphosphate.[13] To test whether a similar mechanism may be present in synaptosomes, we started a search for Ca^{2+}-release channels in membrane vesicles prepared from our highly purified synaptosomal preparation. We were able to incorporate these vesicles into phospholipid bilayers formed at the tip of patch pipettes. Under our conditions, which were designed to observe Ca^{2+}-channel currents, we reconstituted a channel activity that resembles that of the Ca^{2+}-release channel found in muscle.[12,13]

Early Time Course of K$^+$-Evoked ATP Secretion in the Presence of Ca^{2+}

Our assay measures the time course of the accumulation of the ATP secreted in response to a rapid elevation in $[K^+]_0$. Because luciferin is present in excess in the luciferin-luciferase (LL) mixture, from our previous work with medullary chromaffin cells,[7] we expected an exponential increase in the level of ATP reaching steady level after a few minutes. Most of our records in the presence of Ca^{2+}, however, exhibited a rapid increase to a maximum value (at ca 12 s) followed by a slower decay towards the baseline. The constant rate of decay of the signal (FIG. 1, middle panel) indicates that the substrates of the reaction, namely ATP and luciferin, were degraded by the ongoing reaction. Since luciferin is present in excess in the LL mixture, its oxidation could not result in a measurable decrease in emitted light. Thus, ATP degradation by other ATPases not included in LL mixture, such as the nucleotidases present in the external aspect of the synaptosomal membrane,[14] must be responsible for the ATP degradation observed in FIGURE 1 (middle panel). To correct for this effect, we included in our kinetic equation a component with a single time constant (τ_d) to fit the declining part of the signal. Accordingly, we fitted the following function to the original records:

$$ATP(t) = ATP_{max}(1 + \exp(-t/\tau)) \exp(-t/\tau_d), \tag{1}$$

where τ and τ_d represent the time constants for the secretory process and for the ATP hydrolysis due to ATPase activity other than that of the enzyme mixture LL. As shown in FIG. 1 (middle panel) the original record (noisy line) is well-fitted by this empirical function (smooth line). To obtain the corrected time course of the ATP release evoked by a sudden elevation in $[K^+]_0$, we added to the original record a function representing the time course of the ATP hydrolyzed by nucleotidases, that is,

$$ATP(t)^* = [1.0 - \exp(-t/\tau_d)]. \tag{2}$$

This operation generated the corrected record shown in FIGURE 1 (lower panel; $\tau_d = 54.4$ s). The average of the last 10 points of the corrected record (ATP_{max}) represents the maximum ATP that would be detected in the absence of ATP degradation by nucleotidases. For kinetic analysis, each corrected record was normalized by dividing all the values by ATP_{max}. As expected, the time course of the corrected secretory response is well-fitted by a single exponential function with a time constant of 5.3 s (FIG. 1, smooth solid line in the lower panel).

Our interpretation that the decay of the light signal (FIG. 1, middle panel) is caused by nucleotidases present in the synaptosomal preparation was further supported by our observation that $[Ca^{2+}]_0$ has a profound effect on the rate of decay of the signal. In low $[Ca^{2+}]_0$ (<0.01 µM), ATP secretion occurred at a low rate, and the rate of decay detected by our fitting protocol was 3.4×10^{-4} sec^{-1} (FIG. 2, bottom panel). By contrast, the rate of decay increased substantially to 185.2×10^{-4} s^{-1} in the presence of 0.01 mM $[Ca^{2+}]_0$ (FIG. 2, second panel from top). To be able to characterize the $[Ca^{2+}]_0$ dependence of the ATP secretion induced by high $[K^+]_0$, we measured the time constant of decay at different $[Ca^{2+}]_0$ and corrected the individual records using the corresponding time constant (data not shown[10]).

External Calcium-Dependent and Calcium-Independent Secretion Evoked by Membrane Depolarization

Both the extent and the kinetics of ATP secretion depend on $[Ca^{2+}]_0$. The extent of ATP release increased with $[K^+]_0$ up to 7% of the total ATP present in synaptosomes. Lowering $[Ca^{2+}]_0$ from 1 to 0.01 µM decreased the extent of ATP release by nearly 50 percent. The relationship between the extent of release and $[Ca^{2+}]_0$ was sigmoidal, ranging from a lower limit of ca. 10 pmol/mg protein in the

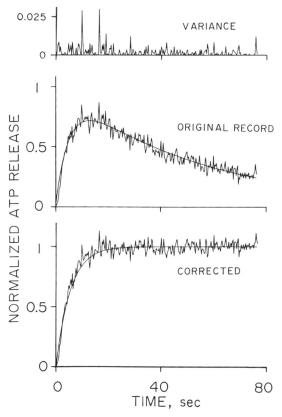

FIGURE 1. Potassium-evoked ATP release from mouse synaptosomes. ATP secretion from synaptosomes was evoked by a rapid elevation of the $[K^+]_o$ and was monitored continuously by including in the reaction mixture a highly purified preparation of luciferin-luciferase (Analytical Luminescence Laboratory, San Diego, CA). The contents of a vial of the LL mixture was resuspended in 2 mL Krebs-Hepes solution (in mM: 145 NaCl, 5 KCl, 1.2 MgSO$_4$, 10 Na-Hepes, 10 glucose, pH 7.4). The reaction medium for the assay contained 20 μL of the enzyme mixture LL, 25 μL of a modified Krebs buffer (mM: 145 NaCl, 1.2 mM MgSO$_4$, and 10 Na Hepes), and 5 μL of synaptosomes. Before the assay, this mixture was incubated for 5 min at 37°C. Changes in $[K^+]_o$ were achieved by the rapid addition of modified high $[K^+]_o$ Krebs buffer (in mM: 150 KCl, 1.2 MgSO$_4$, 10 K-Hepes, pH 7.4). The total content of ATP present in the aliquot of synaptosomes used in the assay was obtained by the addition of Triton X-100 (10 μL, 10%). For this determination the light signal was corrected to take into account some 50% inhibition of the enzyme mixture by Triton. Synaptosomes were resuspended in Krebs-Ringer-Hepes and were preincubated for 5 min at 30°C in the presence of LL. The noisy record shown in the middle panel represents a typical response to a rapid elevation in $[K^+]_o$ from 5 to 75 mM. The noisy record shown in the lower panel represents the normalized ATP secretion after correction for the effects of nucleotidases present in the synaptosomal preparation. The variance of the signal (upper panel) was calculated as

$$\sigma^2 = \{atp(t) - [1 - \exp(-t/\tau)]\}^2.$$

The meaning of this result is that ATP secretion evoked by membrane depolarization is quantal.

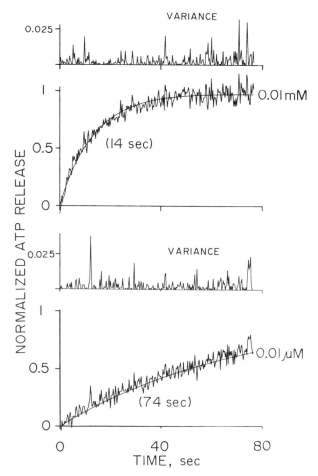

FIGURE 2. ATP secretion evoked by membrane depolarization in the absence of added calcium is quantal. Second and fourth panels (from top to bottom) represent the cumulative ATP secretion from synaptosomes incubated in modified Krebs solutions containing 0.01 mM and 0.01 μM $[Ca^{2+}]_0$, respectively. Noisy lines correspond to the normalized records of the cumulative release of ATP evoked by a rapid elevation of $[K^+]_0$ from 5 to 75 mM. Time constants from the best fit are given next to the fitted smooth curves. The corresponding variance is shown above each record (first and third panel from the top).

absence of Ca^{2+} to an upper limit of 20 pmol/mg protein in the presence of physiological $[Ca^{2+}]_0$ (not shown[10]).

Lowering $[Ca^{2+}]_0$ also had marked effects on the rate constant of ATP secretion. To distinguish between the effects of $[Ca^{2+}]_0$ and $[K^+]_0$ on the kinetics of ATP release, we kept the concentration of K^+ used to depolarize the synaptosomes constant at 75 mM and just varied $[Ca^{2+}]_0$. The kinetics of ATP secretion at two different $[Ca^{2+}]_0$ are compared in FIG. 3. Lowering the concentration of Ca^{2+} from 1 mM (FIG. 3, top panel) to 0.01 mM (lower panel) increased the time constant from 5.3 to 14 seconds.

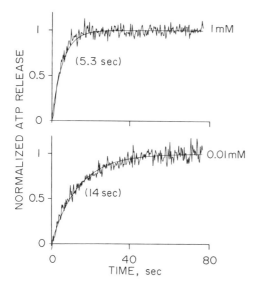

FIGURE 3. Effect of external calcium concentration on the kinetics of ATP release. Synaptosomes were resuspended in a modified Krebs solution with the $[Ca^{2+}]_0$ adjusted to either 1 (upper panel) or 0.01 mM (lower panel) using $CaCl_2/EGTA$ buffer prior to the application of the high $[K^+]_0$ solution. Noisy records represent the time course of the cumulative ATP secreted by the synaptosomes in response to a rapid increase in $[K^+]_0$ from 5 to 75 mM. Both records were corrected as explained in the text. Smooth curves were calculated with equation 3. Time constants are given in parenthesis next to the corresponding fitted curve. Temperature, 30°C.

ATP Secretion Induced by Membrane Depolarization in the Absence of External Ca^{2+} Is Quantal

To verify the quantal nature of the secretion induced by a rapid elevation of $[K^+]_0$, we used noise analysis of the optical signal. In a previous paper[7] we showed that a rapid elevation of $[K^+]_0$ induced ATP secretion from medullary chromaffin cells and that this secretion was always associated with a marked increase in the variance of the light signal. Noise analysis revealed that this excess noise is made up of three components: photomultiplier noise (mainly shot noise), intrinsic noise of the luciferin-luciferase reaction, and noise due to the discrete nature of the ATP release process. It was concluded that the excess noise due to the quantal nature of the ATP secretion was, by and large, the most important component of the variance. The noise content (as measured by the time variance of the signal) during the stimulation of the synaptosomes was significantly higher than during resting conditions. As illustrated in FIGURES 1 (upper panel) and 2 (first and third panel from the top), there is a marked increase in the variance associated with the secretory activity of the synaptosomes. We calculated the variance of the light signal in the presence or absence of external Ca^{2+}. FIGURE 1 shows the calculated variances in the presence of added Ca^{2+} (upper panel), and FIGURE 3 (first and third panels from top) shows the calculated variances in the absence of added Ca^{2+}. The noise content of the initial phase of secretion (< 10 s) was greater in the presence of physiological Ca^{2+} (FIG. 1, upper panel) than in absence of Ca^{2+} (FIG. 2). By contrast, the noise content of the delayed phase of secretion was greater in records made in the absence of Ca^{2+}. Taken together these results support the concept that ATP secretion evoked by membrane depolarization is quantal regardless of the external concentration of Ca^{2+} ($F1$ mM).

The above results prompted us to examine the possibility that the origin of the Ca^{2+} required for the exocytotic secretion of ATP may be intracellular stores, including the endoplasmic reticulum. Our strategy was to search for the presence of Ca^{2+} channels in vesicles prepared by freezing and thawing our highly purified synaptosomal preparation. We were able to incorporate membrane vesicles in bilayer membranes formed at the tip of the patch pipettes. A large proportion (60%) of these incorporated vesicles exhibited the activity of a Ca^{2+}-channel with properties similar to those for the Ca^{2+}-release channel found in the sarcoplasmic reticulum.[12,13]

Calcium Release Channel from Synaptosomal Membranes

FIGURE 4 (left side) depicts six segments of a continuous record of the channel activity incorporated into a phosphatidylserine bilayer. These records were made in the presence of Cl^--free solutions on both sides of the bilayer (in mM: 50 CaHepes, 100 CsPipes at pH 7.4 for the solution in the pipette or *trans* side; 1 CaHepes, 100 CsPipes at pH 6.8 for the solution in the chamber or *cis* side). The pipette potential was varied as indicated by the numbers given above each pair of sample records. The fractional open time was found to be sensitive to pipette potential increasing from 0.2 to 0.8, as the pipet potential was made positive. From bimodal amplitude histograms we obtained two mean amplitudes (for example, -3.9 and -2.9 pA at 60 mV pipette potential in Fig. 5B). FIGURE 4 (right side) shows the current-potential relationship for the events of greater amplitude. To construct this graph we just included the maximum mean values (for example, -3.9 at 60 mV). Each symbol represents a

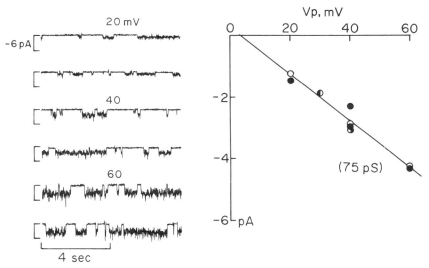

FIGURE 4. Single-calcium channel records reconstituted into a phosphatidylserine bilayer. The methods used have been described in detail elsewhere.[13] Pipettes used to form phosphatidylserine (or phosphatidylinositol) bilayers were coated to near the tips with Sylgard, and the tips were fire polished. Left side: Single-channel activity recorded in the presence of 100 mM Cs^+ on both sides of the bilayer. Three pairs of single-channel records made at pipette potentials of 20 (upper), 40 (middle), and 60 mV (lower). At 60 mV: upper record is the control for the lower record made 10 min after the application of nifedipine (10 μM). Downward deflexions represent openings of the channel. Records were low pass filtered at 1000 Hz. Right side: Right side shows the current-voltage curve obtained from different amplitude histograms for different bilayers (see Fig. 4). Current-voltage relationship for a series of experiments in which two or more amplitude histograms were obtained. Slope conductance is indicated in pS by the number next to the straight line drawn by eye.

series of two or more measurements of single-channel events from different bilayers with the incorporated vesicle from different synaptosomal membrane preparations. The straight line was drawn with a slope of 75 pS. As expected, for a channel preferentially permeable to Cs^+, and in the absence of concentration gradient, the flow of current through the open channel changes direction at a reversal potential close to zero (4 mV).

Examples of our statistical analysis of the properties of the single-channel events shown in FIGURE 4 and 5A are presented in FIG. 5 (B, C, and D). The amplitude

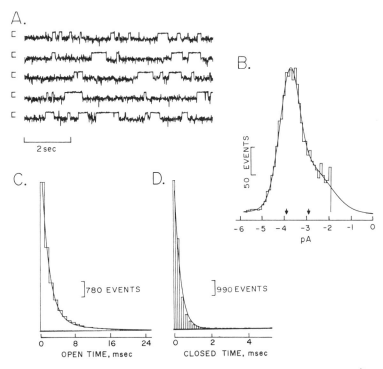

FIGURE 5. Single-channel recording of the putative endoplasmic reticulum (ER) Ca^{2+} release channel reconstituted into a phosphatidylserine bilayer. **A:** Five segments of a continuous single-channel recording. Pipette potential is 60 mV. **B:** Amplitude histogram of the channel activity depicted in A. Smooth curve represents the least squares fit and was calculated using the sum of two Gaussian distributions. Mean values are indicated by the arrows. **C:** Open-time histogram at 60 mV. Smooth curve represents the least squares fit and was calculated as the sum of two exponentials with time constants equal to 1.7 and 8.9 ms. **D:** Closed-time histogram at 60 mV. Time constants for the fitted curve were 0.5 and 1 ms.

histogram (FIG. 5B) was described by a double Gaussian distribution of amplitudes with mean values of -3.9 ± 0.4 and -2.9 ± 1.0 pA. We interpret the presence of two populations of single-channel current amplitudes (FIG. 5B) to indicate the presence of two permeating species (*i.e.* Cs^+ and Ca^{2+}) competing for biding sites within the conduction pore.[12] We also interpret the flickering of the open-channel current from -3.9 to -2.9 pA depicted in FIGURES 4 (left side) and 5A as an indication of blockade of the Cs^+ current by a cation with greater affinity for the site, that is, Ca^{2+}.

Both the open- (FIG. 5C) and closed- (FIG. 5D) time histograms were well-fitted by double exponential distributions (time constants: 1.9 and 8.9 ms for the open-time and 1.0 and 0.6 ms for the closed-time).

The Ca^{2+} channel was activated by ATP (1 mM), caffeine (1 mM), ryanodine (10 μM) and was effectively blocked by La^{3+} (100 μM) and ruthenium red (100 μM; data not shown).

DISCUSSION

We have shown that depolarization of the membrane of mouse brain synaptosomes can evoke ATP release both in the absence or in the presence of external Ca^{2+}. The extent as well as the rate of ATP secretion increases with $[Ca^{2+}]_0$, the rate of ATP release being substantially higher in physiological $[Ca^{2+}]_0$. We interpret these results to indicate that the primary source of the Ca^{2+} required for exocytosis is the extracellular space. Furthermore, noise analysis of the ATP release signal provides compelling evidence to suggest that ATP secretion evoked by a rapid elevation of $[KCl]_0$ is indeed by exocytosis both in physiological and in low external $[Ca^{2+}]$.

Taken together, these results suggest that the Ca^{2+} required for secretion is provided by both extracellular and intracellular pools. Ca^{2+} entry from the external medium is presumably linked to the activation of voltage-gated Ca^{2+} channels known to be present in the presynaptic membrane.[15] In this case Ca^{2+} is rapidly supplied at the most convenient place, that is, near the site for exocytosis, and secretion should proceed at maximum rate.

Calcium Release from Internal Stores: A Possible Mechanism for Secretion in the Absence of External Calcium

As for intracellular Ca^{2+} pools as sources of the Ca^{2+} required for secretion, there is an increasing volume of information that we can use to construct a working hypothesis. This model proposes that, regardless of the $[Ca^{2+}]_0$, membrane depolarization causes the release of second messengers from the membrane and that these messengers act on intracellular Ca^{2+} stores to induce Ca^{2+} release. Proof for this hypothesis would require the demonstration of a number of essential signal transduction steps: (1) Since the stimulus for ATP secretion is the actual depolarization of the synaptosome, the first step of transduction must occur at the level of the plasma membrane. This step requires a membrane potential sensor coupled to an effector protein. (2) The ensuing generation of one or more second messengers will, by a diffusion-limited process, couple the stimulus to target intracellular stores. (3) The membrane defining the confines of the intracellular Ca^{2+} pool should have to be equipped with receptors for the messengers to allow the last step in the signal transduction cycle to occur. Activation of these receptors, at the level of the intracellular membrane, will activate the release of Ca^{2+}. The following two models of signal transduction include the above sequence of steps. Stimulus-secretion coupling in medullary-chromaffin cells involves the activation of muscarinic cholinergic receptors by acetylcholine, which in turn activate phospholipase C with the ensuing generation of inositol 1,2,4 trisphosphate (IP_3) and diacylglycerol (DAG) due to breakdown phosphatydylinositol.[16,17] In the case of excitation-contraction coupling in skeletal muscle, in addition to the identification of the messengers involved as IP_3 and Ca^{2+} and the structural identification of the Ca^{2+} pool as the terminal cisternae of the sarcoplasmic reticulum, a membrane potential sensor acting on phospholipase C has been postulated.[18,19]

We have been able to reconstitute a Ca^{2+}-channel activity by incorporating membrane vesicles prepared from a highly purified preparation of nerve endings.[10] We found that the Ca^{2+} channel was activated by ATP, caffeine, and ryanodine. The three substances are known to be activators of the Ca^{2+}-release channel reconstituted from a sarcoplasmic reticulum membrane,[12,13] and caffeine is known to be a strong potentiator of secretion.[20] These properties, together with the inhibition by ruthenium red, make the Ca^{2+} channel described here the best candidate for the Ca^{2+}-release channel of the intracellular Ca^{2+} pool in the nerve endings.

Although our results in low external Ca^{2+} are in good agreement with previous observations on cholinergic nerve terminals from the electric organ,[21] from mammalian neuromuscular junction,[22] and from highly purified rat brain cholinergic terminals,[23] the possibility that ATP is being released by a mechanism other than exocytosis has to be considered.

For example, membrane depolarization evoked by a rapid elevation of $[KCl]_0$ can induce, at least in principle, swelling of the synaptosomes. This swelling may in turn cause ATP secretion. The bases for this mechanism are as follows. If we assume that K^+ and Cl^- are distributed passively, the concentration ratios and the membrane potential under equilibrium conditions ought to conform to the relation

$$[K^+]_0/[K^+]_i = [Cl^-]_i/[Cl^-]_0 = \exp\{VF/RT\}, \qquad (3)$$

where $[]_0$ and $[]_i$ indicate concentrations outside and inside the cell, V is the intracellular potential, and F, R, and T have their usual meanings.[24]

Although verification of applicability of equation 3 for the synaptosomal membrane requires knowledge of the relative permeabilities for these two ions, the first important consequence of this analysis is that the membrane potential can be calculated using equation 3 only after the concentrations of K^+ and Cl^- inside the cell have come to equilibrium with those in the external solution. The second consequence is that, at equilibrium, the product $[K^+]_0 \times [Cl^-]_0$ is equal to $[K^+]_i \times [Cl^-]_i$. Thus, immediately after the application of a sudden increase in $[K^+]_0$, the product $[K^+]_0 \times [Cl^-]_0$ is substantially greater than $[K^+]_i \times [Cl^-]_i$ and, therefore, the initial ionic and osmotic imbalance will drive both Cl^- and water into the synaptosomes, causing swelling.[20] Thus, it is possible that under our low $[Ca^{2+}]_0$ conditions, high external KCl might cause ATP molecules to leak out of the synaptosomal vesicles. We have repeated the experiments reported in FIGURE 3, however, keeping constant the product $[K^+]_0 \times [Cl^-]_0$ with similar results. For these experiments we used isethionate in place of chloride.[10] It should be mentioned here that our results are in agreement with previous reports demonstrating secretion in the absence of Ca^{2+} under conditions that prevent swelling. Indeed, rat brain synaptosomes, isolated under hyperosmotic gradient, release ATP in response to membrane depolarization, both in the presence or absence of external calcium.[8]

SUMMARY

Depolarization of the synaptosomal membrane by a rapid elevation of $[K^+]_0$ induces secretion of adenosine-5'-triphosphate (ATP) as well as the specific neurotransmitters. In addition to the classical $[Ca^{2+}]_0$-dependent mode, we have found that ATP secretion also occurred in the absence of extracellular calcium ($[Ca^{2+}]_0 < 1$ μM). The extent of both modalities of secretion depended on membrane potential, and the $[Ca^{2+}]_0$-independent secretion proceeded at a rate that was substantially smaller than that of the $[Ca^{2+}]_0$-dependent mode at all membrane potentials examined. We propose that intracellular stores may provide the Ca^{2+} required for exocytosis in the $[Ca^{2+}]_0$-independent mode of ATP secretion. To test this hypothesis, we searched for the presence of Ca^{2+}-release channels gated by intracellular messengers in our synaptosomal preparation. We fused membrane vesicles from lysed synaptosomes with acidic phospholipid bilayers formed at the tip of a patch pipette and found that these membranes contained a Ca^{2+}-selective channel. The properties of this channel resemble those of the Ca^{2+}-release channel reconstituted from sarcoplasmic reticulum membrane vesicles. These include size of the single open-channel conductance (75 pS Cs^+ as the main current carrier), activation by adenine nucleotides (ATP), ryanodine and caffeine, and inhibition by ruthenium red.

REFERENCES

1. STONE, T. W. 1981. Neurosci. **6:** 523–555.
2. POLLARD, H. B. & G. PAPPAS. 1979. Biochem. Biophys. Res. Commun. **88:** 1315–1321.
3. SU, C. 1983. Ann. Rev. Pharmacol. Toxicol. **23:** 397–411.
4. PHILLIS, J. W., G. K. KOSTOPOULOS & J. J. LIMACHER. 1975. Eur. J. Pharmacol. **30:** 125–129.
5. MOREL, N. & F.-M. MEUNIER. 1981. J. Neurochem. **36**(5): 1766–1773.
6. NACHSHEN, D. A. & S. SANCHEZ-ARMASS. 1987. J. Physiol. **387:** 415–423.
7. ROJAS, E., E. FORSBERG & H. B. POLLARD. 1986. Adv. Exp. Med. Biol. **211:** 7–16.
8. WHITE, T. D. 1977. Nature **267:** 67–68.
9. POTTER, P. & T. H. WHITE. 1980. Neurosci. **5:** 1351–1356.
10. FIEDLER, J. L., H. B. POLLARD & E. ROJAS. 1991. Biochim. Biophys. Acta. Submitted.
11. ENDO, M. 1977. Physiol. Rev. **57:** 71–108.
12. SUAREZ-ISLA, B., J. J. MARENGO, V. IRRIBARRA & R. BULL. 1990. *In* Transduction in Biological Systems. C. Hidalgo, J. Bacigalupo, E. Jaimovich & J. Vergara, Eds.: 487–499.
13. SMITH, J. S., R. CORONADO & G. MEISSNER. 1986. J. Gen. Physiol. **88:** 573–588.
14. NAGY, A. K., T. A. SHUSTER & A. V. DELGADO-ESCUETA. 1986. J. Neurochem. **47:** 976–986.
15. TURNER, T. J. & S. M. GOLDIN. 1985. J. Neurosci. **5**(3):841–849.
16. FORSBERG, E., E. ROJAS & H. B. POLLARD. 1988. J. Biol. Chem. **261:** 4915–4922.
17. AZILA, N. & J. N. HAWTHORNE. 1982. Biochem. J. **204:** 291–299.
18. VERGARA, J., R. TSIEN & M. DELAY. 1985. Proc. Natl. Acad. Sci. USA **82:** 6352–6356.
19. VERGARA, J., K. ASOTRA & M. DELAY. 1987. *In* Cell Calcium and the Control of Membrane Transport. L. J. Mandel & D. C. Eaton, Ed. 133–151. Rockefeller University Press. New York.
20. LAMBERT, A. E., Y. KANAZAWA, I. M. BURR, L. ORCI & A. E. RENOLD. 1971. Ann. N.Y. Acad. Sci. **185:** 232–244.
21. MEUNIER, F.-M. 1984. J. Physiol. **354:** 121–137.
22. UNSWORTH, C. D. & R. G. JOHNSON. 1990. Proc. Natl. Acad. Sci. USA **87:** 553–557.
23. RICHARDSON, P. J. & S. J. BROWN. 1987. J. Neurochem. **48:** 622–630.
24. HODGKIN, A. L. & P. HOROWICZ. 1959. J. Physiol. **148:** 127–160.

Primary and Secondary Ca^{2+} Concentration Changes Resulting from Transmitter Stimulation in Dendrites of Neurons from the Mammalian Hippocampus[a]

JOHN A. CONNOR AND WOLFGANG MÜLLER

Roche Institute of Molecular Biology
Roche Research Center
Nutley, New Jersey 07110

INTRODUCTION

It has been only in the last five to six years that successful efforts have been made at recording Ca^{2+} levels and fluctuations in the small neuronal processes characteristic of higher animals. The invention of high-efficiency fluorescent indicators has been of inestimable benefit to these efforts, although such measurements, in a limited sense, were technically possible in mammalian and invertebrate neurons before with the use of absorbance indicators.[1,2] With the recent escalation of interest in phenomena related to synaptic plasticity, such as the different forms of long-term potentiation and depression, and the almost sure involvement of intracellular Ca^{2+} changes in triggering most of these phenomena,[3–6] direct measurements of Ca^{2+} have become of general importance in neurobiology. Results to be reviewed here have shown that dendritic Ca^{2+} changes following either electrical or transmitter-induced stimulus can be large, localized, and under some circumstances quite extended in time after transmitter stimulus. We will discuss observations from two different types of preparations: acutely isolated mammalian neurons[7] and mammalian neurons in brain slice. Some of the observations reviewed here have appeared elsewhere.[8] In all cases the fluorescent indicator, fura-2,[9] has been used in conjunction with a cooled CCD camera system[10] to measure free calcium levels by ratio imaging.[10,11]

CALCIUM CHANGES IN VOLTAGE-CLAMPED CA1 NEURONS

A number of experiments combining whole-cell voltage clamp and fura-2 calcium imaging were carried out using acutely isolated neurons from guinea pig (Connor and Kay, unpublished). Neurons with 50 to 100 μm of dendrite appear to behave as if their interior were isopotential so long as the large transient sodium currents are blocked,[12] and are thus suitable for limited objective voltage clamping. The only technical varient from more or less standard recording configurations[12] was that the

[a]W. Müller was supported in part by a fellowship from the Deutsche Forschungs Gemeinschaft.

recording electrode contained 100 μM fura-2 and no EGTA. Because of the low buffer capacity of this filling solution, it was important to use very clean electrode glass in these experiments. FIGURE 1 illustrates the time course of calcium changes in a CA1 neuron during a depolarization to −20 mV. Tetrodotoxin (TTX, 0.3 mM) was present in the external saline. The Ca^{2+} levels rose rapidly and relatively uniformly in the dendrite with soma levels somewhat lagging (B). This lag most likely results from the small surface-to-volume ratio of the soma compared to the dendrite. The second ratio was made 2 s after the step onset (FIG. 1C), and at that time the calcium levels were relatively uniform throughout the neuron. The ratio of FIGURE 1D was made 1 s after stepping back to −70 mV and shows that recovery is much more rapid in the dendrite than the soma, again probably reflecting surface-to-volume differences. All neurons tested in this manner (n = 10) recovered with a similar time course. Because the whole-cell voltage-clamp technique alters intracellular contents,[13] a second set of undialyzed neurons (n > 20) was examined using high potassium stimulus (50–70 mM KCl, Na replacement) and no voltage recording. The high K saline, containing TTX, was either applied topically over the cell from a 10 μm pipette or by bathing solution changes. Using the faster topical application method, high K quickly dissipated into the surrounding media, and Ca^{2+} levels recovered within a few seconds of stopping the flow. Recoveries were slower where the whole bath was changed. Using either method, the cycle of K depolarization and recovery could be repeated many times, over periods of 15 to 20 minutes with little variation in the responses.

GLUTAMATE-TRIGGERED DENDRITIC GRADIENTS OF CA²⁺: PRIMARY RESPONSE

One of the major experimental advantages offered by acutely isolated neurons is the ability to make controlled presentations of agonists directly to the neuron dendrite, free of glial uptake or secondary modulations. These isolated neurons respond to excitatory amino acids (EAA) such as glutamate and N-methyl-D-aspartate (NMDA).[14] Iontophoretic ejection from a microelectrode (1 to 2 s pulses with the electrode placed approximately 5 μm from the dendrite) has been our preferred method of application. Carefully applied in a chamber with constant flow of saline, the observable effects of EAA application are restricted to a radius of approximately 15 μm. This is illustrated in FIGURE 2 where NMDA was applied (in Mg-free saline) to the midsection of a CA1 neuron apical dendrite. Such stimulation results in local calcium influx that far outlasts the presence of agonist. Here, this influx set up an oscillating "hot spot" of free calcium restricted to the location centered upon the stimulus site.

The application of glutamate to dendrites of CA1 neurons causes a rapid rise in Ca^{2+}. In normal Krebs saline the increase occurs throughout the cell due to action potential invasion of all cellular regions. When action potentials are blocked with TTX, the Ca^{2+} increase is much more restricted to the dendrite. An example of such a response is given in FIGURE 3 where an application of glutamate to the dendrite tip produces a large Ca^{2+} increase in the vicinity of the injection site but only small changes toward the soma. This is to be contrasted to the situation in FIGURE 1 where the neuron was voltage-clamped and where there were large rises in Ca^{2+} all along the initial length of the dendrite. Because the isolated cells appear to be nearly isopotential when Na currents are blocked,[12] it seems reasonable to conclude that a large part of the Ca^{2+} increase at the stimulated site is receptor-activated and not due

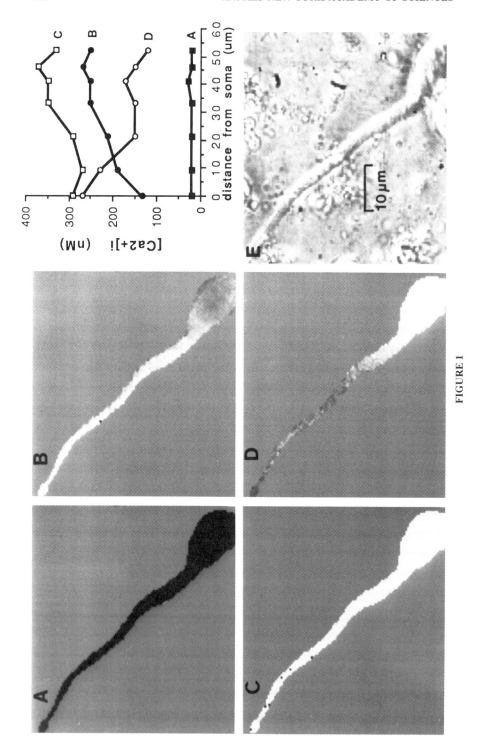

FIGURE 1

to Ca^{2+} influx through voltage-gated channels. The Ca^{2+} response to NMDA (in TTX) was blocked by 2-amino-5-phosphonovaleric acid (APV), (data not shown). The response to EAA receptor agonists was dependent upon the presence of Ca^{2+} in the external medium and in all probability results from flux through the NMDA receptor channel, as has been described for spinal motoneurons,[15] although it is difficult to rule out a component of intracellular release that is observed in tissue-culture neurons.[16,17] This response will be termed a primary Ca response to the EAA agonists in order to differentiate it from the secondary Ca response outlined below.

LONG-LASTING CA^{2+} CHANGES AFTER RECEPTOR ACTIVATION: SECONDARY RESPONSE

Multiple activations of the dendrite by glutamate or NMDA, or in many cases, single activations, produced a secondary, prolonged calcium response that did not depend on the continued presence of the agonist. This is illustrated in FIGURE 4 where the time course of calcium levels is plotted for a dendritic and somatic location. In FIGURE 4A the neuron recovered completely after the first stimulus, but a secondary response was established after the second glutamate application. In FIGURE 4B there was only a partial recovery in the dendrite followed by a slow increase on which subsequent stimulus induced changes were superimposed. In both examples the glutamate stimulus was applied from a microelectrode by iontophoresis. This electrode was always removed to a great distance after the delivery pulse. There was rapid dispersal of the EAA-receptor (R) agonist due to diffusion into the large bath volume as well as bulk flow of the bathing saline. Therefore, it is unlikely that the persistent Ca^{2+} elevations are due to the continued presence of agonist near the cell membrane. It is also unlikely that the agonists remain bound to the membrane receptors for any appreciable length of time, inasmuch as the dissociation constants for receptor activation are in the micromolar range. The variability shown in the responses of the two cells of FIGURE 4 illustrates well that the development of the secondary calcium increase was not a stereotyped response; the responses showed large cell-to-cell variability. In 21 out of 48 neurons from adult guinea pig that were responsive to glutamate or NMDA, a maintained response developed after the first stimulation, whereas in 15 neurons, two stimuli were required. Twelve cells required three or more applications. Data have been pooled from both glutamate and NMDA stimulation. Agonist application in the absence of external Ca^{2+} (buff-

---

FIGURE 1. Ca^{2+} changes in the soma and proximal dendrite of a voltage-clamped CA1 neuron. **A–D:** Grey scale display of Ca^{2+} levels. For these and all Ca^{2+} data, two images of fura-2 fluorescence were made, one using 340 nm wavelength excitation light and the other 380 nm light. Exposure time was 100 ms for each image, and it required approximately 600 ms to read the first picture into the computer so that the total acquisition time for a ratio was 800 ms. After corrections for backround, the 340 nm image was divided, point by point, by the 380 nm image, and the resultant field of ratios was displayed. High ratios were bright and low ratios were dark. Frame **A** was taken prior to a voltage step from −70 to −20 mV; **B** was taken during the 800 ms immediately following the depolarization; **C** was initiated 2 s into the depolarization; and **D** was initiated 2 s after the return to −70 mV. Numerical data for Ca^{2+} levels derived from these images are shown in the upper right inset. Note that the dendrite Ca^{2+} levels are the first up and the first down. **E** shows a transmitted light picture of this neuron. The whole-cell electrode is just out of the field of view to the lower right.

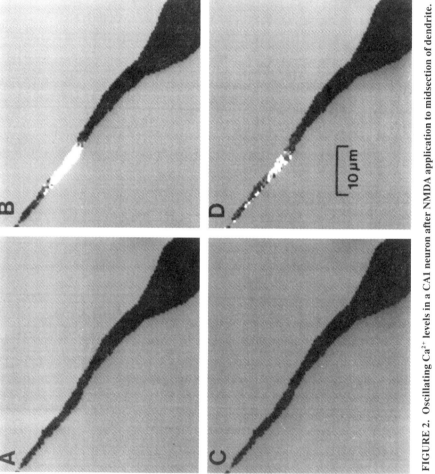

FIGURE 2. Oscillating Ca^{2+} levels in a CA1 neuron after NMDA application to midsection of dendrite.

ered by 0.5 mM EGTA) produced no primary Ca-response and generally no secondary response after restoration of normal external Ca^{2+}. Dendritic gradients were observed in cells loaded with the membrane-permeable fura-2/AM and those microinjected with the nonpermeable free acid. Dendritic gradients were also observed in a few examples of large pyramidal neurons typical of the CA3 region, but these cells were not used routinely because of difficulties in maintaining their viability after isolation.

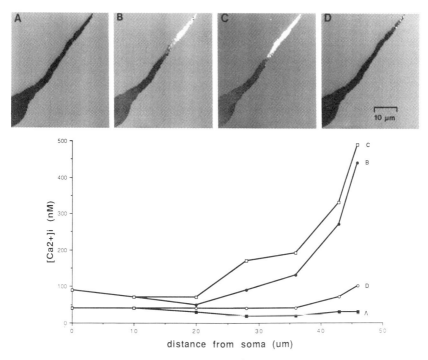

FIGURE 3. NMDA-induced changes in dendrite Ca^{2+} levels: primary response. Top: pictoral records. Bottom: numerical data extracted from each frame. NMDA was applied iontophoretically (1.5 s, 200 nA pulse) from a microelectrode positioned near the tip of the dendrite. The electrode contained 10 mM NMDA, and the saline was nominally Mg^{2+}-free. A: prestimulus, uniform levels of Ca^{2+}. B: during iontophoresis. C: 2–2.8 s after the iontophoretic pulse. Cells often showed such delayed increases after pulse termination, as shown, probably reflecting the time required for diffusion of transmitter away from dendrite.

The total circumstances accompanying the elevation of internal Ca^{2+} by glutamate and NMDA are then very different from those underlying the response to K depolarizations, which were reversible and repeatable. Pretreatment of the neurons with protein kinase inhibitors, however, blocked the onset of the secondary Ca^{2+} rise, and repeated stimuli with glutamate gave results that were much more like the responses to K depolarizations. FIGURE 5 shows an example in which the neuron was treated for a period of 20 minutes before stimulation with sphingosine (10 μM).

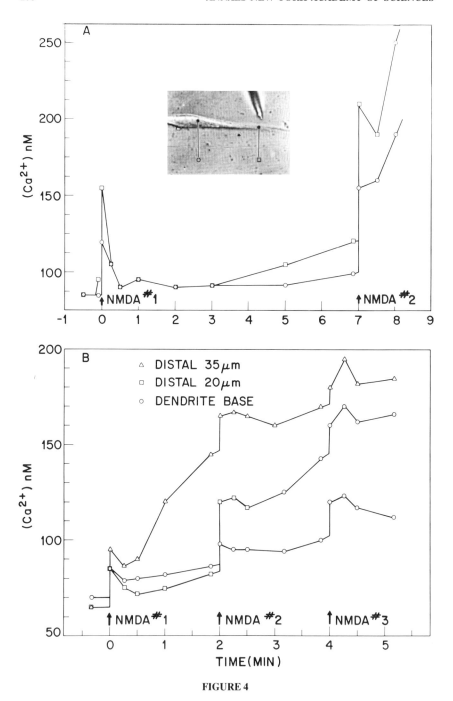

FIGURE 4

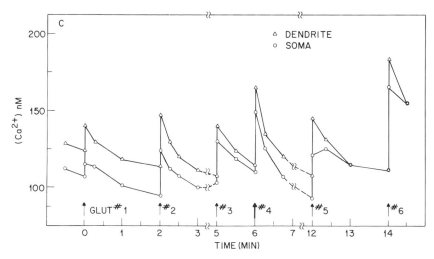

FIGURE 5. Multiple stimulation with glutamate after pretreatment with sphingosine. Neuron recovered completely from the first four stimuli. Recovery from #5 and #6 was incomplete but without soma-dendrite gradient. (Connor *et al.*[8] With permission from *Science.*)

Subsequent Ca^{2+} responses to glutamate recovered to baseline levels. Such observations argue that the secondary Ca response results from protein kinase activation brought about by the combination of glutamate-receptor stimulation and the primary Ca influx. Although sphingosine has a high affinity for members of the C kinase family,[18,19] it is possible that other protein kinases are also blocked by this substance, making it difficult to identify a particular kinase family as the initiator or mediator of the secondary response. Evidence summarized elsewhere[8,19a] shows that the secondary Ca response results from a long-lasting Ca influx that is first localized to the dendrite region stimulated (see FIG. 1).

Once a secondary calcium response was established in the dendrite, it normally spread slowly toward the soma. FIGURE 6 illustrates such a sequence of events, beginning from the time it was clear that the secondary response had been established until uniformly high levels of Ca^{2+} were present throughout the cell. The time course of this spread showed large cell-to-cell variability, occurring over a period as short as 2 to 3 minutes or, as shown, over a greater than 10-minute period. It is

FIGURE 4. Ca^{2+} changes in two neurons responding to multiple applications of NMDA. Top: Ca^{2+} changes are plotted at the stimulation site on the dendrite and in the soma. Neuron recovered from first stimulus and exhibited stable Ca^{2+} level for at least 2.5 min, but slow increase developed in the dendrite. Data acquisition was minimal during this period to limit the exposure to UV excitation. Second stimulus produced a large Ca^{2+} gradient that showed only small initial recovery. Inset: approximate position of stimulating electrode. Bottom: Ca^{2+} changes plotted at 3 locations in a neuron that showed only partial recovery from first stimulus and then strong Ca^{2+} increase in the dendrite. Note that the secondary Ca^{2+} increase begins after the first stimulus at the most distal location, which was nearest the stimulus electrode, but that the more proximal location was hardly affected until the second stimulus. (Connor *et al.*[8] With permission from *Science.*)

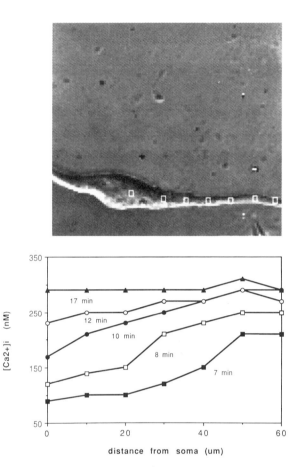

FIGURE 6. Progression, over time, of high Ca^{2+} levels throughout neuron after glutamate stimulation. Top: picture of neuron showing stimulus electrode and locations used in the plots below. Bottom: Ca^{2+} distributions in the neuron beginning 7 min after the last glutamate stimulus until nearly uniformly high levels were reached at 17 min.

unlikely that the spread of the secondary response results simply from a rundown of cellular Ca^{2+} regulatory mechanisms, because the protein kinase inhibitor, 1-(5-isoquinolinylsulfonyl)-2-methyl-piperazine (H7), blocked the spreading aspect of the response when applied after the establishment of a gradient. By contrast, the protein kinase inhibitor sphingosine, applied after stimulation, was ineffective in blocking such spread. Standing gradients of Ca^{2+} were observed for periods as long as 25–30 minutes in neurons treated with 50 μM H7.[19a] In addition to demonstrating the involvement of protein kinase activation in the spread of the secondary response, this result clearly shows that the neurons are capable of handling moderate calcium influx for long periods of time.

The above discussion summarizes some of the evidence for the existence of long-lasting transmembrane fluxes of calcium in neuronal dendrites that are specifically associated with glutamate or NMDA stimulation but are secondary to the actual flux through the receptor-activated channels. This was a new observation when made in these isolated hippocampal neurons and has since been corroborated by calcium flux studies on cerebellar granule neurons in culture[20] and by fura-2 measurements in hippocampal neurons in culture.[21] Activation of this flux by an as-yet-undefined-protein kinase is inferred from the ability to block secondary responses with protein kinase inhibitors such as sphingosine and H7. As it has been used here, the fura-2 imaging method is a sensitive, noninvasive technique for monitoring changes in membrane calcium permeability. Our estimate of the size of the local Ca^{2+} influx required to maintain the 150–250 nM gradients that are seen in pyramidal cell dendrites is only on the order of 1–2 pA.[8] Maximum calcium currents during voltage clamp steps are on the order of 500 pA.[12]

A HYPOTHESIS FOR EXPLAINING THE SECONDARY CALCIUM RESPONSE AND ITS POSSIBLE SIGNIFICANCE

In order to explain these gradients, we have postulated that the protein kinase system activated by the EAA receptor agonists modulates calcium channels in the locality of the application so that opening probability is increased at negative voltages. This modulation also depends on the rapid increase of Ca^{2+} accompanying receptor activation, but a Ca^{2+} change without receptor activation does not seem to be sufficient by itself. FIGURE 7 illustrates two possible modes for such a modification. In FIGURE 7A it is assumed that the kinase recruits previously inactive channels as has been shown by phorbol ester activation of calcium channels in *Aplysia* bag cell neurons.[22] Activation of these channels in neurites and growth cones is capable of generating large, local increases in Ca^{2+} accumulation during action potential firing

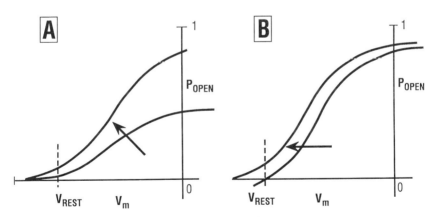

FIGURE 7. Two conceptual schemes for producing Ca^{2+} gradients in a neuron with uniform voltage. Actual membrane resting voltage is unspecified. All measured values in these neurons include some form of distortion. Microelectrodes injure the isolated neurons much more severely than they do in the slice preparation; whole-cell patch electrodes alter internal electrolytes and buffers; perforated patch electrodes alter internal monovalent ion concentration and have an effect on resting potential. Resting voltage under whole-cell recording conditions is between −70 and −60 mV.

or subthreshold depolarizations.[23] The scheme of FIGURE 7B assumes that the voltage dependence of channel gating is shifted to the left, making it more likely that the channel is open at negative voltages after modulation. The action of CaM kinase on calcium channels of GH3 cells, described by David Armstrong (this volume), is a type of modulation that would roughly fit this pattern.

With uniform internal voltage, either of these modulations could, in theory, produce a greater calcium influx at the stimulated site relative to other locations in the neuron and, as a result, produce a Ca^{2+} gradient. Because the isolated CA1 neurons have electrical resistance on the order of 1-3 $G\Omega$[12] it is also possible that the increased calcium influx can generate a small amount of regenerative depolarization. Modulations of this general type would also make the dendrite more excitable inasmuch as EAA receptor activation would result in a larger number of Ca channels available to carry inward current in response to small depolarizations. It has been known for a number of years that calcium currents play a significant role in dendrite responses.[24] Therefore it is possible that this type of channel modulation has a limited function in expressing certain types of neuronal plasticity, such as long-term potentiation (LTP) or the kindling of epileptic foci.[25] There are certainly similarities between the pharmacological sensitivities to protein kinase inhibitors of LTP and the secondary response.[26–30] Spreading responses (FIG. 6) unquestionably hasten neuronal deterioration and death in the isolated cells and could at least in part underly the toxic consequences[31] of sustained EAA stimulation in the brain. At the present time we are attempting to look directly for changes in membrane conductances using nondialyzing recording methods that have been successful in other cell types in combination with fura-2 imaging.[32]

SUSTAINED RESPONSES IN BRAIN SLICE

Although the secondary response has been demonstrated in response to exogenously applied agonists in isolated and tissue culture neurons, it has been an open question as to whether a like response can result from stimuli delivered by way of presynaptic input. For neurons in brain slice, neither CA1[33] nor CA3 neurons (Müller and Connor, unpublished) normally show measurable, long-lasting Ca^{2+} gradients after stimulation. When brief stimuli are applied in the presence of an inhibitory blocker such as picrotoxin (PTX), however, we have observed the establishment of steep, long-lasting gradients in CA3 neurons that are not associated with continued electrical discharge. FIGURE 8 illustrates such an occurrence in dendrites of a CA3 neuron given 3 tetanic stimuli (50 Hz, 2 s) by way of mossy fiber inputs in the presence of 10 μM picrotoxin (PTX). Ca^{2+} levels in 3 of the 4 dendritic branches remained elevated (> 2 μM) for an observation period of one hour, whereas levels in the fourth branch and in the main dendritic shaft were near prestimulus values (80–100 nM). Washout of the PTX was begun immediately after stimulation. Such Ca^{2+} distribution patterns are not indicative of maintained electrical discharge or depolarization as can occur in the presence of PTX. With epileptiform discharge, the whole portion of the dendritic structure in the picture shows elevated Ca^{2+}. Thus the secondary Ca^{2+} response is not an artifact arising from isolation or tissue culture procedures but a phenomenon that can be reproduced when inhibitory inputs (totally absent in the isolated cells and of minor importance in culture where agonists are applied exogenously) are blocked in the slice.

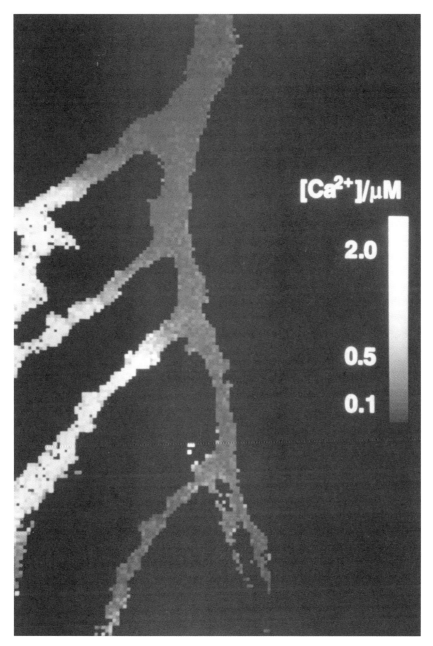

FIGURE 8. Ca^{2+} levels in dendrites of CA3 neuron in brain slice after stimulation of associational-commissural inputs in the presence of picrotoxin. The three upper dendrites have Ca^{2+} levels in excess of 1 μM, whereas the lower dendrite and main shaft are around 100 nM.

ACKNOWLEDGMENTS

We thank David Tank for making available data acquisition software, David Linden for suggesting improvements in the manuscript, and Michelle Smeyne for technical assistance in the brain slice preparation.

REFERENCES

1. Ross, W. & R. Werman. 1987. Mapping calcium transients in the dendrites of Purkinje cells from the guinea-pig cerebellum *in vitro.* J. Physiol. (London) **389:** 319–336.
2. Connor, J. A., R. Kretz & E. Shapiro. 1986. Calcium levels measured in a presynaptic neuron of *Aplysia* under conditions that modulate transmitter release. J. Physiol. (London) **375:** 625–642.
3. Brown, T. H., P. F. Chapman, E. W. Kairiss & C. L. Keenan. 1988. Long-term synaptic potentiation. Science **242:** 724–728.
4. Collingridge, G. L. & W. Singer. 1990. Excitatory amino acid receptors and synaptic plasticity. Trends Pharmacol. Sci. **11:** 290–296.
5. Wigstrom, H. & B. Gustaffson. 1988. Presynaptic and postsynaptic interactions in the control of hippocampal long-term potentiation. *In* Long-Term Potentiation: From Biophysics to Behavior. P. W. Landfield & S. A. Deadwyler. Eds.: 73–107. Alan R. Liss. New York.
6. Zalutsky, R. A. & R. A. Nicoll. 1990. Comparison of two forms of long-term potentiation in single hippocampal neurons. Science **248:** 1619–1624.
7. Kay, A. R. & R. K. S. Wong. 1986. Isolation of neurons suitable for patch-clamping from adult mammalian central nervous system. J. Neurosci. Methods **16:** 227–238.
8. Connor, J. A., W. J. Wadman, P. E. Hockberger & R. K. S. Wong. 1988. Sustained dendritic gradients of Ca^{2+} induced by excitatory amino acids in CA1 hippocampal neurons. Science **240:** 649–653.
9. Grynkiewicz, G., M. Poenie & R. Y. Tsien. 1985. A new generation of Ca indicators with greatly improved fluorescence properties. J. Biol. Chem. **260:** 3440–3450.
10. Connor, J. A. 1986. Digital imaging of free calcium changes and of spatial gradients in growing processes in single, mammalian central nervous system cells. Proc. Natl. Acad Sci. USA **83:** 6179–6183.
11. Connor, J. A. 1988. Fluorescence imaging applied to the measurement of Ca^{2+} in mammalian neurons. *In* Calcium and Ion Channel Modulation. A. Grinnel, D. Armstrong & M. Jackson, Eds.: 395–406. Plenum. New York.
12. Kay, A. R. & R. K. S. Wong. 1987. Calcium current activation kinetics in isolated pyramidal neurones of the CA1 region of the mature guinea-pig hippocampus. J. Physiol. (London) **392:** 603–616.
13. Horn, R. & A. Marty. 1988. Muscarinic activation of ionic currents measured by a new whole cell recording method. J. Gen. Physiol. **92:** 145–159.
14. Kay, A. R. & J. A. Connor. 1990. Preservation of the NMDA response of neurons acutely dissociated from the mature guinea pig hippocampus. J. Neurosci. Methods **33:** 77–79.
15. Mayer, M. L., A. B. MacDermott, G. L. Westbrook, S. J. Smith & J. L. Barker. 1987. Agonist- and voltage-gated calcium entry in cultured mouse spinal cord neurons under voltage clamp measured using arsenazo III. J. Neuroci. **7:** 3230–3244.
16. Murphy, S. N. & R. J. Miller. 1988. A glutamate receptor regulates Ca^{2+} mobilization in hippocampal neurons. Proc. Natl. Acad. Sci. USA **85:** 8737–8741.
17. Mody, I., K. G. Baimbridge, J. A. Shacklock & J. F. MacDonald. 1991. Release of intracellularly stored Ca^{2+} following NMDA receptor activation in hippocampal neurons. Exp. Brain Res. Sers. In press.
18. Hannun, Y. A., C. R. Loomis, A. H. Merill & R. M. Bell. 1986. Sphingosine inhibition of protein kinase C activity and of phorbol dibutyrate binding *in vitro* and in human platelets. J. Biol. Chem. **261:** 12604–12609.
19. Hannun, Y. A. & R. B. Bell. 1989. Functions of sphingolipids and sphingolipid breakdown products in cellular regulation. Science **243:** 500–507.

19a. WADMAN, W. J. & J. A. CONNOR. 1991. Persisting modification of dendritic calcium influx by excitatory amino acid stimulation in isolated CA1 neurons. Neurosci. In press.
20. MANEV, H., M. FARARON, A. GUIDOTTI & E. COSTA. 1989. Delayed increase of Ca^{2+} influx elicited by glutamate: Role in neuronal death. Mol. Pharmacol. **36:** 106–111.
21. GLAUM, S. R., W. K. SCHOLZ & R. J. MILLER. 1990. Acute and long term glutamate mediated regulation of $[Ca^{2+}]$ in rat hippocampal pyramidal neurons *in vitro*. J. Pharmacol. Exp. Ther. **253:** 1293–1302.
22. STRONG, J. A., A. P. FOX, R. E. TSIEN & L. K. KACZMAREK. 1987. Stimulation of protein kinase C recruits covert calcium channels in Aplysia bag cell neurons. Nature **235:** 714–717.
23. KNOX, R. J., E. A. QUATTROCKI, J. A. CONNOR & L. K. KACZMAREK. 1990. The *in vitro* formation of putative peptide release sites using a phorbol ester and cyclic AMP. Soc. Neurosci. (Abstr.) **16:** 457.
24. WONG, R. K. S., D. A. PRINCE & A. I. BASBAUM. 1979. Intradentritic recordings from hippocampal neurons. Proc. Natl. Acad. Sci. USA **76:** 986–990.
25. WADMAN, W. J., U. HEINEMANN, A. KONNERTH & S. NEUHAUS. 1985. Hippocampal slices of kindled rats reveal calcium involvement in epileptogenesis. Exp. Brain Res. **57:** 404–407.
26. LOVINGER, D. M., K. WONG, K. MURAKAMI & A. ROUTTENBERG. 1987. Protein kinase C inhibitors eliminate hippocampal long-term potentiation. Brain Res. **436:** 177–183.
27. MALINOW, R., D. V. MADISON & R. W. TSIEN. 1988. Persistent protein kinase activity underlying long term potentiation. Nature **335:** 820–824.
28. MALINOW, R., H. SCHULMAN & R. W. TSIEN. 1989. Inhibition of postsynaptic PKC or CaMKII blocks induction but not expression of LTP. Science **245:** 862–866.
29. KAUER, J. A., R. C. MALENKA & R. A. NICOLL. 1988. A persistent postsynaptic modification mediates long-term potentiation in the hippocampus. Neuron **1:** 911–917.
30. MALENKA, R. C., J. A. KAUER, D. J. PERKEL, M. D. MAUK, P. T. KELLY, R. A. NICOLL & M. N. WAXMAN. 1989. An essential role for postsynaptic calmodulin and protein kinase activity in long-term potentiation. Nature **340:** 554–557.
31. CHOI, D. W. 1988. Glutamate neurotoxicity and diseases of the nervous system. Neuron **1:** 623–634.
32. KORN, S. J., A. MARTY, J. A. CONNOR & R. HORN. 1990. Perforated patch recording. Methods Neurosci. **4:** 364–373.
33. REGEHR, W. G., J. A. CONNOR & D. W. TANK. 1989. Optical imaging of Ca accumulation in hippocampal pyramidal cells during synaptic activation. Nature **341:** 533–536.

Calcium Channel–Targeted Polypeptide Toxins[a]

BALDOMERO M. OLIVERA,[b] JULITA S. IMPERIAL,[b]
LOURDES J. CRUZ,[b,c] VYTAUTAS P. BINDOKAS,[d]
VIRGINIA J. VENEMA,[d] AND MICHAEL E. ADAMS[d]

[b]*Department of Biology*
University of Utah
Salt Lake City, Utah 84112

[c]*Marine Science Institute*
University of the Philippines
Diliman, Quezon City, Philippines

[d]*Department of Entomology*
University of California
Riverside, California 92521

INTRODUCTION

Animal venoms interfere with the function of key physiological systems. The high potency and selectivity of toxins responsible for such disruption can be used effectively in studies of these key physiological mechanisms. Voltage-sensitive Ca channels at presynaptic terminals are an obvious molecular target for venom components inasmuch as these channels transduce the electrical signals of axons into biochemical events at synapses. Toxins that target voltage-sensitive Ca channels at presynaptic terminals were first described in 1984 with the characterization of the ω-conotoxins.[1-3] At present, the major Ca channel toxins that have been extensively characterized are the ω-toxins of fish-hunting cone snails, and of spiders (in particular *Agelenopsis aperta*). Undoubtedly, more Ca channel toxins await discovery in these and other venom sources.

A continuing theme of ion channel research is the structure/function characterization of different channel subtypes. The availability of dihydropyridine drugs and ω-conotoxins as specific, high-affinity ligands helped Tsien and collaborators to divide the widely used classification of Ca channels into L, N, and T subtypes.[4] Recent molecular genetic evidence, however, suggests that a much larger number of Ca channel subtypes are expressed in the mammalian central nervous system alone.[5] Without doubt, molecular genetics will continue to define different voltage-sensitive Ca channel subtypes and should provide probes for mapping anatomically the locations of these channels. The expected diversity in Ca channel subtypes creates a need for additional pharmacological tools for differentiating one subtype from another. A major theme we will develop is that combinations of Ca channel toxins from the unexpectedly diverse array present in spider and cone snail venoms constitute a powerful pharmacological arsenal for the characterization and classification of Ca channels. In this article, our intention is not to provide a comprehensive

[a]The work of the authors was supported by Grants GM22737 (to B. M. Olivera) and NS24472 (to M. E. Adams).

114

review of the literature, but to use selected examples from our own laboratories to illustrate the potential of channel subtype "toxityping."

HISTORICAL PERSPECTIVE

The ω-conotoxins were first discovered in the venoms of two fish-hunting cone snails, *Conus geographus* and *Conus magus*.[1,3] The first clear-cut identification of ω-conotoxin activity was obtained by Michael McIntosh, then an undergraduate at the University of Utah. He isolated a fraction from *Conus magus* that yielded a highly distinctive symptomatology in mice upon intracranial injection; the intracranial assay was introduced into the Utah laboratory by Craig Clark, another undergraduate.[6] Injected mice exhibited continuous shaking with their limbs splayed (these peptides were originally called "shaker peptides"). The original shaker peptide from *Conus magus* was purified,[3] as well as a homologous peptide from *Conus geographus* venom with similar activity;[1] these are now known as ω-conotoxins MVIIA and GVIA. The mechanisms underlying shaker symptoms remain incompletely understood. It should be noted that although the presently known Ca channel–targeted peptides of *Conus geographus* and *Conus magus* venoms are paralytic to fish, they do not paralyze mice.

An electrophysiological characterization of the peptides, principally using the frog neuromuscular junction, was carried out by Lynn Kerr and Doju Yoshikami.[2] The *Conus magus* toxin (ω-conotoxin MVIIA) did not cause neuromuscular block at nanomolar concentrations; however, ω-conotoxin GVIA from *Conus geographus* venom was a potent inhibitor of transmission at this neuromuscular junction. The block was presynaptic, and the data strongly indicated that the *Conus geographus* peptide inhibited presynaptic voltage-sensitive Ca channels. The same study also revealed that Ca channels in chick dorsal root ganglion neurons in culture were inhibited by this peptide.[2] It is notable that in these initial studies, the identification of voltage-sensitive Ca channels as the macromolecular target of ω-conotoxins specifically required ω-conotoxin GVIA (not MVIIA) and amphibian (not mammalian) neuromuscular junctions. If the peptides had been tested on the neuromuscular junction of mammals, or if the *Conus magus* homologue had been used in the initial amphibian work, it is quite possible that the basic mechanism of action of ω-conotoxins would still be a mystery.

A study of binding competition between the ω-toxins from cone snails and spiders was instrumental in revealing the complexity of Ca channel–targeted toxins in spider venom.[7] An electrophysiological characterization of the polypeptide toxin ω-Aga-IA from venom of the funnel web spider *Agelenopsis aperta* demonstrated a presynaptic block of insect neuromuscular transmission; the data were strongly suggestive that the toxin blocked voltage-sensitive Ca channels.[8] When components from *A. aperta* venom were assayed for their ability to inhibit ω-conotoxin binding to synaptosomal membranes, however, ω-Aga-IA proved to be inactive. Nonetheless, several other fractions from this venom did inhibit ω-conotoxin binding to chick brain membranes. Toxins purified from these fractions have been identified as ω-Aga-IIA[7] and ω-Aga-IIIA.[9] An intriguing new toxin, ω-Aga-IVA, was discovered using voltage-activated ^{45}Ca uptake in mammalian synaptosomes as an assay. This toxin has novel physiological specificity distinct from previously characterized ω-conotoxins and ω-agatoxins. Thus, the characterization of each cone snail and spider toxin not only has provided a new tool for investigating Ca channels, and but has also propelled the search for new toxins with different specificity towards Ca channel subtypes. At this stage, Ca

TABLE 1. Peptide Toxins Specific for Calcium Channels

Toxin	Source	Reference
ω-Conotoxin GVIA	*Conus geographus*	1
ω-Conotoxin MVIIA	*Conus geographus*	3
ω-Agatoxin IA	*Agelenopsis aperta*	7 and 8
ω-Agatoxin IIA	*Agelenopsis aperta*	7
ω-Agatoxin IIIA	*Agelenopsis aperta*	9
ω-Agatoxin IVA	*Agelenopsis aperta*	M. Adams & V. Venema, unpublished results

channel toxinology is an emerging technology that fuels itself. A summary of these Ca channel–targeted peptides is shown in TABLE 1.

ω-CONOTOXINS: GENERAL OVERVIEW

Over 10 peptides have been characterized from venoms of five fish-hunting cone snails so far. These range in size from 25–29 amino acids, and all have three disulfide bonds (refs. 1, 3, and 10; L. J. Cruz, J. Rivier and B. Olivera, unpublished results). The characteristic arrangement of cysteine residues (C...C...CC...C...C) presumably reflects a common disulfide bonding pattern (see TABLE 1).[11] It should be emphasized, however, that for most peptides, the disulfide bonding configuration has not been directly established experimentally. So far, venoms of all fish-hunting species investigated are known to contain ω-conotoxins; by contrast, most fish-hunting *Conus* venoms apparently lack the Na channel–targeted μ-conotoxins.[12] The ω-conotoxins of piscivorous *Conus* may either have evolved *de novo* as the fish-hunting cones evolved from ancestral nonpiscivorous *Conus* species or may be derived from toxins with homologous functions in an ancestral venom.

If all known ω-conotoxin amino acid sequences are compared, there is little absolute sequence conservation, except for the cysteines and one glycine residue. A pair-wise comparison of ω-conotoxins exhibits as little as 30–35% overlap in the sequence of noncysteine amino acids. As shown in TABLE 2, however, some ω-conotoxins from the same venom have sufficient similarity in sequence to be polymorphisms of functionally equivalent peptides (*i.e.,* GVIIA vs. GVIIB). Nevertheless, some of the most divergent pairs of conotoxin sequences are found in the same venom. A case in point is the greater divergence between ω-conotoxins GVIA and GVIIA than that between ω-conotoxin GVIIA and the ω-conotoxins in *Conus magus* venom. This suggests that two functionally different ω-conotoxin subclasses have

TABLE 2. Primary Structures of ω-Conotoxins[a]

ω-Conotoxin	Amino acid sequence
GVIA	CKSOGSSCSOTSYNCCRSCNOYTKRCY*
GVIIA	CKSOGTOCSRGMRDCCTSCLLYSNKCRRY
GVIIB	CKSOGTOCSRGMRDCCTSCLSYSNKCRRY
MVIIA	CKGKGAKCSRLMYDCCTGSCRSGKC*
MVIIB	CKGKGASCHRTSYDCCTGSCNRGKC*

[a]Structures are taken from ref. 10; asterisks indicate toxins for which a C-terminal amide has been established. It is probable that all presently known ω-conotoxins are amidated at the C terminus. O represents hydroxyproline.

been selected in one venom. The significance of two classes of ω-conotoxins in a single fish-hunting cone venom is not understood. Differences, however, in the *in vivo* symptomatology induced by these peptides are readily demonstrable. Although both paralyze fish, GVIA is three orders of magnitude more active than GVIIA against the frog neuromuscular junction; both peptides are ineffective against the mammalian neuromuscular junction.

The ω-conotoxins are in a size range where chemical synthesis is feasible[13]; as a result, these peptides have become widely available from commercial sources. The synthetic peptides can also be modified for various applications. All ω-conotoxins have tyrosine residues that can be readily iodinated to provide radiolabeled ligands. In addition, a number of photoactivatable, fluorescent, and biotinylated derivatives can be made. It should be noted that these modifications generally reduce the affinity of the toxins for target Ca channels, and in certain cases the affinities of modified peptides for different Ca channel subtypes are differentially affected (J. Haack, D. Johnson, and B. Olivera, unpublished results). Thus, some care should be taken to make certain that some of the original targets of the unmodified toxins have not dropped out when the modified peptides are used. Potentially, a chemically modified ω-conotoxin may be a tool for further subdividing the Ca channels targeted by the unmodified peptide.

Finally, it should be emphasized that not only is the specificity of ω-conotoxin-Ca channel interactions dependent on the particular toxin used, but also on the phylogenetic system examined. Thus, the peptides show remarkable phylogenetic variation in their ability to inhibit the neuromuscular junction. Although the affinity of ω-conotoxin for some of its high-affinity target sites is subpicomolar,[14] even micromolar concentrations of the toxins do not block neurotransmitter release at most mammalian neuromuscular junctions. However, even though a specific ω-conotoxin may not inhibit certain Ca channels, the toxin may possibly bind with high affinity to the channel, but not function as an antagonist.

Ca CHANNEL ANTAGONISTS FROM SPIDER VENOMS: THE ω-AGATOXINS

The surprising pharmacological diversity of Ca channel toxins in a cone snail venom such as *Conus geographus* pales in comparison to the diversity of Ca channel–targeted toxins in the venom of the funnel web spider, *Agelenopsis aperta*. Like cone snails, spiders incapacitate prey by injection of venoms containing several types of ion channel–specific toxins. The venom of *A. aperta* targets multiple ion channels located both pre- and postsynaptically at the insect neuromuscular junction.[7,8,15] Three toxin classes have been described: postsynaptic antagonists of glutamate-sensitive ion channels (α-agatoxins),[16] presynaptic Na channel activators (μ-agatoxins),[17] and presynaptic Ca channel antagonists (ω-agatoxins).[7] The ω-agatoxins inhibit neurotransmitter release from motor nerve terminals through antagonism of voltage-sensitive Ca channels.[7,8]

Initial studies of presynaptic Ca channel block showed that ω-Aga-IA, a 7.5 kDa peptide, suppresses evoked synaptic current without affecting spontaneous miniature excitatory junctional current or ionophoretic glutamate potentials, indicating that transmitter release was inhibited.[8] Furthermore, this inhibition occurs even though motor nerve action potentials continue to invade motor nerve terminals. When transmitter release is evoked by direct nerve terminal stimulation in the presence of tetrodotoxin, both ω-Aga-IA or cobalt ions block this release in a similar manner, suggesting that the block involves voltage-sensitive Ca channels. Studies showing that ω-Aga-IA inhibits Ca channels in both insect[8] and rat[18] neuronal cell bodies is in accord with our hypothesis that this toxin blocks neuromuscular transmission by antagonism of presynaptic Ca channels.

It quickly became clear that ω-Aga-IA represented only one component of the Ca channel antagonist activity in funnel web spider venom. In addition to several type I ω-agatoxins similar to ω-Aga-IA in both molecular characteristics and presynaptic antagonist activity, a class of type II toxins was discovered in the venom.[7] Type II toxins are approximately 9.5 kDa and differ significantly in primary amino acid sequence from the type I toxins. Whereas both type I and type II toxins block insect neuromuscular transmission, they proved to be strikingly different in their actions on ω-conotoxin–sensitive Ca channels in chick brain.

Three ω-agatoxins, (ω-Aga-IA, ω-Aga-IB, and ω-Aga-IIA) were tested for ability to inhibit specific, high-affinity binding of $[^{125}I]$ω-conotoxin GVIA to chick brain synaptosomal membranes. Of the three, only ω-Aga-IIA inhibited $[^{125}I]$ω-conotoxin binding,[7] confirming that subtypes of ω-agatoxins have different specificities. Furthermore, the data suggest that ω-agatoxin subtypes recognize binding sites common to both insect and vertebrate Ca channels, indicating that some sites may be evolutionarily conserved. ω-Aga-IIA proved to be a potent inhibitor of ω-conotoxin binding (apparent K_d = 15 nM) and ^{45}Ca flux into K$^+$-depolarized synaptosomes (apparent K_d of about 2 nM).[9] Both ω-Aga-IA and ω-Aga-IB were inactive against both $[^{125}I]$ω-conotoxin binding and ^{45}Ca flux. These data show that type II, but not type I toxins, block synaptosomal Ca channels in chick brain and that this antagonism probably involves interaction with the ω-conotoxin binding site. We now have further evidence for differences between type I and type II blocking mechanisms at the insect neuromuscular junction.[19]

Using the $[^{125}I]$ω-conotoxin binding assay as a screen for *A. aperta* venom fractions, a novel class of type III ω-agatoxins (with primary amino acid sequences similar to type II toxins) was discovered.[9] The type III toxins (ω-Aga-IIIA, ω-Aga-IIIB), however, are of lower molecular mass (8.5 kDa) and, unlike the type II toxins, do not block insect Ca channels. ω-Aga-IIIA inhibits ω-conotoxin binding and ^{45}Ca flux into chick brain synaptosomes with affinities similar to those obtained for ω-Aga-IIA. Recent physiological studies on ω-Aga-IIIA show this toxin to be a potent blocker of high threshold (N and L) Ca currents in primary cultures of frog sympathetic neurons, rat dorsal root ganglion neurons, rat hippocampal neurons, and rat cardiac muscle with apparent K_d values between 1–2 nM.[20] The apparent affinity of ω-Aga-IIIA for Ca channels in these tissues is in good agreement with values obtained from the synaptosome studies.[9] It appears that ω-Aga-IIIA recognizes a common binding site on mammalian N and L type Ca channels, whereas ω-conotoxin antagonism is largely confined to N-type channels alone.

Further evidence that ω-Aga-IIIA is active in the vertebrate brain comes from results of intracranial injections in mice. These studies show that this toxin induces lethal convulsions, an effect very different from the shaker syndrome produced by ω-conotoxin. The above studies show that ω-Aga-IIIA and ω-conotoxin recognize overlapping populations of Ca channels in the chick brain and should prove useful as tools for studies of the anatomical distribution and functional significance of N and L Ca channels in the central nervous system.

Although ω-Aga-IIIA and ω-conotoxin are potent antagonists of ^{45}Ca flux in chick brain synaptosomes, these toxins are comparatively inactive against rat brain ^{45}Ca flux under identical conditions. In hopes of discovering an antagonist of rat brain Ca channels, we used ^{45}Ca flux to screen *A. aperta* venom fractions. This approach was successful in identifying several potent antagonists of rat brain Ca channels. One of these is ω-Aga-IIA, which was shown previously to inhibit [^{125}I]ω-conotoxin binding and [45]Ca flux in chick brain synaptosomes. In addition, we discovered a fourth type of ω-agatoxin, the type IV toxins, (ω-Aga-IVA, ω-Aga-IVB). ω-Aga-IVA blocks [45]Ca flux into rat brain synaptosomes, with an apparent K_d of 20 nM, and blocks a comparatively small component of [45]Ca flux into chick brain synaptosomes. ω-Aga-IVA, like ω-Aga-IIIA, appears to be inactive against insect Ca channels.

The foregoing account demonstrates that although the ω-agatoxins are Ca channel antagonists, considerable heterogeneity exists in their receptor specificity. Our ability to recognize this diversity of spider toxin Ca channel antagonists was greatly assisted by several screening assays. The use of radiolabeled ω-conotoxin as a differentiating probe allowed for the first clear demonstration of different binding specificities between type I and type II ω-agatoxins.[7] Using the same assay, we discovered the type III toxins,[9] which had been completely overlooked due to lack of activity against insect Ca channels.[7,18] Finally, using [45]Ca flux through rat brain synaptosomal Ca channels as an assay, we discovered the type IV toxins.

Ca CHANNEL "TOXITYPING": USING OVERLAPPING SPECIFICITIES FOR CHANNEL SUBTYPING

We expect that the major future challenge in Ca channel toxinology will be to expand the battery of cone snail and spider venom Ca channel–targeted toxins for classifying the anticipated multitude of channel subtypes revealed by cloning polymerase chain reaction (PCR) techniques. It is unclear at this time how many different Ca channels occur in a tissue such as rat brain, but present indications are that the number will be large.[5] The outline above provides evidence that the ω-agatoxins and the ω-conotoxins have overlapping specificities. In principle, overlapping specificities could be used to advantage in defining Ca channel subtypes. For example, two toxins (A and B) that overlap but are not identical in their receptor-targeting specificity could define up to four subtype classes of Ca channels (A^+B^+, A^+B^-, A^-B^+, A^-B^-). This assumes that binding to Ca channel subtypes is an all or none phenomenon; if a toxin had multiple receptor targets with distinguishable affinities, even more subclasses could, in principle, be defined. Given the diversity in Ca channel specificity discovered in toxins from venoms of one spider and several *Conus* species so far, it seems reasonable to expect that an expanding set of toxins with overlapping receptor specificity can be obtained.

The use of ω-agatoxins and ω-conotoxins in combination should be an immediately fruitful approach. Because of the divergent evolutionary history of *Agelenopsis aperta* and *Conus geographus,* the selective pressures operating on their toxins were undoubtedly different. Thus, if a large set of Ca channel subtypes in a tissue such as mammalian brain is presented to any ω-agatoxin/ω-conotoxin pair, it seems unlikely that the two toxins will exhibit an identical receptor subtype specificity. Consequently, a collection of ω-agatoxin/ω-conotoxin pairs with overlapping specificities should prove particularly useful for distinguishing Ca channel subtypes. Such an approach already has been initiated using the ω-agatoxin IIIA/ω-conotoxin GVIA pair on rat dorsal root ganglion cells by Mintz *et al.*[19] The use of such toxin combinations to define which Ca channel subtypes are present (Ca channel toxityping) may become a routine diagnostic procedure in defining biological roles for Ca channels in particular neuronal circuits or cells.

DETERMINANTS OF ω-TOXIN SPECIFICITY

Two subtypes of ω-conotoxins from the venom of *Conus geographus* have been defined so far (ω-conotoxins GVIA and GVIIA are examples). Preliminary evidence has shown that multiple subtypes of ω-conotoxins exist in other *Conus* species as well (B. Olivera, G. Zafaralla, M. McIntosh, and L. J. Cruz, unpublished results). The heterogeneity of the ω-agatoxins is much more striking, with at least four major toxin types that are both pharmacologically and biochemically distinguishable. The ω-agatoxins thus appear to have a relatively broader phylogenetic spectrum of activity against Ca channels as compared to the *Conus* toxins. This may relate, in part, to the fact that spiders evolved much earlier than the cone snails and hence may have encountered ancestral forms of Ca channels. Second, a greater phylogenetic diversity of prey animals envenomated by a single spider species may have led to evolutionary strategies favoring broader recognition of common binding sites on phylogenetically distinct Ca channels. By contrast, the presynaptic Ca channel diversity of teleost fish on which the cone snails prey may be more limited. This may also explain why, in contrast to the ω-conotoxins that target only neuronal Ca channels, several ω-agatoxins exhibit broader tissue specificity. It is also remarkable that some ω-agatoxins (*i.e.* ω-Aga-IIA) are high-affinity inhibitors of Ca channels at the insect neuromuscular junction as well as in avian and mammalian brain, indicating that some toxin-binding sites on Ca channels are highly conserved.

The fact that the spider toxins are roughly twice the molecular weight of the cone toxins may facilitate a broad phylogenetic recognition strategy. Recognition of an ω-agatoxin binding site may involve a larger number of binding determinants on the extracellular domain of Ca channel proteins (FIG. 1). The smaller ω-conotoxins could bind only to a subset of these determinants. Small changes in ω-conotoxin binding sites would be more likely to alter the affinity of the cone snail toxins than of spider toxins. This might help to explain the comparatively broad spectrum of activity of ω-Aga-IA[8,18] and ω-Aga-IIA,[7,9] which recognize Ca channels in both insects and vertebrates, whereas ω-conotoxin GVIA antagonism is confined largely to the vertebrates. It remains unclear why both ω-Aga-IIIA, a large toxin, and ω-conotoxin GVIA, a relatively small toxin, both fail to recognize Ca channels in insects and mammals. ω-Aga-IIA, which is apparently quite similar to ω-Aga-IIIA, retains activity in both animal groups. One possible rationale is illustrated by the model in FIGURE 1; amino acid substitutions at key determinants near the binding domain could affect the binding of one toxin, but not another.

Although the phylogenetic target diversity of ω-conotoxins may generally be narrower than for ω-agatoxins, for *Conus* toxins we can nevertheless expect to find novel pharmacological variants of Ca channel–targeted toxins in new *Conus* venoms. The ω-conotoxins sequenced from five different *Conus* venoms make it clear that each venom has its own distinctive spectrum of ω-conotoxin sequences; indeed, of the 100 biologically active peptides (of all types) from *Conus* venoms that have been sequenced, not a single one has been found in venoms of two different species. The underlying biological reason for this appears to be the unique mechanism that cone snails have evolved for hypervarying their toxins.[6,21] In addition, although there are approximately 50 species of fish-hunting *Conus,* these constitute only a minor fraction (ca. 10%) of the total. If venoms of the *Conus* species that prey on other snails, or on polychaete and hemichordate worms, also contain Ca channel–targeted polypeptide toxins, then the total diversity of Ca channel toxins in cone snails should be a very significant pharmacological resource. Because only one species of spider

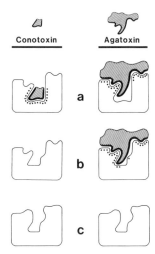

FIGURE 1. A cartoon illustrating possible interactions of an ω-conotoxin (left) and an ω-agatoxin (right) with three different Ca channel subtypes (labeled a, b, and c). The smaller size of the ω-conotoxins suggests that they interact with a smaller receptor epitope than the ω-agatoxins. It is therefore conceivable that small changes in the "receptor target pocket," with which ω-conotoxin interacts, would prevent its binding, but not necessarily affect the binding of ω-agatoxins (a, b). Multiple changes in the binding epitope (compare a and c) would be needed to alter the binding of the ω-agatoxins. Whereas the presynaptic Ca channels at teleost fish neuromuscular junctions may constitute a more conserved set of epitopes to which the ω-conotoxins bind, the ω-agatoxins could bind to a larger variety of Ca channels, thus permitting spiders to paralyze a greater diversity of prey.

(*Agelenopsis aperta*) has been studied intensively, the venoms of the thousands of spider species not yet examined may have even greater pharmacological potential for yielding Ca channel–targeted toxins of diverse specificity.

REFERENCES

1. OLIVERA, B. M., J. M. MCINTOSH, L. J. CRUZ, F. A. LUQUE & W. R. GRAY. 1984. Purification and sequence of a presynaptic peptide toxin from *Conus geographus* venom. Biochemistry **23**: 5087–5090.
2. KERR, L. M. & D. YOSHIKAMI. 1984. A venom peptide with a novel presynaptic blocking action. Nature **308**: 282–284.
3. OLIVERA, B. M., L. J. CRUZ, V. DE SANTOS, G. LECHEMINANT, D. GRIFFIN, R. ZEIKUS, J. M. MCINTOSH, R. GALYEAN, J. VARGA, W. R. GRAY & J. RIVIER. 1987. Neuronal Ca channel antagonists. Discrimination between Ca channel subtypes using ω-conotoxin from *Conus magus* venom. Biochemistry **26**: 2086–2090.
4. NOWYCKY, M. C., A. P. FOX & R. W. TSIEN. 1985. Three types of neuronal calcium channel with different calcium agonist sensitivity. Nature **316**: 440–443.
5. SNUTCH, T. P., J. P. LEONARD, M. M. GILBERT, H. A. LESTER, N. DAVIDSON. 1990. Rat brain expresses a heterogeneous family of calcium channels. Proc. Natl. Acad. Sci. USA **87**: 3391–3395.
6. OLIVERA, B. M., J. RIVIER, C. CLARK, C. A. RAMILO, G. P. CORPUZ, F. C. ABOGADIE, E. E.

MENA, S. R. WOODWARD, D. R. HILLYARD & L. J. CRUZ. 1990. Diversity of *Conus* neuropeptides. Science **249:** 257–263.

7. ADAMS, M. E., V. P. BINDOKAS, L. HASEGAWA & V. J. VENEMA. 1990. ω-Agatoxins: novel calcium channel antagonists of two subtypes from funnel web spider (*Agelenopsis aperta*) venom. J. Biol. Chem. **265:** 861–867.

8. BINDOKAS, V. P. & M. E. ADAMS. 1989. ω-Aga-I: A presynaptic calcium channel antagonist from venom of the funnel web spider, *Agelenopsis aperta.* J. Neurobiol. **20:** 171–188.

9. VENEMA, V. J. & M. E. ADAMS. Synaptosomal calcium channel antagonism by ω-agatoxins from funnel web spider venom. To be submitted.

10. OLIVERA, B. M., W. R. GRAY, R. ZEIKUS, J. M. MCINTOSH, J. VARGA, J. RIVIER, V. DE SANTOS & L. J. CRUZ. 1985. Peptide neurotoxins from fish-hunting cone snails. Science **230:** 1338–1343.

11. NISHIUCHI, Y., K. KUMAGAYE, Y. NODA, T. X. WATANABE & S. SAKAKIBARA. 1986. Synthesis and secondary structure determination of ω-conotoxin GVIA: A 27-peptide with three intramolecular disulfide bonds. Biopolymers **25:** 561–568.

12. CRUZ, L. J., W. R. GRAY, B. M. OLIVERA, R. D. ZEIKUS, L. KERR, D. YOSHIKAMI & E. MOCZYDLOWSKI. 1985. *Conus geographus* toxins that discriminate between neuronal and muscle sodium channels. J. Biol. Chem. **260:** 9280–9288.

13. RIVIER, J., R. GALYEAN, W. R. GRAY, A. AZIMI-ZONOOZ, J. M. MCINTOSH, L. J. CRUZ & B. M. OLIVERA. 1987. Neuronal calcium channel inhibitors: Synthesis of ω-conotoxin GVIA and effects on ⁴⁵Ca-uptake by synaptosomes. J. Biol. Chem. **262:** 1194–1198.

14. FEIGENBAUM, P., M. L. GARCIA & G. J. KACZOROWSKI. 1988. Evidence for distinct sites coupled to high affinity ω-conotoxin receptors in rat brain synaptic plasma membrane vesicles. Biochem. Biophys. Res. Commun. **154:** 298–305.

15. ADAMS, M. E., E. E. HEROLD & V. J. VENEMA. 1989. Two classes of channel-specific toxins from funnel web spider venom. J. Comp. Physiol. A. **164:** 333–342.

16. QUISTAD, G. B., S. SUWANRUMPHA, M. A. JAREMA, M. J. SHAPIRO, W. S. SKINNER, G. C. JAMIESON, A. LUI & E. W. FU. 1990. Structures of paralytic acylpolyamines from the spider, *Agelenopsis aperta.* Biochem. Biophys. Res. Commun. **169:** 51–56.

17. SKINNER, W. S., M. E. ADAMS, G. B. QUISTAD, H. KATAOKA, B. J. CESARIN, F. E. ENDERLIN & D. A. SCHOOLEY. 1989. Purification and characterization of two classes of neurotoxins from the funnel web spider, *Agelenopsis aperta.* J. Biol. Chem. **264:** 2150–2155.

18. SCOTT, R. H., A. C. DOLPHIN, V. P. BINDOKAS & M. E. ADAMS. 1990. Inhibition of neuronal Ca^{2+} channels by the funnel web spider toxin ω-Aga-IA. Mol. Pharmacol. **38:** 711–718.

19. BINDOKAS, V. P., V. J. VENEMA & M. E. ADAMS. 1991. Differential presynaptic antagonism by subtypes of ω-agatoxins. J. Neurophysiol. In press.

20. MINTZ, I. M., V. J. VENEMA, M. E. ADAMS & B. P. BEAN. 1991. Inhibition of N- and L-type Ca^{2+} channels by the spider venom toxin, ω-Aga-IIIA. Proc. Natl. Acad. Sci. USA. In press.

21. WOODWARD, S. R., L. J. CRUZ, B. M. OLIVERA & D. R. HILLYARD. 1990. Constant and hypervariable regions in conotoxin propeptides. EMBO Journal **1:** 1015–1020.

Synthetic Organic Ligands Active at Voltage-Gated Calcium Channels[a]

D. J. TRIGGLE, M. HAWTHORN, M. GOPALAKRISHNAN,
A. MINARINI, S. AVERY, A. RUTLEDGE, R. BANGALORE,
AND W. ZHENG

Department of Biochemical Pharmacology
School of Pharmacy
State University of New York
Buffalo, New York 14260

INTRODUCTION

The calcium channel antagonists, including verapamil, nifedipine, and diltiazem, are a major class of drugs active in cardiovascular medicine.[1-3] Since their discovery (reviewed by Fleckenstein[4]) a number of questions have been posed that have served to define the sites and mechanisms of action of these agents. These questions may be summarized as follows:[5] (1) Are the specific sites of action discrete or multiple? What are the structure-activity relationships? (2) Are mobilization and currents involved in a relationship to Ca^{2+}? (3) Is the specificity of action in specific tissues or organs? What is the basis for the specificity? (4) How are membranes and sidedness involved in multiple sites of action? (5) Are the mechanisms single or multiple?

There is now quite general agreement that, consistent with their chemical and pharmacologic heterogeneity, verapamil, nifedipine, and diltiazem (FIG. 1), as representatives of the phenylalkylamine, 1,4-dihydropyridine, and benzothiazepine chemical classes, respectively, interact at three distinct sites that are located on a major protein, the nonglycosylated alpha$_1$ subunit of the voltage-gated L class of channel.[1,5-7] These sites are linked allosterically one to the other and to the functional machinery of the channel (FIG. 1). The 1,4-dihydropyridine structure, including Bay K 8644 and PN 202 791, and possibly the phenylalkylamine and benzothiazepine structures also, expresses potent activator properties (FIG. 1).[8] Furthermore, within the 1,4-dihydropyridine structure potent activator and antagonist properties may exist within the enantiomers of a single structure.[9] Expression of the alpha$_1$ protein shows that it possesses the major properties of the Ca^{2+} channel[10,11] and that it exists in several subclasses.[12]

Although these agents all interact at a single category of Ca^{2+} channel and although these channels are widespread in excitable tissues, there is considerable selectivity of drug action. The actions of current therapeutically available agents dominate in the cardiovascular system, and they exhibit also a significant range of cardiac:vascular selectivity (FIG. 1). Furthermore, the selectivity of the agents may be distinguished not only between groups, but also within groups. Thus, the 1,4-dihydropyridine structure embraces a range of activity from the normal vascular selective agents to more recently described cardiac selective agents (TABLE 1).[13]

[a]Original work described in this paper was supported by a Grant from the National Institutes of Health (HL 16003). Additional support from The Miles Institute for Preclinical Pharmacology is gratefully acknowledged.

123

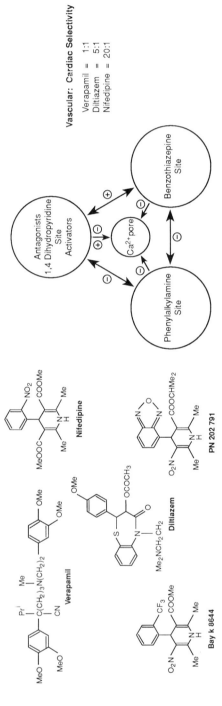

FIGURE 1. Structural formulas of Ca^{2+} channel antagonists and activators, the schematic representation of binding sites associated with the Ca^{2+} channel, and the vascular:cardiac selectivity of verapamil, diltiazem, and nifedipine.

Although these agents do not show major neuronal actions under many pharmacologic and therapeutic circumstances, this is not because of an absence of neuronal L channels as measured by electrophysiologic and radioligand binding techniques.[14] Furthermore, under some circumstances the Ca^{2+} channel antagonists do exhibit neuronal effects. Thus, the 1,4-dihydropyridine nimodipine (FIG. 2) protects neurons against death induced by the AIDS virus glycoprotein gp-120[15] and facilitates memory acquisition in a rabbit-associative learning model.[16] The neuronal effects of nimodipine have been reviewed recently.[17]

In principle this selectivity arises from a variety of causes either alone or in combination:[1-3] (1) pharmacokinetic features, including distribution and absorption; (2) mode of Ca^{2+} mobilization: voltage-gated channels versus other pathways; (3) class of voltage-gated channel: the existence of different classes of channels with differing pharmacologic characteristics; (4) state-dependent interactions: frequency and voltage-dependent interaction; and (5) pathologic state of tissue: numbers and function of channels are regulated according to disease state.

TABLE 1. Selectivity of Action of 1,4-Dihydropyridines X R R' Vascular:Cardiac Ratio

	X		R'	
[Felodipine]	$2,3Cl_2$	Et	$-Me$	~ 100:1
[Nifedipine]	$-2NO_2$	Me	$-Me$	~ 20:1
[Amlodipine]	$-2Cl$	Et	$-CH_2OCH_2CH_2NH_2$	~ 10:1
	2-Cl	Et	$-CH_2OCH_2CH_2NHCH_2$ $H_2NCH_2CH_2NHCO$	1:1
	2-Cl	Et	-NHCONH (pyrimidinyl-OH)	1:10

Three factors are of particular importance to the determination of selectivity at the molecular level. It is now clear that at least three, and probably more, major classes of Ca^{2+} channel exist, L, N, and T, each with its own electrophysiologic and pharmacologic characteristics (TABLE 2). The antagonists exhibit frequency-dependent (verapamil and diltiazem) and voltage-dependent (nifedipine) interactions, whereby potency increases with increasing frequency of depolarization or with decreased membrane potential, respectively.[18,19] Ca^{2+} channels are regulated both in number and function in a number of experimental and clinical states, including cardiomyopathy, ischemia, drug treatment, and hormone actions.[20]

In many respects, the Ca^{2+} channel may be viewed as a pharmacologic receptor. It possesses specific drug-binding sites where both activators and antagonists interact. These binding sites are linked to the functions of the Ca^{2+} channel, and they are regulated by homologous and heterologous influences. To strengthen this analogy, at least some Ca^{2+} channels are linked to G proteins: in the heart this may be important in contributing a cAMP-independent component of the Ca^{2+} current.[21]

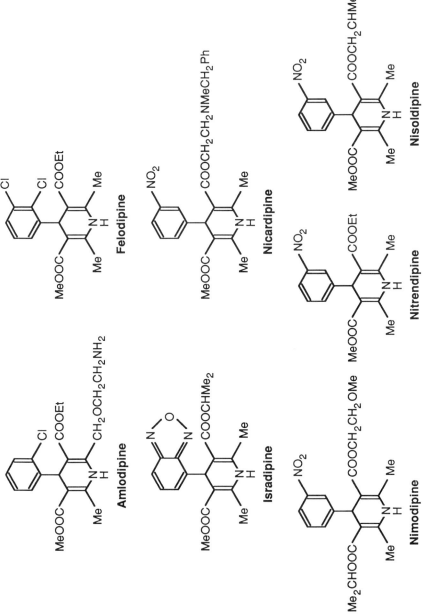

FIGURE 2. Structural formulas of 1,4-dihydropyridines.

There is no reason why other drug-binding sites associated with the L class of channel should not exist.[22] Similar arrays of binding sites should, in principle, exist for the other classes of voltage-gated Ca^{2+} channels. Considerable activity is, in fact, occurring both with respect to the development of new members of existing major drug classes and to the development of new structures for new channels. It remains true, however, that the great majority of synthetic drugs active at voltage-gated Ca^{2+} channels have been developed for and examined in the cardiovascular system.[2,3]

DEVELOPMENTS IN EXISTING DRUG CLASSES

Among the existing structures, the 1,4-dihydropyridine nucleus has been the focus of most synthetic exploitation.[23] A summary of structural requirements for

TABLE 2. Classification of Voltage-Dependent Calcium Channels

Property	L	T	N
Conductance, pS	25	8	12–20
Activation threshold	high	low	high
Inactivation rate	slow	fast	moderate
Permeation	$Ba^{2+} > Ca^{2+}$	$Ba^{2+} = Ca^{2+}$	$Ba^{2+} > Ca^{2+}$
Function	E-coupling cardiovascular system, smooth muscle, endocrine cells, and some neurons	Cardiac SA node: repetitive spike activity in neurons and endocrine cells	Neuronal only: neurotransmitter release
Pharmacologic sensitivity:			
1,4-Dihydropyridines (Activators/ antagonists) Phenylalkylamines Benzothiazepines	Sensitive	Insensitive	Insensitive
ω-Conotoxin	Sensitive? (some)	Insensitive	Sensitive
Octanol, amiloride	Insensitive?	Sensitive	Insensitive

antagonism and activation around this nucleus is depicted in FIGURE 3. Recently developed structures are summarized in FIGURE 2. Particular interest is attached to amlodipine and to related agents, including tiamdipine, because they reveal significantly different properties from the neutral 1,4-dihydropyridines. Amlodipine[13,24] and its tiamdipine analogues[25] reveal slow onset and offset of action and a stereoselectivity of action, approximately 1000-fold, that is significantly higher than the 5- to 50-fold revealed with other agents. Additionally, the phenyl ring substituent influence is muted in tiamdipine,[25] suggesting that the two series may interact in different manners with the binding site (FIG. 4). Whether these agents exert specific neuronal actions is not known.

Few studies are available for 1,4-dihydropyridine Ca^{2+} channel activators. For a small series, we observed, in common with the 1,4-dihydropyridine antagonists, very similar binding properties in cardiac muscle, smooth muscle, and neuronal prepara-

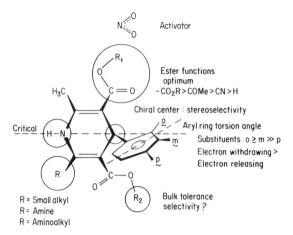

FIGURE 3. Structural features of 1,4-dihydropyridines associated with channel activation and antagonism.

tions.[26] We further observed that the influence of aryl ring substituents was differently expressed in both activator and antagonist series (TABLE 3).

It is generally considered that the 1,4-dihydropyridine (nifedipine) and benzothiazepine (diltiazem) structures are independent and interact at separate binding sites. Hybrid 2,5-dihydro-4-methyl-2-phenyl-1,5-benzothiazepine-3-carboxylic acid esters can, however, according to the nature of the N substituent, interact with the dihydropyridine site or with both the dihydropyridine and the diltiazem site (FIG. 5).[27]

The 1,4-dihydropyridine nucleus has proved to be a flexible structure with which to design agents that have dual functions of channel and receptor antagonism. These agents include (FIG. 6) CD-349, a nitrovasodilator;[28,29] BMY 20064, an alpha$_1$-adrenoceptor antagonist;[30] WY 27569, a thromboxane synthetase inhibitor;[31] compound 6 that combines alpha$_1$- and alpha$_2$-adrenoceptor antagonism;[32] and YM-16151-1, a beta$_1$-adrenoceptor antagonist.[33]

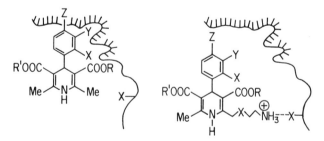

FIGURE 4. Schematic representation of binding of nifedipine and tiamdipine derivatives at the Ca^{2+} channel. This representation accommodates the importance of the 2-substituent interaction and the diminished phenyl ring interaction in the timadipine series.

TABLE 3. Influence of Aryl Ring Substituent on Pharmacologic and Radioligand Binding Activities in Nifedipine and Bay K 8644 Series[26]

Phenyl substituent	Nifedipine series				Bay K 8644 series		
	$-\log K_1$ ileum	binding heart	$-\log IC_{50}$ ileum	pharmacology heart	$-\log K_1$ ileum	binding heart	$-\log EC_{50}$ pharmacology ileum
2-NO$_2$	9.08	9.64	9.52	6.43	7.29	7.68	6.68
3-NO$_2$	9.97	8.92	9.05	6.24	8.11	8.31	7.06
4-NO$_2$	6.52	6.42	6.72	5.50	6.45	6.82	6.35

NEW STRUCTURAL CLASSES OF COMPOUNDS

A number of new structures have been introduced quite recently (FIG. 7). For the most part they share little obvious structural resemblance to existing agents and likely define new sites associated with the L category of Ca^{2+} channel.[22]

The benzothiazinone HOE 166 binds with high affinity in a voltage-dependent manner to Ca^{2+} channels in a variety of preparations.[34-36] Although the binding site density appears to be equivalent in skeletal muscle to that defined by the major structural classes of agent, kinetic experiments indicate that HOE 166 defines a separate site that is allosterically linked to those for verapamil, nifedipine, and diltiazem. A good correlation was observed between the binding affinities for HOE 166 and a series of analogues and their ability to inhibit depolarization-induced ^{45}Ca^{2+} uptake into A7r5 smooth muscle cells and RINm5F insulinoma cells, consistent with the HOE binding site being linked to the functional machinery of the Ca^{2+} channel.

The indolizine SR33557 likely also defines a novel and functional binding site, because it, like HOE 166, heterotropically modulates the binding of other channel ligands, defines an identical number of binding sites,[37,38] and reveals good correlation to functional inhibition of dopamine release and ^{45}Ca^{2+} uptake in PC12 cells.

McN5691 and McN6186 are members of the ethynylbenzenealkaneamine series whose pharmacological properties have not been explored in neuronal systems.[39-41] Existing data, however, suggest a substantial selectivity in other systems, including heart, vascular muscle, and secretory cells. An identification of a discrete binding site remains to be made. Similarly, the lactamimides, including MDL 12330A, interact at peripheral sites[42,43] and reveal a good correlation between binding and pharmacologic properties. It is not established, however, that these effects are exerted at a unique site.

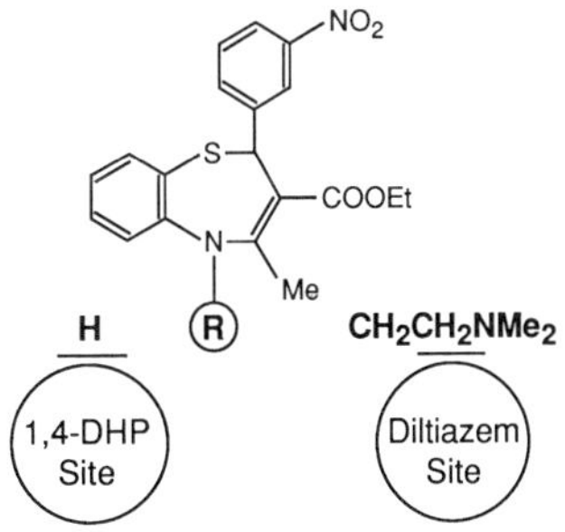

FIGURE 5. Dual interaction of benzothiazepines at 1,4-dihydropyridine and diltiazem sites at the Ca^{2+} channel.[27]

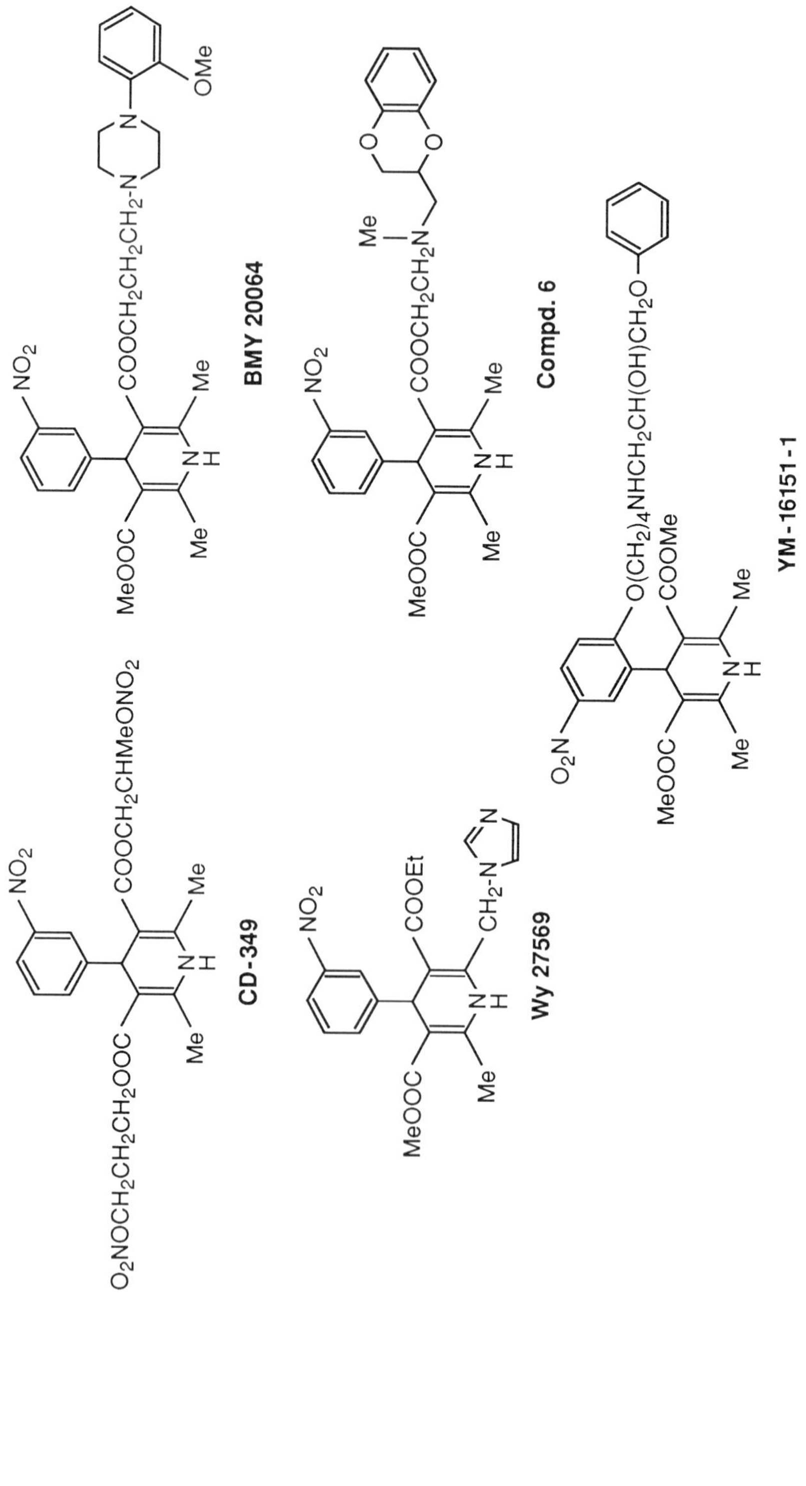

FIGURE 6. Structural formulas of 1,4-dihydropyridines with dual Ca^{2+} channel and receptor blocking activities.

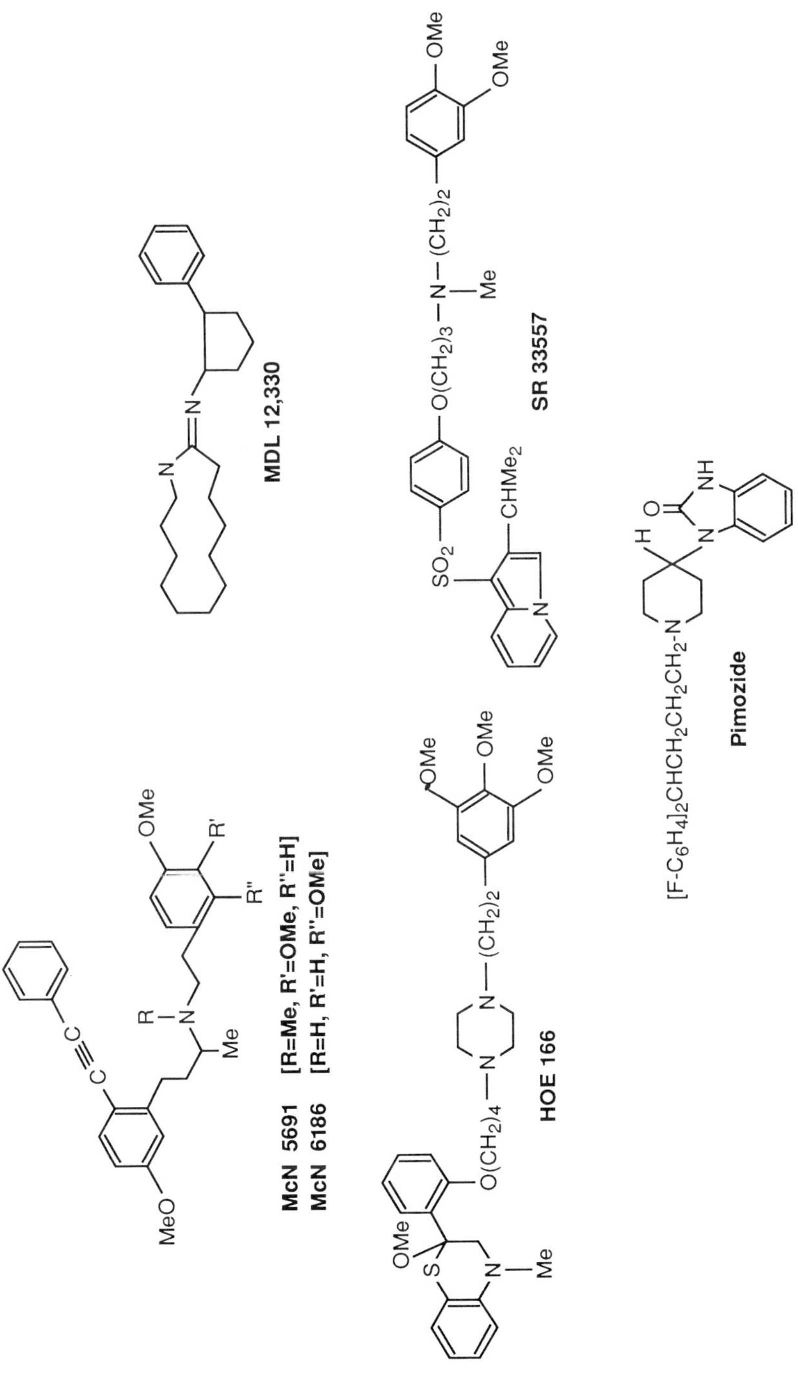

FIGURE 7. Formulas of new structures active at voltage-gated L channels.

The diphenylbutylpiperidines including pimozide, fluspirilene, and penfluridol define high-affinity binding sites in excitable cells.[44,45] These sites are distinct from those defined by nifedipine, verapamil, and diltiazem but are present in equal amounts. The ability of these agents to block the negative symptoms of schizophrenia may reflect a unique interaction at neuronal Ca^{2+} channels.[45]

Few studies are available on new synthetic agents mediating activator responses at the L channel. FPL 64176[46] produces large tension increases in vascular smooth muscle, remarkably in excess of those mediated by Bay K 8644 or K^+ depolarization (FIG. 8), which are blocked by concentrations of verapamil, nifedipine, and diltiazem consistent with an interaction mediated through a voltage-gated L channel. This agent does not interact with conventional binding sites and may define a novel activator binding site.

A schematic representation of the possible arrangements of the major and minor drug binding sites at the L class of voltage-gated Ca^{2+} channel is depicted in FIG-URE 9.

DRUGS ACTIVE AT T AND N CLASSES OF CA^{2+} CHANNELS

There are currently no synthetic agents known with a potency and selectivity for T or N channels comparable to that exhibited by the 1,4-dihydropyridines for the L

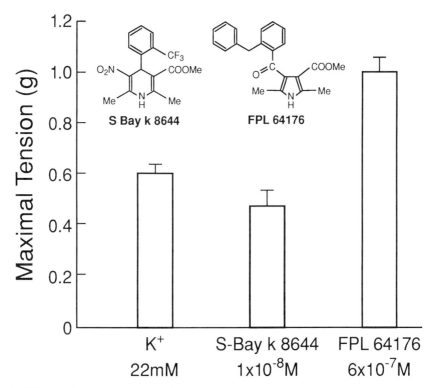

FIGURE 8. Tension responses to K^+ depolarization, S-Bay K 8644, and FPL 64176 in rat tail artery.

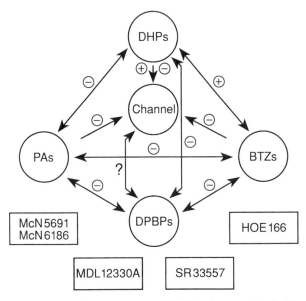

FIGURE 9. Proposed schematic arrangement of binding sites associated with the L class of Ca^{2+} channel.

channel. A number of synthetic structures have proved of utility, particularly in electrophysiologic studies, for characterization of non-L Ca^{2+} channels. A need for potent, small molecule antagonists, however, is apparent to evaluate the therapeutic potential of T and N channel blockade.

T channel drugs include amiloride,[47,48] chlorpromazine,[49] valproic acid,[50] and tetramethrin[51] (FIG. 10). None of these agents is specific, and all have well-documented effects on other ion channel or receptor systems.

Although the 1,4-dihydropyridines are conventionally viewed as L channel–selective,[23] an increasing weight of evidence suggests that they act at other types of voltage-gated Ca^{2+} channels as well as at other classes of voltage-gated cation channels. Ca^{2+} current in adrenal glomerulosa cells show both L- and T-type characteristics.[52] T channel current and aldosterone secretion is stimulated by angiotensin II and by low concentrations of K^+ to which adrenal glomerulosa cells are very sensitive. T channel current was blocked by nitrendipine with calculated affinities for the resting and inactivated states of 1.3×10^{-5} and 1.9×10^{-7}M, respectively. These values are some two orders of magnitude higher than those for L channel inhibition. Similar sensitivities of T channel current to 1,4-dihydropyridines have been reported in other systems. In rat hypothalamic neurons[53] several 1,4-dihydropyridines, including nicardipine, nifedipine, and nimodipine, blocked current in use-dependent fashion with K_D values of 3.5×10^{-6}M, 5×10^{-6}M, and 7×10^{-6}M, respectively. The most potent antagonist, however, was flunarizine with a K_D value of 7×10^{-7}M. This high sensitivity of hypothalamic neurons to 1,4-dihydropyridines contrasts to the insensitivity of DRG neurons.[54] High sensitivity of T channel current to Ca^{2+} antagonists is also revealed in vascular smooth muscle.[55] The comparison of nicardipine (and flunarizine) activities at T and L channels (TABLE 4) reveals that the inactivated state of the T channels is more sensitive to these antagonists than the resting state of the L channels. There are obvious and important pharmacologic implications to this relative sensitivity.

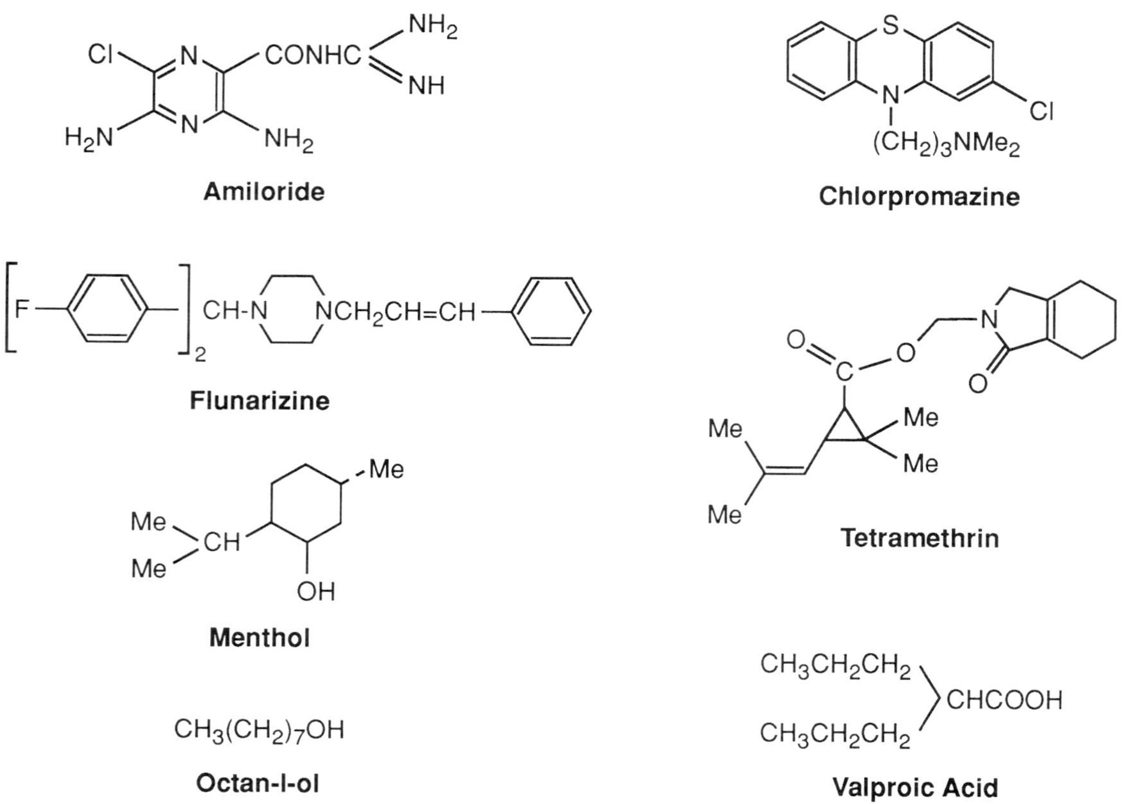

FIGURE 10. Structural formulas of drugs active at the T class of Ca^{2+} channel.

1,4-DIHYDROPYRIDINES AS GENERAL MODULATORS OF
VOLTAGE-GATED CHANNELS

That 1,4-dihydropyridines are effective at both T and L Ca^{2+} channel classes is plausible given the likely homology existing. It is likely that 1,4-dihydropyridines will be discovered that have activity at N channels. An important consideration will be whether the 1,4-dihydropyridine structure can be discretely optimized for each channel class.

By the same criterion it is also not unexpected that 1,4-dihydropyridines also serve as modulators of other classes of voltage-gated cation channels. Yatani and Brown[56] reported that nitrendipine blocked Na^+ channels in cardiac myocytes with a K_D value of 3×10^{-6}M at -80 mV. Of particular interest, the S and R enantiomers of Bay K 8644 behaved on Na^+ channels as activator and antagonist respectively, thus paralleling their behavior on Ca^{2+} channels.[57] The 1,4-dihydropyridine PD 122860 (ethyl-5-cyano-1,4-dihydro-6-methyl-2-[(4-pyridylsulfonyl) methyl]-4-(2-(trifluoro-

TABLE 4. Calculated Affinities of Nicardipine and Flunarizine for the Resting (R) and Inactivated (I) States of the L and T Channels of Vascular Smooth Muscle[55]

	L Channel			T Channel		
	R	K_D, nM	I	R	K_D, nM	I
Nicardipine	160		9	710		48
Flunarizine	90		11	137		19

methyl)phenyl)-3-pyridine carboxylate) exhibits Ca^{2+} channel blocking activity in the $(+)$-enantiomer and sodium channel, stimulating activity in both the $(+)$ and $(-)$ enantiomers.[58] Similarly, 1,4-dihydropyridines also modulate K^+ channels.[59-61] Niguldipine (3-methyl-5-[3-(4,4-diphenyl-1-piperidinyl)propyl]-1,4-dihydro-2,6-dimethyl-4-(3-nitrophenyl)-pyridine-3,5-dicarboxylate) is of particular interest because the $(+)$ and $(-)$ enantiomers are Ca^{2+} channel antagonists while serving as K^+ channel activator and antagonist, respectively.

REFERENCES

1. JANIS, R. A., P. SILVER & D. J. TRIGGLE. 1987. Drug action and cellular calcium regulation. Adv. Drug Res. **16:** 309–591.
2. TRIGGLE, D. J. 1990. Calcium antagonist drug development. Current Patents **1:** 365–384.
3. TRIGGLE, D. J. 1990. Calcium antagonists: history and perspective. Stroke. **21**(Suppl. IV): IV-49–IV-58.
4. FLECKENSTEIN, A. 1983. Calcium Antagonism in Heart and Smooth Muscle. Experimental Facts and Therapeutic Prospects. J. Wiley & Sons. New York.
5. TRIGGLE, D. J. & R. A. JANIS. 1987. Calcium channel ligands. Annu. Rev. Pharmacol. Toxicol. **27:** 347–369.
6. GLOSSMANN, H. & J. STRIESSNIG. 1989. Molecular properties of calcium channels. Rev. Physiol. Biochem. Pharmacol. **114:** 1–105.
7. CATTERALL, W. A. 1988. Structure and function of voltage-sensitive ion channels. Science **242:** 50–62.
8. SCOTT, R. H. & A. C. DOLPHIN. 1987. Activation of a G protein promotes agonist response to calcium channel ligands. Nature **330:** 760–762.

9. RAMPE, D. & D. J. TRIGGLE. 1989. 1,4-Dihydropyridine activators and antagonists: structural and functional distinctions. Trends Pharmacol. Sci. 10: 507–511.

10. PEREZ-REYES, E., H. S. KIM, A. E. LACERDA, W. HORNE, X. Y. WEI, D. RAMPE, K. P. CAMPBELL, A. M. BROWN & L. BIRNBAUMER. 1989. Indication of calcium currents by the expression of the alpha₁-subunit of the dihydropyridine receptor from skeletal muscle. Nature 340: 233–236.

11. MIKAMI, A., K. IMOTO, T. TANABE, T. NIIDOME, Y. MORI, H. TAKESHIMA, S. NARUMIYA & S. NUMA. 1989. Primary structure and functional expression of the cardiac dihydropyridine-sensitive calcium channel. Nature 340: 230–233.

12. SNUTCH, T. P., J. P. LEONARD, M. M. GILBERT, H. A. LESTER & N. DAVIDSON. 1990. Rat brain expresses a heterogeneous family of calcium channels. Proc. Natl. Acad. Sci. USA 87: 3391–3395.

13. ALKER, D., S. F. CAMPBELL, P. E. CROSS, R. A. BURGES, A. J. CARTER & D. G. GARDINER. 1990. Long-acting dihydropyridine calcium antagonists. 4. Synthesis and structure-activity relationships for a series of basic and nonbasic derivatives of 2-[(2-aminoethoxy)methyl]-1,4-dihydropyridine calcium antagonists. J. Med. Chem. 33: 585–591.

14. MILLER, R. J. 1987. Multiple calcium channels and neuronal function. Science 235: 46–52.

15. DREYER, E. B., P. K. KAISER, J. T. OFFERMANN & S. A. LIPTON. 1990. HIV-1 coat protein neurotoxicity prevented by calcium channel antagonists. Science 248: 364–367.

16. DEYO, R. A., K. T. STRAUBE & J. F. DISTERHOFT. 1989. Nimodipine facilitates trace conditioning of the eye-blink response in aging rabbits. Science 243: 809–811.

17. SCRIABINE, A., T. SCHUURMAN & J. TRABER. 1989. Pharmacological basis for the use of nimodipine in central nervous system disorders. FASEB J. 3: 1799–1806.

18. HONDEGHEM, L. M. & B. G. KATZUNG. 1985. Antiarrhythmic agents: the modulated receptor mechanisms of action of sodium and calcium channel blocking drugs. Annu. Rev. Pharmacol. Toxicol. 24: 387–423.

19. TRIGGLE, D. J. 1989. Structure-function correlations of 1,4-dihydropyridines calcium channel antagonists and activators. In Molecular and Cellular Mechanism of Antiarrhythmic Agents. L. Hondeghem, Ed.: 269–292. Futura Press. Mt. Kisco, NY.

20. FERRANTE, J. F. & D. J. TRIGGLE. 1990. Drug- and disease-induced regulation of voltage-dependent Ca^{2+} channels. Pharmacol. Rev. 42: 29–44.

21. BROWN, A. M. & L. BIRNBAUMER. 1990. Ionic channels and their regulation by G protein subunits. Annu. Rev. Physiol. 52: 197–214.

22. RAMPE, D. & D. J. TRIGGLE. 1990. New ligands for L-type Ca^{2+} channels. Trends Pharmacol. Sci. 11: 112–115.

23. TRIGGLE, D. J., D. A. LANGS & R. A. JANIS. 1989. Ca^{2+} channel ligands: structure-function relationship of the 1,4-dihydropyridines. Med. Res. Rev. 9: 123–180.

24. ARROWSMITH, J. E., S. F. CAMPBELL, P. E. CROSS, J. K. STUBBS, R. A. BURGES, D. G. GARDINER & K. J. BLACKBURN. 1986. Long acting dihydropyridine calcium antagonists. I. 2-Alkoxymethyl derivatives incorporating basic substituents. J. Med. Chem. 29: 1696–1702.

25. KWON, Y.-Y., X.-Y. ZONG, W. ZHENG & D. J. TRIGGLE. 1990. The interactions of 1,4-dihydropyridines bearing a 2-(2-aminoethylthio)-methyl substituent at voltage-dependent Ca^{2+} channels of smooth muscle, cardiac muscle and neuronal tissues. Naunyn-Schmiedeberg's Arch. Pharmakol. 341: 128–136.

26. KWON, Y. W., G. FRANCKOWIAK, D. A. LANGS, M. HAWTHORN, A. JOSLYN & D. J. TRIGGLE. 1989. Pharmacologic and radioligand binding analysis of 1,4-dihydropyridine activators related to Bay K 8644 in smooth muscle, cardiac muscle and neuronal preparations. Naunyn-Schmiedeberg's Arch. Pharmakol. 339: 19–30.

27. ATWAL, K. S., J. L. BERGER, A. HEDBERG & S. MORELAND. 1987. Synthesis and biological activity of novel calcium channel blockers: 2,5-dihydro-4-methyl-2-phenyl-1,5-benzothiazepine-3-carboxylic acid esters and 2,5-dihydro-4-methyl-2-ophenyl-1,5-benzodiazepine-3-carboxylic acid esters. J. Med. Chem. 30: 635–640.

28. TSUCHIDA, K., R. YAMAZAKI, K. KANBEKO & H. AIHARA. 1987. Effects of the new calcium antagonist 2-nitratopropyl-3-nitratopropyl-2,6-dimethyl-4-(3-nitrophenyl)-1,4-dihydropyridine-3,5-dicarboxylate on cerebral circulation in dogs. Arzheim. Forsch. 57: 1239–1243.

29. MURAMATSU, M., A. FUJITA-TOMINAGA, M. TANAKA, Y. ISHII & H. AIHARA. 1988. A new Ca antagonist, CD-349, binding to the Ca channel of rat myocardium and brain and hog coronary artery. Jpn. J. Pharmacol. **48:** 453–462.

30. STANTON, H. C., L. B. ROSENBERGER, R. C. HANSON, J. B. FLEMING & G. S. POINDEXTER. 1988. Pharmacology of BMY 20064, a potent Ca^{2+} entry blocker and alpha$_1$-adrenoceptor antagonist. J. Cardiovasc. Pharmacol. **11:** 387–395.

31. ENNIS, C., S. E. GRANGER, V. C. MIDDLEFELL, M. E. PHILPOT & N. B. STEPPERSON. 1989. Pharmacological effects of WY 27569: a combined calcium channel blocker and thromboxane synthetase inhibitor. J. Cardiovasc. Pharmacol. **13:** 511–519.

32. MARCINIAK, G., A. DELGADO, G. LECLERC, J. VELLY, N. DECKER & J. SCHWARTZ. 1989. New 1,4-dihydropyridine derivatives combining calcium antagonism and adrenolytic properties. J. Med. Chem. **32:** 1402–1407.

33. ASANO, M., W. VCHIDA, K. SHIBASAKI, M. TERAI, O. INAGAKI, T. TAKENAKA, Y. MATSU-MOTO & T. FUJIKURA. 1990. Pharmacological profiles of YM 16151-1 and its optical isomers: a novel calcium entry blocking and selective beta-1 adrenoceptor blocking agent. J. Pharmacol. Exp. Ther. **254:** 204–211.

34. STRIESSNIG, J., E. MEUSBURGER, M. GRABNER, H.-G. KNAUS, H. GLOSSMANN, J. KAISER, B. SCHOLKENS, R. BECKER, W. LINZ & R. HENNING. 1988. Evidence for a distinct Ca^{2+} antagonist receptor for the novel benzothiazinone compound HOE 166. Naunyn-Schmiedeberg's Arch. Pharmakol. **337:** 331–340.

35. QAR, J., J. BARHANIN, G. ROMEY, R. HENNING, U. LERCH, R. OEKONOMOPULOS, H. URBACH & M. LAZDUNSKI. 1988. A novel high affinity class of Ca^{2+} channel blocker. Mol. Pharmacol. **33:** 363–369.

36. GRASSEGER, A., J. STRIESSNIG, M. WEILER, H.-G. KNAUS & H. GLOSSMANN. 1989. [3H]HOE 166 defines a novel calcium antagonist drug receptor—distinct from the 1,4-dihydropyridine binding domain. Naunyn-Schmiedeberg's Arch. Pharmakol. **340:** 752–759.

37. NOKIN, P., M. CLINET, P. POLSTER, P. BEAUFONT, L. MEYSMANS, J. GOURGAT & P. CHATELAIN. 1989. SR 33557 a novel calcium antagonist: interaction with [3H]-(+)-nitrendipine and [3H]-(−)-desmethoxyverapamil binding sites in cerebral membranes. Naunyn-Schmiedeberg's Arch. Pharmakol. **339:** 31–36.

38. SCHMID, A., G. ROMEY, J. BARHANIN & M. LAZDUNSKI. 1989. SR 33557, an indolizine-sulfone blocker of Ca^{2+} channels: identification of receptor sites and analysis of its mode of action. Mol. Pharmacol. **35:** 766–773.

39. CARSON, J. R., H. R. ALMOND, M. D. BRANNAN, R. J. CARMOSIN, S. F. FLAIM, A. GILL, M. M. GLEASON, S. L. KEEL, D. W. LUDOVICI, P. M. PITIA, M. C. REBARCHAK & F. J. VILLANI. 1988. 2-Ethynylbenzenealkanamines. A new class of Ca^{2+} entry blocker. J. Med. Chem. **31:** 630–636.

40. RAMPE, D., A. SKATTEBOL, D. J. TRIGGLE & A. M. BROWN. 1988. Effects of McN 6186 on voltage-dependent Ca^{2+} channels in heart and pituitary cells. J. Pharmacol. Exp. Ther. **248:** 164–170.

41. FLAIM, S. F., M. T. STRANIERI, A. GILL, J. R. CARSON & M. D. BRANNAN. 1990. Effects of the novel coronary selective calcium channel blocker, McN 6186, on cardiocirculatory dynamics, coronary vascular resistance, and cardiac output distribution in normal conscious rats. J. Cardiovasc. Pharmacol. **15:** 780–790.

42. RAMPE, D., D. J. TRIGGLE & A. M. BROWN. 1987. Electrophysiologic and biochemical studies on the putative Ca^{2+} channel blocker MDL 12330A in an endocrine cell. J. Pharmacol. Exp. Ther. **243:** 402–407.

43. PALFREYMAN, M. G., M. W. DUDLEY, H. C. CHENG, A. K. MIR, S. YAMADA, W. R. ROESKE, T. OBATA & H. I. YAMAMURA. 1989. Lactamimides: a novel chemical class of calcium antagonists with diltiazem-like properties. Biochem. Pharmacol. **38:** 2459–2465.

44. KING, V. F., M. L. GARCIA, J. L. SHEVELL, R. S. SLAUGHTER & G. J. KACZOROWSKI. 1989. Substituted diphenylbutylpiperidines bind to a unique high affinity site on the L-type calcium channel. J. Biol. Chem. **264:** 5633–5641.

45. GOULD, R. J., K. M. M. MURPHY, I. J. REYNOLDS & S. H. SNYDER. 1983. Antischizo-

phrenic drugs of the diphenylbutylpiperidine type act as calcium channel antagonists. Proc. Natl. Acad. Sci. USA **80:** 5122–5125.

46. McKechnie, K., P. G. Killingback, I. Naya, S. E. O'Connor, G. W. Smith, D. G. Wattam, E. Wells, Y. M. Whitehead & G. E. Williams. 1989. Calcium channel activator properties in a novel non-dihydropyridine FBL 64176. Br. J. Pharmacol. **98:** 673P.

47. Tang, C.-M., F. Presser & M. Morad. 1988. Amiloride selectively blocks the low threshold (T) calcium channel. Science **240:** 213–215.

48. Tytgat, J., J. Vereeke & E. Carmeliet. 1990. Mechanism of cardiac T-type Ca channel blockade by amiloride. J. Pharmacol. Exp. Ther. **254:** 546–551.

49. Ogata, N. & T. Narahashi. 1990. Potent blocking action of chlorpromazine on two types of calcium channels in cultured neuroblastoma cells. J. Pharmacol. Exp. Ther. **252:** 1142–1149.

50. Kelly, K. M., R. A. Gross & R. L. Macdonald. 1990. Valproic acid selectively reduces the low threshold (T) calcium current in rat nodose neurons. Neurosci. Lett. **116:** 233–238.

51. Yoshii, M., A. Tsunoo & T. Narahashi. 1985. Effects of pyrethroids and veratridine on two types of Ca^{2+} channels in neuroblastoma cells. Soc. Neurosci. Abstr. **11:** 518.

52. Cohen, C. J., R. T. McCarthy, P. Q. Barrett & H. Rasmussen. 1988. Ca channels in adrenal glomerulosa cells: K^+ and angiotensin II increase T-type Ca channel current. Proc. Natl. Acad. Sci. USA **85:** 2142–2146.

53. Akaike, N., P. G. Kostyuk & Y. V. Osipchik. 1989. Dihydropyridine-sensitive low-threshold calcium channels in isolated rat hypothalamic neurons. J. Physiol. **412:** 181–195.

54. Fox, A. P., M. C. Nowycky & R. W. Tsien. 1978. Kinetics and pharmacological properties distinguishing three types of calcium currents in chick sensory neurons. J. Physiol. **394:** 149–172.

55. Kuga, T., J. I. Sadoshima, H. Tomoike, H. Kanaide, N. Akaike & M. Nakamura. 1990. Actions of Ca^{2+} antagonists on two types of Ca^{2+} channels in rat aorta smooth muscle cells in primary culture. Circ. Res. **67:** 469–480.

56. Yatani, A. & A. M. Brown. 1985. The calcium channel blocker nitrendipine blocks sodium channels in neonatal rat cardiac myocytes. Circ. Res. **57:** 868–875.

57. Yatani, A., D. L. Kunze & A. M. Brown. 1988. Effects of dihydropyridine calcium channel modulators on cardiac sodium channels. Am. J. Physiol. **254:** H140–147.

58. Haleen, S. J., R. P. Steffen, I. Sircar, T. C. Major, M. D. Taylor, T. A. Pugsley & R. E. Weishacr. 1989. PD 122860: A novel 1,4-dihydropyridine with sodium channel stimulating and calcium channel blocking properties. J. Pharmacol. Exp. Ther. **250:** 22–30.

59. Hume, J. R. 1985. Comparative interactions of organic Ca^{++} antagonists with myocardial Ca^{++} and K^+ channels. J. Pharmacol. Exp. Ther. **234:** 134–140.

60. Nerbonne, J. M. & A. M. Gurney. 1987. Blockade of Ca^{2+} and K^+ currents in hog cell neurons of *Aplysia californica* by dihydropyridine Ca^{2+} antagonists. J. Neurosci. **7:** 882–893.

61. Klockner, U. & G. Isenberg. 1989. The dihydropyridine niguldipine modulates calcium and potassium currents in vascular smooth muscle cells. Br. J. Pharmacol. **97:** 957–967.

G Protein Modulation of Calcium Entry and Transmitter Release[a]

ANNETTE C. DOLPHIN, ELAINE HUSTON,
HUGH PEARSON, ANATOLE MENON-JOHANSSEN,
MARVA I. SWEENEY, MICHAEL E. ADAMS,[b]
AND RODERICK H. SCOTT[c]

Department of Pharmacology
Royal Free Hospital School of Medicine
London NW3 2PF, United Kingdom

[b]Department of Entomology
University of California
Riverside, California 92521

[c]Department of Physiology
St. George's Hospital Medical School
London, W17 ORE, United Kingdom

MULTIPLE CLASSES OF VOLTAGE-DEPENDENT CALCIUM CHANNEL IN NEURONS

In many types of excitable cells, there are several classes of voltage-dependent calcium channel (VDCC) as determined by the characteristic properties of the single channel activity. There is a clear distinction between a low conductance channel activated by moderate depolarizations (low voltage–activated, LVA) and a high conductance channel activated by large depolarizations (high voltage–activated, HVA).[1,2] These have been termed T and L channels, respectively, and are pharmacologically, as well as biophysically, distinct.[2] Because of this they can also be clearly differentiated in whole-cell current recordings.[2,3] There is also evidence for a third class of single channel conductance (N-type), whose properties are intermediate between T and L, that appears to be expressed only in cells of neuronal origin.[3–5] Because of the lack of pharmacological tools, it remains difficult to distinguish the exact contribution of this channel to whole cell currents, although it is defined as an HVA current, insensitive to dihydropyridines. The sensitivity of N-type channels to ω-conotoxin,[4] and the large number of ω-conotoxin binding sites in neuronal tissue, indicates that they are likely to be important for neuronal function.[6] High threshold Ca^{2+} channels, however, insensitive to either ω-conotoxin or dihydropyridines have been reported,[4,7] and it is clear that new pharmacological agents are necessary to categorize VDCCs.

In an attempt to study new VDCC antagonists we have used purified peptide toxins from *Agelenopsis aperta* and examined their ability to block VDCCs in cultured rat dorsal root ganglia (DRG).[8] ω-Aga-IA (10 nM) inhibited by 80 ± 7% (n = 9) both dihydropyridine-sensitive and -insensitive components of high threshold cur-

[a]We thank the MRC and Wellcome Trust for support. M. I. Sweeney holds a Canadian MRC fellowship, and A. S. Menon-Johanssen is an MRC PhD student. We thank I. Pullar, Lilly Research (UK) Ltd., for providing the FTX analogue, arginine polyamine.

139

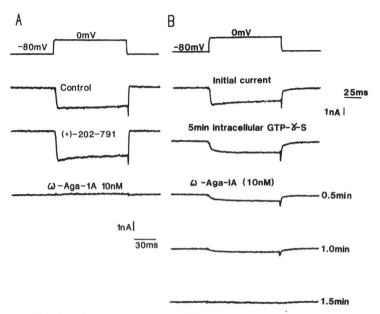

FIGURE 1. Blockade by ω-Aga-1A of the dihydropyridine-sensitive component of I_{Ba} and GTPγS-modified I_{Ba} in cultured rat DRGs. **A:** Control I_{Ba} activated at V_c 0 mV by 100 ms depolarizing voltage step commands. The dihydropyridine-sensitive component of I_{Ba} was enhanced by the agonist (+)-202-791 (5 μM) applied under conditions of low illumination. In the same cell ω-Aga-1A (10 nM) was then applied and, in this case, completely abolished I_{Ba} after 2 minutes. **B:** I_{Ba} was recorded 30 s after establishing whole-cell clamp (initial current) and after 5 min equilibration with the pipette containing 200 μM GTPγS. ω-Aga-1A (10 nM) was then applied and abolished the current over 1.5 minutes.

rent (FIG. 1A)[8] while having much less effect on T current[8] (46 $\pm$ 5% inhibition (n = 6)). It also inhibited I_{Ba} following G protein activation with GTPγS (FIG. 1B). We have also tested the synthetic arginine polyamine analogue of the polyamine toxin FTX[9] and found that it differentially inhibits T currents in rat DRG. At 10 nM it inhibited T current by 51 $\pm$ 1% (n = 4) over 3–5 min application while having no effect on high threshold current in the same cells (FIG. 2). At 100 nM, it reduced low threshold current by 58 $\pm$ 4% (n = 4) and high threshold current by 12 $\pm$ 3% (n = 6). At 10 μM a greater inhibition of high threshold current was produced (62 $\pm$ 4%, n = 5), but it was not specific for VDCCs in this concentration range, also affecting Ca^{2+} independent K^+ conductances. It is likely that toxins from *Agelenopsis aperta,* including ω-agatoxins, will be useful tools in defining functional roles for different subtypes of VDCC.

INHIBITION OF VDCCs BY PTX SUBSTRATE G PROTEINS

The direct interaction of PTX substrate G proteins with ion channels is now well-established. Evidence is fairly strong that G_i and G_o activate K^+ channels in a manner independent of any second messenger (for review, see ref. 11). Experiments have been performed with excised patches and purified and recombinant activated α

subunits in several tissues, including cardiac myocytes and hippocampal neurons. In the former, all species of α_i are effective, whereas in the latter, α_o is more effective than α_i.[12] Despite this evidence, the controversy concerning whether or not there is an additional involvement of $\beta\gamma$ and phospholipase A_2 has not yet been resolved.[9] As regards the direct interaction of VDCCs with these same G proteins, the situation remains much less clear. Although there is evidence from whole cell studies that calcium current inhibition by neurotransmitters in various neuronal and secretory cell types involves a PTX-sensitive G protein, there is no conclusive single channel data that a second messenger is not required.

Initial evidence came from studies of calcium currents in DRG neurons, in which noradrenaline acting at α_2-adrenergic receptors GABA and the GABA$_B$ analogue baclofen inhibit the current, and this can be mimicked by GTPγS (FIG. 1B) and inhibited by GDPβS and PTX.[14–16] Similarly, in the pituitary cell line At-T-20, the calcium current is inhibited by somatostatin and by GTP analogues.[17] The most marked effect, particularly of GTP analogues, is to slow current activation,[16] which was interpreted as an inhibition of N current (for review, see ref. 5), although pituitary cells have not been shown to possess N current.[17] More recently, it has been suggested that this slowed current activation is a result of voltage-dependent interaction between the activated G protein and the calcium channel (FIG. 3A and B).[18]

In the presence of internal GTPγS the calcium current often still has an initial rapidly activating, as well as a slowly activating, component, the fast component having a similar time constant to that in control cells, and probably representing channels that are not associated with, or modified by activated G protein.[19,20] In support of this idea, it is found that the slowly activating component increases in proportion with time after the start of dialysis with GTPγS, at the expense of the rapidly activating component.[16,20] The slowly activating component may represent channels that are associated with activated G protein and open with a slower time course upon depolarization. In some well-perfused cells the fast component is completely lost in the presence of GTPγS, indicating that all the VDCCs are potentially able to interact with activated G protein (Dolphin, unpublished results). The proportion of total current showing rapid, relative to slow, activation is not dependent on holding potential (V_H) between -30 and -90 mV;[20] in addition, Marchetti and Robello[20] and ourselves[21] have observed that the rate of activation of the slowly activating component is not dependent on holding potential between V_H -80 and -30 mV. These results suggest that the interaction of the closed resting

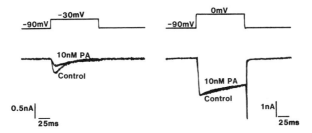

FIGURE 2. Differential inhibition by arginine-polyamine of low- compared to high-threshold I_{Ba}. The low-threshold T current (left) was activated at V_c -30 mV and the high-threshold current at 0 mV (right), in the same cell, held at -90 mV. Arginine polyamine (PA) was applied at 10 nM for 3 min and reduced T current with no effect on high-threshold current.

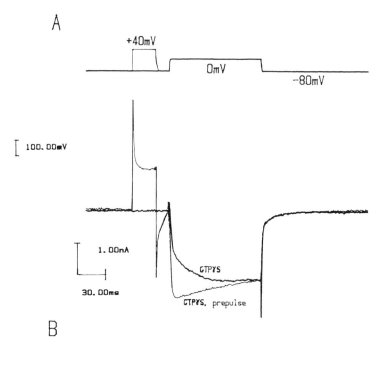

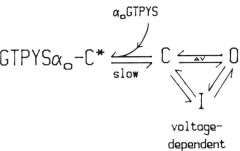

FIGURE 3. The effect of a 20 ms prepulse to +40 mV given 10 ms before the test pulse on the kinetics of activation of the test current. **A:** Recordings were performed in the presence of 200 μM GTPγS in the patch pipette. **B:** Scheme of activated G protein (α_0 GTPγS) binding to a closed state of the channel C to form C*.

state of the channel (C) with activated G protein (FIG. 3B) is not itself voltage-dependent,[19] and there is potentially a large excess of activated G protein.

We have hypothesized that activated G protein interacts with closed resting VDCCs to form a modified closed state C*, which may be unavailable to open with depolarization.[19] This complex, C*-G-GTPγS, can dissociate with a slow rate constant, and the free closed state C is then available to open as normal. Depolarization increases the rate of $C \rightarrow 0$, thus diminishing the pool of free C, and increasing the net rate of G-GTPγS-$C^* \rightarrow C$. From this model it is not necessary to postulate that this reaction is itself affected by voltage. In the experiments of Grassi and Lux[18] and Scott and Dolphin,[22] a brief prepulse to a large depolarizing voltage reversed the GTPγS- or agonist-induced slowing of current activation in a subsequent test pulse activated immediately afterwards (FIG. 3A). During the prepulse, the equilibrium $C^* \rightleftharpoons C \rightleftharpoons 0$ is shifted towards 0. At the end of the prepulse, $0 \rightarrow C$ occurs rapidly, but the rate of $C \rightarrow C^*$ is sufficiently slow that most of the channels remain as C at the time the test pulse is delivered. Thus current activation due to the test pulse occurs rapidly with this voltage paradigm.

Although the G protein involved in the inhibition of calcium currents is PTX-sensitive, the finding that PTX blocks the response to GTPγS[16] is controversial, in that PTX has been regarded as preventing receptor G protein interaction, but not GTPγS activation. It may be that a proportion of G proteins are associated with an empty receptor or with GAP-43, which has recently been shown to enhance GTPγS binding to G_o.[23] This interaction may allow GTPγS to activate the G protein and affect calcium currents in a PTX-sensitive manner. Indeed PTX also reduces basal GTP-ase activity in several systems.[24] The identification of the G protein involved in coupling receptors to Ca^{2+} current inhibition has been aided by experiments in which G proteins are included in the patch pipette when recording Ca^{2+} currents in PTX-treated cells. Exogenously added G proteins can restore the ability of neurotransmitters to inhibit Ca^{2+} currents. These experiments have generally suggested that G_o or its α subunit is more effective than G_i in restoring coupling.[25] In several systems the use of anti-G protein antibodies that inhibit function have confirmed that a G_o protein mediates inhibition of neuronal calcium currents by neurotransmitters.[26,27] We have investigated the ability of anti-G protein antibodies to prevent the effect of GTPγS in cultured rat DRG. The cells were replated before use by nonenzymatic removal from the culture dish. When this was done in the presence of IgG, it resulted in their entry into the cells by a form of scrape-loading. This was confirmed immunocytochemically. We have shown that an anti-G_o antipeptide antibody (OC1, provided by G. Milligan, Glasgow), when loaded into cells in this way, prevents the GTPγS-inducing slowing of the activation rate of Ca^{2+} channel currents in DRG (Menon-Johanssen *et al.*, in preparation). The activation time constant fitted to a single exponential was 1.7 ± 0.3 ms in control neurons, 3.0 ± 0.6 ms in the presence of GTPγS (200 μM) in the patch pipette, and 1.8 ± 0.2 ms in the presence of GTPγS in cells preloaded with OC1 antibody, (mean $\pm$ SEM, n = 5–8).

In several experiments it was observed that α_i species and anti-α_i antibodies were effective, although to a lesser extent than α_o[25,27] in reconstituting or blocking receptor-mediated VDCC inhibition. It has also been observed, however, that in a rat pituitary tumor cell line that possesses no G_o, dopamine does not inhibit prolactin release, whereas in another cell line containing G_o, dopamine is effective.[28] Thus it does not appear that G_i plays a major role in coupling to VDCCs.

POSSIBLE INVOLVEMENT OF A SECOND MESSENGER IN THE INHIBITION OF VDCCs BY PTX-SUBSTRATE G PROTEINS

There is no unequivocal evidence that the inhibition of neuronal VDCCs by neurotransmitters occurs by direct interaction with activated G protein α subunits, in an analogous way to G_s interaction with heart and skeletal muscle VDCCs, as well as G_i (and G_o) interaction with K^+ channels. Neither is there any universally accepted evidence, however, that a second messenger is involved in this process. Most evidence suggests that despite the fact that a PTX-sensitive G protein is involved, inhibition of adenylyl cyclase is not essential for the observation of a response, because it will still occur when cyclic AMP levels are elevated.[29] Nevertheless, the activity of L-type VDCCs in neurons, as in heart, is increased by cAMP-dependent phosphorylation,[30] and we have recently observed that forskolin is particularly able to increase Ca^{2+} channel currents in DRG by a process involving cyclic AMP–dependent phosphorylation following inhibition of the current by internal GTPγS.[31]

Several pieces of evidence suggest that, if there is a second messenger involved in the response to neurotransmitters, it is not readily diffusible, because the effect can be observed for baclofen and noradrenaline in cell-attached patches when the agonist is present in the patch pipette, but not when it is present in the bathing solution but excluded from the patch pipette.[32,33] It has been proposed that protein kinase C (PKC) activation may be involved in the neurotransmitter-mediated inhibition of calcium current.[34] PKC would be activated by diacylglycerol (DAG) formed by phospholipase C (PLC) activation. Receptor-mediated activation of PLC, however, is largely mediated by non-PTX sensitive G proteins in neuronal cells, and the neurotransmitters that activate PLC do not generally belong to the same subset as those inhibiting calcium currents.

Rane and Dunlap[34] demonstrated an inhibition of the sustained (L-type) Ca^{2+} current in chick DRG by phorbol esters and the synthetic DAG, although other groups have observed either no effect of PKC activators[29,35,36] or an activation of calcium currents[37] and single calcium channels.[38,39] In addition, PKC inhibitors, including H7 and staurosporine, were not observed to prevent neurotransmitter-mediated inhibition of calcium currents,[29] although Rane et al.[40] have shown peptide inhibitors of PKC to prevent noradrenaline-mediated inhibition of calcium currents. Hockberger et al.,[41] however, have suggested that a major effect of phorbol esters and synthetic DAGs is to inhibit calcium currents by an effect on the external cell membrane not involving PKC activation. Another complicating factor is that prolonged application of phorbol ester causes down-regulation of PKC by enhanced proteolysis of activated PKC.[42] This may be the reason why an initial increase in the open probability of VDCCs by phorbol esters was followed by an inhibition after a few minutes, suggesting a basal permissive effect of PKC-induced phosphorylation on VDCCs.[38]

Positive evidence that there is no second messenger involved in the G protein–mediated inhibition of VDCCs can only come from examining the effects of agonists on cell-free outside-out patches or GTP analogues on inside-out patches. This has been proven difficult because of the instability of HVA VDCCs from neuronal and secretory cells in cell-free systems. Even under these conditions, lipid-derived second messengers or processes such as dephosphorylation might still be implicated. More rigorous proof will come from systems in which cloned receptors, G proteins, and channels are reconstituted into lipid bilayers.

It is now clear that several other mechanisms for neurotransmitter-mediated inhibition of calcium currents are available, with an obligatory role for Ca^{2+}. Bradykinin inhibits Ca^{2+} but not Ba^{2+} currents, possibly by liberation of internal Ca^{2+} and Ca^{2+}-dependent inactivation of the current (McGuirk and Dolphin, unpublished results and ref. 29). Similarly, glutamate and quisqualate, acting at the G protein–coupled glutamate receptor, inhibit Ca^{2+} but not Ba^{2+} currents in hippocampal neurons.[43] The exact mechanism of this effect is unclear because both raised internal Ca^{2+} and activation of a G protein are required.

SECOND MESSENGER REGULATION OF VDCCs: CYCLIC AMP-DEPENDENT PHOSPHORYLATION

In several of the original studies of the properties of calcium currents in cardiac muscle, a very marked enhancement by cAMP was observed.[44,45] This is the major mechanism whereby β-adrenergic agonists enhance cardiac contractility, although evidence has now also been obtained for direct G_s-Ca channel coupling at the whole-cell level.[46] The second messenger effect results from a cascade consisting of G_s activation of adenylyl cyclase, cAMP activation of cAMP-dependent protein kinase (PKA), and phosphorylation of components associated with the Ca^{2+} channel. Following purification and reconstitution experiments using skeletal muscle VDCCs, several groups have come to the conclusion that L-type VDCCs must be phosphory-

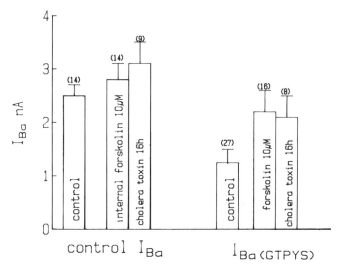

FIGURE 4. The amplitude of control calcium channel currents (I_{Ba}) or those in the presence of 200 μM GTPγS ($I_{Ba(GTPγS)}$) is shown under control conditions and in the presence of forskolin (10 μM) or following pretreatment of cells with cholera toxin (0.5 μg/mL for 16 h). Results are mean ± SEM of the number of experiments shown in parentheses.

lated to be functional,[47,48] as previously suggested from work on GH_3 cells by Armstrong and Eckert,[49] and that the residual activity of purified channels is due to incomplete channel dephosphorylation during the purification procedure. This is in contrast to the finding that a peptide inhibitor of cAMP-dependent protein kinase did not affect basal calcium currents, although it prevented the effect of β-adrenergic agonists.[50] It is extremely difficult, however, to abolish cAMP-dependent phosphorylation completely, and basal phosphorylation might also be subserved by PKC.[38]

Neuronal Ca^{2+} currents recorded at the whole-cell level are little affected by agents that increase cAMP[29,35,51] (FIG. 4), although at the single channel level, effects have been observed on hippocampal and sympathetic L-type channels.[30,39] These findings may indicate either that the channels are fully phosphorylated under control conditions, or that the structure of the majority of neuronal Ca^{2+} channels is sufficiently different not to be modulated by cAMP-dependent phosphorylation. A corollary of this latter hypothesis would be that there are few classical L-type channels in neurons. There are a large number of dihydropyridine (DHP) binding sites in neuronal tissue, however,[6] and antibodies to skeletal muscle DHP receptors precipitate a DHP receptor complex from neuronal tissue.[52] It has not yet been reported whether neuronal DHP receptors are substrates for PKA.

We have evidence supporting the hypothesis that neuronal VDCCs may normally be fully phosphorylated (particularly in the absence of Ca^{2+} to activate calcineurin). Forskolin, cholera toxin, and cAMP analogues normally produce only a small enhancement of the Ca^{2+} channel current in cultured rat DRG.[29] Following G protein activation with GTPγS in DRG, however, forskolin, and other means of enhancing intracellular cAMP, all increased the amplitude of the calcium channel current[29] (FIG. 4). The reason for this may be that activation of all neuronal G proteins by GTPγS results in some inhibition of adenylyl cyclase because GTPγS-activated $α_i$ will be in excess of $α_s$. This may result in a reduction in cyclic AMP–mediated phosphorylation, manifested as a reduction in the current amplitude.[29] This effect would be in addition to G_o-induced slowing of current activation (compare FIG. 3 with FIG. 5a). Forskolin, because of its ability to enhance G_s-GTPγS coupling to adenylyl cyclase,[53] would then markedly increase cAMP levels and possibly cause phosphorylation of a "difficult-to-phosphorylate" site on the calcium channel. We have also observed the increase in current amplitude caused by forskolin to be blocked by a peptide inhibitor of PKA.[31]

EFFECTS OF CALCIUM CHANNEL LIGANDS ON VDCCs

All DHP calcium channel ligands appear to have some ability to function both as agonists and as antagonists.[54] Even agonist optical isomers such as (+)-202-791 and (−)-Bay K8644 cannot be considered as pure agonists. Agonist activity is promoted at hyperpolarized membrane potentials,[54,55] whereas antagonist activity is promoted by depolarization and results from an increase in the proportion of time that channels remain in the closed state.[56] This has been interpreted as the binding of DHP antagonists to the inactivated state of the channel, resulting in its stabilization.[47,49,56]

Although the effects of DHP ligands and cAMP-dependent phosphorylation were initially thought to result from functionally different modifications of channel activity, there are now several pieces of evidence that suggest that there is an interaction between the two responses and a similarity between the effects of DHP agonists and cAMP-dependent phosphorylation at the single-channel level.[57] Armstrong and Eckert[49] showed Bay K8644 to increase VDCC activity only following channel phosphorylation and suggested that Ca^{2+} channel agonists bind only to phosphorylated channels and function by preventing dephosphorylation. Armstrong[58] has further suggested that DHP antagonists promote dephosphorylation by calcineurin and stabilize the dephosphorylated inactivated state of the channel.

At the whole-cell level, interactions have also been observed. Bay K8644 alone was found to enhance Ca^{2+} channel current amplitude, but also to accelerate inactivation, the latter probably being a reflection of its antagonist properties.[59] When cAMP levels were elevated, Bay K8644 not only further enhanced the current amplitude but also slowed the decay of the whole-cell current.

We have observed that the Ca^{2+} channel ligands (including nifedipine and (−)-202-791) showed marked agonist properties in the presence of internal GTPγS.[21,55] These agonist responses mimicked those of forskolin (FIG. 5B and C), and both were

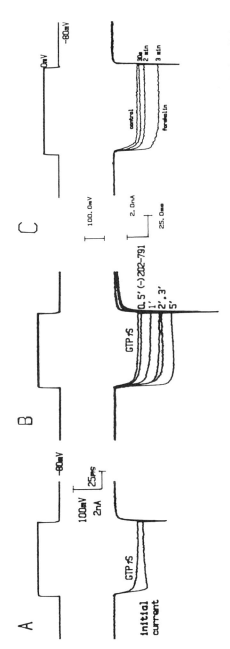

FIGURE 5. A comparison of the effect of (−)-202-791 and forskolin on $I_{Ba(GTP\gamma S)}$. **A:** The initial I_{Ba} is shown within 30 s of obtaining whole-cell clamp. The effect of 200 μM internal GTPγS is shown after 2 minutes. **B:** Application of (−)-202-791 (5 μM) to the same cell caused a slow increase in $I_{Ba(GTP\gamma S)}$ over 5 minutes. Scale bars refer to **A** and **B**. **C:** In a different cell, application of forskolin (10 μM) caused an increased in $I_{Ba(GTP\gamma S)}$ over 3 minutes. Scale bars on right refer to C.

blocked by Walsh inhibitor.[31] A possible explanation is that the calcium channel ligand alters the conformation of the channel such that a difficult-to-phosphorylate site becomes exposed. Further studies showed that both of these phosphorylation-dependent effects occurred only transiently or not at all at depolarized membrane potentials,[21,31] possibly because a larger proportion of channels are in the inactivated state under these conditions and are not available for phosphorylation.[49] Armstrong and Kalman[60] also attributed the voltage-dependence of binding of DHP antagonists to a voltage-dependent dephosphorylation of the channel.

WHICH TYPES OF VDCC CHANNEL MEDIATE TRANSMITTER RELEASE?

The release of neurotransmitters from presynaptic terminals is dependent on an influx of Ca^{2+} through VDCCs. Evidence concerning the subtype(s) of VDCC involved in transmitter release remains equivocal. It has been suggested that N channels are the most important[5,61] primarily because transmitter release is not markedly sensitive to DHP Ca^{2+} channel antagonists, although it is sensitive to agonists.[62] Because of the marked voltage-sensitivity of DHP antagonists,[54-56] however, they are poorly effective at hyperpolarized membrane potentials,[63] which may preclude their action on any L-type channels opening briefly at the nerve terminal. Indeed, we have recently observed that when cultured cerebellar neurons are maintained in a depolarized state in 50 mM K^+ and Ca^{2+}-free medium, and when glutamate release is stimulated by a brief pulse of 5 mM Ca^{2+}, this release is almost completely inhibited by DHP antagonists (FIG. 6A), the IC_{50} for $(-)$-202-791 being about 1 nM.[64] Thus these results indicate that L-type VDCCs are present at these glutamate-releasing terminals and are able to subserve transmitter release. It remains unclear whether release is normally poorly sensitive to DHP antagonists because it relies on Ca^{2+} entry through N channels that are unaffected by DHPs, or whether L channels are also involved in some systems but show little response to DHP antagonists during brief depolarizations.

The other agent that has been used to dissect out the channels involved in transmitter release is ω-conotoxin. This inhibits transmitter release in many, but by no means all, systems that have been investigated, but there is disagreement as to whether it selectively inhibits N channels[4] or whether L channels are also affected.[65] Although ω-conotoxin labels a different protein band from the DHPs, antibodies that immunoprecipitate 64% of brain DHP receptors also recognise 13% of ω-conotoxin binding sites.[52] Thus the diagnostic use of ω-conotoxin remains limited, and there is a need for a battery of other pharmacological tools, among which are likely to be the agatoxins.[8]

A further argument for the prime importance of N channels in the mediation of transmitter release is that "N current" can be inhibited by various neurotransmitters that also subserve presynaptic inhibition.[61] As discussed above, however, there is also evidence that inhibition of the transient component of whole-cell Ca current is due to a slow recovery from voltage-dependent block of the current, and that L current can also be inhibited by neurotransmitters. In addition, in recent experiments we have shown that $(-)$-baclofen is capable of inhibiting neurotransmitter release evoked by a pulse of 5 mM Ca^{2+} from cerebellar neurons maintained in a depolarized state in 50 mM K^+, Ca^{2+}-free medium. Under these conditions, the Ca channels involved are entirely nonvoltage-inactivated DHP-sensitive L-type channels[64] (FIG. 6B). Thus the involvement of different Ca channel types in physiological synaptic transmission and its inhibition by neurotransmitters remains an open question.

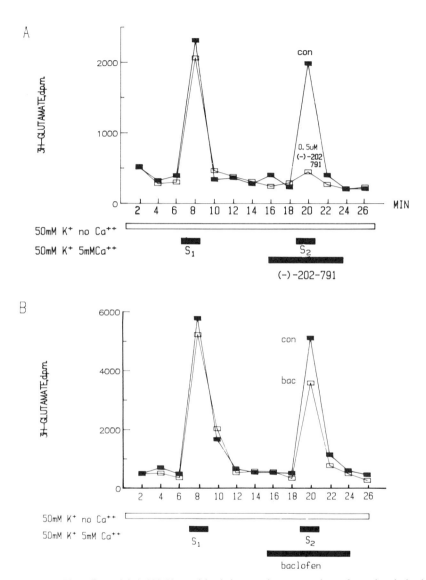

FIGURE 6. The effect of $(-)$-202-791 and baclofen on glutamate release from depolarized cerebellar granule neurons. Granule neurons were grown on coverslips for 7–15 days, and glutamate release was measured by preincubation of the neurons with [³H]glutamate as previously described.[66] Neurons were then maintained in a depolarizing medium containing 50 mM K^+ in the absence of Ca^{2+}. Glutamate release was then stimulated by 2 min incubation in a medium containing 50 mM K^+ together with 5 mM Ca^{2+}. Drugs were included before and during S_2. **A:** $(-)$-202-791 (0.5 μM) almost completely prevented glutamate release in S_2. **B:** Baclofen (100 μM) produced a 30% reduction of release in S_2.

THE ROLE OF G PROTEINS IN MEDIATING PRESYNAPTIC INHIBITION

In biochemical studies of neurotransmitter release, there are many examples of the ability of pertussis toxin to prevent presynaptic inhibition, particularly in cultured cells but also in brain slices.[66-69] By contrast, there is less electrophysiological evidence that presynaptic inhibition of synaptic potentials is prevented by pertussis toxin, although an early study showed that presynaptic inhibition of the twitch response in guinea pig ileum by opiates and the α_2 agonist clonidine was inhibited by pertussis toxin.[70] Colmers and Williams[71] showed that the 5HT inhibition of the excitatory postsynaptic potential recorded in dorsal raphe neurons upon local stimulation of slices was prevented by pertussis toxin. In addition Silinsky et al.[72] showed that pertussis toxin prevented adenosine inhibition of the mammalian motor nerve excitatory junction potential. The contradictory data relates particularly to $GABA_B$-mediated events. Whereas pertussis toxin has been shown to block the baclofen-mediated inhibition of noradrenaline, substance P, and glutamate release,[64,69] several studies have shown no effect of pertussis toxin on baclofen-mediated presynaptic inhibition of excitatory and inhibitory postsynaptic potentials.[71,73,74]

These findings suggest that biochemical measurements of the modulation of transmitter release, evoked either by elevated K^+ depolarization or by electrical stimulation by pulse trains, do not mimic well the process of synaptic release of transmitter. There are several possible explanations for the discrepancies outlined above. It may be that there is a large excess of G proteins in synaptic boutons, and only a small proportion of these are required to mediate a presynaptic inhibitory effect on the synaptic potential resulting from a single action potential. Because pertussis toxin treatment rarely results in complete ADP-ribosylation of all its substrate G proteins, particularly when applied to intact tissues, it is possible that sufficient G proteins remained unaffected. Penetration of pertussis toxin into presynaptic terminals may be less efficient than into postsynaptic elements. Another reason for the ineffectiveness of pertussis toxin might be that a proportion of G proteins in presynaptic terminals are tonically GTP-activated, and thus not substrates for pertussis toxin. The observation of an effect of pertussis toxin on presynaptic inhibitory responses may be favored in biochemical studies of neurotransmitter release because of the prolonged and repeated depolarizations used. It is likely that these studies will benefit from direct intraterminal recording of presynaptic currents.

REFERENCES

1. NILIUS, B., P. HESS, J. B. LANSMAN & R. W. TSIEN. 1985. Nature 316: 443–446.
2. BEAN, B. P. 1985. J. Gen. Physiol. 86: 1–30.
3. FOX, A. P., M. C. NOWYCKY & R. W. TSIEN. 1987. J. Physiol. (Lond.) 394: 149–172.
4. PLUMMER, M. R., D. E. LOGOTHETIS & P. HESS. 1989. Neuron 2: 1453–1463.
5. TSIEN, R. W., D. LIPSCOMBE, D. V. MADISON, K. R. BLEY & A. P. FOX. 1988. Trends Neurosci. 11: 431–438.
6. MARTIN-MOUTOT, N., M. SEAGAR & F. COURAUD. 1990. Neurosci. Lett. 115: 300–306.
7. LLINÁS, R., M. SUGIMORI, J. W. LIN & B. CHERKSEY. 1989. Proc. Natl. Acad. Sci. USA 86: 1689–1693.
8. SCOTT, R. H., A. C. DOLPHIN, V. P. BINDOKAS & M. E. ADAMS. 1990. Mol. Pharmacol. 38: 711–718.
9. CHERKSEY, B., R. LLINAS, M. SUGIMORI & J-W. LIN. 1989. Biol. Bull. (Woods Hole) 177: 121.

10. SCOTT, R. H., M. I. SWEENEY, A. C. DOLPHIN, G. H. TIMMS & I. A. PULLAR. 1991. J. Physiol. (Lond.) **434:** 29.
11. CODINA, J., A. YATANI, A. M. J. VAN DONGEN, E. PADRELL, D. CARTY, R. MATTERA, A. M. BROWN, R. IYENGAR & L. BIRNBAUMER. 1990. *In* G proteins. R. Iyengar & L. Birnbaumer, Eds.: 268–295. Academic Press.
12. VAN DONGEN, A., J. CODINA, J. OLATE, R. MATTERA, R. JOHO, L. BIRNBAUMER & A. M. BROWN. 1988. Science **242:** 1433–1437.
13. KIM, D., D. L. LEWIS, L. GRAZIADEI, E. J. NEER, D. BAR-SAGI & D. E. CLAMPHAM. 1989. Nature **337:** 557–560.
14. HOLZ, G. G., S. G. RANE & K. DUNLAP. 1986. Nature **319:** 670–672.
15. SCOTT, R. H. & A. C. DOLPHIN. 1986. Neurosci. Lett. **56:** 59–64.
16. DOLPHIN, A. C. & R. H. SCOTT. 1987. J. Physiol. (Lond.) **386:** 1–17.
17. LEWIS, D. L., F. F. WEIGHT & A. LUINI. 1986. Proc. Natl. Acad. Sci. USA **83:** 9035–9039.
18. GRASSI, F. & H. D. LUX. 1989. Neurosci. Lett. **105:** 113–117.
19. DOLPHIN, A. C. 1990. Biochem. Soc. Symp. **56:** 43–60.
20. MARCHETTI, C. & M. ROBELLO. 1989. Biophys. J. **56:** 1267–1272.
21. DOLPHIN, A. C. & R. H. SCOTT. 1989. J. Physiol. (Lond.) **413:** 271–288.
22. SCOTT, R. H. & A. C. DOLPHIN. 1990. Br. J. Pharmacol. **99:** 629–630.
23. STRITTMATTER, S. M., D. VALENZUELA, T. E. KENNEDY, E. J. NEER & M. C. FISHMAN. 1990. Nature **334:** 836–841.
24. MCLEISH, K., P. GIERSCHIK, T. SCHEPERS, D. SIDIROPOULOS & K. H. JAKOBS. 1989. Biochem. J. **260:** 427–434.
25. HESCHELER, J., W. ROSENTHAL, W. TRAUTWEIN & G. SCHULTZ. 1987. Nature **325:** 445–447.
26. HARRIS-WARWICK, R. M., C. HAMMOND, D. PAUPARDIN-TRITSCH, V. HOMBURGER, B. ROUOT, J. BOCKAERT & H. M. GERSCHENFELD. 1988. Neuron **1:** 27–32.
27. MCFADZEAN, I., I. MULLANEY, D. A. BROWN & J. MILLIGAN. 1989. Neuron **3:** 177–182.
28. COLLU, R., C. BOUVIER, G. LAGACE, C. UNSON, G. MILLIGAN, P. GOLDSMITH & A. SPEIGEL. 1988. Endocrinology **122:** 1176–1178.
29. DOLPHIN, A. C., S. M. MCGUIRK & R. H. SCOTT. 1989. Br. J. Pharmacol. **97:** 263–273.
30. GRAY, R. & D. JOHNSON. 1987. Nature **327:** 620–622.
31. DOLPHIN, A. C. 1991. J. Physiol. (Lond.) **432:** 23–43.
32. GREEN, K. A. & G. A. COTTRELL. 1987. Br. J. Pharmacol. **94:** 235–246.
33. LIPSCOMBE, D., S. KONGSAMUT & R. W. TSIEN. 1989. Nature **340:** 639–642.
34. RANE, S. G. & K. DUNLAP. 1986. Proc. Natl. Acad. Sci. USA **83:** 184–188.
35. MCFADZEAN, I. & R. J. DOCHERTY. 1989. Eur. J. Neurosci. **1:** 141–147.
36. WANKE, E., A. FERRONI, A. MALGAROLI, A. AMBROSINI, T. POZZAN & J. MELDOLESI. 1987. Proc. Natl. Acad. Sci. USA **84:** 4313–4317.
37. DOSEMECI, A., R. S. DHALLAN, N. M. COHEN, W. J. LEDERER & T. B. ROGERS. 1988. Circ. Res. **62:** 347–357.
38. LACERDA, A. E., D. RAMPE & A. M. BROWN. 1988. Nature **335:** 249–251.
39. LIPSCOMBE, D., K. BLEY & R. W. TSIEN. 1988. Soc. Neurosci. Abs. **14:** 64–12.
40. RANE, S. G., M. P. WALSH, J. R. MCDONALD & K. DUNLAP. 1989. Neuron **3:** 239–245.
41. HOCKBERGER, P., M. TOSELLI, D. SWANDULLA & H. D. LUX. 1989. Nature **319:** 670–672.
42. SHENOLIKAR, S., C. W. KARBON & S. J. ENNA. 1986. Biochem. Biophys. Res. Commun. **139:** 251–258.
43. LESTER, R. A. J. & C. E. JAHR. 1990. Neuron **4:** 741–749.
44. REUTER, H. 1983. Nature **301:** 569–574.
45. BRUM, G., W. OSTERRIEDER & W. TRAUTWEIN. 1984. Pflügers Arch. **401:** 111–118.
46. SHUBA, Y. M., B. HESSLINGER, W. TRAUTWEIN, T. F. MCDONALD & D. PELTZER. 1990. J. Physiol. **424:** 205–228.
47. TSIEN, R. W., B. P. BEAN, P. HESS, J. B. LANSMAN, B. NILIUS & M. C. NOWYCKY. 1986. J. Mol. Cell Cardiol. **18:** 691–710.
48. NUNOKI, K., V. FLORIO & W. A. CATTERALL. 1989. Proc. Natl. Acad. Sci. USA **86:** 6816–6820.
49. ARMSTRONG, D. & R. ECKERT. 1987. Proc. Natl. Acad. Sci. USA **84:** 2518–2522.

50. KAMEYAMA, M., J. HESCHELER, F. HOFMANN & W. TRAUTWEIN. 1986. Pflügers Arch. **405:** 285–293.
51. BLEY, K. R. & R. W. TSIEN. 1990. Neuron **4:** 379–391.
52. AHLIJANIAN, M. K., R. E. WESTENBROEK & W. A. CATTERALL. 1990. Neuron **4:** 819–832.
53. YAMASHITA, A., T. KUROKAWA, K. HIGASHI, I. DANURA & S. ISHIBASHI. 1986. Biochem. Biophys. Res. Commun. **137:** 190–194.
54. BROWN, A. M., D. L. KUNZE & A. YATANI. 1986. J. Physiol. (Lond.) **379:** 495–514.
55. SCOTT, R. H. & A. C. DOLPHIN. 1987. Nature **330:** 760–762.
56. HESS, P., J. B. LANSMAN & R. W. TSIEN. 1984. Nature **311:** 538–544.
57. YUE, D. T., S. HERZIG & E. MARBAN. 1990. Proc. Natl. Acad. Sci. USA **87:** 753–757.
58. ARMSTRONG, D. 1989. Trends Neurosci. **12:** 117–122.
59. TIAHO, F., S. RICHARD, P. LORY, J. M. NERBONNE & J. NARGEOT. 1990. Pflügers Arch. **417:** 58–66.
60. ARMSTRONG, D. & D. KALMAN. 1990. Biophys. J. **57:** 516a.
61. HIRNING, D., A. P. FOX, E. W. MCCLESKEY, B. M. OLIVERA, S. A. THAYER, R. J. MILLER & R. W. TSIEN. 1988. Science **239:** 57–61.
62. RANE, S. G., G. G. HOLZ & K. DUNLAP. 1987. Pflügers Arch. **409:** 361–366.
63. SANGUINETTI, M. C. & R. S. KASS. 1984. Circ. Res. **55:** 336–348.
64. HUSTON, E., R. H. SCOTT & A. C. DOLPHIN. 1990. Neurosci. **38:** 721–729.
65. MCCLESKEY, E. W., A. P. FOX, D. FELDMAN, L. Y. CRUZ, B. M. OLIVERA, R. W. TSIEN & D. YOSHIKAMI. 1987. Proc. Natl. Acad. Sci. USA **84:** 4327–4331.
66. DOLPHIN, A. C. & S. A. PRESTWICH. 1985. Nature **316:** 148–150.
67. ALLGAIER, C., T. J. FEUERSTEIN, R. JAKISCH & G. HERTTING. 1985. Naunyn-Schmiedeberg's Arch. Pharmakol. **331:** 235–239.
68. KAWATA, K. & Y. NOMURA. 1987. Neurosci. Res. **4:** 236–240.
69. HOLZ, G. G., R. M. KREAM, A. SPIEGEL & K. DUNLAP. 1989. J. Neurosci. **9:** 657–666.
70. TUCKER, J. F. 1984. Br. J. Pharmacol. **83:** 326–328.
71. COLMERS, W. F. & J. T. WILLIAMS. 1988. Neurosci. Lett. **93:** 300–306.
72. SILINSKY, E. M., C. SOLSONA & J. K. HIRSH. 1989. Br. J. Pharmacol. **97:** 16–18.
73. HARRISON, N. 1990. J. Physiol. (Lond.) **422:** 433–446.
74. DUTAR, P. & R. A. NICOLL. 1988. Neuron **1:** 535–538.

Inositol Trisphosphate/ Calcium-Dependent Acetylcholine Release Evoked by Bradykinin in NG108-15 Rodent Hybrid Cells

HARUHIRO HIGASHIDA[a] AND AKIHIKO OGURA[b]

[a]Department of Biophysics
Neuroinformation Research Institute
Kanazawa University School of Medicine
Kanazawa 920, Ishikawa, Japan

[b]Department of Neuroscience
Mitsubishi Kasei Institute of Life Sciences
Machida 194, Tokyo, Japan

INTRODUCTION

It is now generally agreed that the physiological stimuli for neurotransmitter secretion are Ca^{2+} ions that enter the cytoplasm through voltage-dependent Ca^{2+} channels (VDCCs) in the surface membrane activated by depolarization.[1,2] Little is known, however, about the mechanism(s) for the receptor-mediated facilitation of transmitter release. Recently a possibility has been suggested that a sustained increase of the cytosolic free Ca^{2+} concentration ($[Ca^{2+}]_i$) due to a Ca^{2+} release from intracellular Ca^{2+} storage sites by inositol-1,4,5-trisphosphate ($InsP_3$) plays a crucial role.[3]

In an NG108-15 cell,[4] a hybrid cell line derived from mouse neuroblastoma and rat glioma cells, the external application of bradykinin (BK) produces a biphasic change in membrane potential (a hyperpolarization followed by a depolarization) accompanied by an increase in acetylcholine (ACh) secretion.[5-8] BK also increases phosphatidylinositol-4,5-bisphosphate (PIP_2) degradation leading to the production of $InsP_3$ and diacylglycerol (DG).[6,9,10] The biphasic membrane potential change is due to the sequential activation and suppression of two membrane K^+-currents: a Ca^{2+}-dependent K^+-current and a so-called M current.[11,12] Previous examinations indicate that these effects of BK are mediated by $InsP_3$ and DG, respectively.[7,13,14]

The release of ACh from NG108-15 cells has several features advantageous for the study of the regulation of neurotransmitter secretion. (1) The hybrid cells have a low quantal content, so that the contribution of a Ca^{2+} influx accompanied by each individual action potential to ACh secretion does not much interfere receptor-operated secretion. (2) Because the ACh release from cell somata or from short neurites of NG108-15 cells is essentially the same nature as that from synapses formed at the terminals of long neurites, release processes in the cell soma can be considered equivalent to those at the terminals.[8] (3) A considerably large perikaryon of the cell allows experimental manipulations such as intracellular injections of chemicals.

Taking those advantages, we investigated physiological and biochemical consequences in the receptor-mediated regulation of neurotransmitter release at a single-cell level. In the present report, we added a further line of evidence to the above-mentioned hypothesis[15]: the neuromodulator presynaptically regulates the transmitter release by way of phosphoinositide turnover and cytoplasmic Ca^{2+} homeostasis.

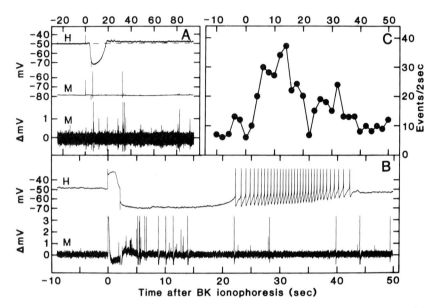

FIGURE 1. ACh release from NG108-15 cells in response to BK. **A:** Membrane potentials recorded simultaneously from the hybrid cell (H) and a paired myotube (M). Upper and lower recordings from M are DC- and AC-coupled recordings, respectively. BK was applied extracellularly to the hybrid cell soma by iontophoresis (20 nA for 5 s) at time zero. Hyperpolarization followed by depolarization was elicited with a delay of ca. 3 seconds. Note that a series of MEPPs were generated in M. **B:** Another hybrid cell exposed to BK (20 nA for 2 s; an initial depolarization is a recording artifact). Action potentials were elicited in M (AC-coupled recording) during the recovery phase of BK-induced hyperpolarization in H. Note that MEPPs were elicited during the hyperpolarization. **C:** MEPPs as a function of time after the application of BK. Data from 28 hybrid-myotube pairs that have one-to-one connections are plotted. Microelectrodes contained 3M KCl. Recordings were done with standard salt solution composed of (mM) NaCl (130), KCl (5.4), $CaCl_2$ (2), $MgCl_2$ (1), glucose (5.5), and Hepes-NaOH (10), pH 7.2, supplemented with additional 2 mM $CaCl_2$ and 0.1 mM choline chloride in this and following synapse assay experiments unless otherwise noted.

RESULTS

BK-Induced Transmitter Release

An iontophoretic application of BK to the extracellular surface of the cell soma of an NG108-15 cell produced a hyperpolarization of membrane potential followed by a depolarization (FIG. 1A). During this biphasic response, a series of miniature end-plate potentials (MEPPs) were recorded from the striated muscle cell that had been cocultured and paired with the NG108-15 cell for more than 2 weeks in the presence of 0.25–1.0 mM dibutyryl cyclic AMP.[6,8]

The BK-induced MEPP frequency increased 1.3–27-fold (6.9 ± 1.2; mean ± SEM, n = 29). The frequency increase started 2–5 s after the iontophoretic application of BK and peaked at 2–14 s when most of the hybrid cells underwent hyperpolarization (FIG. 1B) (due to the activation of Ca^{2+}-dependent K$^+$ channels); then the frequency gradually returned to the prestimulus level. This time course of the increase of MEPPs in response to iontophoretically applied BK in 28 hybrid/myotube pairs is shown in FIGURE 1C.

Though the frequency was lower than the initial phase, MEPPs were evoked at a higher rate than prestimulus level over the period of 20–50 s after the BK application (FIG. 1C). This period corresponds to the phase of depolarization where a train of action potentials were superposed in some of the specimens (FIG. 1B), indicating that it is due to a suppression of the M-current.[7,13]

BK-Induced ACh Release in the Absence of Potential Changes in Hybrid Cells

To examine whether the membrane potential changes induced by BK contribute to the ACh secretion, especially in their early phase, synaptic activities were assayed under conditions where the membrane hyperpolarization was modified by pharmacological means.

First we used phorbol-12,13-dibutyrate (PDBu) to potentiate the BK-induced hyperpolarization, because it is known that PDBu itself induces a depolarization in unclamped membrane leading to the suppression of the BK-induced depolarization.[13,14,16] In FIGURE 2, the BK application elicited MEPPs in the myotube during the initial hyperpolarization phase of the hybrid cell, which had been treated with 1 μM PDBu for 30 minutes. No apparent change was seen in the MEPP frequency, although the hyperpolarization was prolonged and enhanced (compare FIG. 2A with 2B).

On the other hand, the BK-induced hyperpolarization of the hybrid cell was suppressed by 4 mM Ba^{2+}, a K$^+$-channel blocker[12,17] (FIG. 2C and D). The MEPP frequency increased beginning 2–10 s after the BK application and lasted for 10–30 seconds. The mean latency and duration of the MEPP appearance in the presence of Ba^{2+} was 7.2 ± 5.1 and 20 ± 9 s, respectively. These values correspond well to the mean latency and duration of the BK-induced hyperpolarization in its absence (8.1 ± 3.2 and 21 ± 10 s, respectively). No increase was observed in MEPP frequency during the late phase with (FIG. 2C) or without (FIG. 2D) the BK-induced depolarization under the presence of Ba^{2+}. These observations strongly suggest that the initial facilitation induced by BK normally accompanied by hyperpolarization of the hybrid cell does not depend on the membrane potential change per se.

BK-Induced Increase of [Ca^{2+}]$_i$

Fura-2 is a fluorescent Ca^{2+} indicator applicable to the study on a single-cell level.[18] With a digital processing of fluoromicroscopic images, it is possible to reveal the intracellular spatial distribution of [Ca^{2+}]$_i$ in parallel with the monitoring membrane potential.[19] As was already mentioned, NG108-15 hybrid cells responded to an external perfusion of BK with a transient rise in [Ca^{2+}]$_i$,[15,20,21] and the [Ca^{2+}]$_i$ rise in response to BK was observed whether the membrane potential was clamped (FIG. 3A and B) or unclamped (FIG. 3D; see also FIG. 3 in ref. 15). The mean peak level of $[Ca^{2+}]_i$ in 61 individual unclamped NG108-15 cells challenged to 1 μM BK was 227 ± 9 nM in contrast to 75 ± 2 nM of the resting state, when monitored at the cells' central parts.

The rise reached the peak in 2.8 ± 0.2 s, followed by a gradual decay. The time for recovery to the half level of the peak $[Ca^{2+}]_i$ was 11.1 ± 0.5 seconds. The state of

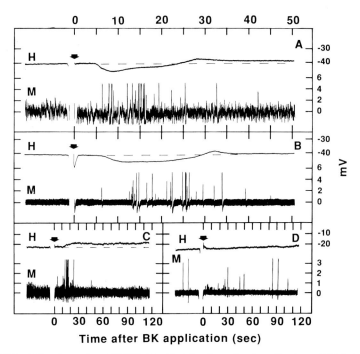

FIGURE 2. ACh release from NG108-15 cells following a focal application of BK before (**A**) and after (**B**) treatment with PDBu or Ba^{2+} (**C,D**). Each panel shows membrane potentials recorded from a pair of a hybrid cell (H) and a myotube (M) connected by a short neurite (<20 μm). The resting potentials of H and M were −41 and −53 mV, respectively, for **A** and **B**, and both of those were −22 mV for **C** and **D**. Recordings in H and M were done in a DC-coupled and a high-gain AC-coupled mode, respectively. BK (3 μL of 10 mM solution) was applied at the timings indicated by arrows. Recording **B** was done in the same specimen as in **A** after a 30 min treatment with 1 μM PDBu. In **C** and **D**, two different cell pairs were exposed to a medium supplemented with 4 mM $BaCl_2$, where the BK-induced hyperpolarization of the hybrid cells was abolished, whereas MEPPs were evoked at the "right" time point in muscle cells.

raised $[Ca^{2+}]_i$ thus lasted for approximately 30 seconds. The rise was transient so that the decay of $[Ca^{2+}]_i$ began even in the presence of BK. The hyperpolarization always started after the rise in $[Ca^{2+}]_i$; the mean latency was 0.5 ± 0.2 s (n = 10). The time course of hyperpolarization nearly paralleled that of the $[Ca^{2+}]_i$ rise; however, the duration of the hyperpolarization was shorter in most cases because the hyperpolarization was overridden by the subsequent depolarization.

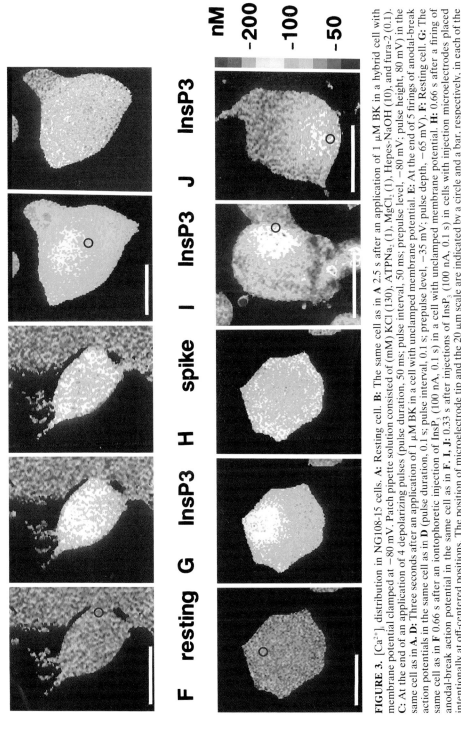

FIGURE 3. [Ca²⁺]ᵢ distribution in NG108-15 cells. **A:** Resting cell. **B:** The same cell as in **A** 2.5 s after an application of 1 μM BK in a hybrid cell with membrane potential clamped at −80 mV. Patch pipette solution consisted of (mM) KCl (130), ATPNa₂ (1), MgCl₂ (1), Hepes-NaOH (10), and fura-2 (0.1). **C:** At the end of an application of 4 depolarizing pulses (pulse duration, 50 ms; pulse interval, 50 ms; prepulse level, −80 mV; pulse height, 80 mV) in the same cell as in **A**. **D:** Three seconds after an application of 1 μM BK in a cell with unclamped membrane potential. **E:** At the end of 5 firings of anodal-break action potentials in the same cell as in **D** (pulse duration, 0.1 s; pulse interval, 0.1 s; prepulse level, −35 mV; pulse depth, −65 mV). **F:** Resting cell. **G:** The same cell as in **F** 0.66 s after an iontophoretic injection of InsP₃ (100 nA, 0.1 s) in a cell with unclamped membrane potential. **H:** 0.66 s after a firing of anodal-break action potential in the same cell as in **F**. **I, J:** 0.33 s after injections of InsP₃ (100 nA, 0.1 s) in cells with injection microelectrodes placed intentionally at off-centered positions. The position of microelectrode tip and the 20 μm scale are indicated by a circle and a bar, respectively, in each of the cells.

The topographical distribution of $[Ca^{2+}]_i$ rise on the application of BK differed from that due to the activity of VDCCs (FIG. 3C and E; see also FIG. 3 in ref. 15). The $[Ca^{2+}]_i$ elevation began from the deep compartment of the cell in response to BK, whereas the action potential–induced $[Ca^{2+}]_i$ rise began from the submembranous compartment. (Note that the fluorograph is a two-dimensional projection of a cell of hemispheric shape so that a shell-formed distribution of a high $[Ca^{2+}]_i$ layer should result in a ring-formed image of a high $[Ca^{2+}]_i$ area). The results indicate that BK-receptor stimulation is converted to an intracellular signal in the term of Ca^{2+}.

Intracellular Ca^{2+} Injection Mimics MEPP Facilitation

To test the role of Ca^{2+}, the divalent cation was iontophoretically injected into the cytoplasm of NG108-15 cells through a second glass capillary filled with 0.5 M $CaCl_2$. A train of MEPPs was evoked during the current passage (FIG. 4). This persisted only for a few seconds, probably because of rapid diffusion of Ca^{2+}. Then the cell was hyperpolarized, which results from the activation of Ca^{2+}-dependent K^+ channels.[22,23] Hence this indicates effective release of Ca^{2+} from the pipette into the cytoplasm.

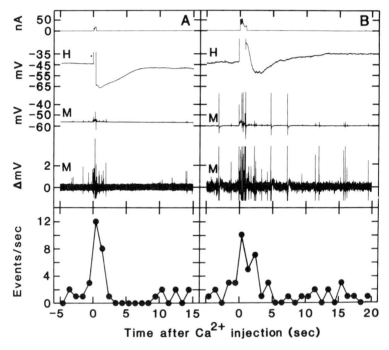

FIGURE 4. MEPPs evoked by intracellular injections of Ca^{2+} into NG108-15 cells. Recordings **A** and **B** were obtained from two different pairs. Uppermost traces indicate iontophoretic currents for Ca^{2+} iontophoresis, which were +20 nA for 0.5 s in **A** and +50 nA for 1 s in **B**. The second traces (H) from the top are membrane potentials of the hybrid cells. The third and fourth traces (M) are membrane potentials of myotubes recorded in DC- and AC-modes, respectively. Bottom histograms show the numbers of MEPPs plotted for 1 s sampling intervals after the Ca^{2+} injections.

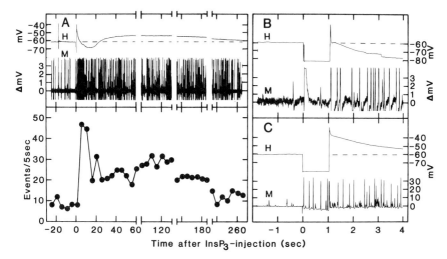

FIGURE 5. MEPPs triggered by InsP$_3$ injections into NG108-15 cells. Recordings in **A, B,** and **C** were obtained from separate pairs between a hybrid cell (H) and a myotube (M). In **A,** InsP$_3$ was injected by a negative current pulse (-50 nA, 1 s) at time zero. Prolonged depolarization was elicited in the hybrid cell preceded by an initial depolarization and a transient hyperpolarization. Histogram at bottom shows the occurrence of MEPPs sampled for 5 s intervals. Note two phases in the InsP$_3$-induced increase in MEPP frequency. **B** and **C:** MEPP occurrence immediately after the InsP$_3$ injection. **B** represents the case with no initial depolarizing phase, whereas **C** indicates the case with a significant initial depolarization. Note that MEPPs were generated in M during either the depolarizing or the hyperpolarizing phase in presynaptic hybrid cells (H).

The mean MEPP frequency increased by 3.9 $\pm$ 0.6-fold (n = 6) following Ca^{2+} injections. Similar iontophoretic injections of K$^+$ cations (from a pipette filled with 3 M KCl) did not produce any comparable effect.

Microinjection of InsP$_3$ Induces ACh Release

Because BK stimulates the conversion of InsP$_3$ and DG from PIP$_2$ in NG108-15 cells[9,10] and because injected InsP$_3$ raises [Ca^{2+}]$_i$,[24] intracellular injections of InsP$_3$ are expected to result in ACh secretion. The expectation was confirmed (FIG. 5). The InsP$_3$ injection into an NG108-15 cell initiated a burst of MEPPs in the muscle cell during the hyperpolarization in the NG108-15 cell (FIG. 5A and B). The frequency increase of MEPPs was 3.1 $\pm$ 0.35-fold (n = 17) over the preinjection frequency. The minimum latency for the appearance of MEPPs after InsP$_3$ injections was 0.2–0.5 s, which was shorter than that by BK receptor stimulation and longer than that by Ca^{2+} injection. In addition to this, MEPPs persisted during the subsequent depolarization that occasionally followed the hyperpolarization.

Injection of InsP$_3$ with a large current often produced a long-lasting depolarization first rather than a hyperpolarization, which presumably was due to an activation of Ca^{2+}-dependent nonspecific cation channels[13,23] (see next section). MEPPs were vigorously evoked in the muscle cell during the initial depolarizing phase of the hybrid cell (FIG. 5C). The results again indicate that facilitation of ACh release from

NG108-15 cells, induced by InsP$_3$ injection in this case, does not largely depend upon cell membrane potentials.

$[Ca^{2+}]_i$ Rise from the InsP$_3$ Injection Site

When InsP$_3$ was intracellularly introduced into an NG108-15 cell by iontophoresis, a $[Ca^{2+}]_i$ elevation occurred up to 200–500 nM (FIG. 3F and G) as shown previously.[23,24] The magnitude of the elevation depended upon the dose of injected InsP$_3$: twenty nM of $[Ca^{2+}]_i$ per nC of iontophoresing current (FIG. 6B). Similarly, injected inositol-4,5-bisphosphate (InsP$_2$) (FIG. 6A) or inositol-1,3,4,5-tetrakisphosphate (InsP$_4$) (FIG. 6C) produced no comparable $[Ca^{2+}]_i$ elevation, confirming the previous observation that InsP$_4$ failed to activate Ca^{2+}-dependent K$^+$ channels in NG108-15 cells.[23]

Sites of the preferred $[Ca^{2+}]_i$ rise upon InsP$_3$ injection differed from those following action potentials as well (FIG. 3H). In all specimens examined, the $[Ca^{2+}]_i$ rise began at the location of a pipette tip (FIG. 3G, I, and J), whether the tip was placed at the center or periphery of the cell. This suggests that InsP$_3$ receptors, which were recently demonstrated in NG108-15 cells[25] and Ca^{2+}-storage sites, distribute rather homogeneously over the cytoplasm in the cells. This is in contrast to the

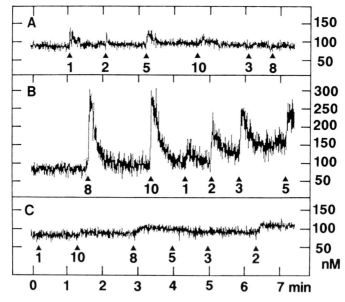

FIGURE 6. $[Ca^{2+}]_i$ rises accompanied by the injections of inositol polyphosphates (InsP$_x$) into NG108-15 cells. InsP$_x$s were iontophoretically injected into the cells from microelectrode pipettes filled with 1 mM aqueous solutions of InsP$_x$ (Boehringer) at the timings indicated by arrows. Digits indicate the amount of iontophoresed charge in 10^{-8} coulombs ($0.1 \mu A \times 0.1$–1 s). Injected InsP$_x$ was inositol-4,5-bisphosphate (**A**), inositol-1,4,5-trisphosphate (**B**), and inositol-1,3,4,5-tetrakisphosphate (**C**). Note the dose-dependent $[Ca^{2+}]_i$ rise for InsP$_3$. Small dose-independent Ca^{2+} rises in the cases of InsP$_2$ and InsP$_4$ were due to firings of anodal-break action potentials.

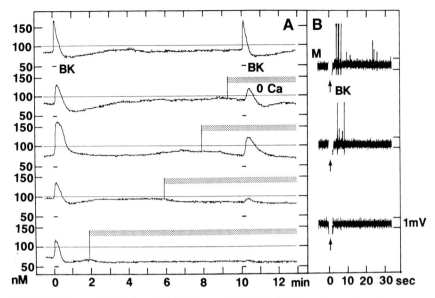

FIGURE 7. Loss of BK-induced $[Ca^{2+}]_i$ rise and MEPP facilitation after prolonged exposures to Ca^{2+}-depleted medium. **A:** Ca^{2+}-depleted medium ($CaCl_2$ was withdrawn from, and 0.1 mM EGTA was supplemented to, the standard salt solution) was perfused in the periods indicated by dotted bars. BK was applied at 0 min and 10 min for 15 s each. Note that the second response to BK was gradually diminished with a progress of external Ca^{2+} deprivation. All records were carried out in one NG108-15 cell. **B:** From top to bottom, BK-induced MEPP facilitation before, and 5 and 15 min after exposure to the Ca^{2+}-free medium. BK was applied at 0 seconds.

situation of chromaffin cells, where the possible Ca^{2+} storage sites localize in the limited compartment of the cell.[26]

The rising phase of $[Ca^{2+}]_i$ induced by InsP₃ injections with an appropriate dose coincided in time with the cell's hyperpolarization, whereas an injection of InsP₃ with a relatively large current occasionally produced the initial membrane depolarization (FIG. 5A). The $[Ca^{2+}]_i$ rise had already started in the period of the InsP₃ injection and developed markedly during the initial depolarization. This, however, should give an explanation for the facilitation during the InsP₃-induced initial depolarization (FIG. 5C), assuming the causal relationship of the $[Ca^{2+}]_i$ rise in ACh secretion.

If BK exerts its facilitatory effect on ACh release by way of InsP₃ production, downstream from the receptor stimulation, a cross-talk (mutual desensitization) is observable between InsP₃ injection and BK application. This was ascertained (cf. FIG. 6B in ref. 15). The magnitude of the InsP₃-induced $[Ca^{2+}]_i$ rise and hyperpolarization immediately after the BK application was smaller than the average of isolated injections. The reverse was also true: the BK receptor stimulation was less effective when applied immediately after the InsP₃ injection (data not shown).

Effects of Extracellular Ca^{2+} on BK-Induced ACh Release

Although the source of Ca^{2+} in the BK-induced $[Ca^{2+}]_i$ elevation appeared to be intracellular storage,[27] the responsiveness to BK diminished when external Ca^{2+} was removed. As seen in FIGURE 7A, the BK-induced $[Ca^{2+}]_i$ elevation significantly diminished by an 8-min exposure to a Ca^{2+}-free milieu and mostly disappeared in 12 minutes. Reintroduction of Ca^{2+} in the medium partially restored the responsiveness (cf. FIG. 7A in ref. 15). In accordance to that, the removal of external Ca^{2+} (replaced with Mg^{2+}) suppressed the BK-induced increase of MEPP frequency in 15 min (FIG. 7B).

Do these results suggest that an entry of Ca^{2+} through VDCCs contributes to the BK response? The following evidence, however, led us to see that the intracellularly stored Ca^{2+} could be easily emptied by depletion of external Ca^{2+}; in other words, there would be a rapid exchange of internal and external Ca^{2+}.[27]

Depletion of Ca^{2+} for a shorter period (5 min) produced little effect, although Ca^{2+}-dependent action potentials were quickly suppressed. Perfusion with 0.5 mM Cd^{2+} in a dose effective to block VDCCs did not inhibit the BK-induced facilitation of MEPPs (data not shown).

A rapidly inactivating low-threshold VDCC and a slowly inactivating high-threshold VDCC were activated by depolarization steps from a holding potential of -50 to -70 mV before and during the application of BK to NG108-15 cells. The Ca^{2+} currents through both VDCCs were suppressed during the period where the BK-induced outward current persisted (FIG. 8). The examination of current-voltage

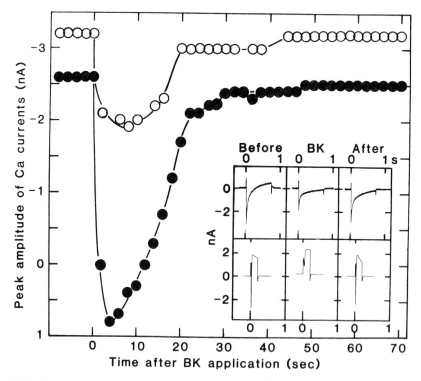

FIGURE 8. Inhibition in two types of Ca^{2+} currents after BK application in NG108-15 cells. Low-threshold Ca^{2+} currents (● and lower panel in the inset) were evoked by 200 ms voltage steps to -30 mV from a holding potential of -70 mV. High threshold Ca^{2+} currents (○ and upper panel in the inset) were evoked by 700 ms voltage commands to $+20$ mV from the same holding potential. Recording solutions for the high-threshold current are identical to those reported.[29]

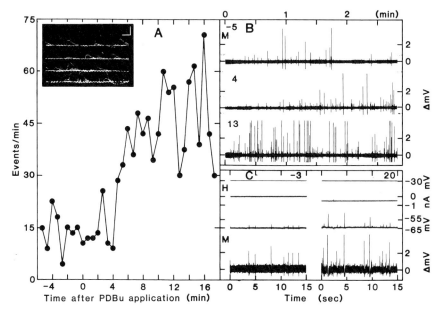

FIGURE 9. Effect of phorbol dibutyrate (PDBu) on MEPPs. An NG108-15/myotube pair was exposed to 1 μM PDBu at time zero. **A:** Increase in MEPP frequency after the PDBu treatment. Representative MEPPs 9 min after PDBu are shown in inset. Calibration, 20 ms, 5 mV. **B:** MEPPs recorded from other myotubes at different times as indicated (5 min before, 4 and 13 min after the PDBu treatment). The membrane potential of the presynaptic hybrid cell was not clamped. **C:** Effect of PDBu on MEPPs when the hybrid cell's potential was clamped at −30 mV. Records were obtained 3 min before and 20 min after the PDBu treatment. The second trace from the top shows a PDBu-induced inward current.

curves revealed that the degree of suppression was approximately proportional to the peak Ca^{2+} current (cf. FIG. 11 of ref. 12). Although the mechanism of the BK-induced suppression of VDCCs is unknown, this result again excludes the view that BK would increase the Ca^{2+} influx through VDCCs.

Late Effect of BK

The BK-receptor activation leading to the production of InsP$_3$ should be accompanied by the equimolar production of DG. Assuming the late effects of BK, the slow membrane depolarization and the sustained facilitation of MEPPs (FIG. 1), as the causal effects of DG, we applied PDBu, a protein kinase C activator,[28] on the present NG108-15/myotube system to see whether the drug mimics the late effects of BK. Within 3–5 min after perfusion with PDBu, the frequency of MEPPs started to increase and reached a plateau after 8–10 min (FIG. 9A). Some MEPPs after PDBu exposure are shown in FIGURE 9B. The frequency increase was also observed when the cell was voltage-clamped at −30 mV (FIG. 9C), indicating that the increase of synaptic responses after PDBu treatment is not simply due to the cell depolarization.

Then the next question raised is whether this PDBu facilitation of MEPPs is caused also by an elevation of [Ca^{2+}]$_i$. We found that PDBu failed to elevate [Ca^{2+}]$_i$ in

NG108-15 cells regardless of how the membrane potential was clamped (FIG. 10) or unclamped (cf. FIG. 6 in ref. 15), confirming the previous report.[21]

In the cells after the PDBu exposure, it might be expected that the Ca^{2+} influx through the VDCC was much enhanced due to, for example, a possible phosphorylation of the channel molecule; thereby the coupling between Ca^{2+} influx and ACh release would be enhanced. FIGURE 10 shows, however, that this was not the case. Rather, both the influx of Ca^{2+} and the magnitude of $[Ca^{2+}]_i$ elevation per depolarizing pulse decreased during the PDBu response. As a consequence, it is suggested that DG directly influences the machinery of ACh release to enhance the probability of exocytosis.

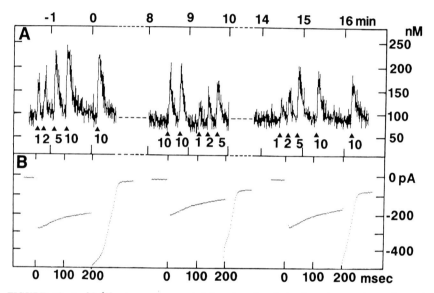

FIGURE 10. A: $[Ca^{2+}]_i$ rises accompanied by step depolarizations in a voltage-clamped NG108-15 cell before, during, and after application of 1 μM PDBu. PDBu was included in the perfusion medium at 0 min and washed out at 10 minutes. The cell was depolarized by a command pulse to 0 mV for various periods at the timings indicated by triangles from a holding potential of −60 millivolts. The duration of applied pulses in 10^{-1} s is shown under each triangle. Traces are intersected twice for saving space. B: Inward Ca^{2+} currents were elicited by test pulses to 0 mV for 0.2 s before, during, and after the application of PDBu in the same cell shown in A. External solution contained (mM) NaCl (120), $CaCl_2$ (5), KCl (5), tetraethylammonium chloride (10), 4-aminopyridine (0.1), tetrodotoxin (0.001), and Hepes-NaOH (10), pH 7.2. Patch pipette solution consisted of (mM) CsCl (130), $ATPNa_2$ (1), $MgCl_2$ (1), Hepes-NaOH (10), pH 7.2 and fura-2 (0.1).

CONCLUSION

The present results indicate that the increased level in $InsP_3$ following the activation of BK receptors leads to the enhancement of ACh exocytosis from the NG108-15 neuroblastoma × glioma hybrid cell. The data suggest that the facilitation of ACh release is due primarily to an increase in cytoplasmic free Ca^{2+}, mobilized from InsP$_3$-sensitive intracellular Ca^{2+}-storage sites. The BK-induced membrane potential change, either depolarization or hyperpolarization, is not the cause of [Ca^{2+}]$_i$ elevation but rather its result. The direct administration of InsP$_3$ into the cytoplasm of the presynaptic hybrid cell thus replicates the BK-induced facilitation of MEPP in the postsynaptic muscle cell, regardless of the accompanying changes of presynaptic membrane potential. The proposed consequence is

$$BK \rightarrow Ins\ P_3 \rightarrow [Ca^{2+}]_i\ rise \underset{Hyperpolarization}{\overset{ACh\ release}{\lessgtr}}.$$

If the late effect of BK is integrated in this scheme, a slight modification is to be added:

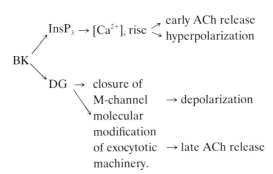

The mechanism underlying presynaptic facilitation after a repetitive nerve excitation (posttetanic potentiation) is thought to be mediated by a maintenance of the elevated [Ca^{2+}]$_i$ level due to a large influx of Ca^{2+} that surpasses a limited rate of sequestration. This is a so-called *residual Ca^{2+} hypothesis.*[1,2] In the case of BK-induced facilitation, the sustained elevation of [Ca^{2+}]$_i$ is crucial as well, but it is caused not by an influx of Ca^{2+} but by an InsP$_3$-dependent liberation of stored Ca^{2+}. We like to designate this mechanism as an *InsP$_3$-mediated residual Ca^{2+} hypothesis.*

REFERENCES

1. KATZ, B. & R. MILEDI. 1968. The role of calcium in neuromuscular facilitation. J. Physiol. (Lond.) **195:** 481–492.
2. LLINÁS, R. R. & J. E. HEUSER. 1977. Depolarization-release coupling systems in neurons. Neurosci. Res. Program Bull. **15:** 563–687.
3. BERRIDGE, M. J. 1986. Cell signalling through phospholipid metabolism. J. Cell Sci. (Suppl.) **4:** 137–153.
4. NIRENBERG, M., S. WILSON, H. HIGASHIDA, A. ROTTER, K. KRUEGER, N. BUSIS, R. RAY, J. G. KENIMER & M. ADLER. 1983. Modulation of synapse formation by cyclic adenosine monophosphate. Science **222:** 794–799.
5. REISER, G. & B. HAMPRECHT. 1982. Bradykinin induced hyperpolarizations in rat glioma cells and in neuroblastoma x glioma hybrid cells. Brain Res. **239:** 191–199.
6. YANO, K., H. HIGASHIDA, R. INOUE & Y. NOZAWA. 1984. Bradykinin-induced rapid breakdown of phosphatidylinositol 4,5-bisphosphate in neuroblastoma x glioma hybrid NG108-15 cells. J. Biol. Chem. **259:** 10201–10207.
7. HIGASHIDA, H., R. A. STREATY, W. KLEE & M. NIRENBERG. 1986. Bradykinin-activated transmembrane signals are coupled via No or Ni to production of inositol 1,4,5-trisphosphate, a second messenger in NG108-15 neuroblastoma-glioma hybrid cells. Proc. Natl. Acad. Sci. USA **83:** 942–946.

8. HIGASHIDA, H. 1988. Acetylcholine release by bradykinin, inositol 1,4,5-trisphosphate and phorbol dibutyrate in rodent neuroblastoma cells. J. Physiol. (Lond.) **397:** 209–222.

9. YANO, K., H. HIGASHIDA, H. HATTORI & Y. NOZAWA. 1985. Bradykinin-induced transient accumulation of inositol trisphosphate in neuron-like cell line NG108-15 cells. FEBS Lett. **181:** 403–406.

10. FU, T., Y. OKANO & Y. NOZAWA. 1988. Bradykinin-induced generation of inositol 1,4,5-trisphosphate in fibroblasts and neuroblastoma cells: effects of pertussis toxin, extracellular calcium, and down-regulation of protein kinase C. Biochem. Biophys. Res. Commun. **157:** 1429–1435.

11. BROWN, D. A. & H. HIGASHIDA. 1988. Voltage- and calcium-activated potassium currents in mouse neuroblastoma x rat glioma hybrid cells. J. Physiol. (Lond.) **397:** 149–165.

12. BROWN, D. A. & H. HIGASHIDA. 1988. Membrane current responses of NG108-15 mouse neuroblastoma x rat glioma hybrid cells to bradykinin. J. Physiol. (Lond.) **397:** 167–184.

13. BROWN, D. A. & H. HIGASHIDA. 1988. Inositol 1,4,5-trisphosphate and diacylglycerol mimic bradykinin effects on mouse neuroblastoma x rat glioma hybrid cells. J. Physiol. (Lond.) **397:** 185–207.

14. HIGASHIDA, H. & D. A. BROWN. 1986. Two polyphosphatidylinositide metabolites control two K$^+$ currents in a neuronal cell. Nature **323:** 333–335.

15. OGURA, A., Y. MYOJO & H. HIGASHIDA. 1990. Bradykinin-evoked acetylcholine release via inositol trisphosphate-dependent elevation in free calcium in neuroblastoma x glioma hybrid NG108-15 cells. J. Biol. Chem. **265:** 3577–3584.

16. HIGASHIDA, H. & D. A. BROWN. 1987. Bradykinin inhibits potassium (M) currents in N1E-115 neuroblastoma cells. FEBS Lett. **220:** 302–306.

17. ADAMS, P. R., D. A. BROWN & A. CONSTANTI. 1982. Pharmacological inhibition of the M-current. J. Physiol. (Lond.) **332:** 223–262.

18. GRYNKIEWICZ, G., M. POENIE & R. Y. TSIEN. 1985. A new generation of Ca^{2+} indicators with greatly improved fluorescence properties. J. Biol. Chem. **260:** 3440–3450.

19. KUDO, Y. & A. OGURA. 1986. Glutamate-induced increase in intracellular Ca^{2+} concentration in isolated hippocampal neurones. Br. J. Pharmacol. **89:** 191–198.

20. OSUGI, T., T. IMAIZUMI, A. MIZUSHIMA, S. UCHIDA & H. YOSHIDA. 1987. Phorbol ester inhibits bradykinin-stimulated inositol trisphosphate formation and calcium mobilization in neuroblastoma × glioma hybrid NG108-15 cells. J. Pharmacol. Exp. Ther. **240:** 617–622.

21. REISER, G. & B. HAMPRECHT. 1985. Bradykinin causes a transient rise of intracellular Ca^{2+}-activity in cultured neuronal cells. Pflügers Arch. **405:** 260–264.

22. HIGASHIDA, H. & D. A. BROWN. 1988. Ca^{2+}-dependent K$^+$ channels in neuroblastoma hybrid cells activated by intracellular inositol trisphosphate and extracellular bradykinin. FEBS Lett. **238:** 395–400.

23. HIGASHIDA, H. & D. A. BROWN. 1986. Membrane current responses to intracellular injections of inositol 1,3,4,5-tetrakisphosphate and inositol 1,3,4-trisphosphate in NG108-15 hybrid cells. FEBS Lett. **208:** 283–286.

24. OSUGI, T., S. UCHIDA, T. IMAIZUMI & H. YOSHIDA. 1986. Bradykinin-induced intracellular Ca^{2+} elevation in neuroblastoma x glioma hybrid NG108-15 cells; relationship to the action of inositol phospholipid metabolites. Brain Res. **379:** 84–89.

25. FURUICHI, T., S. YOSHIKAWA, A. MIYAWAKI, K. WADA, N. MAEDA & K. MIKOSHIBA. 1989. Primary structure and functional expression of the inositol 1,4,5-trisphosphate-binding protein P$_{400}$. Nature **342:** 32–38.

26. O'SULLIVAN, A. J., T. R. CHEEK, R. B. MORETON, M. J. BERRIDGE & R. D. BURGOYNE. 1989. Localization and heterogeneity of agonist-induced changes in cytosolic calcium concentration in single bovine adrenal chromaffin cells from video imaging of fura-2. EMBO J. **8:** 410–411.

27. BERRIDGE, M. J. & R. F. IRVINE. 1989. Inositol phosphates and cell signalling. Nature **341:** 197–205.

28. NISHIZUKA, Y. 1986. Studies and perspectives of protein kinase C. Science **233:** 305–312.

29. FISHMAN, M. C. & I. SPECTOR. 1981. Potassium current suppression by quinidine reveals additional calcium currents in neuroblastoma cells. Proc. Natl. Acad. Sci. USA **78:** 5245–5249.

Inhibition of Synaptic Transmission and Calcium Currents in Cultured Hippocampal Neurons[a]

KENNETH P. SCHOLZ AND RICHARD J. MILLER

Department of Pharmacological and Physiological Sciences
The University of Chicago
Chicago, Illinois 60637

The inhibition of excitatory junction potentials at the crayfish neuromuscular junction was analyzed by application of the principles of quantal analysis by Dudel and Kuffler[1] and found to arise from a presynaptic mechanism. Since then, the inhibition of neurotransmitter release at presynaptic nerve terminals has been studied at many synapses ranging from crayfish neuromuscular junction to mammalian central synapses. At the crayfish neuromuscular junction, the release of an inhibitory neurotransmitter from a nearby inhibitory motor neuron is believed to open Cl-permeable channels in or near the terminal of the excitor neuron, thereby leading to shunting of the action potential and inhibition of calcium influx and transmitter release from the excitatory neuron.[2] Presynaptic inhibition that follows fundamentally similar principles is found throughout the nervous system.

At many synapses, a fundamentally different form of presynaptic inhibition occurs. For example, presynaptic inhibition of excitatory synaptic potentials (EPSPs) or currents (EPSCs) following activation of type B gamma-aminobutyric acid (GABAb) receptors occurs at the synapses between CA3 and CA1 hippocampal pyramidal neurons.[3] Similar examples have been observed throughout the central and peripheral nervous system. This latter form of presynaptic inhibition does not involve the direct neurotransmitter gating of a membrane ion channel. Rather, the neurotransmitter involved often has multiple actions (see ref. 4).

Due to the numerous actions of transmitters that induce the second type of presynaptic inhibition, the precise mechanisms that are responsible for the inhibition of transmitter release are unknown. At least three major hypotheses exist, which are not mutually exclusive. These are discussed below with regard to presynaptic inhibition induced by adenosine receptors in the hippocampus.

(1) Many neurotransmitters that induce presynaptic inhibition, including adenosine, activate a membrane K^+ channel.[4] This action has been studied in considerable detail. Furthermore, inhibition of labeled rubidium efflux has been observed to occur concomitant with inhibition of neurotransmitter release in synaptosome preparations.[5] Thus, it has been proposed that this K^+ current may act by decreasing the presynaptic spike, thereby decreasing the influx of Ca^{2+} into the terminal and reducing transmitter release.

(2) Adenosine agonists have been shown to inhibit voltage-gated calcium currents in peripheral neurons[6,7] that undergo presynaptic inhibition by these same agents. Whether this also occurs in central neurons has been controversial. The

[a]Address correspondence to Kenneth P. Scholz, Department of Pharmacological and Physiological Sciences, The University of Chicago, 947 E. 58th St. Chicago, IL 60637.

inhibition of calcium channels at the presynaptic terminal has been postulated to be involved in presynaptic inhibition.

(3) An undefined intracellular component of the vesicle release process has also been postulated to be involved in the inhibition of transmitter release.[8] The best evidence for this to date has been obtained in invertebrate neurons in culture. Release of vesicles from several types of endocrine cells and brain synaptosomes, however, can also be regulated by a mechanism that occurs "downstream" from Ca^{2+} influx across the plasma membrane.[9] Unfortunately, very little is known about the molecular mechanisms involved in this process.

This chapter describes some of our recent attempts to address some of these issues in hippocampal pyramidal neurons in cell culture. Because the K^+ currents in the soma have been studied in detail in the past, we will focus on the inhibition of Ca^{2+} currents (I_{Ca}) in the soma. This will be followed by a description of experiments in which single monosynaptic connections were observed. Finally, we will turn to recordings of spontaneous miniature excitatory synaptic currents (mEPSCs) used to begin assessing the roles of I_{Ca} inhibition and intracellular mechanisms in the inhibition of transmitter release. These discussions will focus on the actions of adenosine receptor agonists.

Whole-cell voltage clamp recordings of somatic membrane currents in cultured hippocampal pyramidal neurons revealed that adenosine receptor agonists were capable of inducing inhibition of I_{Ca}. FIGURE 1A shows the current responses of a neuron to depolarizing pulses from a holding potential of -80 mV to test potentials ranging from -70 to $+40$ mV with 2 mM Ba^{2+} as the charge carrier through Ca channels. The addition of the A1 selective adenosine receptor agonist cyclopentyl-adenosine (CPA, 100 nM) reduced the current (FIG. 1B). This agent also slowed the rate of activation of I_{Ca} at intermediate test potentials. For example, at a test potential of -20 mV, CPA shifted the time to peak from 23 ± 2.2 ms in control traces to 59 ± 6.5 milliseconds. This effect was much more evident when Ba^{2+} was used as the charge carrier than when Ca^{2+} was used. The inhibition of I_{Ca} by CPA has been shown to be due to inhibition of I_{Ca} and not to activation of K^+ current in poorly clamped neuronal processes.[10]

CPA is a selective A1 adenosine receptor agonist. The results of FIGURE 1 give strong support to the conclusion that the inhibition of I_{Ca} by adenosine in these cells is due to the activation of A1 receptors. Further support for this conclusion was obtained by using the A1 selective antagonist cyclopentyltheophylline (CPT). FIG-URE 2 shows the inhibition of I_{Ca} obtained in the presence of 1 μM 2-cl-adenosine (a non-selective adenosine agonist) in the presence of CPT (0.1 μM). These results indicate that the inhibition of I_{Ca} by adenosine receptors in these cells is due to activation of A1 type receptors.

As an initial examination of the role of intracellular messengers in the generation of a cellular response following activation of the cell-surface receptor, we treated the neurons with pertussis toxin (PTX) several hours prior to the experiments. PTX was able to completely abolish the actions of CPA (FIG. 3), indicating that a G protein of the G_i or G_o subclass is involved in this action.

In order to compare the inhibition of I_{Ca} in the soma to the inhibition of transmitter release at the presynaptic terminal, we began by investigating the properties of synaptic transmission between pyramidal neurons in culture. FIGURE 4 shows a whole-cell current clamp recording of a pyramidal neuron in culture. Stimulation of an action potential by passing depolarizing current through the pipette produced a prolonged depolarization arising from excitatory synaptic input back onto the cell under observation. This indicated that the cell participated in an excitatory neuronal circuit that may synapse onto itself. Addition of the excitatory

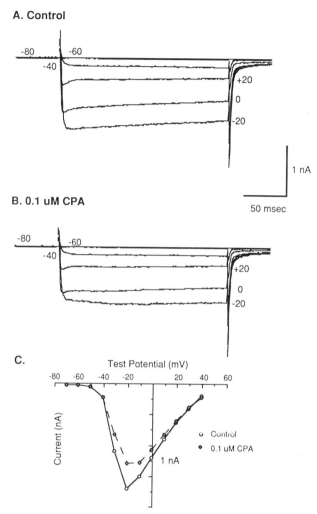

FIGURE 1. Inhibition of barium currents by the A1-selective adenosine agonist CPA (0.1 μM). Current responses in a voltage-clamped pyramidal neuron to the indicated test potentials from a holding potential of -80 mV in the absence (**A**) and presence (**B**) of CPA. **C:** Plot of inward current at 10 ms after initiation of the test pulse under control and experimental conditions (from traces in **A** and **B**).

amino acid receptor antagonists CNQX and APV abolished the synaptic input onto this cell and revealed that the same depolarizing stimulus could now elicit several spikes. These results indicate that the cells form excitatory synapses that release an amino acid neurotransmitter.

When the cultures are exposed to solutions deprived of Mg^{2+}, the cells begin to fire bursts of action potentials that can be monitored noninvasively by recording the resulting Ca^{2+} elevations using the Ca^{2+} indicator dye fura-2.[11] This activity arises, at

0.1 uM CPT

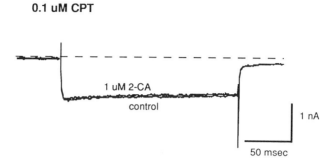

FIGURE 2. Inhibition of the actions of adenosine receptor agonists by the A1 selective antagonist cyclopentyltheophylline (CPT). In the presence of 0.1 μM CPT, 2-cl-adenosine (2-CA) was without effect.

least in part, from enhanced current flowing through NMDA receptor channels at the postsynaptic membrane following release of an excitatory amino acid from the presynaptic terminal. We have used this property to begin an investigation of presynaptic inhibition in this system. Addition of 2-CA reduces the elevations of Ca^{2+} induced by Mg^{2+}-deprived solutions (FIG. 5a). In addition, this action is blocked by preincubation of the cells with PTX (FIG. 5B).

Whole-cell voltage-clamp recordings of evoked monosynaptic currents also revealed that 2-CA inhibited synaptic potentials, as has been shown in hippocampal slice preparations. This action was shown to arise from presynaptic inhibition of transmitter release.[10,12] In addition, this action has pharmacological properties that are identical to those found for inhibition of I_{Ca} in the soma. There has been considerable controversy concerning the sensitivity of this action to PTX.[13,14] We have found that the presynaptic inhibition of transmitter release by adenosine in cultured hippocampal pyramidal neurons is inhibited by pretreatment with PTX.[10] These results indicate that inhibition of I_{Ca} at the presynaptic terminal cannot be ruled out as a major player in the inhibition of transmitter release in this system. Indeed, the results suggest that this process may be very important for presynaptic inhibition.

PTX

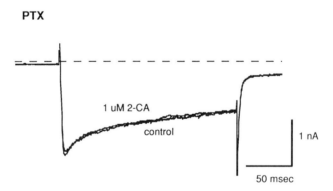

FIGURE 3. The inhibition of calcium current by adenosine analogues is blocked by pretreatment of the cells with pertussis toxin (PTX, 250 ng/mL).

To examine further the role of inhibition of I_{Ca}, as well as the possible role of inhibition of an intracellular component of the release process in presynaptic inhibition, we have turned to whole-cell recordings of spontaneous mEPSCs. This phenomenon was first described by Katz and his colleagues[15] at the neuromuscular junction and is widely believed to reflect release of single synaptic vesicles into the synaptic cleft. These events have a number of useful properties. For example, the frequency of occurrence of mEPSCs is independent of the properties of the postsynaptic membrane,[16] and can thus be used to obtain specific information about the

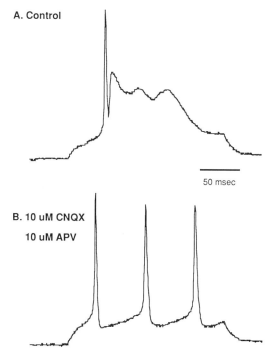

FIGURE 4. Whole-cell current clamp recording of evoked action potentials in a cultured pyramidal neuron. **A:** In control conditions, a 200 ms current stimulus evokes a single action potential that is followed by numerous synaptic potentials. **B:** Addition of the glutamate receptor antagonists CNQX and APV at the indicated concentrations blocks the synaptic potentials allowing for multiple spikes in response to the current stimulus.

vesicle release process at the presynaptic terminal. In addition, although influx of Ca^{2+} at the presynaptic terminal can stimulate the release of vesicles, mEPSCs can still be observed even after blockade of Ca^{2+} influx.[17] This may be a result of the basal Ca^{2+} levels in the terminal setting a specific probability of release, or possibly from cytosolic fluctuations of intracellular Ca^{2+} resulting from release from a Ca^{2+} store. Nevertheless, these events can be used to assay the efficacy of the release process in the absence of Ca^{2+} influx across the plasma membrane. FIGURE 6A demonstrates that mEPSCs can be recorded in cultured pyramidal neurons and that the frequency

A. Control

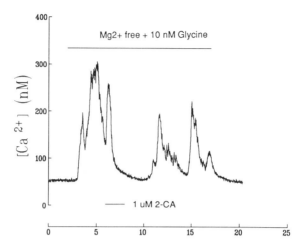

B. PTX

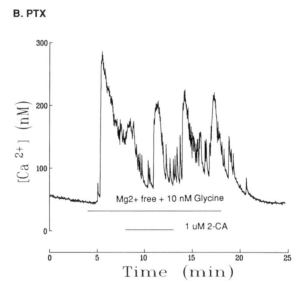

Time (min)

FIGURE 5. Removal of extracellular Mg^{2+} in the presence of glycine causes an increase in the activity of synaptically coupled pyramidal neurons as monitored with the Ca^{2+}-indicator dye fura-2. **A:** Addition of 2-CA to the chamber reduces the synaptic activity of the cells. **B:** Pretreatment of the cultures with PTX blocks the actions of 2-CA.

of occurrence is reduced in the presence of CPA (FIG. 6B). To begin examining if the release process itself is affected independent of Ca^{2+} influx, these experiments were repeated while the cells were bathed in 2 mM Mn^{2+} to block Ca^{2+} influx. Under these conditions, CPA was still able to reduce the frequency of mESPCs, but to a lesser degree. Although Mn^{2+} is generally considered to inhibit Ca^{2+} influx through voltage-gated channels, there is one report suggesting that it may permeate and activate vesicle release.[18] Clearly, further experiments with other Ca^{2+} channel antagonists will be necessary to clarify this issue. These results suggest, however, that CPA may inhibit a component of the release apparatus, possibly by altering the sensitivity to Ca^{2+} (see ref. 8). These experiments also indicate, however, that other events are likely to be important for the inhibition of transmitter release.

The results presented here demonstrate that activation of adenosine A1 receptors in hippocampal pyramidal neurons in cell culture leads to inhibition of I_{Ca} in these cells. This action requires the presence of a PTX-sensitive G protein. Likewise,

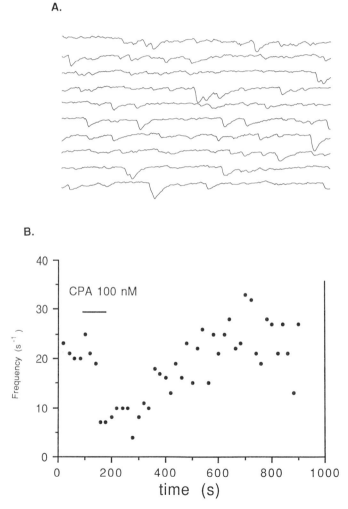

FIGURE 6. Adenosine analogues reduce the frequency of mEPSCs. **A:** Whole-cell voltage clamp recording of spontaneous mEPSCs. **B:** Frequency versus time plot of mEPSC occurrence. Application of CPA reduces the frequency in a reversible manner.

presynaptic inhibition of transmitter release by activation of the same receptors also requires a PTX-sensitive G protein. It has been demonstrated previously that activation of a K^+ current in hippocampal neurons by adenosine also requires a PTX-sensitive G protein.[19] It is unclear whether an additional second messenger is required for these actions. Some evidence suggests, however, that G proteins may couple directly to K^+ channels to mediate this action of adenosine.[20] Whether this may also be true for reduction of I_{Ca} or synaptic transmission will require further experiments to address. It should be noted, however, that receptor-mediated inhibition of I_{Ca} in several types of neurons does not require a cytoplasmic second messenger.[21,22]

The mechanisms underlying presynaptic inhibition produced by adenosine have been studied in many preparations. This has lead to different conclusions regarding the mechanisms of action of adenosine. Although it is possible that different mechanisms may operate at different synapses, some of the confusion may arise from the use of many different preparations to study I_{Ca} and synaptic transmission. Therefore, we have chosen a single preparation in which to study the adenosine receptors involved in reducing I_{Ca} and in producing presynaptic inhibition. In addition, effects of neurotransmitters on unknown cell types (as may occur in the hippocampal slice preparation) can be eliminated by choosing appropriately sparse cultures. Furthermore, because the cultures contain very few glial cells, the neurons are accessible for fluorescent measurements of intracellular Ca^{2+}.

Although it might seem reasonable that a reduction in I_{Ca} may underly presynaptic inhibition mediated by adenosine (cf. 7), to date, no definitive conclusion has been reached regarding the actions of adenosine on I_{Ca} in hippocampal neurons. Our experiments have shown that adenosine analogues can reduce I_{Ca} and Ca^{2+} influx into the cell bodies of pyramidal neurons.

Some reports on motor nerve terminals[23] and from paired-pulse potentiation experiments in hippocampal slices[12] suggest that inhibition of I_{Ca} is not responsible for presynaptic inhibition mediated by adenosine. By contrast, several reports have concluded that inhibition of I_{Ca} is important for presynaptic inhibition. Our results strongly support this latter conclusion. Adenosine analogues appear to have only very small effects on K^+ currents in culture preparations either in the cell body or processes.[19] Although we feel that inhibition of I_{Ca} at the presynaptic terminal is involved in presynaptic inhibition, it is clear that further experiments will be necessary to clarify this issue.

An additional mechanism that may be involved in presynaptic inhibition stems from the findings of Man-Son-Hing et al.[8] These authors observed that presynaptic inhibition at a molluscan synapse is mediated, at least in part, by mechanisms downstream from modulation of membrane currents. This raises the possibility that adenosine or other agents that induce presynaptic inhibition may alter properties of the vesicle release process in addition to altering I_{Ca}.

Recent reports, based on the use of pharmacological tools, have shown that N-type I_{Ca} plays a major role in mediating neurotransmitter release from presynaptic terminals,[24] although it is clear that this may be variable between different cell types.[25] Based on these results, it has been postulated that reduction of N-type calcium current in the cell body may reflect a mechanism for presynaptic inhibition of neurotransmitter release at the presynaptic terminal. Although our results also show a similar correlation, ultimate proof of this hypothesis will depend upon characterization of the Ca^{2+} channels that exist at the presynaptic terminal and how they are regulated by neurotransmitters.

REFERENCES

1. DUDEL, J. & S. W. KUFFLER. 1961. Presynaptic inhibition at the crayfish neuromuscular junction. J. Physiol. (Lond.) **155:** 543–562.
2. NICOLL, R. A. & B. E. ALGER. 1979. Presynaptic inhibition: transmitter and ionic mechanisms. Int. Rev. Neurobiol. **21:** 217–258.
3. LANTHORN, T. H. & C. W. COTMAN. 1981. Baclofen selectively inhibits excitatory synaptic transmission in the hippocampus. Brain Res. **225:** 171–178.
4. NICOLL, R. A. 1988. The coupling of neurotransmitter receptors to ion channels in the brain. Science **241:** 545–551.
5. ZOLTAY, G. & J. R. COOPER. 1990. Ionic basis of inhibitory presynaptic modulation in rat cortical synaptosomes. J. Neurochem. **55:** 1008–1012.
6. MACDONALD, R. L., J. H. SKERRITT & M. A. WERZ. 1986. Adenosine agonists reduce voltage-dependent calcium conductance of mouse sensory neurones in cell culture. J. Physiol. (Lond.) **370:** 75–90.
7. DOLPHIN, A. C., S. R. FORDA & R. H. SCOTT. 1986. Calcium-dependent currents in cultured rat dorsal root ganglion neurones are inhibited by an adenosine analogue. J. Physiol. (Lond.) **373:** 47–61.
8. MAN-SON-HING, H., M. J. ZORAN, K. LUKOWIAK & P. G. HAYDON. 1989. A neuromodulator of synaptic transmission acts on the secretory apparatus as well as on ion channels. Nature **341:** 237–239.
9. ALMERS, W. 1990. Exocytosis. Annu. Rev. Physiol. **52:** 607–624.
10. SCHOLZ, K. P. & R. J. MILLER. 1991. Analysis of adenosine actions on calcium currents and synaptic transmission in cultured rat hippocampal pyramidal neurones. J. Physiol. (Lond.) **435:** 373–393.
11. ABELE, A. E., K. P. SCHOLZ, W. K. SCHOLZ & R. J. MILLER. 1990. Excitotoxicity induced by enhanced excitatory neurotransmission in cultured hippocampal pyramidal neurons. Neuron **4:** 413–419.
12. DUNWIDDIE, T. V. & H. L. HAAS. 1985. Adenosine increases synaptic facilitation in the *in vitro* rat hippocampus: evidence for a presynaptic site of action. J. Physiol. (Lond.) **369:** 365–377.
13. FREDHOLM, B. B., W. PROCTOR, I. VAN DER PLOEG & T. V. DUNWIDDIE. 1989. *In vivo* pertussis toxin treatment attenuates some, but not all, adenosine A1 effects in slices of the rat hippocampus. Eur. J. Pharmacol. **172:** 249–262.
14. STRATTON, K. R., A. J. COLE, J. PRITCHETT, C. U. ECCLES, P. F. WORLEY & J. M. BARABAN. 1989. Intrahippocampal injection of pertussis toxin blocks adenosine suppression of synaptic responses. Brain Res. **494:** 359–364.
15. DEL CASTILLO, J. & B. KATZ. 1954. Quantal components of the end-plate potential. J. Physiol. (Lond.) **124:** 560–573.
16. REDMAN, S. J. 1990. Quantal analysis of synaptic potentials in neurons of the central nervous system. Physiol. Rev. **70:** 165–198.
17. DEL CASTILLO, J. & B. KATZ. 1954. The effect of magnesium on the activity of motor nerve endings. J. Physiol. (Lond.) **124:** 553–559.
18. DRAPEAU, P. & D. A. NACHSHEN. 1984. Manganese fluxes and manganese-dependent neurotransmitter release in presynaptic nerve endings isolated from rat brain. J. Physiol. (Lond.) **348:** 493–510.
19. TRUSSELL, L. O. & M. B. JACKSON. 1987. Dependence of an adenosine-activated potassium current on a GTP-binding protein in mammalian central neurons. J. Neurosci. **7:** 3306–3316.
20. VANDONGEN, A. M. J., J. CODINA, J. OLATE, R. MATTERA, R. JOHO, L. BIRNBAUMER & A. M. BROWN. 1988. Newly identified brain potassium channels gated by the guanine nucleotide binding protein Go. Science **242:** 1433–1437.
21. FORSCHER, P., G. S. OXFORD & D. C. SCHULTZ. 1988. Noradrenaline modulates calcium channels through tight receptor channel coupling. J. Physiol. **379:** 131–144.
22. LIPSCOMBE, D., S. KONGSAMUT & R. W. TSIEN. 1989. a-Adrenergic inhibition of sympathetic neurotransmitter release mediated by modulation of N-type calcium channel gating. Nature **340:** 637–642.

23. SILINSKY, E. M. 1984. On the mechanism by which adenosine receptor activation inhibits the release of acetylcholine from motor nerve endings. J. Physiol. **346:** 243–256.

24. HIRNING, L. D., A. P. FOX, E. W. MCCLESKEY, B. M. OLIVERA, S. A. THAYER, R. J. MILLER & R. W. TSIEN. 1988. Dominant role of N-type Ca^{2+} channels in evoked release of norepinephrine from sympathetic neurons. Science **239:** 57–60.

25. HOLZ, IV, G. G., K. DUNLAP & R. M. KREAM. 1988. Characterization of the electrically-evoked release of substance P from dorsal root ganglion neurons: methods and dihydropyridine sensitivity. J. Neurosci. **8:** 463–471.

Amount and Time-Course of Release

The Calcium Hypothesis and the Calcium-Voltage Hypothesis

I. PARNAS, H. PARNAS, AND B. HOCHNER

The Otto Loewi Center for Cellular and Molecular Neurobiology
The Hebrew University
Jerusalem, Israel 91904

INTRODUCTION

Secretion of cellular constituents by means of exocytosis is a fundamental step in intercellular communication. For most of the exocytotic processes identified to date, irrespective of their exact nature, elevation of intracellular calcium concentration, $[Ca^{2+}]_i$, is an absolute requirement for exocytosis to take place. The time-course of release can vary greatly. For example, after stimulation, hormone release proceeds with a slow rate of rise and decay.[1] On the other hand, release from nerve terminals at neuromuscular junctions is very brief, starting after a delay as short as 0.2 ms and ending by about 2 ms (at room temperature).[2-7] Despite the great variation in time-course of release in different systems, a common theory, the Ca^{2+}-hypothesis, was formulated. Entry of Ca^{2+} following an activating signal was seen as the trigger that initiates release, and removal of Ca^{2+} was seen as the mechanism to stop release. It follows that at least for nerve terminals, Ca^{2+} must be removed from below the release sites in less than 2 milliseconds.[8-12]

Ca^{2+} indicators such as Arsenazo III[13-15] or Fura II[16,17] have been used to show that Ca^{2+} signals last for tens of milliseconds to seconds in somata, dendrites, and even nerve terminals.[18] Such findings must be explained if we are to adhere to the notion of rapid (<2 ms) removal of Ca^{2+} in nerve terminals in order to stop release. To meet this demand, the Ca^{2+} hypothesis was refined to include detailed spatial distribution of Ca^{2+} channels and release sites that resulted in highly localized Ca^{2+} domains in the vicinity of the release sites.[10,19] It was also assumed that near the release sites, which must be very close to the Ca^{2+} channels, Ca^{2+} reaches high levels for only a brief period due to fast diffusion away from the release sites. Hence, it was argued that the Ca^{2+} indicators measure the total Ca^{2+} concentration in the cytoplasm but not the rapid changes at the small Ca^{2+} domains.

In the first part of this article we show that the refined Ca^{2+} models, as well as the older conventional one, fail to account for the most crucial experimental observations, namely that the time-course of evoked release is insensitive to variations in the spatiotemporal distribution of $[Ca^{2+}]_i$. We further show that adding a slow process following the entry and binding of Ca^{2+} to the release sites [such slow processes are not included in the models of Simon and Llinás[10] and Fogelson and Zucker[19]] does not alter the most fundamental prediction of the Ca^{2+} hypothesis, namely that the time-course of release should be highly sensitive to temporal variations in intracellular Ca^{2+} concentration.

The second part of the article summarizes evidence indicating that, in addition to Ca^{2+}, another factor, which is sensitive to changes in membrane potential, must be

177

present for release to occur. Thus Ca^{2+} is essential but insufficient to trigger the processes leading to release. The putative additional factor, denoted S, is produced with depolarization and has a short life span after the membrane repolarizes. When the action potential arrives at the nerve terminal, Ca^{2+} enters and S is formed. The Ca^{2+} and the S together induce release. Upon repolarization, S inactivates with a certain time-constant, and because Ca^{2+} cannot act without S, release ceases even though $[Ca^{2+}]_i$ is still high. According to the Ca^{2+}-voltage hypothesis,[20–24,7] there is a clear distinction between the amount of release and the time-course of release. The amount of release is determined by both $[Ca^{2+}]_i$ and the level of S. The time-course of release is determined by the kinetics of activation/inactivation of the S, a process that is voltage-dependent.

WHY EXISTING CA^{2+} MODELS CANNOT ACCOUNT FOR THE TIME-COURSE OF RELEASE

Theoretical Considerations

Existing mathematically formulated Ca^{2+} models vary in different aspects. They all, however, share the following common principles: Ca^{2+} is both necessary and sufficient to evoke release, and the main process dominating the spatiotemporal distribution of intracellular Ca^{2+} is diffusion.[8–10,19] Fogelson and Zucker[19] and Simon and Llinás[10] also consider 3D diffusion and provide a nonhomogenous spatial distribution of the Ca^{2+} channels and the adjacent release sites. In the models cited above, the time-course of release is simply obtained by raising $[Ca^{2+}]_i$ to a power that represents Ca^{2+} cooperativity. In the model of Simon and Llinás,[10] a linear relation is assumed. In the other models cooperativity is taken as four or five. Consequently these models predict most of the release process to occur during the entry of Ca^{2+} and especially for a brief depolarizing pulse. Experiments show, however, that most of the release occurs after the pulse, with the peak of the release occurring significantly after the end of the stimulus (see, for example, FIG. 2). To overcome this shortcoming in the Ca^{2+} models, a slower process must be included after entry and binding of Ca^{2+}, while keeping other features of the models unaltered.

For definiteness, the model of Fogelson and Zucker,[19] extended to include a slow step, was analyzed. A detailed account of this refined model, its parameters and the numeric procedures involved, has been provided earlier.[25]

Simulations of the time-course of release elicited by the first and second pulses of a pair are given in FIGURE 1A. It is clear that release evoked by the second pulse has a much shorter minimal delay and that the peak of release shifted to the right. Increasing intracellular Ca^{2+} buffering caused reduction in the quantal content, with release beginning later and ending later (FIG. 1B). In the Fogelson and Zucker[19] model buffering is introduced as a denominator in the diffusion equation. Accordingly, when buffering is increased diffusion is slowed and it takes longer for Ca^{2+} to diffuse from the channels onto the release sites. If fast buffering is introduced as a term that accelerates removal of Ca^{2+}, a different prediction is obtained. In this case the quantal content is also reduced, but release stops sooner[26] (not shown in FIG. 1).

FIGURE 1 demonstrates that the 3D diffusion model of Fogelson and Zucker[19] predicts the time-course of release to be sensitive to temporal changes in $[Ca^{2+}]_i$. Similar sensitivity is shared by the other models mentioned above.

Experimental Results

One method of measuring time-course of release is by constructing a synaptic delay histogram.[2,3] When working under experimental conditions in which the quantal content is low, excitation of the nerve terminal results mostly in release of single quanta that appear after a variable delay from the stimulus (FIG. 2B). Measuring the delay of many such events and constructing a synaptic delay histogram (FIG. 2A) gives the time-course of release, or in other words the probability of distribution over time for quantal release. The following features characterize the time-course of release: (a) There is always a minimal delay, that outlasts short pulses, during which no release is seen irrespective of the number of pulses given. (b) The peak of the delay histogram appears appreciably later than the end of the pulse. (c)

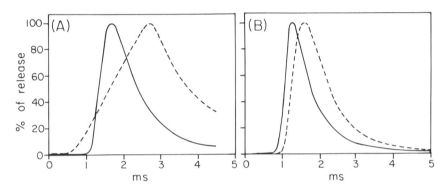

FIGURE 1. Computer simulations, using the Fogelson and Zucker[19] Ca^{2+} domain model, to compute the time-course of release for twin pulses (**A**) and after increasing intracellular buffering (**B**). Ca^{2+} profiles were calculated using the Fogelson and Zucker equations. $X = 1$; $D = 0.6 \, \mu m^2/ms$; $B = 500$ and 1000; $p = 0.08 \, ms^{-1}$; cooperativity was taken as 4. To include the slow step the following scheme was adopted:

$$Ca + X \underset{k_{-1}}{\overset{k_1}{\rightleftharpoons}} Q; \quad 4Q \overset{k_2}{\rightarrow} \text{Release}; \quad K_1 = 1.0; K_{-1} = 0.5; K_2 = 0.5.$$

For all simulations the pulse duration was 1 ms. Depolarization was strong so that all 64 Ca^{2+} channels were activated. Distance between channels was 0.1 μm. For further details see Fogelson and Zucker[19] and Parnas *et al.*[25]

Within a few milliseconds (depending on temperature) the probability of release drops to very low levels.

Synaptic delay histograms were measured under different experimental conditions that presumably alter the temporal distribution of $[Ca^{2+}]_i$. An example of such a result is seen in FIGURE 3. Delay histograms of the first and second pulses of a pair, when normalized, are practically identical. Most notable is the identical minimal delay and time of peak, despite facilitation. The difference between the experimental result in FIGURE 3 and the prediction seen in FIGURE 1A is evident. Intra-axonal injection of BAPTA or nitr-5 (fast Ca^{2+} buffers) reduced the quantal content by 70% without any effect on the time-course of release.[26] In addition to the result given in FIGURE 3, other experimental manipulations that are known to affect entry, accumu-

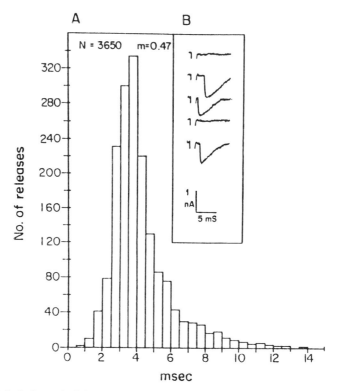

FIGURE 2. A. Synaptic delay histogram for crayfish neuromuscular junction in the opener muscle. Temperature 9°C; normal ringer; direct nerve terminal depolarization (macropatch technique[41]). N, number of pulses; m, quantal content. **B.** Sample records of single quanta (modified from Parnas *et al.*[31]). Notice failures of release in the first and fourth traces.

lation within the terminal and removal of Ca^{2+}, had no effect on the synaptic delay histogram[4,5,27-30] (see also FIG. 4 in ref. 31).

By contrast, in all the cases listed above, other aspects of release, such as the quantal content and facilitation, were strongly affected in the expected direction according to the experimental conditions. In contrast to the experimental findings indicating dissociation between the dependence of the amount of release and that of the time-course of release on $[Ca^{2+}]_i$, the various existing Ca^{2+} hypotheses predict that variations in quantal content or facilitation should coincide with changes in the time-course of evoked release.

In view of the disagreement between predictions of the Ca^{2+} hypothesis and experiments, it must be concluded that the time-course of release is not determined by $[Ca^{2+}]_i$. Hence one of the most basic postulates of the Ca^{2+} hypothesis must be wrong. As Ca^{2+} was found to be necessary for evoked release to take place, the assumption that must be erroneous is that Ca^{2+} is also sufficient.

It follows that at least one other factor, apart from Ca^{2+}, becomes available upon stimulation. As the natural stimulus for evoked release in nerve terminals is normally the rapid-action potential, this other factor is probably activated by depolarization. The resulting hypothesis, which extends the Ca^{2+} hypothesis, was therefore denoted as the Ca^{2+}-voltage hypothesis for neurotransmitter release. A detailed discussion of the Ca^{2+}-voltage hypothesis is given in a recent review.[31]

THE CA²⁺-VOLTAGE HYPOTHESIS FOR NEUROTRANSMITTER RELEASE

The Ca^{2+}-voltage hypothesis postulates that evoked release in nerve terminals is controlled by, at least, two events. One is elevation of intracellular Ca^{2+} concentration. The second is activation of a molecule (or a complex) rendering it sensitive to Ca^{2+}. Combination of Ca^{2+} with the active molecule sets in motion the chain of events leading to exocytosis.

Under natural conditions, that is, upon arrival of the action potential at the nerve terminals, the two factors become independently available as a result of the common stimulus, membrane depolarization. Release starts only subsequent to the depolarization-induced activation of the molecule, termed in its active form as S, and terminates only following repolarization when S undergoes inactivation (termed T in its inactive form).

As these transformations

$$T \underset{\text{hyp}}{\overset{\text{dep}}{\rightleftarrows}} S$$

comprise the main regulation of the time-course of release, it is not surprising that the Ca^{2+}-voltage hypothesis predicts the time-course of release to be insensitive to any experimental treatment that varies the temporal distribution of intracellular Ca^{2+}.[32]

Second in importance are other facets of the Ca^{2+}-voltage hypothesis, for example, the exact location of the S molecule. Simplicity would require that it be

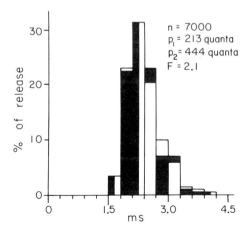

FIGURE 3. Synaptic delay histograms for twin pulses 10 ms apart. Crayfish opener muscle. Pulse duration 1.5 ms; pulse amplitude -0.8 μA. Temperature 12°C; normal Ringer, $5 \cdot 10^{-7}$ M TTX. Repetition rate 2 Hz. 7000 pulses were given; 213 quanta were released after the first pulse and 444 quanta after the second pulse (Fisher and Ravin, unpublished results, our laboratory).

located in the cell membrane, to detect changes in membrane potential. Also for simplicity we perceive S to be the molecule that binds Ca^{2+}. Other variations, however, are possible. For example, the voltage sensor can be located in the cell membrane and in its active form can recognize a vesicular protein that binds the Ca^{2+}. The exact location of the Ca^{2+}-binding protein, as well as other details, must of course be clarified in the future. They are not, however, crucial at this stage for the hypothesis to be tested as to whether membrane potential affects release by a mechanism other than entry of Ca^{2+}. One possible version of the Ca^{2+}-voltage hypothesis is schematically depicted in FIGURE 4.

EXPERIMENTAL TESTING OF THE CA²⁺-VOLTAGE HYPOTHESIS

The synthesis of caged Ca^{2+} compounds such as nitr-5[33] or DM-nitrophen[34] can be used to test the Ca^{2+}-voltage hypothesis. Intracellular injection of a caged Ca^{2+} compound makes it possible to increase $[Ca^{2+}]_i$ after photolysis without activating Ca^{2+} channels. According to the Ca^{2+}-voltage hypothesis, depolarization of the membrane after such photolysis, but under experimental conditions that do not allow entry of Ca^{2+}, should produce synchronized evoked release. Experiments of this nature were carried out by Hochner et al.[35] FIGURE 5 shows recordings from the crayfish opener muscle in which the axon was injected with nitr-5. In controls (FIG. 5A), before photolysis, but with Ca^{2+} present in the extracellular fluid, nerve stimulation produced synaptic potentials. The external solution was then replaced with one containing only 0.2 mM Ca^{2+} and Ca^{2+} entry blockers. Evoked release was

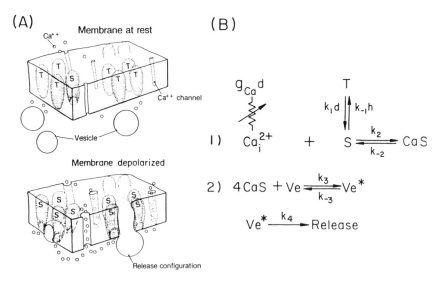

FIGURE 4. A. Diagrammatic representation of the Ca^{2+}-voltage hypothesis. **B.** Formal representation of the Ca^{2+}-voltage equations. Upon depolarization g_{Ca} increases and T transforms to S with a K_1 rate constant that increases with depolarization. K_{-1} is the rate constant of transformation of S to T, and it increases with hyperpolarization. Ca binds to S to form the complex CaS, rate constants K_2 and K_{-2}. Four complexes of CaS are required to activate a vesicle (see Parnas et al.[6] for reasons), rate constant K_3 and K_{-3}. The activated vesicle fuses with the membrane, rate constant K_4. K_3 and K_4 may represent more than one actual step.

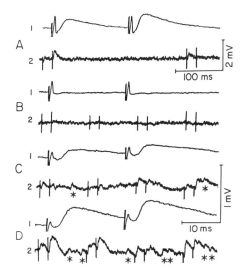

FIGURE 5. Release is obtained after CCCP treatment and nitr-5 photolysis. Intracellular recording from crayfish opener muscle; nerve stimulation. **A.** Normal ringer, 12 mM Ca^{2+}. Stimulation, two pulses, 20 ms apart; repetition rate, 3.3 Hz 75 min after injection of nitr-5. A_1, average of 100 sweeps. A_2, single trace at a slower speed. Note evoked release; no spontaneous release. **B.** The external solution replaced with one containing 0.2 mM Ca^{2+}, 12.5 mM Mg^{2+} (5 times normal), and 2 mM Mn^{2+}. B_1, averaging of 100 sweeps. All responses blocked, even though repetition rate was increased to 10 Hz. B_2, single sweep, same conditions. **C.** Eleven minutes after application of 10 μM CCCP. C_1, average of 100 sweeps now shows evoked release. MEPPs (miniature end-plate potentials) are seen in C_2 asterisks. **D.** Nitr-5 photolysis caused a further increase in MEPP frequency and evoked release. D_1, average of only 50 sweeps. The average response in D_1 is four times larger than in C_1. D_2, evoked release is clear and large. For further details see Hochner *et al*.[35]

evidently blocked as no excitatory postsynaptic potential (EPSP) could be recorded even at a higher rate of stimulation (FIG. 5B). At this stage the uncoupler CCCP (carbonyl cyanide m-chlorophenyl hydrazone) was added. This treatment by itself was sufficient to increase intracellular Ca^{2+} concentration, as is evidenced by the appearance of spontaneous release. Note that at times nerve stimulation produced evoked release (FIG. 5C). Photolysis of the injected nitr-5 produced a further increase in the rate of spontaneous release. Concurrently, evoked release was now seen to occur after each nerve impulse (FIG. 5D). These experimental results support the Ca^{2+}-voltage hypothesis.

THE USE OF DM-NITROPHEN

DM-nitrophen is considered to be more efficient than nitr-5 in increasing Ca^{2+} concentration upon photolysis.[34] Hence, DM-nitrophen was employed instead of nitr-5 in the following experiments. FIGURE 6A shows EPSPs recorded in the crayfish opener muscle in which the axon was injected with DM-nitrophen and the bathing solution contained normal Ca^{2+}. A brief flash of light produced significant release presumably without membrane depolarization (FIG. 6B). Nerve stimulation produced additional evoked release that summated with the flash-evoked response (FIG. 6B). Interestingly, the flash-evoked release declined in 40 ms while the evoked

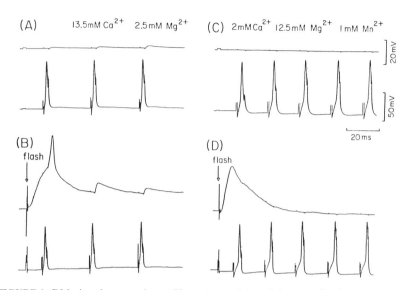

FIGURE 6. DM-nitrophen experiment. Upper traces, intracellular recording from a postsynaptic crayfish opener muscle cell. Lower traces, intracellular recording with the DM-nitrophen microelectrode from the axon. The microelectrode contained 20 mM DM-nitrophen; 100 mM KCl, 15 mM CaCl$_2$, 10 mM Tris (pH 7.4), and 0.5% fast green. The axon was stimulated by the intracellular microelectrode. **A.** Normal Ringer, 12 mM Ca^{2+}. Three pulses are given at intervals of 33 ms; repetition rate 2 Hz. Note release after each stimulus. **B.** Flash of light produced large release. Nerve stimulation produced an electrogenic response when it coincided with the flash response. The second and third pulses produced facilitated EPSPs. **C** and **D.** Another preparation in which responses like those in **A** were obtained after DM-nitrophen injection in normal Ringer. **C.** External solution replaced with one containing 2 mM CaCl$_2$, 12.5 mM Mg^{2+}, and 1 mM Mn^{2+}. Less severe blocking conditions than those used in FIG. 5, nevertheless no release was seen for 5 pulses 20 ms apart and repetition rate of 2 Hz. **D.** DM-nitrophen photolysis produced a "flash response" but no evoked release upon nerve stimulation.

release continued to be facilitated. The experiment, the results of which are depicted in FIGURE 6C and D, was designed to test the Ca^{2+}-voltage hypothesis. Again the axon was injected with DM-nitrophen. The bathing solution contained 2 mM Ca^{2+}, and calcium blocking conditions were less severe (12.5 mM Mg^{2+}, 1 mM Mn^{2+}). Even with these less severe conditions, no release was seen upon nerve stimulation (FIG. 6C). At this point a flash of light produced a large response, but nerve stimulation was not followed by evoked release (FIG. 6D). This result does not support the Ca^{2+}-voltage hypothesis.

DM-NITROPHEN AND CCCP

In view of the inconsistent results obtained with the two-caged Ca^{2+} compounds, we repeated the experiments seen in FIGURE 5 with DM-nitrophen and CCCP. The axon was injected with DM-nitrophen. As in FIGURES 5B and 6C, the external solution was replaced with one blocking entry of Ca^{2+}, but with only 0.2 mM Ca^{2+} and a higher concentration of entry blockers. Thus the experimental conditions are similar to those of FIGURE 5 and more severe than those of FIGURE 6. Indeed evoked release was not seen (FIG. 7A). CCCP was then added, and the rate of spontaneous release increased (FIG. 7B, left). Nerve stimulation produced some evoked release similar to the responses seen in FIGURE 5C. Photolysis produced a large postsynaptic response. In the presence of CCCP, however, nerve stimulation did produce additional evoked release. This result supports the Ca^{2+}-voltage hypothesis. It is puzzling that in the presence of a higher extracellular Ca^{2+} concentration (2 mM) nerve stimulation did not support release (FIG. 6D), and the mere addition of CCCP produced evoked release (FIG. 7B) in the presence of the lower extracellular Ca^{2+} concentration (0.2 mM).

We must conclude that at this stage the results obtained with DM-nitrophen are inconclusive and need further research.

THE USE OF CA^{2+} IONOPHORE

We explored the possibility of raising $[Ca]_i$ by other means and without membrane depolarization. Such experiments involved the use of a Ca^{2+} ionophore, together with a buffered external solution, resulting in very low (in the μM range) controlled $[Ca^{2+}]_o$.

The advantages of such a procedure are that if the ionophore and $[Ca^{2+}]_o$ are fixed at low levels, equilibrium between $[Ca^{2+}]_i$ and $[Ca^{2+}]_o$ is expected to be achieved in time. $[Ca^{2+}]_i$ will be higher than at rest, though still at very low levels. Low $[Ca^{2+}]_i$ is important as it has been suggested that high $[Ca^{2+}]_i$ might be toxic for the cell.[36] Furthermore, after equilibration, entry of Ca^{2+} (due to depolarization) through Ca^{2+} channels will be minimal (if not completely abolished).

In several experiments where ionomycin (1 μM) was employed and $[Ca^{2+}]_o$ was buffered to the range of 500 nM to 2 μM, we observed the following results: Initially, the level of spontaneous release was low (about 1/min), and there was no evoked

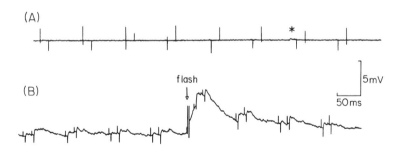

0.2mM Ca^{2+}, 12.5mM Mg^{2+}, 2 mM Mn^{2+}, 0.1mM 3.4 DAP, 10 μM CCCP

FIGURE 7. DM-nitrophen-CCCP experiment. Same techniques as in FIGURE 5 and 6. The external solution was replaced with one containing 0.2 mM Ca^{2+}, 12.5 mM Mg^{2+}, and 2 mM Mn^{2+}. More severe blocking conditions than in the experiment of FIG. 6 and same conditions as the nitr-5 experiment in FIG. 5. **A.** No release seen with 2 pulses 20 ms apart, repetition rate 10 Hz. **B.** After application of 10 μM CCCP, MEPPs appeared together with some evoked release. Photolysis produced large release. Note that now, however, evoked release is also superimposed on the flash response and is facilitated.

release. As time elapsed (> 20 min) and ionomycin took effect, spontaneous release occurred more frequently (starting from 1–2/s and ending with barrages), and a brief depolarizing pulse, either by means of an action potential or by direct nerve-terminal depolarization, triggered evoked release. The time-course of this evoked release, in the presence of persisting elevated levels of $[Ca^{2+}]_i$, was indistinguishable from normal release at the same temperature (manuscript in preparation).

These last results provide strong support for the Ca^{2+}-voltage hypothesis. In addition, they cast heavy doubt on one central issue raised by recent versions of the Ca^{2+} hypothesis—a need for localized high concentrations of Ca^{2+} in the vicinity of the releasing zone. The exact level of $[Ca^{2+}]_i$ obtained with the application of ionomycin in the presence of 500 nM $[Ca^{2+}]_o$ cannot accurately be estimated. Localized high concentrations of Ca^{2+}, however, can certainly be ruled out.

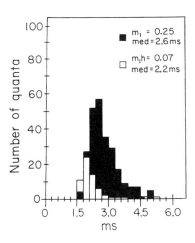

FIGURE 8. Postpulse hyperpolarization experiment (from Arechiga et al.[30]). Crayfish abdominal extensor preparation. Direct nerve terminal depolarization. Ringer contained $5 \cdot 10^{-7}$ M TTX. Depolarizing pulse 1 ms duration, -0.8 μA in amplitude. Hyperpolarizing postpulse, 0.5 ms duration, $+0.6$ μA in amplitude. The hyperpolarizing pulse followed the depolarizing pulse with zero delay.

MODULATING RELEASE BY HYPERPOLARIZING PULSES

Another line of experiments to test the Ca^{2+}-voltage hypothesis concerns its main assumption, that it is the life span of the depolarization dependent factor that determines the time-course of release.

Recall that according to the Ca^{2+}-voltage hypothesis, release starts due to, and following, the transformation of T to S (FIG. 4). The rate of formation of S increases with depolarization. Release subsequently terminates due to, and following, the conformational change of S back to the inactive form of T upon repolarization. The rate of this latter process increases with stronger hyperpolarizations. Hence, it should be possible to accelerate termination of release by brief hyperpolarization following the depolarizing pulse.[22,30]

FIGURE 8 depicts the result of such a hyperpolarizing postpulse experiment. A delay histogram was established as a control for a depolarizing pulse alone (filled bars). The same depolarizing pulse was then followed by brief hyperpolarization. It is evident that the postpulse hyperpolarization not only reduced the quantal content but definitely accelerated termination of release (FIG. 8, empty bars). Note also that the peak of the delay histogram shifted to the left. A postpulse hyperpolarization similarly reduced release and shortened its time-course to the same degree as when the $[Na^+]_o \leftrightarrow [Ca^{2+}]_i$ exchanger was blocked.[30]

Similar results concerning reduction in release and shortening of its time-course were obtained in the presence of Ca^{2+} ionophore and normal $[Ca^{2+}]_o$. The quantal content with the ionophore increased by a factor of 4, but a hyperpolarizing postpulse reduced the quantal content to the same proportional extent (manuscript in preparation).

The effect of postpulse hyperpolarization on the time-course of release is of particular importance in view of the invariance of the latter, despite alterations in the temporal distribution of $[Ca^{2+}]_i$. Simulations of the Ca^{2+}-voltage hypothesis reveal that postpulse hyperpolarization is expected, as in the experiments, to reduce the quantal content, shorten the time-course of release, and shift the peak of release to the left.[37]

In the mathematical formulation of the Ca^{2+}-voltage hypothesis, the slowest step (hence the rate-limiting one) was assigned to be the last one. It follows that the rate-limiting step takes place subsequent to the fast processes, which include entry and binding of Ca^{2+} as well as the transformation $T \rightarrow S$. Yet, the time-course of release is highly sensitive to changes in one of the fastest steps ($S \rightleftarrows T$), because this step determines termination of release.

DISCUSSION

The importance of Ca^{2+} and its involvement in the release process is beyond dispute. Also, there is no doubt that other factors are involved in the chain of events leading to release. More and more information is accumulating on Ca^{2+}-binding proteins[38] that affect or modulate release,[39] and on activation of enzymes that may be involved in fusion of vesicles.[40]

One question that has emerged in recent years is whether, in face of the many constituents involved, Ca^{2+} is the only limiting factor that controls evoked release.[31] The experiments described, as well as many others that have been mentioned here, suggest otherwise.

Refinements of the simple version of the Ca^{2+} hypothesis that include detailed spatial distribution of Ca^{2+} channels and release sites and consider 3D diffusion of $[Ca^{2+}]_i$ fail to breach the gap between predictions and experimental findings.

The key assumption that is responsible for the serious discrepancy between the various versions of the Ca^{2+} hypothesis and experiments is that Ca^{2+} is the only limiting factor controlling evoked release.

We have suggested extending the Ca^{2+} hypothesis to become the Ca^{2+}-voltage hypothesis, according to which evoked release is controlled by two factors, both of which become available as a result of the natural stimulus.

The requirement that key biological processes be controlled by more than one factor may be of general importance. An obvious example of a key process is synaptic transmission. It is difficult to accept that transmission may be determined solely by perturbations in $[Ca^{2+}]_i$ that can result from a number of sources. Certainly a machine as sophisticated as the brain would require additional safeguards to control its synaptic activity.

The Ca^{2+}-voltage hypothesis provides for such an additional safeguard. In the case of the neuromuscular junction, release is accordingly controlled by a depolarization-dependent $T \rightleftarrows S$ transformation. In other systems the controlling factor could obviously be different.

CONCLUSION

The amount of transmitter released from nerve terminals is highly sensitive to treatments known to affect depolarization-mediated entry of Ca^{2+} or its subsequent removal. The time-course of release, however, is unaffected by such treatments. Specifically, the time-course of release in fast synapses (1–2 ms at 20°C) has been shown to be insensitive to changes in extracellular calcium concentration ($[Ca^{2+}]_o$), to Ca^{2+} entry blockers, and to increase of intracellular Ca^{2+} by Ca^{2+} ionophore and repeated stimulation. When fast Ca^{2+} buffers were injected into the axon, the amount of release was reduced, but the time-course of release did not change. These findings are inconsistent with the Ca^{2+} hypothesis that assumes Ca^{2+} to be the only limiting factor in the release process. Versions of the Ca^{2+} hypothesis that include Ca^{2+} domains and 3D diffusion, and also a slow step following Ca^{2+} entry, predict that the time-course of release should be highly sensitive to variations in the temporal distribution of Ca^{2+} near the release sites. By contrast, the Ca^{2+}-voltage hypothesis, an extension of the Ca^{2+} hypothesis, predicts that the time-course of release is insensitive to the treatments described above. Experiments supporting the Ca^{2+}-voltage hypothesis are presented.

REFERENCES

1. SALZBERG, B. M., A. L. OBAID & H. GAINER. 1985. Large and rapid changes in light scattering accompany secretion by nerve terminals in the mammalian neurohypophysis. J. Gen. Physiol. **86:** 395–411.
2. KATZ, B. & R. MILEDI. 1965. The measurement of synaptic delay, and the time course of acetylcholine release at the neuromuscular junction. Proc. R. Soc. London Ser. **161:** 483–495.
3. KATZ, B. & R. MILEDI. 1965. The effect of temperature on the synaptic delay at the neuromuscular junction. J. Physiol. (Lond.) **181:** 656–670.
4. DATYNER, N. B. & P. W. GAGE. 1980. Phasic secretion of acetylcholine at the mammalian neuromuscular junction. J. Physiol. (Lond.) **303:** 299–314.
5. ANDREU, R. & E. F. BARRETT. 1980. Calcium dependence of evoked transmitter release at very low quantal contents at the frog neuromuscular junction. J. Physiol. (Lond.) **308:** 79–97.
6. PARNAS, H., I. PARNAS & L. SEGEL. 1986. A new method for determining cooperativity in neuromuscular release. J. Theor. Biol. **119:** 481–499.
7. DUDEL, J. 1989. Nerve terminal depolarization, calcium inflow and transmitter release. *In* Neuromuscular Junction. L. C. Sellin, R. Sibelius & S. Thesleff, Eds. Elsevier Science Publishers (Biomedical Division).
8. ZUCKER, R. S. & N. STOCKBRIDGE. 1983. Presynaptic calcium diffusion and the time courses of transmitter release and synaptic facilitation at the squid giant synapse. J. Neurosci. **3:** 1263–1269.
9. STOCKBRIDGE, N. & J. W. MOORE. 1984. Dynamics of intracellular calcium and its possible relationship to phasic transmitter release and facilitation at the frog neuromuscular junction. J. Neurosci. **4:** 803–811.
10. SIMON, S. M. & R. R. LLINÁS. 1985. Compartmentalization of the submembrane calcium activity during calcium influx and its significance in transmitter release. Biophys. J. **48:** 485–498.
11. AUGUSTINE, G. J., M. P. CHARLTON & S. J. SMITH. 1987. Calcium action in synaptic transmitter release. Annu. Rev. Neurosci. **10:** 633–693.
12. BLAUSTEIN, M. P. 1988. Calcium transport and buffering in neurons. TINS **11:** 438–443.
13. ROSS, W. N., L. L. STOCKBRIDGE & N. L. STOCKBRIDGE. 1986. Regional properties of

calcium entry in barnacle neurons determined with Arsenazo III and a photodiode array. J. Neurosci. **6:** 1148–1159.

14. ROSS, W. M., H. ARECHIGA & J. G. NICHOLLS. 1987. Optical recording of calcium and voltage transients following impulses in cell bodies and processes of identified leech neurons in culture. J. Neurosci. **7(12):** 3877–3887.

15. ROSS, W. N. & R. WERMAN. 1987. Mapping calcium transients in dendrites of Purkinje cells from the guinea pig cerebellum *in vitro*. J. Physiol. (Lond.) **389:** 319–336.

16. CONNOR, J. A., R. KRETZ & E. SHAPIRO. 1986. Calcium levels measured in a presynaptic neuron of Aplysia under conditions that modulate transmitter release. J. Physiol. (Lond.) **375:** 625–642.

17. CONNOR, J. A., W. J. WADMAN, P. E. HOCKBERGER & R. K. S. WONG. 1988. Sustained dendritic gradients of Ca^{2+} induced by excitatory amino acids in CA1 hippocampal neurons. Science **240:** 649–653.

18. DELANEY, K. R., R. S. ZUCKER & D. W. TANK. 1989. Calcium in motor nerve terminals associated with posttetanic potentiation. J. Neurosci. **9(10):** 3558–3567.

19. FOGELSON, A. L. & R. S. ZUCKER. 1985. Presynaptic calcium diffusion from various arrays of single channels. Implications for transmitter release and synaptic facilitation. Biophys. J. **48:** 1003–1017.

20. DUDEL, J., I. PARNAS & H. PARNAS. 1983. Neurotransmitter release and its facilitation in crayfish muscle. VI. Release determined by both intracellular calcium and depolarization of the nerve terminal. Pflügers Arch. **399:** 1–10.

21. DUDEL, J. 1984. Control of quantal transmitter release at frog's nerve terminals. II. Modulation by de- or hyperpolarizing pulses. Pflügers Arch. **402:** 235–243.

22. PARNAS, H., J. DUDEL & I. PARNAS. 1986. Neurotransmitter release and its facilitation in crayfish. VII. Another voltage dependent process besides Ca entry controls the time course of phasic release. Pflügers Arch. **406:** 121–130.

23. PARNAS, I. & H. PARNAS. 1986. Calcium is essential but insufficient for neurotransmitter release: the calcium-voltage hypothesis. J. Physiol. (Paris) **81:** 289–305.

24. PARNAS, I. & H. PARNAS. 1988. The 'Ca-voltage' hypothesis for neurotransmitter release. Biophys. Chem. **29:** 85–93.

25. PARNAS, H., G. HOVAV & I. PARNAS. 1989. The effect of Ca^{2+} diffusion on the time course of neurotransmitter release. Biophys. J. **55:** 859–874.

26. HOCHNER, B., H. PARNAS & I. PARNAS. Effects of intracellularly injected Ca^{2+} chelator on evoked release and on facilitation in the crayfish neuromuscular junction. Submitted.

27. BARRETT, E. F. & C. F. STEVENS. 1972. Quantal independence and uniformity of presynaptic release kinetics at the frog neuromuscular junction. J. Physiol. (Lond.) **227:** 665–689.

28. BARRETT, E. F. & C. F. STEVENS. 1972. The kinetics of transmitter release at the frog neuromuscular junction. J. Physiol (Lond.) **227:** 691–708.

29. MATZNER, H., H. PARNAS & I. PARNAS. 1988. Presynaptic effects of d-tubocurarine on neurotransmitter release at the neuromuscular junction of the frog. J. Physiol. (Lond.) **398:** 109–121.

30. ARECHIGA, H., A. CANNONE, H. PARNAS & I. PARNAS. 1990. Blockage of synaptic release by brief hyperpolarizing pulses. J. Physiol. (Lond.) **430:** 119–133.

31. PARNAS, H., I. PARNAS & L. A. SEGEL. 1990. On the contribution of mathematical models to the understanding of neurotransmitter release. Int. Rev. Neurobiol. **32:** 1–50.

32. LUSTIG, C., H. PARNAS & L. SEGEL. 1989. Neurotransmitter release: Development of a theory for total release based on kinetics. J. Theor. Biol. **136:** 151–170.

33. ADAMS, S. R., J. P. Y. KAO, G. GRYNKIEWICZ, A. MINTA & R. Y. TSIEN. 1988. Biologically useful chelators that release Ca^{2+} upon illumination. J. Am. Chem. Soc. **110:** 3212–3220.

34. KAPLAN, J. H. & G. C. R. ELLIS-DAVIS. 1988. Photolabile chelators for the rapid photorelease of divalent cations. Proc. Natl. Acad. Sci. USA **85:** 6571–6575.

35. HOCHNER, B., H. PARNAS & I. PARNAS. 1989. Membrane depolarization evokes neurotransmitter release in the absence of calcium entry. Nature **342:** 433–435.

36. ADAMS, O. J., K. TAKEDA & J. A. UMBACH. 1985. Inhibitors of calcium buffering depress evoked transmitter release at the squid giant synapse. J. Physiol. (Lond.) **369:** 145–159.

37. PARNAS, I., H. PARNAS & J. DUDEL. 1986. Neurotransmitter release and its facilitation in crayfish. VIII. Modulation of release by hyperpolarizing pulses. Pflügers Arch. **406:** 131–137.
38. ATLAS, D. 1990. The role of calcium in neurotransmitter release: Existing models and new approaches to evaluate possible mechanisms. Curr. Top. Cell. Regul. **31:** 129–159.
39. LLINÁS, R., T. L. McGUINNESS, C. S. LEONARD, M. SUGIMORI & P. GREENGARD. 1985. Intraterminal injection of synapsin I or calcium/calmodulin-dependent protein kinase II alters neurotransmitter release at the squid giant synapse. Proc. Natl. Acad. Sci. USA **82:** 3035–3039.
40. KARLI, U. O., T. SCHAFER & M. BURGER. 1990. Fusion of neurotransmitter vesicles with target membrane is calcium independent in a cell free system. Proc. Natl. Acad. Sci. USA **87:** 5912–5951.
41. DUDEL, J. 1981. The effect of reduced calcium on quantal unit current and release at the crayfish neuromuscular junction. Pflügers Arch. **391:** 35–40.

Presynaptic Calcium in Transmitter Release and Posttetanic Potentiation[a]

ROBERT S. ZUCKER, KERRY R. DELANEY,
ROSEL MULKEY, AND DAVID W. TANK

Department of Molecular and Cell Biology
University of California
Berkeley, California 94720
and
Molecular Biophysics Research Department
A T & T Bell Laboratories
Murray Hill, New Jersey 07974

Until recently, study of the role of calcium in transmitter release has been limited to electrophysiological recording of postsynaptic responses while altering the calcium influx into presynaptic terminals, either by changing external calcium concentration or by manipulating the presynaptic potential.[1-3] Now it is possible to monitor calcium concentration ($[Ca^{2+}]_i$) changes at single presynaptic boutons during synaptic transmission, and to rapidly alter presynaptic $[Ca^{2+}]_i$ in nerve terminals with photolabile calcium chelators. We present here some of our recent observations on the relationship between presynaptic $[Ca^{2+}]_i$ and transmitter release.

LOCALIZATION OF CALCIUM ACCUMULATION AT PRESYNAPTIC NERVE TERMINALS

We have focused on transmitter release at motor nerve terminals at crayfish neuromuscular junctions. The claw opener muscle is innervated by a glutamate-releasing excitor motor neuron and a γ-aminobutyric acid (GABA)–releasing inhibitor motor neuron, which branch together and release transmitter from varicosities and boutons about 1–5 μm in diameter.[4,5] Changes in presynaptic $[Ca^{2+}]_i$ can be followed by injecting the calcium-sensitive dye fura-2[6] into the preterminal axon. Using a sensitive video camera, we form images of the fluorescence of fura when excited by 350 and 385 nm light.[7] Ratios of emitted light intensities at each pixel are color-coded to generate an image of the spatial distribution of $[Ca^{2+}]_i$. The time resolution of our measurements is on the order of 1 s, whereas the spatial resolution is limited by the wavelength of light and related optical properties. We are therefore unable to measure the local high submembrane $[Ca^{2+}]_i$ after single action potentials, but instead measure the average $[Ca^{2+}]_i$ in nerve processes during repetitive stimulation. Because equilibration of $[Ca^{2+}]_i$ across the small volume of the terminal occurs rapidly, measurements of residual $[Ca^{2+}]_i$ following electrical activity probably reflect accurately $[Ca^{2+}]_i$ at sites of transmitter release.

FIGURE 1 (on the color plate) shows two regions of presynaptic terminals of a single excitor motor neuron. During repetitive presynaptic stimulation, $[Ca^{2+}]_i$ rises

[a]This work was supported by NIH Grant NS 15114 and by A T & T Bell Laboratories. K. Delaney is the recipient of a Canadian MRC Fellowship.

191

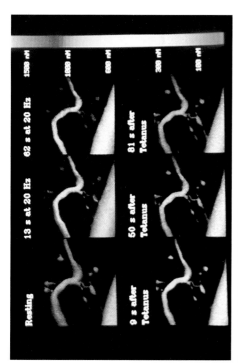

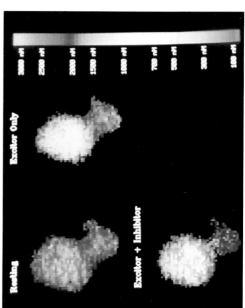

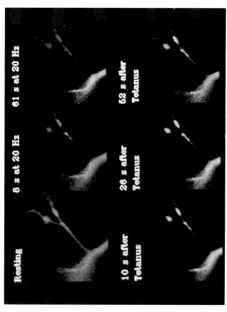

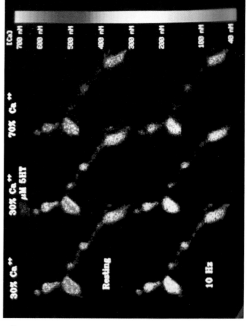

rapidly in boutons and small processes, and more slowly in major axonal branches. After cessation of stimulation, $[Ca^{2+}]_i$ drops more rapidly in the boutons and fine processes than in larger branches. This data is shown graphically in FIGURE 2.

The spatial distribution of the tetanic rise in $[Ca^{2+}]_i$ shows clearly that calcium accumulation occurs locally into boutons and small processes where synaptic vesicles and synaptic "active zones" are located.[5] The rapid posttetanic drop in $[Ca^{2+}]_i$ in boutons and small branches suggests that calcium is locally removed from cytoplasm in these regions as well. We may ask whether these rapid localized $[Ca^{2+}]_i$ changes reflect a high density of calcium channels and removal equipment locally, or simply the larger surface-to-volume ratio of small processes. One indication that calcium channel density may be higher at release sites comes from panel B of FIGURE 2. Point A measures a bouton of similar dimensions to a rather narrow region of an axonal branch marked point C. The faster $[Ca^{2+}]_i$ changes at point A suggest a real concentration of calcium influx and of sequestering or extruding capabilities near synaptic release sites. Differences in cytoplasmic calcium buffering, however, (greater in axonal branches) might also account for our observations.

INCREASING CALCIUM INFLUX NONLINEARLY INCREASES TRANSMITTER RELEASE

Doubling external $[Ca^{2+}]$ increases $[Ca^{2+}]_i$ accumulation about 30%, by increasing the calcium influx through each channel opened by an action potential. The small increase in calcium accumulation is probably due to saturation of influx through channels as external $[Ca^{2+}]$ is raised[8] and to local extracellular buffering of $[Ca^{2+}]$.[9] This modest rise in calcium influx increases transmission about four times (FIG. 3). If we suppose that the 30% increase in calcium accumulation reflects a 30% increase in calcium influx per channel, this suggests a highly nonlinear relationship between $[Ca^{2+}]_i$ at release sites and transmitter release.

At 5 mM, the potassium channel blocker tetraethylammonium (TEA) prolongs action potentials[10] and increases tetanic $[Ca^{2+}]_i$ accumulation about 70 percent. But this larger rise in calcium influx (compared to what we got by increasing external $[Ca^{2+}]_i$) is correlated with increased transmission only about twofold (FIG. 3). Thus

---

FIGURE 1. Ratiometric fluorescent images of two regions of crayfish excitor motor nerve terminals filled with fura-2. Colors correspond to $[Ca^{2+}]_i$ levels indicated by the color bar on the right. The motor neuron was stimulated at 20 Hz for 70 s. The time before, during, or after stimulation is marked on each panel. Scale bar (see FIG. 8) corresponds to 4 μm.

FIGURE 7. Effect of 5 μM 5HT on presynaptic $[Ca^{2+}]_i$ in excitor terminals. The top three images show resting $[Ca^{2+}]_i$, and the bottom images show $[Ca^{2+}]_i$ during 10 Hz stimulation. The left column shows controls, the middle column shows effects of 5 μM 5HT, and the right column shows effects of increasing extracellular $[Ca^{2+}]$ from 30% to 70% of its normal level of 13.5 mM. The average resting $[Ca^{2+}]_i$ in the large central bouton was 98 nM in low $[Ca^{2+}]$, 112 nM in 5 μM 5HT, and 98 nM in high $[Ca^{2+}]$. During stimulation, $[Ca^{2+}]_i$ rose to 305 nM, 295 nM, and 376 nM in these solutions, respectively. Scale bar (see FIG. 8) corresponds to 12 μm.

FIGURE 8. Effect of inhibitor stimulation on tetanic $[Ca^{2+}]_i$ accumulation in excitor terminals. Both motor neurons were injected with fura-2; the excitor terminal is the larger circle on the upper left. The images show resting $[Ca^{2+}]_i$, stimulation of the excitor alone at 10 Hz, and concurrent stimulation of the excitor and inhibitor, with each excitor stimulus preceded by 4 inhibitor stimuli. Scale bar corresponds to 3 μm.

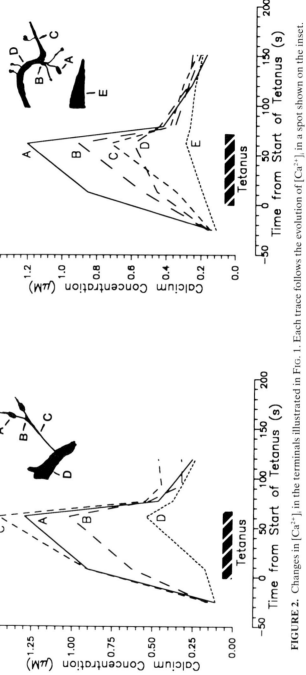

FIGURE 2. Changes in $[Ca^{2+}]_i$ in the terminals illustrated in FIG. 1. Each trace follows the evolution of $[Ca^{2+}]_i$ in a spot shown on the inset.

increasing calcium influx by prolonging action potentials is less efficient in enhancing transmitter release than is increasing calcium influx by raising $[Ca^{2+}]_i$ in the medium.

We explain these results by recognizing that transmitter release occurs in the immediate neighborhood of calcium channels opened by action potentials, before the sharp gradients of $[Ca^{2+}]_i$ near channel mouths have had time to collapse.[11-13] Increasing calcium influx per channel by raising extracellular $[Ca^{2+}]$ simply scales up the highly nonuniform submembrane distribution of $[Ca^{2+}]_i$ and captures much of the stoichiometry of the nonlinear activation of exocytosis by $[Ca^{2+}]_i$. By contrast, TEA prolongs action potentials and allows for the desynchronized opening of calcium

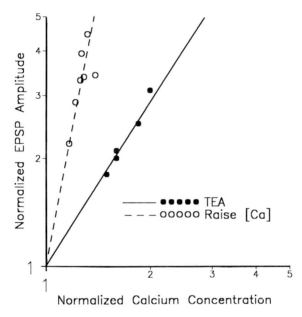

FIGURE 3. Relationship between changes in EPSP amplitude and changes in $[Ca^{2+}]_i$. Each point represents a different experiment. In each case, the excitor was stimulated at 8–10 Hz for at least 20 s before the EPSP and $[Ca^{2+}]_i$ values were recorded in control solution to provide the normalizing levels. In some experiments, 5 mM TEA was added, whereas in others, external $[Ca^{2+}]$ was raised (from 50% to 100% normal or from 30% to 70% normal); then the tetanus was repeated to obtain changes under the experimental condition. The results are plotted on double logarithmic coordinates, and lines are drawn with the average slope for each type of experiment.

channels early and late in the spike. This leads to shifting clusters of open calcium channels and shifting domains of high $[Ca^{2+}]_i$ that trigger transmitter release. In an extreme case, an action potential of doubled duration might evoke transmitter release from two nonoverlapping sets of high $[Ca^{2+}]_i$ domains occurring early and late in the action potential. Then both calcium influx (and $[Ca^{2+}]_i$ accumulation) and transmitter release would double, and the change in the two would be linearly related. Because the observed relationship between the increase in transmission and increase in $[Ca^{2+}]_i$ accumulation has an apparent power of about 2, this suggests that some overlap occurs between $[Ca^{2+}]_i$ domains early and late in a TEA-prolonged action potential, which is hardly surprising. A low power dependence of transmitter release on calculated calcium influx in TEA-prolonged action potentials was recently observed at the squid giant synapse and explained in a similar manner.[14]

ROLE OF RESIDUAL CALCIUM IN POSTTETANIC POTENTIATION

Stimulation of the excitor motor neuron at 20–35 Hz for 10–20 min is accompanied by a rise in transmitter released per impulse that takes several minutes to develop and that lasts for 10–50 min after the end of the tetanus.[15] This phase of potentiated release depends on calcium ions. Blocking calcium influx by stimulation in a calcium-free medium results in substantially reduced posttetanic potentiation (PTP).[5,16]

We have followed the time course of $[Ca^{2+}]_i$ accumulation and removal during the development and decay of excitatory postsynaptic potential (EPSP) potentiation and have found them to be similar (FIG. 4). The posttetanic decay of $[Ca^{2+}]_i$ matched closely the decay of PTP,[7] suggesting that the PTP was directly caused by the elevated residual $[Ca^{2+}]_i$. Transmission during a tetanus was greater for a given level of $[Ca^{2+}]_i$ than after the tetanus, partly because a tetanus $[Ca^{2+}]_i$ does not have enough time to fully equilibrate. Then the local submembrane $[Ca^{2+}]_i$ will be slightly higher than the volume average $[Ca^{2+}]_i$ that we measure and should more effectively potentiate release. During the tetanus, additional short-term facilitatory processes add to longer-lasting potentiation. These decay within a few seconds of the offset of stimulation and so do not contribute to transmitter release when comparing posttetanic potentiation to posttetanic changes in $[Ca^{2+}]_i$.

How does increased $[Ca^{2+}]_i$ potentiate release? PTP could be a direct consequence of the nonlinear relationship between $[Ca^{2+}]_i$ and transmitter release.[17] Transmitter release would be very sensitive to a small increase in the peak $[Ca^{2+}]_i$ achieved near calcium channels during action potentials in the presence of increased residual $[Ca^{2+}]_i$ from prior activity. Calculations of such a model, however, predict a significantly more rapid decay of PTP than observed experimentally (FIG. 4). Therefore, the linear relationship between EPSP PTP and $[Ca^{2+}]_i$ suggests that $[Ca^{2+}]_i$ operates in some other way to potentiate release. Possibilities include mobilizing vesicles into docking positions at release sites and sensitizing the release apparatus to sudden large changes in $[Ca^{2+}]_i$.

ROLE OF SODIUM ACCUMULATION IN POSTTETANIC POTENTIATION

PTP is reduced when $[Na^+]_i$ accumulation is prevented, and it is enhanced when $[Na^+]_i$ accumulation is boosted with ouabain to block sodium extrusion by sodium/potassium exchange.[5,15,16] Sodium might act internally to directly potentiate transmitter release. Alternatively, sodium could affect the amount of $[Ca^{2+}]_i$ accumulation in a tetanus and thereby influence PTP.

There are two ways that $[Na^+]_i$ could elevate $[Ca^{2+}]_i$: by release of calcium from internal stores, or by entry from the external medium through Na/Ca exchange. To test these possibilities, we looked at the effect of elevating $[Na^+]_i$ on the level of $[Ca^{2+}]_i$ (FIG. 5). $[Na^+]_i$ was raised either by injection from a micropipette placed in an excitor branch on the surface of the claw opener muscle, or by exposure to veratridine, a drug that shifts the activation curve for sodium channels so that they are partially open at resting membrane potential. In either case, we found that $[Ca^{2+}]_i$

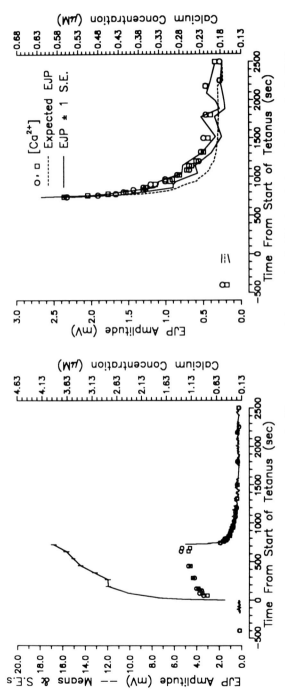

FIGURE 4. EPSP from the muscle fiber (solid lines) and $[Ca^{2+}]_i$ in two presynaptic boutons (symbols) before, during, and after a 12 min 20 Hz tetanus. The vertical bars on the left show SEs for mean EPSPs, whereas the two solid lines on the right represent the mean EPSPs ± 1 SE. EPSP means were calculated using a running average of 10 responses to smooth EPSP fluctuations. The dotted line was calculated from $V = K (P + R)$,[5] where V represents EPSP amplitude, R is the corresponding value of $[Ca^{2+}]_i$, and P is the peak rise in $[Ca^{2+}]_i$ at active zones caused by an action potential. P and K were determined from V and R at rest and shortly after the tetanus, and these were used to predict the posttetanic EPSP decay from the observed decay in $[Ca^{2+}]_i$.

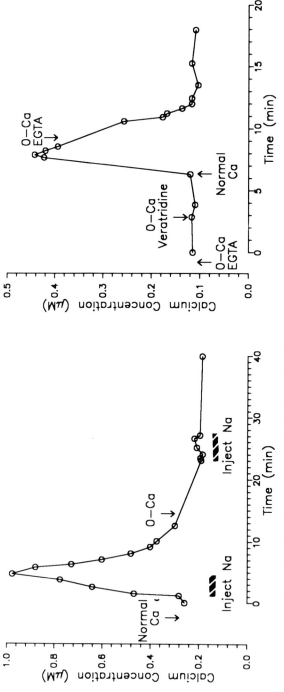

FIGURE 5. The left panel monitors changes in $[Ca^{2+}]_i$ during iontophoretic injection of Na^+ (10 nA) into a major branch of the excitor motor neuron, in normal Ringer and with 13.5 mM Co^{2+} substituted for the calcium. The right panel shows effects of 0.5 μM veratridine on $[Ca^{2+}]_i$ in a calcium-free medium and after changing to normal Ringer.

increased, but only when calcium was present in the external medium. This suggests that increased $[Na^+]_i$ can cause an elevation of $[Ca^{2+}]_i$, but only by way of changes in Na/Ca exchange, and not by release from intracellular stores.

Next we asked, What does a physiological sodium load do to $[Ca^{2+}]_i$? FIGURE 6A shows that stimulating the motor neuron tetanically in a calcium-free medium had no effect on $[Ca^{2+}]_i$. Following the tetanus, the bathing solution was changed to one containing normal $[Ca^{2+}]$; there was still no rise in $[Ca^{2+}]_i$. Apparently sodium accumulation in a tetanus neither releases calcium from intracellular stores nor admits calcium from outside by significantly altering the function of Na/Ca exchange. There is a third way in which $[Na^+]_i$ and $[Ca^{2+}]_i$ might interact in producing PTP. During a normal tetanus, presynaptic terminals would be loaded with both sodium and calcium. Perhaps the concomitant rise in $[Na^+]_i$ slows the extrusion of the increased $[Ca^{2+}]_i$ by reducing the sodium gradient that drives Ca extrusion by the Na/Ca pump.

To test this idea, we asked what effect a sodium load has on the extrusion of a calcium load. Preparations were depolarized with high potassium to admit both sodium and calcium through voltage-dependent channels while monitoring the rise in $[Ca^{2+}]_i$. Then normal potassium was restored, and the decay of $[Ca^{2+}]_i$ was followed. This provided a measure of the rate of removal of extra internal calcium in the presence of an elevated sodium load. The preparation was again depolarized by high potassium with choline in place of sodium. Again removing excess potassium, the decay of $[Ca^{2+}]_i$ was followed when no sodium load had developed. We found (FIG. 6B) that an intracellular sodium load slows the removal of calcium, consistent with the idea that $[Na^+]_i$ operates to reduce the extrusion of $[Ca^{2+}]_i$ and therefore increases and prolongs PTP. In other experiments, we used ouabain to increase sodium loading during a tetanus by blocking the active extrusion of sodium, and therefore to increase the sodium load during a tetanus. FIGURE 6C shows that this treatment increases the amount of EPSP potentiation and $[Ca^{2+}]_i$ accumulation during a tetanus and prolongs the posttetanic decay of both. These results all suggest that presynaptic sodium loading augments PTP by slowing the extrusion of calcium by Na/Ca exchange.

SEROTONIN-ACTIVATED ENHANCEMENT OF TRANSMITTER RELEASE

Serotonin (5-hydroxytryptamine, 5HT) is a naturally occurring hormone in crayfish, which increases the amount of transmitter release to action potentials at neuromuscular junctions.[18] Because the frequency of spontaneously released quanta, or miniature EPSPs, is also increased, it seemed possible that 5HT's effects were mediated by a rise in $[Ca^{2+}]_i$. This is especially possible because 5HT depolarizes presynaptic axons by up to 10 mV, which might open some calcium channels.[19] We found (FIG. 7, on the color plate) that even 5 μM 5HT, however, which augments EPSPs approximately fourfold, has little or no effect on resting $[Ca^{2+}]_i$ levels in presynaptic boutons. We doubt that the small increases in nerve terminals, typically under 25 nM, could be responsible for 5HT's augmentation of transmitter release, because a similar amount of PTP requires a $[Ca^{2+}]_i$ increase of about 100 nM.[7] Apparently the presynaptic depolarization caused by 5HT is insufficient to open many calcium channels; motor nerve terminals had to be depolarized by at least 15 mV (using elevated potassium) before a detectable increase in $[Ca^{2+}]_i$ could be observed. Such a depolarization decreases transmitter release slightly,[20] so it is unlikely to be involved in the augmentation of transmitter release by 5HT.

Instead, 5HT might increase voltage-dependent calcium current in crayfish

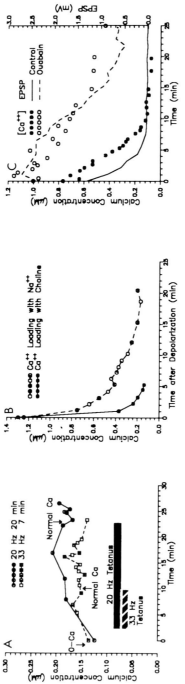

FIGURE 6. **A:** The excitor was stimulated tetanically in calcium-free Ringer in two experiments; normal calcium was restored at the end of each tetanus. **B:** Excitor nerve terminals were calcium-loaded two times by depolarizing the terminals in a solution with [K⁺] increased by 35 mM. In one case, they were also sodium-loaded with normal [Na⁺]; in the other, sodium was replaced by choline. **C:** The excitor was stimulated with two tetani (33 Hz for 5 min): once in normal Ringer and once in the presence of 0.5 mM ouabain to block sodium extrusion.

motor terminals, as it does in molluscan neurons.[21] 5HT, however, caused no increase in tetanic $[Ca^{2+}]_i$ accumulation; on the contrary, we usually saw about a 10% decrease in $[Ca^{2+}]_i$ accumulation in the presence of 5 μM 5HT (FIG. 7). Nevertheless, the EPSPs were increased about fourfold. We contrast this result with the effect of increasing calcium influx by either raising extracellular $[Ca^{2+}]$ or prolonging action potentials: a fourfold increase in transmitter release is accompanied by a 30%–70% increase in $[Ca^{2+}]_i$, depending upon how the calcium influx is increased (FIGURES 3 and 7). We conclude that serotonin does not enhance transmitter release by modulating the calcium influx through calcium channels or by increasing the number of open channels, the way raising extracellular $[Ca^{2+}]$ or adding TEA does. Rather, our results suggest an effect independent of presynaptic $[Ca^{2+}]_i$ action. Perhaps transmitter stores are mobilized, or the secretory machinery is made more sensitive to $[Ca^{2+}]_i$.

PRESYNAPTIC INHIBITION REDUCES TETANIC $[CA^{2+}]_I$ ACCUMULATION

At the claw opener neuromuscular junction, GABA released from inhibitory nerve terminals reduces the number of quanta released by excitor nerve impulses while simultaneously shunting EPSPs postsynaptically. We have now observed changes in $[Ca^{2+}]_i$ accumulation in excitor nerve terminals during presynaptic inhibition. We injected both excitor and inhibitor nerves with fura-2. By stimulating either neuron alone and looking for increases in $[Ca^{2+}]_i$, we identified excitatory and inhibitory nerve terminals. FIGURE 8 (on the color plate) shows a case of an excitatory and inhibitory bouton making contact with each other on the muscle surface. When the excitor was stimulated at 10 Hz, $[Ca^{2+}]_i$ rose in this excitor terminal by 475 nM. When each excitatory action potential was preceded by 4 inhibitory spikes at 50 Hz, with the last one preceding the excitatory action potential by the optimal interval for presynaptic inhibition[22] (2.3 ms at this synapse), then $[Ca^{2+}]_i$ in the excitor terminal rose by only 270 nM. If this reflects a similar reduction (to 57%) in calcium influx per excitatory action potential, this would have a profound effect on the amount of transmitter released by this particular bouton. Such a reduction in the number of calcium channels opened by an action potential might be expected to reduce transmitter release to about 18% at this particular synapse,[23] well within the range of presynaptic inhibition observed physiologically.[22]

ROLE OF PRESYNAPTIC POTENTIAL IN TRANSMITTER RELEASE

It has been suggested that presynaptic depolarization might play a direct role in neurosecretion, beyond simply opening calcium channels. In recent experiments by Hochner *et al.*,[24] supporting this hypothesis, the excitor axon was injected with the photolabile caged calcium chelator nitr-5. When the medium contained little calcium (12.5 mM magnesium with no added calcium), action potentials (10 Hz pairs separated by 20 ms) evoked no detectable transmitter release. Photolysis of nitr-5 increased the spontaneous release of transmitter fourfold, presumably by release of $[Ca^{2+}]_i$. Now, action potentials caused a slight increase in transmitter release within 5 ms of the spikes. In other experiments, calcium influx was blocked by 2 mM manganese with 0.2 mM calcium, and mitochondrial inhibitors were used to elevate $[Ca^{2+}]_i$. Again, action potentials evoked phasic release of transmitter.

These results were taken to show that when $[Ca^{2+}]_i$ is already high, membrane depolarization evokes neurotransmitter release in the absence of calcium entry. The solutions used, however, did not include chelators to remove extracellular calcium, which is known to leak out of muscles and collect in the bath,[17] and was already present at 0.2 mM in the manganese solution. We used fura-2 to check whether these solutions really block presynaptic calcium entry. FIGURE 9 shows that $[Ca^{2+}]_i$ more than doubled in these solutions when the excitor was stimulated with 10 Hz pairs. This small calcium influx was apparently insufficient to release transmitter at detectable levels, not surprising in view of the nonlinear dependence of release on calcium. Stimulation at 100 Hz revealed massive calcium influx and very large EPSPs in these solutions.[25] Such experiments, therefore, allow no conclusion about a direct effect of membrane depolarization on release.

We found that solutions in which all of the calcium is replaced by either cobalt or manganese, or in which calcium is chelated with 2 mM EGTA, show absolutely no rise in $[Ca^{2+}]_i$ to stimulation with 10 Hz pairs, and only 10–20 nM increase at 100 Hz. No transmitter release was observed at all in these solutions. These solutions may be used to test for an effect of presynaptic potential on transmitter release. Instead of nitr-5 we used DM-nitrophen,[26] a photolabile EDTA analogue that causes a much larger rise in $[Ca^{2+}]_i$ and displays none of the toxic effects of nitr-5 on neurosecretion.[27]

FIGURE 10 illustrates our results. Action potentials elicited normal EPSPs in normal Ringer. Photolysis of nitrophen caused a massive increase in transmitter release (the miniature EPSP frequency increased from 1 s^{-1} to over 3,000 s^{-1}), and the EPSPs were facilitated about 10-fold. After a few seconds, transmitter release subsided to a lower but nearly constant level (probably due to depletion of the most readily releasable store of quanta), and spikes still evoked strongly facilitated EPSPs. We performed similar experiments on preparations bathed in a solution containing cobalt instead of calcium. This blocked spike-evoked release. Nitrophen photolysis still accelerated miniature EPSP frequency, but now action potentials caused no additional release of transmitter. A nerve terminal field potential recorded from the muscle fiber indicated that the motor axon still conducted action potentials. When

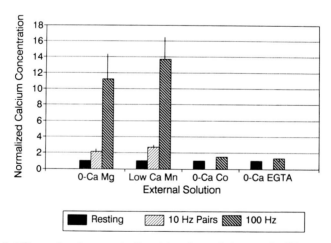

FIGURE 9. Effects of various nominally calcium-free solutions on $[Ca^{2+}]_i$ accumulation in presynaptic boutons, measured at rest, after stimulation with 10 Hz pairs separated by 20 ms, or stimulation at 100 Hz.

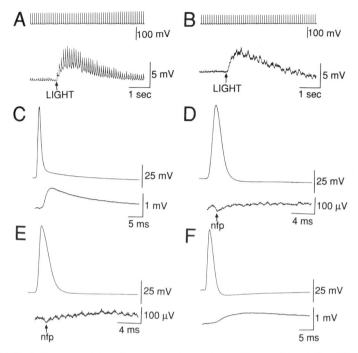

FIGURE 10. Action potentials evoke no transmitter release without calcium influx. The excitor axon was injected with DM-nitrophen 30% bound to calcium. In each panel, the top trace shows intracellularly recorded presynaptic action potentials, and the bottom trace shows intracellularly recorded postsynaptic potentials. Panel **A** shows results from an experiment in which nitrophen was photolyzed (with a 10 s exposure to UV light beginning at the arrow) while stimulating the motor nerve at 10 Hz in normal Ringer. Miniature EPSP frequency increased and evoked EPSPs were facilitated. The remaining panels are from a different experiment in which nitrophen was photolyzed while stimulating the nerve in a zero-calcium medium containing 13.5 mM Co^{2+}. Panel **B** shows that photolysis still increased miniature EPSP frequency, but that action potentials evoked no EPSPs either before or after the photolysis. The remaining panels show computer averages of 50 responses from the experiment of panel **B**. In panel **C**, spikes evoke EPSPs before injection of nitrophen while still in normal Ringer. In panel **D**, spikes evoke no EPSPs in the calcium-free cobalt Ringer after nitrophen injection. In panel **E**, spikes still evoke no EPSPs in the calcium-free Ringer even after photolysis increased the miniature EPSP frequency. Panel **F** shows the recovery of EPSPs after replacement of the solution with normal Ringer.

the medium was replaced with normal Ringer, spike-evoked transmission was restored. We think these results demonstrate that action potentials cannot evoke transmitter release in the absence of calcium influx, even when presynaptic $[Ca^{2+}]_i$ has been elevated to directly activate transmitter release at high levels.

We have also explored this question at the giant synapse in the stellate ganglion of the squid, a fast glutaminergic central nervous system synapse.[28] When the presynaptic terminal is injected with DM-nitrophen, action potentials evoke transmitter release with calcium present in the medium[27] (FIG. 11). Replacement of calcium with 10 mM EGTA completely blocked transmitter release to action potentials. Nitrophen photolysis by an intense light flash triggered transmitter release by

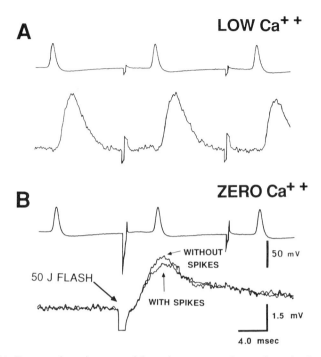

FIGURE 11. Presynaptic action potentials evoke no transmitter release in the absence of calcium entry at the squid giant synapse. The presynaptic terminal has been injected with DM-nitrophen 32% loaded with calcium. In each panel, the top trace shows the presynaptically recorded action potential, while the bottom trace shows postsynaptic potentials. In panel **A,** spikes evoke small EPSPs in low calcium medium (while replacing calcium with 10 mM EGTA). In panel **B,** extracellular $[Ca^{2+}]$ has been fully chelated, and spikes now evoke no transmitter release, even after flash photolysis of nitrophen elevates $[Ca^{2+}]_i$ to activate transmitter release directly. Two postsynaptic traces are superimposed showing responses to two flashes, but presynaptic action potentials were present during only one of the flashes.

elevating presynaptic $[Ca^{2+}]_i$, but action potentials failed to have any effect on this release. We conclude that at these synapses, as at crayfish neuromuscular junction, the only effect of the depolarization of an action potential is to open calcium channels and admit calcium ions, and that calcium alone triggers exocytosis at active zones.

A striking property of phasic spike-evoked release is that its time course is virtually unaffected by changes in extracellular $[Ca^{2+}]$, when comparing facilitated to unfacilitated release, or when release is triggered by pulses of different amplitude. A recent theoretical paper[29] used simulations of calcium diffusion from calcium channel mouths to nearby active zones to test the possibility that calcium could evoke transmitter release with a constant time-course under all these conditions. These simulations showed that, even when calcium was made to bind to a sensor that subsequently triggered exocytosis, changes in pulse amplitude, external $[Ca^{2+}]$, and state of facilitation all should affect the time-course of transmitter release. This was taken as proof that calcium entering through channel mouths and acting locally to trigger release and then quickly diffusing away cannot explain the constancy of the time-course of release.

We have repeated and confirmed these simulations.[30] We discovered, however, that the parameters chosen would saturate the presynaptic calcium receptor even at low extracellular [Ca^{2+}], contrary to observation. Furthermore, the binding step was taken as being the rate-limiting step, rather than exocytosis. When binding constants (on and off rates) more similar to BAPTA were used for the calcium receptor, transmitter release became rate-limited by the exocytosis step, and its time-course was as invariant as shown by experimental result. Thus, this objection to the calcium hypothesis of transmitter release is easily overcome.

TRANSMITTER RELEASE BY SUDDEN ELEVATION OF PRESYNAPTIC [CA^{2+}]$_I$

FIGURES 11 and 12 illustrate a surprising property of transmitter release evoked by flash photolysis of DM-nitrophen at the squid giant synapse: the postsynaptic response is quite transient, dropping to half its peak in 5–10 milliseconds. A prolonged tail of release continues for several seconds. Part of this transience in the response arises from the chemical properties of DM-nitrophen. When this chelator is partially photolyzed by a light flash, the calcium released re-equilibrates with the remaining unphotolyzed nitrophen. Because nitrophen is an EDTA derivative, it also binds magnesium tightly, absorbing the several millimolar present in cytoplasm. Photolytically liberated calcium rebinds to unphotolyzed nitrophen only after displacing hydrogen and magnesium. But the unbinding of magnesium is slow, and this leads to a period during which the calcium liberated from photolyzed nitrophen remains free. This leads to a transient rise in [Ca^{2+}]$_i$ following partial flash photolysis of nitrophen. This behavior was confirmed by co-injecting fura-2 with nitrophen into squid giant synapses.[27] Measurement of [Ca^{2+}]$_i$ revealed a transient rise to the low micromolar range and a subsequent fall to about half this level with a time-constant of 65 milliseconds. A nonlinear dependence of transmitter release upon [Ca^{2+}]$_i$

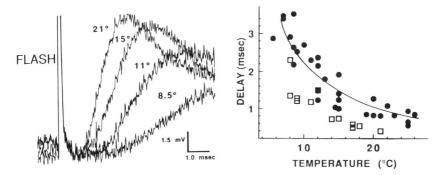

FIGURE 12. Effect of temperature on the postsynaptic responses to flash photolysis of DM-nitrophen injected into a squid presynaptic terminal. Sample responses are on the left, while the graph plots the delay to the beginning of postsynaptic potentials following nitrophen photolysis (filled circles) as well as synaptic delays from the peak of presynaptic spikes to the foot of the EPSP (open squares). The photolysis response delays have been corrected for the expected time between the flash and photolysis of nitrophen. The curve is a least squares fit of the logarithm of the delay from photolysis to changes in temperature.

would largely account for the rapidly decaying (15–20 ms time-constant) transient phase of transmitter release, followed by a smaller long-lasting tail. Depletion of releasable transmitter may also contribute to the decay of release.

Nitrophen photolysis also releases intracellular magnesium. We have found that a $[Mg^{2+}]_i$ jump alone evokes no transmitter release, because nitrophen injected without calcium evokes no transmitter release upon photolysis.

A measured rise of $[Ca^{2+}]_i$ to a few μM evokes transmitter release at a rate that resembles that caused by action potentials. Spikes are thought to release transmitter from very near calcium channels at concentrations well above 10 μM.[12-14] How, then, can a few μM $[Ca^{2+}]_i$ elicit such powerful transmitter release? Although we do not have a quantitative answer to this question, we believe that one factor is that calcium released by nitrophen acts uniformly on every single releasable vesicle. Action potentials open a small fraction of the available calcium channels and release transmitter quanta at only a few of the many release sites, so a higher local $[Ca^{2+}]_i$ is needed at these sites to release as many quanta as calcium released from nitrophen, acting globally.

Another factor may be that we have underestimated the peak calcium rise. Photolysis of 20% of the 10 or so mM of injected nitrophen 30% loaded with calcium releases 600 μM of calcium, most of which will be rapidly rebound by unphotolyzed free nitrophen. To protect our photomultiplier tube from damage, we could begin to measure $[Ca^{2+}]_i$ only 3–5 ms after the flash. Thus an initial intense peak in $[Ca^{2+}]_i$, lasting until the calcium binds to free nitrophen, would be missed in our measurements (and in any case would be blunted by the noninstantaneous association of calcium with fura-2). If the displacement of hydrogen from nitrophen takes longer than the binding of calcium to the receptor for releasing transmitter, then this undetected calcium spike could contribute significantly to the amount of transmitter released by a flash of light.

Postsynaptic responses following nitrophen photolysis show a "synaptic delay" consisting of the time to photolyze nitrophen (about 100 μs in vitro) plus the time for exocytosis to occur. The latter step is highly temperature-dependent, with a Q_{10} of about 3.5 between 5 and 15°C (FIG. 12). This is similar to the temperature sensitivity of the evoked synaptic delay following presynaptic impulses,[31] suggesting that some step in exocytosis following calcium entry has a high activation energy and is rate-limiting in determining the initial delay and subsequent time-course of transmitter release.

SUMMARY

This review gives some indication of the progress that has been made in understanding synaptic transmission by use of new methods for measuring and controlling presynaptic $[Ca^{2+}]_i$. Many unsolved problems remain. We still do not have a clear idea of the exact relationship between $[Ca^{2+}]_i$ and transmitter release and whether this relationship is the same under all circumstances. The apparently different $[Ca^{2+}]_i$-dependence of evoked transmitter release and of PTP suggest multiple molecular sites of calcium action that remain to be identified. A complete and comprehensive model of transmitter release has yet to be devised, and questions raised by our experiments may indicate that it is still too early to try to construct a precise model. We also do not know just how serotonin acts to modulate transmitter release, only that it does not appear to alter either resting or entering calcium. Some of these questions may be approachable with the techniques described here; others are not and require different methods for their resolution. The work continues.

REFERENCES

1. KATZ, B. 1969. The Release of Neural Transmitter Substances. Charles C. Thomas. Springfield, Ill.
2. LLINÁS, R., I. Z. STEINBERG & K. WALTON. 1981. Biophys. J. **33**: 323–352.
3. AUGUSTINE, G. J. & M. P. CHARLTON. 1986. J. Physiol. (Lond.) **381**: 619–640.
4. BITTNER, G. D. 1989. J. Neurobiol. **20**: 386–408.
5. ATWOOD, H. L. & J. M. WOJTOWICZ. 1986. Int. Rev. Neurobiol. **28**: 275–362.
6. GRYNKIEWICZ, G., M. POENIE & R. Y. TSIEN. 1985. J. Biol. Chem. **260**: 3440–3450.
7. DELANEY, K. R., R. S. ZUCKER & D. W. TANK. 1989. J. Neurosci. **9**: 3558–3567.
8. HAGIWARA, S. & L. BYERLY. 1981. Annu. Rev. Neurosci. **4**: 69–125.
9. GINSBURG, S. & R. RAHAMIMOFF. 1983. Nature **306**: 62–64.
10. WOJTOWICZ, J. M. & H. L. ATWOOD. Unpublished.
11. SIMON, S. M. & R. R. LLINÁS. 1985. Biophys. J. **48**: 485–498.
12. FOGELSON, A. L. & R. S. ZUCKER. 1985. Biophys. J. **48**: 1003–1017.
13. SMITH, S. J. & G. J. AUGUSTINE. 1988. Trends Neurosci. **11**: 458–464.
14. AUGUSTINE, G. J. 1990. J. Physiol. (Lond.) **431**: 343–364 .
15. WOJTOWICZ, J. M. & H. L. ATWOOD. 1985. J. Neurophysiol. **54**: 220–230.
16. MISLER, S., FALKE, L. & S. MARTIN. 1987. Am. J. Physiol. **252**: C55–C62.
17. MILEDI, R. & R. THIES. 1971. J. Physiol. (Lond.) **212**: 245–257.
18. GLUSMAN, S. & E. A. KRAVITZ. 1982. J. Physiol. (Lond.) **325**: 223–241.
19. DIXON, D. & H. L. ATWOOD. 1985. J. Neurobiol. **16**: 409–424.
20. ZUCKER, R. S. 1974. J. Physiol. (Lond.) **241**: 111–126.
21. PAUPARDIN-TRITSCH, D., C. HAMMOND & H. M. GERSCHENFELD. 1986. J. Neurosci. **6**: 2715–2723.
22. DUDEL, J. & S. W. KUFFLER. 1961. J. Physiol. (Lond.) **155**: 543–562.
23. ZUCKER, R. S. & A. L. FOGELSON. 1986. Proc. Natl. Acad. Sci. USA **83**: 3032–3036.
24. HOCHNER, B., H. PARNAS & I. PARNAS. 1989. Nature **342**: 433–435.
25. MULKEY, R. M. & R. S. ZUCKER. 1991. Nature **350**: 153–155.
26. KAPLAN, J. H. & G. C. R. ELLIS-DAVIES. 1988. Proc. Natl. Acad. Sci. USA **85**: 6571–6575.
27. DELANEY, K. R. & R. S. ZUCKER. 1990. J. Physiol (Lond.) **426**: 473–498.
28. ZUCKER, R. S. 1991. *In* Presynaptic Regulation of Neurotransmitter Release. J. Feigenbaum & M. Hanani, Eds.: 153–195. Freund. Tel Aviv.
29. PARNAS, H., G. HOVAV & I. PARNAS. 1989. Biophys. J. **55**: 859–874.
30. YAMADA, W. M. & R. S. ZUCKER. 1991. In preparation.
31. CHARLTON, M. P. & H. L. ATWOOD. 1979. Brain Res. **170**: 543–546.

Changes in Presynaptic Function during Long-Term Potentiation

RICHARD W. TSIEN AND ROBERTO MALINOW[a]

Department of Molecular and Cellular Physiology
Beckman Center
Stanford University Medical Center
Stanford, California 94305

Long-lasting changes in synaptic function are thought to be essential for learning and memory in both vertebrates[1,2] and invertebrates.[3,4] Long-term potentiation (LTP) is the most widely studied example of such synaptic plasticity in the mammalian brain.[5-19] The remarkable feature of LTP is that a short burst of synaptic activity can trigger persistent enhancement of synaptic transmission lasting for at least several hours, and possibly weeks or longer.[5] First found in the hippocampus[6,7] (where selective damage in humans can result in defects in memory acquisition[8]), LTP is now known to exist in cerebral cortex and other areas of the mammalian central nervous system (CNS).[9,10] Thus, there is intense interest in understanding the cellular and molecular mechanisms that underly LTP.[11-19] This paper is a brief summary of our recent studies of LTP.[20-26] The emphasis is on new evidence that expression of LTP involves changes in presynaptic signaling. [21-27]

Most studies on LTP focus on the synapse between Schäffer collaterals and hippocampal CA1 neurons. In this system, a brief burst of afferent stimulation leads to induction of LTP in postsynaptic CA1 cells through a combination of (1) membrane depolarization and (2) activation of glutamate receptors of the N-methyl-D-aspartate (NMDA) type.[12-17] It is generally agreed that the depolarization relieves Mg^{2+} block of NMDA receptor channels and allows a Ca^{2+} influx into dendritic spines that somehow triggers LTP.[28,29] The key question is how a rise in $[Ca^{2+}]_i$ can lead to a long-lasting enhancement of synaptic function. A generic working hypothesis, favored by many investigators,[18,19] is that Ca^{2+} acts through a signal transduction pathway that involves a Ca^{2+}-dependent protein kinase such as protein kinase C (PKC) or multifunctional Ca/calmodulin-dependent protein kinase (CaMK). Specific conclusions about the nature of the Ca^{2+}-dependent signaling were derived from our experiments with various inhibitors of PKC and CaMK, including highly selective pseudosubstrate peptides.[21,25] These observations, and parallel experiments from other groups,[30,31] have indicated that postsynaptic PKC and CaMK may both be essential for the establishment of LTP.

PURELY POSTSYNAPTIC EXPRESSION?

A major question concerns the expression of enhanced synaptic efficacy during LTP. Is synaptic transmission strengthened by increased transmitter release or enhanced postsynaptic receptivity? This issue has been keenly debated for several years.[13-16] Evidence in favor of a strictly postsynaptic mechanism for the expression of

[a] Present address: Department of Physiology and Biophysics, University of Iowa, Iowa City, IA 52242.

LTP has come from the groups of Lynch[32,33] and Nicoll.[34] Their results indicated that the expression of LTP was associated with a selective enhancement of the response of only one class of glutamate receptors, the α-amino-3-hydroxy-5-methyl-4-isoxazole proprionate (AMPA)-sensitive type, but not the NMDA-sensitive type. Both AMPA- and NMDA-sensitive components might be expected to increase if transmitter release were increased. Thus, they concluded that the locus of expression must be entirely postsynaptic.[32-34]

The experimental basis for this conclusion is controversial. We have found a significant potentiation of NMDA-mediated transmission.[24] Using 1– 10 μM 6-cyano-7-nitroquinoxaline-2,3-dione (CNQX) to block AMPA receptors, we found clear and significant increases in the NMDA component during LTP in tetanized pathways but not control pathways (FIG. 1). The potentiated epsps were completely blocked by the NMDA receptor blocker 2-amino-5-phosphonovalerate (APV). Thus, an enhancement of the NMDA-receptor component can be detected. Bashir et al. have also reported LTP of the NMDA component.[35] Both of these studies run counter to the previous arguments[32-34]; thus, the hypothesis of a purely postsynaptic locus of LTP expression has not been firmly substantiated.

ANY PRESYNAPTIC EXPRESSION?

Studies of Skrede and Malthe-Sorenssen,[36] and Bliss and colleagues[37] provided early suggestions of an enhancement of presynaptic release. Using a push-pull cannula system in vivo, Dolphin, Errington and Bliss[37] found evidence for increased release of [³H]glutamate in the dentate gyrus in association with LTP and proposed that presynaptic release was elevated (see also ref. 36). Bliss et al.,[38] however, were careful to point out that some questions remain unanswered. Which type of cell is the source of the increase? Could the increased concentration of glutamate in the perfusate be due to decreased uptake? If presynaptic glutamate release is truly increased, is this evoked by action potentials or merely an increase in nonquantal leakage? Having discussed these questions, Bliss and Lynch[13] concluded that the available evidence provided "plausible though not conclusive reasons for attributing the enhanced release to an increase in the amount of transmitter released per action potential from potentiated terminals." They suggested that quantal analysis would be needed to settle the issue of whether the locus of LTP expression was postsynaptic or presynaptic (see also refs. 15 and 16).

WHOLE CELL RECORDINGS AND LTP

A major obstacle to a statistical analysis of synaptic events has been the poor signal-to-noise ratio of conventional intracellular microelectrode recordings. Recently, we have succeeded in applying the whole-cell voltage clamp technique to study LTP in conventional hippocampal slices.[22] Our analysis of changes in the statistical properties of transmitter release before and during LTP supports an increased likelihood of presynaptic transmitter release.[22-24,26] Similar results have been reported by Bekkers and Stevens.[27]

We have found that whole cell recordings can be obtained from CA1 neurons 2–3 cell diameters below the surface in conventional slices of rat hippocampus. This method allows recordings from cells with largely intact dendritic structures, while also providing much better signal resolution and biochemical access than recordings

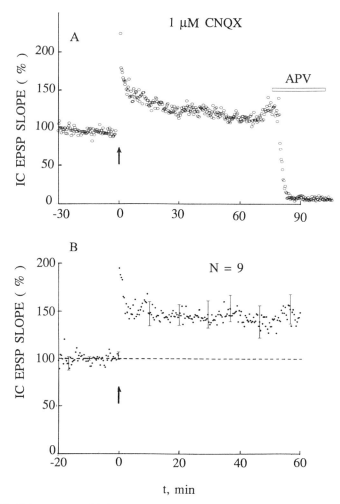

FIGURE 1. Enhancement of NMDA-receptor response during LTP. **A:** Representative experiment in the presence of 1 μM CNQX to block AMPA-sensitive glutamate receptors. Relative amplitude of excitatory postsynaptic potential (epsp), recorded with an intracellular microelectrode plotted against time. Tetanic stimulation was applied at the arrow. Abolition of epsp by 50 μM APV demonstrates that epsp was mediated by NMDA receptors. **B:** Collected results from similar experiments in a total of nine slices. Epsp amplitudes were normalized to control values before tetanic stimulation, then ensemble averaged. Bars indicate SEM. Note significant and long-lasting potentiation of the NMDA receptor–mediated response. (Tsien & Malinow.[24] With permission from Cold Spring Harbor Laboratory.)

with conventional microelectrodes. The recordings are generally very stable, lasting many hours, although occasionally whole cell access is lost because of sealing over.

We have carried out a number of experiments in which a single CA3 neuron was directly stimulated by an intracellular microelectrode while, simultaneously, recordings were carried out in a CA1 neuron.[23,26] In most of the experiments, synaptic currents were elicited by minimal extracellular stimulation, only slightly stronger than the highest stimulus that gives all failures. Under these conditions, activation is thought to be restricted to a single synapse onto the monitored neuron.[39,40] With either type of stimulation, the synaptic currents showed a large intertrial variability that was much greater than the background noise, but similar time courses (FIG. 2a and b), supporting the view that they originated from the same synapse. There were occasional clear failures (FIGURES 2a and 5a and b), and sporadic spontaneous events that resembled the elicited response, ranging in amplitude from <1 pA up to ~ 10 pA (FIG. 1b, inset).

To optimize the chances of obtaining LTP under whole-cell recording conditions, we used internal solutions with minimal Ca^{2+} buffering to avoid block of LTP, and with Cs^+ as the main cation to enhance voltage control of the postsynaptic membrane. We also included ATP and GTP in the internal solution to allow activity of protein kinases or GTP-binding proteins. Following a stable baseline period of 10–15 minutes, we were able to induce LTP by pairing a steady postsynaptic depolarization to ~ 0 mV with continued activation of the test pathway (40 stimuli at 2 Hz). This pairing procedure resulted in LTP in the majority of experiments (FIGURES 2c, 5c, and 4 (top panel)). By contrast, no potentiation was found in transmission through a simultaneously monitored control pathway that did not receive presynaptic stimuli during the postsynaptic depolarization (FIGURES 2d and 4 (top, open symbols). Furthermore, synaptic stimulation at 2 Hz without postsynaptic depolarization did not give synaptic enhancement. Thus, the potentiation was synapse-specific and required a combination of presynaptic activity and postsynaptic depolarization, just as seen in conventional recordings of LTP.

To investigate whether diffusible cytoplasmic factors are involved in potentiation, we attempted to trigger LTP at different times after gaining whole-cell access (FIG. 2 d). Pairing soon after beginning whole-cell recording (~ 20 min or less) consistently resulted in LTP lasting > 1 h (FIGURES 2, 4, 5). Little or no potentiation, however, was found with pairing > 30 min after whole-cell access. One possibility is that some diffusible postsynaptic component is needed to trigger LTP, but not to maintain the potentiation.

ANALYSIS OF PRESYNAPTIC AND POSTSYNAPTIC FACTORS

To understand the basis of the synaptic variability and its possible relation to fluctuations in transmitter release, we modified presynaptic or postsynaptic functions by changing the bathing medium (FIG. 3). Elevating $[Ca^{2+}]_o$ to increase presynaptic release enhanced the synaptic currents (FIG. 3a). The amplitude histogram changed from a highly skewed distribution (FIG. 3b) to a nearly symmetrical bell shape (FIG. 3c). By contrast, when we added low concentrations of the glutamate receptor antagonist CNQX to modify postsynaptic responsiveness, the average synaptic current was dramatically reduced (FIG. 3a,e), but the shape of the distribution remained unchanged (FIG. 3c,d). Thus, the distributions before and after CNQX matched closely when normalized by their means (FIG. 3d).

To obtain a simple and revealing index of synaptic variability, we computed $CV^{-2} = M^2/\sigma^2$ where CV is the coefficient of variation, M is the mean synaptic current, and σ^2 is the variance about M, for a given epoch of consecutive responses from t to t + τ. This kind of analysis has often been applied to synaptic transmission in other systems.[41–43] We can compute the expected behaviour of M^2/σ^2 if we make assumptions regarding the mechanisms underlying synaptic transmission. In the simplified case of a binomial distribution of transmitter release, where p is the

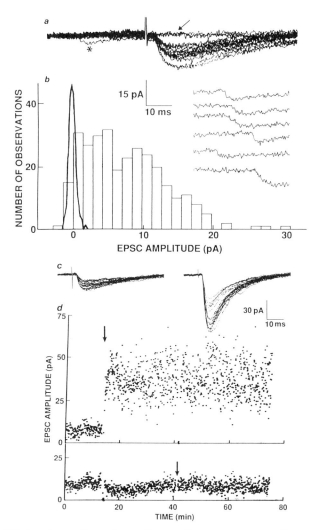

FIGURE 2. Whole-cell recordings of synaptic transmission in conventional hippocampal slices show large intertrial variability, synapse-specific LTP, and loss of induction but not expression with prolonged dialysis. The method of recording is described in ref. 22 (see also refs. 58–61). *a:* Sixteen consecutive records of synaptic currents, superimposed. Note spontaneous event in baseline period (*) and synaptic failures (arrow). *b:* Amplitude distribution histograms for 200 consecutive synaptic currents (bars) and baseline noise (smooth curve). Inset: representative spontaneous synaptic currents. Note the variability in amplitude and time course but general similarity to evoked responses. *c* and *d:* Plots of synaptic responses against time in a postsynaptic cell receiving two independent inputs. *c:* LTP was selectively induced in one pathway by a pairing procedure 15 min following break-in (arrow); in the other pathway (*d*), the pairing procedure was applied 25 min later, but failed to induce LTP, in contrast to the maintenance of LTP in *c*. In the pairing procedure, the cell was depolarized from −70 mV to ∼0 mV, whereas the paired (conditioned) pathway was stimulated 40 times at 2 Hz with no change in stimulus strength. Nonconditioned pathway received no stimuli during the postsynaptic depolarization. Inset: families of consecutive current records showing excitatory postsynaptic currents (epsc) of conditioned pathway, collected before (left) and 30 min after pairing (right). (Malinow & Tsien.[22] With permission from *Nature.*)

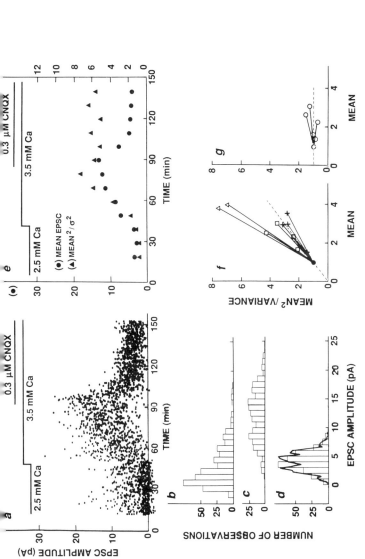

FIGURE 3. Selective changes in presynaptic and postsynaptic function produce expected changes in mean and variance of synaptic currents. Agents acting through presynaptic mechanisms affect shape of distribution histograms and M^2/σ^2, whereas inhibition of postsynaptic receptors does not. *a*: Epsc amplitude plotted against time. Bathing calcium was elevated from 2.5 mM to 3.5 mM, and 0.3 μM CNQX was applied where shown. *b–d*: Amplitude distribution histograms for 300 epscs before manipulation (*b*), after elevation of calcium (*c*), and after subsequent addition of CNQX (*d*). Continuous line in *d* shows data from *c*, normalized to mean epsc amplitude in *d*. Note close agreement of normalized histograms. *e*: Plot of mean epsc amplitude, M (circles) and M^2/σ^2 (triangles) for the experiment shown in *a*, with θ = 10 min (150 trials). *f*: Plot of M^2/σ^2 against M for several presynaptic manipulations: Ca increased from 2.5 to 3.5 mM (triangles); Mg decreased from 1.3 to 0.65 mM in the presence of 50 μM APV (squares); Mg increased stimulus strength to recruit more fibers (cross). *g*: Plot of M^2/σ^2 against M for experiments in which CNQX (0.2–0.3 μM) was bath-applied. For each experiment in *f* and *g*, lines connect points obtained before and after manipulation. M and M^2/σ^2 were computed for 300 trials prior to the manipulation, and 300 trials at the peak of the effect, and normalized by the values corresponding to the smaller M for that experiment. Note that presynaptic manipulations that are thought to increase p affect M^2/σ^2 more than the mean, whereas increasing stimulus strength, which increases N, affects M^2/σ^2 as much as M. These findings are expected for a binomial release process (see text). (Malinow & Tsien.[22] With permission from *Nature*.)

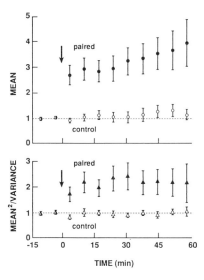

FIGURE 4. A synapse-specific increase in M^2/σ^2 associated with LTP; results from the 14 of 18 experiments that showed LTP with pairing. In the other 4 experiments with no LTP, M^2/σ^2 remained unchanged (not shown). Top panel: ensemble averages and SEMS of M for the paired pathway (filled circles) and the control pathway (open circles, n = 10; in 4 experiments this pathway was not monitored). Arrow marks time of pairing procedure (as in FIGURES 1 and 2). Bottom panel: ensemble averages of M^2/σ^2 for paired (filled triangles) and nonpaired (open triangles) pathways for the same experiments as in the top graph. (Malinow & Tsien.[22] With permission from *Nature.*)

probability of release for each of N available quanta, v is the vesicular content, and z is the postsynaptic response to a fixed amount of transmitter,

$$M^2/\sigma^2 = (Npvz)^2/Np(1-p)(vz)^2 = Np/(1-p). \qquad (1)$$

Thus, M^2/σ^2 is independent of changes in z and is a useful measure of some changes in presynaptic function, but not all factors (*e.g.* v). It increases in proportion to N, and at least linearly with p, as experimentally confirmed at the neuromuscular junction.[41] The lack of dependence of M^2/σ^2 on the postsynaptic responsiveness (z), holds for more general cases (not necessarily binomial) as long as z does not vary from trial to trial within a given epoch.[22]

Assuming z is constant for an epoch, the theory predicts that changes in M^2/σ^2 between epochs will result from changes in release characteristics but not postsynaptic modifications. This was tested by examining changes in M^2/σ^2 following interventions known to affect presynaptic or postsynaptic mechanisms. As FIGURE 3e illustrates, raising extracellular calcium dramatically increased M^2/σ^2. This was found for all experimental maneuvers expected to affect presynaptic release: lowering magnesium, application of the potassium channel blocker 4-aminopyridine (not shown), or increasing the stimulus strength to recruit more afferent fibers (FIG. 3f). In general, M^2/σ^2 increased at least as much as the mean synaptic current. By contrast, addition of CNQX produced no significant change in M^2/σ^2, despite its large effect on synaptic transmission (see FIG. 3e and g).

CHANGES IN SYNAPTIC VARIABILITY DURING LTP

Does M^2/σ^2 change with LTP? FIGURE 4b compares M^2/σ^2 of the test pathway with that of the control (unpaired) pathway, for a group of experiments showing potentiation of mean synaptic current (FIG. 4a). Following pairing, M^2/σ^2 increased significantly in the test pathway, with no change in the control pathway. The increase in M^2/σ^2 with LTP could arise from various presynaptic mechanisms: an increase in the number of available vesicles; an increase in the probability of release of some or all vesicles; or changes in nonvesicular release. It would not be expected from uniform changes in the number, sensitivity, or conductance of glutamate receptor channels, or in the effectiveness of charge transfer from spines to dendrites.

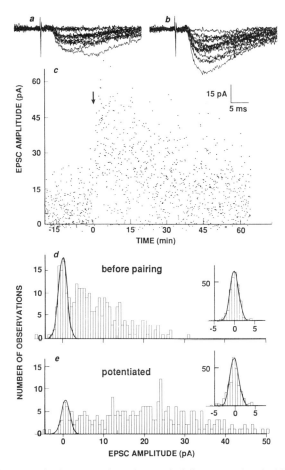

FIGURE 5. Decreases in the proportion of synaptic failures associated with LTP. *a* and *b*: Groups of 16 consecutive epscs taken before (*a*) and 40 min after (*b*) a pairing procedure to induce LTP. *c*: Amplitude of epscs elicited by minimal stimulation plotted against time. Arrow marks pairing procedure (see FIG. 2). *d* and *e*: Amplitude distribution histograms for 17 min epochs prior to pairing (*d*, from t = −17 to t = 0) and after pairing (*e*, from t = 5 to t = 22 min). Smooth curves are gaussians whose height was adjusted to fit the first peak in the amplitude distribution. The half of the gaussians, 2.5 pA, was obtained by fitting amplitude histograms of the baseline noise during the same epochs (insets). The proportion of failures was estimated as the area under the gaussian curve. (Malinow & Tsien.[22] With permission from *Nature.*)

ANALYSIS OF FAILURES

If the expression of LTP involves an increased probability of release or a greater number of available quanta, one would expect fewer failures of transmission during LTP. FIG. 5 illustrates an experiment where failures and responses were clearly resolvable. The amplitude distribution histogram displayed a distinct peak at zero amplitude that matched the amplitude distribution of the noise (inset). The area under the zero amplitude peak was used to estimate the percentage of failures. In this experiment, the proportion of failures was 27% prior to pairing (*d*), falling to 11% between 5 and 22 min after pairing (*e*). This change accompanied a 2.8-fold increase in mean synaptic current.

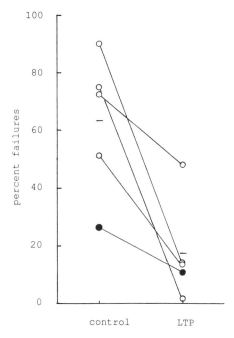

FIGURE 6. Consistent decrease in proportion of synaptic failures during LTP. Collected results from five experiments. Horizontal lines show mean percentage of failures (63 ± 11% in control before pairing, 17 ± 8% during LTP after pairing). Filled symbols show results from experiment illustrated in FIG. 5. The two experiments with the highest percentage of failures in control were recordings of one-to-one transmission from presynaptic CA3 neurons, stimulated with an intracellular microelectrode.[23,26]

This decrease in the proportion of failures was a consistent finding.[22] FIGURE 6 shows collected results from five experiments where failures could be clearly resolved. Two of the experiments in FIGURE 6 were obtained with intracellular microelectrode stimulation of a CA3 neuron in cell-pair recordings.[23,26] The collected data from all five experiments showed a mean (± SEM) decrease in failures from 63 ± 11% in control to 17 ± 8% after pairing, consistent with a greater likelihood of transmitter release during LTP. This conclusion is supported by the overall amplitude distribution, which changes from a skewed shape in control (FIG. 5*d*) to a bell-shape during LTP (FIG. 5*e*), as with increasing extracellular Ca (FIG. 3*b* and *c*). Very similar observations for LTP have been reported by Bekkers and Stevens.[27]

OTHER APPROACHES FOR LOCALIZING THE MECHANISMS
OF LTP EXPRESSION

Additional approaches are currently in use to localize mechanisms of synaptic potentiation. Besides analysis of coefficient of variation (or $CV^{-2} = M^2/\sigma^2$) and observations of failures of transmission, reviewed above, it is also possible to carry out direct measurements of quantal spacing,[43,44] (4) analysis of the amplitude and frequency of miniature epscs[45] (cf. ref. 46), and assays of postsynaptic responsiveness by local application of transmitter.[45,47] So far, most,[22,23,26,27] but not all,[40] of the experiments in area CA1 support the view that enhancement of presynaptic transmitter release is a predominant factor in LTP.

NEW QUESTIONS ABOUT SYNAPTIC SIGNALING DURING LTP

The evidence for significant presynaptic modifications is striking, given the compelling arguments that induction of LTP is postsynaptic.[12–19,48] The combination of postsynaptic induction and (largely or wholly) presynaptic expression leads to the conclusion that a retrograde message must travel from the postsynaptic cell back to the presynaptic terminal. Although the nature of the retrograde signal is not known, two popular candidates include nitric oxide (EDRF),[49,50] or arachidonic acid or one of its metabolites.[51,52]

How is the retrograde signal linked to presynaptic function? Presynaptic GTP-binding proteins and protein kinases are possible mediators of the communication between the retrograde messenger and changes in presynaptic function. The involvement of presynaptic GTP-binding proteins was suggested by Goh and Pennefather[53] who showed that LTP requires a pertussis toxin–sensitive G-protein (G_{LTP}) whose action was not occluded by postsynaptic injection of GTPγS. The results imply that the G-protein is localized in a site outside the postsynaptic cell.

Participation of presynaptic protein kinase activity in LTP was suggested some time ago by Routtenberg.[54] A number of protein kinases are known to enhance transmitter release, including PKC[55,56] and CaMKII.[57] Participation of presynaptic kinase would fit with our finding that established LTP cannot be extinguished by postsynaptic intracellular injection of H-7 or peptide inhibitors of CaM KII and PKC, even though it remains responsive to bath application of H-7.[21,25] The effect of H-7 is quite selective for the potentiated pathway.[20,24] The implication is that the bath-applied H-7 acts outside the postsynaptic spine, possibly presynaptically. This interpretation could be tested by seeing if H-7 reverses the increased likelihood of transmitter release seen with LTP, by restoring synaptic failures and amplitude distributions to their original state before induction of LTP. It will also be important to see if LTP can be selectively prevented by intracellular delivery of protein kinase inhibitors from whole cell recording pipettes on the presynaptic cell body. The retrograde signaling pathway must work quickly: synaptic failures are drastically reduced within 1 min after the pairing procedure.

CONCLUSION

Many gaps remain in our understanding of signal transduction during long-term potentiation. Nevertheless, considerable progress has been made in demonstrating that a change in presynaptic function is a predominant mechanism of LTP expression. This opens the way for further work on presynaptic signaling in the hippocampus. There is little doubt that clarification of fundamental mechanisms of Ca^{2+} entry and control of exocytosis in a variety of systems will help our understanding of LTP and other long-term synaptic changes in the CNS.

REFERENCES

1. ECCLES, J. C. 1953. The Neurophysiological Basis of Mind. Clarendon Press. Oxford.
2. HEBB, D. O. 1949. The Organization of Behavior. Wiley. New York.
3. GOELET, P., V. F. CASTELLUCCI, S. SCHACHER & E. R. KANDEL. 1985. The long and short of long-term memory—a molecular framework. Nature 322: 419–422.
4. ALKON, D. L. & T. J. NELSON. 1990. Specificity of molecular changes in neurons involved in memory storage. FASEB J. 4: 1567–1576.
5. BLISS, T. V. P. & A. GARDNER-MEDWIN. 1973. Long-lasting potentiation of synaptic transmission in the dentate area of the unanaesthetized rabbit following stimulation of the perforant path. J. Physiol. (London) 232: 357–74.
6. LOMO, T. 1966. Frequency potentiation of excitatory synaptic activity in the dentate area of the hippocampal formation. Acta Physiol. Scand. Suppl. 277: 128.
7. BLISS, T. V. P. & T. LOMO. 1973. Long-lasting potentiation of synaptic transmission in the dentate area of the anaesthetized rabbit following stimulation of the perforant path. J. Physiol. (London) 232: 331–56.
8. SQUIRE, L. R. & E. LINDENLAUB, EDS. 1990. The Biology of Memory. Shattauer. Stuttgart.
9. ARTOLA, A. & W. SINGER. 1987. Long-term potentiation and NMDA receptors in rat visual cortex. Nature 330: 649–652.
10. IRIKI, A., C. PAVLIDES, A. KELLER & H. ASANUMA. 1989. Long-term potentiation in the motor cortex. Science 246: 1385–1387.
11. LYNCH, G. & M. BAUDRY. 1984. The Biochemistry of Memory: A new and specific hypothesis. Science 224: 1057–1063.
12. COLLINGRIDGE, G. L. & T. V. P. BLISS. 1987. NMDA receptors—their role in long-term potentiation. TINS 10: 288–293.
13. BLISS, T. V. P. & M. LYNCH. 1988. Long-term potentiation of synaptic transmission in the hippocampus: properties and mechanisms. In Long-term potentiation: From Biophysics to Behavior. P. W. Landfield & S. A. Deadwyler, Eds.: 3–72. Alan R. Liss. New York.
14. NICOLL, R. A., J. A. KAUER & R. C. MALENKA. 1988. The current excitement in long-term potentiation. Neuron 1: 97–103.
15. STEVENS, C. F. 1989. Strengthening the synapses. Nature 338: 460–461.
16. BROWN, T. H., P. F. CHAPMAN, E. W. KAIRISS & C. L. KEENAN. 1988. Long-term synaptic potentiation. Science 242: 724–728.
17. COTMAN, C. W., R. J. BRIDGES, J. S. TAUBE, A. S. CLARK, J. W. GEDDES & D. T. MONAGHAN. 1989. The role of the NMDA receptor in central nervous system plasticity and pathology. J. NIH Res. 1(2): 65–74.
18. KENNEDY, M. B. 1989. Regulation of synaptic transmission in the central nervous system: long-term potentiation. Cell 59: 777–787.
19. MALENKA, R. C., J. A. KAUER, D. J. PERKEL & R. A. NICOLL. 1989. The impact of postsynaptic calcium on synaptic transmission—its role in long term potentiation. Trends. Neurosci. 12: 444–450, 1989.
20. MALINOW, R., D. V. MADISON & R. W. TSIEN. 1988. Persistent protein kinase activity underlying long-term potentiation. Nature 335: 820–824.
21. MALINOW, R., H. SCHULMAN & R. W. TSIEN. 1989. Inhibition of postsynaptic PKC or CaMKII blocks induction but not expression of LTP. Science 245: 862–866.
22. MALINOW, R. & R. W. TSIEN. 1990a. Presynaptic enhancement revealed by whole cell recordings of long-term potentiation in rat hippocampal slices. Nature 346: 177–180.
23. MALINOW, R. & R. W. TSIEN. 1990b. Long-term potentiation of synaptic transmission between individual CA3 and CA1 neurons in rat hippocampal slices. Soc. Neurosci. (Abst) 16: 145.

24. TSIEN, R. W. & R. MALINOW. 1990c. Long-term potentiation: presynaptic enhancement following postsynaptic activation of Ca^{2+}-dependent protein kinases. Cold Spring Harbor Symp. Quant. Biol. **55**. In press.

25. TSIEN, R. W., H. SCHULMAN & R. MALINOW. 1990. Peptide inhibitors of PKC and CaMK block induction but not expression of long-term potentiation. *In* The Biology and Medicine of Signal Transduction. ed. Y. Nishizuka, M. Endo & C. Tanaka, Eds.: **24**: 101–107. Raven Press. New York.

26. MALINOW, R. 1991. Synaptic transmission between individual hippocampal slice neurons shows quantal levels, oscillations and LTP. Science **252**: 722–724.

27. BEKKERS, J. & C. F. STEVENS. 1990. Presynaptic mechanism for long-term potentiation in the hippocampus. Nature **346**: 724–729.

28. ASCHER, P. & L. NOWAK. 1988. Electrophysiological studies of NMDA receptors. Trends Neurosci. **10**: 284–288.

29. MAYER, M. L. & G. L. WESTBROOK. 1987. The physiology of excitatory amino acids in the vertebrate central nervous system. Prog. Neurobiol. **28**: 197–276.

30. MALENKA, R. C., J. A. KAUER, D. J. PERKEL, M. D. MAUK, P. T. KELLY, R. A. NICOLL & M. N. WAXHAM. 1989. An essential role for postsynaptic calmodulin and protein kinase activity in long-term potentiation. Nature **340**: 554–7.

31. ANDERSEN, P., J. M. GODFRAIND, P. GREENGARD, O. HVALBY, A. NAIRN, M. RAASTAD & J. F. STORM. 1990. Injection of a peptide inhibitor of protein kinase C blocks the induction of long-term potentiation in rat hippocampal cells *in vitro*. J. Physiol. (London) **429**: 25P.

32. MULLER, D., M. JOLY & G. LYNCH. 1988. Contributions of quisqualate and NMDA receptors to the induction and expression of LTP. Science **242**: 1694.

33. MULLER, D. & G. LYNCH. 1988. Long-term potentiation differentially affects two components of synaptic responses in hippocampus. Proc. Natl. Acad. Sci. USA **85**: 9346–9350.

34. KAUER, J. A., R. C. MALENKA & R. A. NICOLL. 1988. A persistent postsynaptic modification mediates long-term potentiation in the hippocampus. Neuron **1**: 911–917.

35. BASHIR, Z. I., S. ALFORD, S. N. DAVIES, A. D. RANDALL & G. L. COLLINGRIDGE. 1991. Long-term potentiation of NMDA receptor-mediated synaptic transmission in the hippocampus. Nature **369**: 156–158.

36. SKREDE, K. K. & D. MALTHE-SORENSSEN. 1981. Increased resting and evoked release of transmitter following repetitive electrical tetanization in hippocampus: a biochemical correlate to long-lasting synaptic potentiation. Brain Res. **208**: 436.

37. DOLPHIN, A. C., M. L. ERRINGTON & T. V. P. BLISS. 1982. Long-term potentiation of the perforant path *in vivo* is associated with increased glutamate release. Nature **297**: 496.

38. BLISS, T. V. P., R. M. DOUGLAS, M. L. ERRINGTON & M. A. LYNCH. 1986. Correlation between long-term potentiation and release of endogenous amino acids from dentate gyrus of anaesthetized rats. J. Physiol. (London) **377**: 391–408.

39. MCNAUGHTON, B. L., C. A. BARNES & P. ANDERSEN. 1981. Synaptic efficiacy and EPSP summation in granule cells of rat fascia dentat studied *in vitro*. J. Neurophysiol. **46**: 952–966.

40. FOSTER, T. C. & B. L. MCNAUGHTON. 1991. Long-term synaptic enhancement in CA1 is due to increased quantal size, not quantal content. Hippocampus. **1**: 79–91.

41. DEL CASTILLO, J. & B. KATZ. 1954. Quantal components of the end-plate potential. J. Physiol. (London) **124**: 560–573.

42. MARTIN, A. R. 1977. Junctional transmission II. Presynaptic mechanisms. *In* Handbook of Physiology: The Nervous System. Sect. 1, vol. I, Chpt. 10: 329–355. American Physiological Society. Bethesda, MD.

43. LARKMAN, A., K. STRATFORD & J. J. B. JACK. 1991. Quantal analysis of excitatory synaptic action and depression in hippocampal slices. Nature **350**: 344–347.

44. KAUER, J. A., F. SCHWEIZER, D. D. FRIEL & R. W. TSIEN. 1991. Quantal amplitude remains constant with long-term potentiation in rat hippocampal slices. Soc. Neurosci. Abstr. In press.

45. MALGAROLI, A. & R. W. TSIEN. 1991. Glutamate-induced long-term potentiation of miniature epsp frequency in cultured hippocampal neurons. Biophys. J. **59**: 19a.

46. BAXTER, D. A., G. D. BITTNER & T. H. BROWN. 1985. Quantal mechanisms of long-term synaptic potentiation. Proc. Natl. Acad. Sci. USA **82:** 5978–5982.
47. DAVIES, S. N., R. A. J. LESTER, K. G. REYMANN & G. L. COLLINGRIDGE. 1989. Temporally distinct pre- and post-synaptic mechanisms maintain long-term potentiation. Nature **330:** 500.
48. LYNCH, G., J. LARSON, S. KELSO, G. BARRIONUEVO & F. SCHOTTLER. 1983. Intracellular injections of EGTA block induction of hippocampal long-term potentiation. Nature **305:** 719–721.
49. GARTHWAITE, J., S. L. CHARLES & R. CHESS-WILLIAMS. 1988. Endothelium-derived relaxing factor release on activation of NMDA receptors suggests role as intercellular messenger in the brain. Nature **336:** 385–388.
50. SHIBUKI, K. & D. OKADA. 1991. Endogenous nitric oxide release required for long-term synaptic depression in the cerebellum. Nature **349:** 326–328.
51. WILLIAMS, J. H. & T. V. P. BLISS. 1988. Induction but not maintenance of calcium-induced long-term potentiation in dentate gyrus and area CA1 of the hippocampal slice is blocked by nordihydroguaiaretic acid. Neurosci. Lett. **88:** 81–85.
52. WILLIAMS, J. H., M. L. ERRINGTON, M. A. LYNCH & T. V. P. BLISS. 1989. Arachidonic acid induces a long-term activity-dependent enhancement of synaptic transmission in the hippocampus. Nature **341:** 739–742.
53. GOH, J. W. & P. A. PENNEFATHER. 1989. Pertussis toxin-sensitive G protein in hippocampal long-term potentiation. Science **244:** 980–983.
54. ROUTTENBERG, A. 1985. Protein kinase C activation leading to protein F1 phosphorylation may regulate synaptic plasticity by presynaptic terminal growth. Behav. Neural Biol. **44:** 186–200.
55. BITTNER, M. A. & R. W. HOLZ. 1990. Phorbol esters enhance exocytosis from chromaffin cells by two mechanisms. J. Neurochem. **54:** 205–210.
56. FINCH, D. M. & M. B. JACKSON. 1990. Presynaptic enhancement of synaptic transmission in hippocampal cell cultures by phorbol esters. Brain Res. **518:** 269–273.
57. LIN, J.-W., M. SUGIMORI, R. R. LLINÁS, T. L. MCGUINNESS & P. GREENGARD. 1990. Effects of synapsin I and calcium/calmodulin-dependent protein kinase II on spontaneous neurotransmitter release in the squid giant synapse. Proc. Natl. Acad. Sci. USA **87:** 8257–8261.
58. BARNES, S. & F. WERBLIN. 1987. Gated currents generate single spike activity in amacrine cells of the tiger salamander retina. Proc. Natl. Acad. Sci. USA **83:** 1509–1512.
59. BLANTON, M. G., J. J. LO TURCO & A. R. KRIEGSTEIN. 1989. Whole cell recording from neurons in slices of reptilian and mammalian cerebral cortex. J. Neurosci. Methods **30:** 203–210.
60. COLEMAN, P. A. & R. F. MILLER. 1989. Measurement of passive membrane parameters with whole-cell recordings from neurons in the intact amphibian retina. J. Neurophysiol. **61:** 218–230.

The Hair Cell as a Presynaptic Terminal[a]

WILLIAM M. ROBERTS,[b] R. A. JACOBS,[c]
AND A. J. HUDSPETH[c,d]

[b]Institute of Neuroscience
University of Oregon
Eugene, Oregon 97403

[c]Department of Cell Biology and Neuroscience
University of Texas Southwestern Medical Center
Dallas, Texas 75235-9039

INTRODUCTION

The hair cell, the sensory receptor of the internal ear, is an excellent subject for electrophysiological studies because it manifests the neuronal characteristics needed to process and transmit electrical signals in the experimentally tractable form of an epithelial cell. The hair cell's compact shape, essentially that of a short, smooth cylinder with a bundle of mechanically sensitive stereocilia at one end, endows it with an isopotential interior ideal for voltage clamping. Because it lacks entangling axonal and dendritic processes, an individual hair cell is easily dissociated from the sensory epithelium. After dissociation, the entire cellular surface is free of glial vestments and is accessible to extracellular patch electrodes. These and other morphological features have facilitated detailed analyses of mechanoelectrical transduction and the subsequent electrical events leading to chemical transmission across afferent synapses.[1-3]

In several important respects, hair cells resemble nonspiking neurons. Because they do not need action potentials to transmit signals over long distances, they are free to use graded potentials to perform sophisticated signal-processing tasks involving ion channels that interact with the receptor current and the membrane capacitance. In addition, hair cells both make and receive chemical synapses. In contrast to the situation with most neurons, all of these important cellular processes can be studied using intracellular and extracellular voltage-clamp methods.

In this paper we shall focus on presynaptic mechanisms. Each hair cell in the ear makes synaptic contacts onto one or more afferent fibers of the eighth cranial nerve. Intraaxonal recordings have shown that transmission is quantal and requires Ca^{2+} in the extracellular medium.[4] Depolarization of the hair cell increases the release of an excitatory neurotransmitter, probably glutamate, and hyperpolarization diminishes the steady release that occurs in the absence of stimulation.[5] As at most other chemical synapses, transmitter release evidently occurs by exocytosis at discrete active zones, which can be recognized by their distinctive morphological features. In hair cells, these include the features common to conventional chemical synapses: a synaptic cleft separating densely stained pre- and postsynaptic membranes, and

[a]This work was supported by National Institutes of Health Grants NS27142, NS07904, NS22389, and DC00317; by a Sloan Fellowship (W. M. Roberts); and by the Perot Family Foundation (R. A. Jacobs and A. J. Hudspeth).
[d]To whom correspondence should be addressed.

small (30–60 nm), clear-cored vesicles in the presynaptic cytoplasm. Each active zone additionally possesses an osmiophilic presynaptic body 200–400 nm in diameter,[6] which is surrounded by a shell of synaptic vesicles that appear attached to it by filaments. Filamentous links also connect the synaptic body to the presynaptic membrane. Hair cells bear several morphological and physiological similarities to retinal photoreceptors, including three that pertain to afferent synapses: both types of cells have prominent presynaptic bodies of unknown function, release transmitter continuously in response to graded changes in membrane potential, and apparently employ amino acid neurotransmitters.

Depending on the species and the auditory or vestibular organ in which it is situated, a hair cell may make as few as one or as many as 50 synaptic contacts onto afferent axons.[7] Even when many active zones are present, however, they occupy only a small fraction of the cell's basolateral surface. A saccular hair cell from a grassfrog (*Rana pipiens*) has about 20 active zones, scattered at an average density of one per 50 μm^2 of the basolateral membrane. Each active zone is associated with an array of voltage-gated Ca^{2+} channels that controls the local concentration of free Ca^{2+} ($[Ca^{2+}]_i$) in the cytoplasm independently of other active zones and of the cell as a whole.[8]

Our results indicate that there is a steep spatial gradient of $[Ca^{2+}]_i$ in the vicinity of each active zone. To account for this gradient, one needs only consider free diffusion of Ca^{2+} away from a cluster of Ca^{2+} channels. A similar situation probably obtains in the presynaptic terminals of many neurons, which contain several active zones that release transmitter onto one or more postsynaptic cells. Although some terminals may behave electrically as single compartments, synaptic transmission and other processes that involve diffusion or chemical intermediates may be subject to local control acting over distances of tens to hundreds of nanometers.

The local nature of Ca^{2+} action has been a major impediment to understanding the role of this ion in synaptic transmission.[9–11] Although several techniques are available to measure the $[Ca^{2+}]_i$ within a cell's interior, such measurements reveal no more about the $[Ca^{2+}]_i$ at an active zone than a thermometer in the living room tells about the temperature in the fireplace. More localized measurements of $[Ca^{2+}]_i$ have been made with confocal microscopy and Ca^{2+}-sensitive dyes,[11,12] but even the best optical techniques fall short by a factor of ten in the spatial resolution needed to assess accurately the $[Ca^{2+}]_i$ that mediates exocytosis.

By using an endogenous Ca^{2+} detector that colocalizes with active zones, we have achieved better spatial resolution in the measurement of local $[Ca^{2+}]_i$. In the course of investigating the ion channels responsible for electrical tuning in the frog's saccular hair cells, we discovered an intimate association between Ca^{2+}-activated K^+ channels and presynaptic active zones. After characterizing the dual dependence of these K^+ channels' open probability on the membrane potential and $[Ca^{2+}]_i$, we used them as *in situ* indicators of $[Ca^{2+}]_i$ at active zones. We are unaware of any direct involvement of the Ca^{2+}-activated K^+ channels in synaptic transmission. Their proximity to active zones may instead be a coincidence of their association with Ca^{2+} channels that, along with the K^+ channels and the membrane capacitance, produce an electrical resonance that tunes each hair cell to respond best to vibrations at a particular frequency. We propose that both types of channels are located at active zones so that the same Ca^{2+} channels can participate in both electrical resonance and synaptic transmission.

Most of the experimental procedures and results discussed in this paper were reported previously.[8]

ELECTRICAL RESONANCE

A principal function of the voltage-gated ion channels in many hair cells is to produce electrical resonance, which can be observed experimentally as a damped, sinusoidal oscillation of the membrane potential following injection of a step or pulse of current into the cell.[2,13] A depolarizing stimulus opens Ca^{2+} channels that have a biphasic effect on the membrane potential. The immediate effect is to generate an inward Ca^{2+} current that augments the depolarization. After a delay, determined in part by the rate of Ca^{2+} accumulation in the cytoplasm, the increased $[Ca^{2+}]_i$ opens K^+ channels that counteract the depolarization. The outward K^+ current repolarizes the cell, leading to closure of some Ca^{2+} channels, return of $[Ca^{2+}]_i$ toward its resting level, and finally closure of the K^+ channels in preparation for the next cycle of the oscillation. Oscillations can occur only if the time-courses of activation and deactivation of the Ca^{2+} and K^+ currents fall within certain limits. In addition, the magnitudes of both currents and of the membrane resistance and capacitance must be appropriate; the membrane potential otherwise reaches a constant level without oscillating.

Similar mechanisms have been proposed to generate oscillating membrane potentials in a variety of cell types. Pancreatic islet cells, for example, may generate low-frequency bursts of action potentials using a related mechanism.[14] Interactions between Ca^{2+} currents and Ca^{2+}-activated K^+ currents may also be important for bursting in hippocampal[15] and thalamic[16] neurons, although several additional types of ion channels are also involved in these cells. The best-known examples of bursting neurons are from *Aplysia* and other mollusks. It was in these cells that Ca^{2+}-activated K^+ currents were initially described, and that their importance in generating oscillating membrane potentials was first proposed.[17] A decade of intense experimentation in several laboratories has led to a new model, however, in which Ca^{2+}-activated K^+ channels are no longer thought responsible for the hyperpolarization between bursts.[18] This revision raises the possibility that the simple mechanism proposed for hair cells also may fail the test of time. There are, however, good reasons to be more confident in the hair-cell model. Voltage-clamp studies of molluscan neurons have always been confounded by the cells' complex geometries and varied complements of ionic conductances; hair cells are much smaller and simpler. The slow oscillations in molluscan neurons, at frequencies below 0.1 Hz, are also difficult to study because they are governed by small, slow currents. To produce oscillations at frequencies above 100 Hz, hair cells by contrast require currents nearly as large and fast as the currents that underlie action potentials. Although it is likely that additional ion channels, for example, other types of K^+ channels, have secondary functions in the frog's saccular hair cells, the Ca^{2+} and Ca^{2+}-dependent K^+ currents[19,20] are clearly the most important for resonance. Pharmacological experiments[21] and computer modeling[22] demonstrate that, in conjunction with membrane capacitance and leak resistance, these currents are both necessary and sufficient to produce resonance.

The electrical oscillations in hair cells are 100–10,000 times as fast as those in other cells that use similar ionic mechanisms. The highest resonant frequencies reported (350–450 Hz)[13,23] probably approach the limit that can be achieved in a process involving diffusion of an intracellular messenger.[2] If $[Ca^{2+}]_i$ controls the opening and closing of K^+ channels during each cycle of the oscillation, then $[Ca^{2+}]_i$ must alternate between its minimal and maximal values in about one millisecond. Because there is insufficient time for Ca^{2+} ions to diffuse far from their point of entry during each cycle, it would be difficult for the $[Ca^{2+}]_i$ deep in the cellular interior to undergo substantial high-frequency oscillations.

To explain how Ca^{2+} channels participate in the hair cell's resonance, Hudspeth and Lewis[22] assumed that Ca^{2+} is confined within a small cytoplasmic compartment near the plasma membrane, where it rapidly accumulates to concentrations exceeding 100 μM when Ca^{2+} channels are open. Although this notion of a small submembrane compartment was a convenient contrivance for the initial model of resonance, we thought it unlikely that there were physical barriers to cytoplasmic diffusion. Instead, we hypothesized that local accumulation of Ca^{2+} could be explained simply by the simultaneous openings of many Ca^{2+} channels located in a tight cluster. To test this hypothesis, we studied the spatial distribution of the Ca^{2+} channels and Ca^{2+}-activated K^+ channels on the cellular surface. Our measurements showed that the channels are indeed clustered, and that the time needed for Ca^{2+} to diffuse away from these densely packed channels accounts for the local accumulation of Ca^{2+} required for resonance.[8]

ELECTRICAL MEASUREMENT OF CHANNEL DISTRIBUTIONS

We sought channel clustering by recording the currents through regions of various size and position on the cellular surface simultaneously with the current through the entire cell membrane. Saccular hair cells from grass frogs were dissociated and studied *in vitro*.[19,24] Voltage steps were imposed through a tightly sealed, whole-cell pipette[25] that recorded the whole-cell current, while patch currents were measured through a second pipette sealed loosely to the surface[26] and maintained at the same voltage as the bath by a separate voltage-clamp amplifier. We took considerable care to ensure that the patch pipette did not damage or distort the membrane beneath its tip. By measuring simultaneously the whole-cell and patch currents, we could be certain that the lack of ionic current observed in many small patches was due to a highly nonuniform distribution of Ca^{2+} channels and K^+ channels on the cellular surface, rather than to the poor physiological condition of some cells. Each current amplitude was converted to a current density by dividing it by the area of membrane from which the recording was made; the area was in turn determined from capacitance measurements. The average current density from many patches was the same as the average basolateral current density, which indicates that the patch pipette did not damage the membrane or systematically under- or overestimate the local current density. The whole-cell recordings showed that the Ca^{2+} current enters through noninactivating, dihydropyridine-sensitive, L-type Ca^{2+} channels.[27]

In the first series of experiments, we used recording pipettes that engulfed large membrane patches to seek differences between the hair cell's apical and basolateral surfaces. Pipettes covering the entire apical surface, including the hair bundle, recorded no voltage-activated ionic currents, whereas pipettes covering large regions of the basolateral surface recorded currents with the same voltage dependence and time-course as the whole-cell current. The apical surface was thus devoted entirely to mechanoelectrical transduction, whereas all of the voltage- and Ca^{2+}-gated channels involved in electrical resonance and synaptic transmission occurred on the basolateral surface. The basal half of the basolateral surface usually had a higher current density than the apical half.

To delineate still finer variations in channel density, we next focused our recordings on smaller patches of basolateral membrane. Based on previous experience with other types of cells,[28-31] we were not surprised to find large patch-to-patch differences in the densities of Ca^{2+} channels and Ca^{2+}-activated K^+ channels. Because Ca^{2+} channels in hair cells are involved in two separate processes, synaptic transmission and resonance, we expected to encounter some patches holding presynaptic active zones, in which Ca^{2+} channels predominated, and other patches that contained both types of channels. To our surprise, we found no patches that contained solely Ca^{2+} channels; all patches with significant currents held both channel types in the same ratio as in the whole cell. The variation between patches was extreme, with half of the patches that covered less than 5% of the basolateral surface containing no measurable currents, while the other half contained up to 23% of the whole-cell current.

The most interesting finding was a close correspondence between the densities of Ca^{2+} channels and Ca^{2+}-activated K^+ channels. Although it was not practical in these patch recordings to separate the two currents pharmacologically, we could estimate their relative amplitudes because the currents commenced at different rates. In a few patches, we blocked the K^+ current to demonstrate that the Ca^{2+} currents in basolateral patches had the same rapid time-course and lack of inactivation as the whole-cell Ca^{2+} current. Under the usual conditions, in which both currents were active, the amplitude of the Ca^{2+} current could be measured during the initial 0.5 ms following a depolarization, before the Ca^{2+}-activated K^+ channels opened. The amplitude of the K^+ current could then be estimated by subtracting the Ca^{2+} current. In all patches in which the amplitudes of the two currents were large enough to estimate, their ratio was similar to that in the whole cell. In particular, we found no patches that contained a significant steady-state inward current, which we anticipated would occur if active zones were associated with dense clusters of Ca^{2+} channels. Given the number (57) and sizes of patches studied, it is highly likely that our sample included many recordings from active zones. We were therefore left with two possibilities: either the Ca^{2+} currents at active zones were too small to measure, or both Ca^{2+} channels and Ca^{2+}-activated K^+ channels were associated with active zones. We have no direct evidence to refute the first possibility, but have four lines of evidence that support the second.

CLUSTERING OF CA^{2+} AND K^+ CHANNELS AT ACTIVE ZONES

The first piece of evidence suggesting that clusters containing both Ca^{2+} and Ca^{2+}-activated K^+ channels are associated with active zones was their similar numbers. We counted 19 ± 2 active zones per cell (mean $\pm$ SEM; $n = 5$) in electron micrographs of serially sectioned hair cells. Because we could rarely record from more than one membrane patch on a given cell, it was more difficult to quantify channel clustering electrophysiologically. We therefore resorted to statistical analysis of the distribution of current densities encountered in patches of different sizes on many cells. In essence, we determined how large a patch had to be to have a good chance of containing a channel cluster. The actual analysis involved a maximum-likelihood fit to a model with two free parameters: the number of channel clusters per cell and the amount of measurement error in the current density. The best fit had 20 clusters per cell, in agreement with the number of active zones counted in electron micrographs. Any number between 16 and 27 gave a satisfactory fit, with a likelihood of at least 10% of the maximum.

The second piece of evidence was the finding that both active zones and channel clusters occurred at higher densities near the basal cellular pole than elsewhere on the basolateral surface. In the electron micrographs used to count active zones, we noted whether each was below (towards the basal pole) or above (towards the apical surface) the level of the nucleus. The density of active zones below the nucleus was 2.4 ± 0.9 times the density above the nucleus (mean $\pm$ SEM; $n = 5$). We similarly noted in electrical recordings whether each patch was located below or above the nucleus, and found the ratio of the average current densities in these two regions to be 2.1. Both active zones and channel clusters are thus approximately twice as dense below the nucleus as above.

The third piece of evidence came from counting the number of ion channels per cell and intramembrane particles per active zone. Channel counts, obtained from ensemble-variance analysis of whole-cell currents, gave estimates of 1800 ± 400 Ca^{2+} channels (mean $\pm$ SEM; $n = 6$ cells) and approximately 700 Ca^{2+}-activated K^+ channels (550 ± 70, $n = 8$; 810 ± 80, $n = 19$; measured under two different conditions). Assuming that these channels were apportioned equally among the 19 or so active zones per cell, these numbers corresponded to roughly 90 Ca^{2+} channels and 40 Ca^{2+}-activated K^+ channels per active zone. In freeze-fracture electron micrographs, we found 133 ± 15 large particles (mean $\pm$ SEM; $n = 13$ synapses) packed in a tight array at the center of each active zone. The number of large intramembrane particles at each active zone therefore closely matched the combined number of Ca^{2+} and K^+ channels determined physiologically.

The final piece of evidence for colocalization of Ca^{2+} channels and Ca^{2+}-activated K^+ channels at active zones was the good agreement between the measured accumulation of cytoplasmic Ca^{2+} near Ca^{2+}-activated K^+ channels, inferred from their probability of being open, and the accumulation expected at an active zone where 5% of the whole-cell current entered through 90 Ca^{2+} channels packed into a space the size of the particle array. These experiments and calculations are described in detail below.

Taken together, these four pieces of evidence strongly support the hypotheses that most or all of the hair cell's Ca^{2+} and Ca^{2+}-activated K^+ channels occur in clusters, and that these clusters are the arrays of intramembrane particles seen at the active zones. Because whole-cell recordings provide information about the ionic currents and local $[Ca^{2+}]_i$ at active zones, the hair cell is thus uniquely suited for studying synaptic physiology.

INTRACELLULAR CA^{2+} CONCENTRATION AT ACTIVE ZONES

Before we could use Ca^{2+}-activated K^+ channels to assay the local $[Ca^{2+}]_i$, we had to calibrate their response to Ca^{2+}. Most Ca^{2+} indicators bind Ca^{2+} at a single site with a fixed affinity, and are therefore most sensitive to concentration changes when $[Ca^{2+}]_i$ is close to the binding site's dissociation constant (K_d). At Ca^{2+} concentrations much lower or higher than the K_d, the indicator is less sensitive because the binding site is respectively vacant or occupied nearly all of the time. Ca^{2+}-activated K^+ channels could be used to indicate $[Ca^{2+}]_i$ over a much wider range because their apparent affinity for Ca^{2+} decreased when the membrane was hyperpolarized. Within the range of membrane potentials easily applied to a hair cell, the K^+ channels' apparent affinity for Ca^{2+} varied from below 1 μM to above 1 mM. The channels' dual sensitivity to membrane potential and $[Ca^{2+}]_i$ made them excellent indicators of $[Ca^{2+}]_i$ over the range of physiological interest.

Although information regarding the K^+ channels' Ca^{2+} sensitivity was already available from single-channel studies in a related species,[20] we considered it prudent to calibrate their sensitivity under conditions closer to those used when measuring $[Ca^{2+}]_i$. In whole-cell, voltage-clamp experiments, we blocked Ca^{2+} entry from the extracellular solution and replaced the cytoplasm with an internal solution containing known, highly buffered concentrations of free Ca^{2+}. These conditions of constant $[Ca^{2+}]_i$ unmasked the channels' intrinsic voltage dependence, which we characterized at three free Ca^{2+} concentrations: 10, 100, and 1000 μM. At each $[Ca^{2+}]_i$, we estimated the steady-state probability of a Ca^{2+}-activated K^+ channel's being open as a function of membrane potential by measuring the amplitudes of K^+ tail currents following depolarizing voltage steps to various levels. For each measurement, the membrane potential was held depolarized for 10 ms (long enough for the K^+ current to reach its steady maximum) and then stepped to -40 mV. The initial amplitude of the K^+ current at -40 mV, which was proportional to the number of channels opened by the previous depolarization, was plotted against the membrane potential during the depolarization. As found for Ca^{2+}-activated K^+ channels in other cells,[32] the relation between membrane potential and tail-current amplitude was sigmoidal and could be fit by a Boltzmann equation. These measurements did not directly indicate the channels' open probability (p), but we knew from ensemble-variance experiments that large depolarizations opened nearly all of the Ca^{2+}-activated K^+ channels at the three Ca^{2+} concentrations tested. We therefore assumed that the sigmoidal curves approached maxima corresponding to $p = 1$. The three curves had midpoints (voltages for which $p = 0.5$) of 15 mV, -28 mV, and -65 mV at Ca^{2+} concentrations respectively of 10, 100, and 1000 μM. These whole-cell measurements agreed well with the previous single-channel experiments.[20] The Ca^{2+}-activated K^+ channels were found in both instances to display a surprisingly low affinity for Ca^{2+}, requiring approximately 100 μM $[Ca^{2+}]_i$ to be kept open 50% of the time at potentials within the cells' normal operating range.

When $[Ca^{2+}]_i$ was kept constant, the Ca^{2+}-activated K^+ channel's shallow voltage dependence, with a Boltzmann slope coefficient of 26 mV, contrasted sharply with its steep apparent voltage dependence when activated by the cell's Ca^{2+} current. With the Ca^{2+} current intact, depolarization from -58 mV to -42 mV increased the fraction of K^+ channels open from 5 to 70 percent. To obtain the same open probabilities at these membrane potentials, with the Ca^{2+} current blocked, required respectively 10 μM and 1 mM $[Ca^{2+}]_i$. At membrane potentials positive to -42 mV, even 1 mM free Ca^{2+} did not open as many Ca^{2+}-activated K^+ channels as did the Ca^{2+} current. By measuring the Ca^{2+} current at these membrane potentials, we inferred the relation between the size of the whole-cell Ca^{2+} current and the local $[Ca^{2+}]_i$ at the K^+ channels' Ca^{2+}-binding sites. This relation fit a straight line through the origin, with a slope of -1.8 $\mu M/pA$. Assuming that the whole-cell current was equally divided among 19 active zones, the slope of the relation between local $[Ca^{2+}]_i$ and local Ca^{2+} current was therefore -34 $\mu M/pA$. Unless the procedure for calibrating the K^+ channels seriously underestimated their affinity for Ca^{2+}, these experiments demonstrated that the Ca^{2+}-activated K^+ channels were exposed to a cytoplasmic Ca^{2+} concentration that exceeded 10 μM at the normal resting potential near -55 mV, and that surpassed 1 mM during depolarizations positive to -40 millivolts.

Our claim that the Ca^{2+}-activated K^+ channels' open probability reveals the local $[Ca^{2+}]_i$ at active zones obviously rests upon the assumption that the channels reside there. The patch recordings were consistent with this hypothesis, and the similar numbers and spatial distributions of channel clusters and active zones suggested an association between the two. The patch recordings did not have sufficient spatial resolution, however, to localize channel clusters to regions smaller than 20 μm^2. Although the patch recordings indicated that over 5% of the whole-cell current was sometimes concentrated into an area of 20 μm^2, they did not reveal how the channels were spread within this area. The first evidence suggesting that channels were tightly packed into a 300-nm-diameter region at the center of each active zone was the concordance between the numbers of channels per cluster and of intramembrane particles at an active zone. Based upon similar circumstantial evidence, several investigators earlier proposed that particle arrays in presynaptic membranes of other cells are clusters of Ca^{2+} channels.[33–35] In hair cells, the case was greatly strengthened by the observation that the Ca^{2+}-activated K^+ channels experience an extraordinarily high $[Ca^{2+}]_i$. Based upon the diffusion model described below, we concluded that tens or hundreds of Ca^{2+} channels had to be clustered together to produce such a high local $[Ca^{2+}]_i$. Dense clusters containing this many channels should have been apparent as arrays of intramembrane particles in freeze-fracture electron micrographs. Aside from particle clusters at presynaptic active zones and postsynaptic to efferent synaptic contacts,[36] however, we observed no organized arrays of intramembrane particles that could have corresponded to the channel clusters.

CA^{2+} DIFFUSION FROM CLUSTERED CHANNELS

To investigate how clustering of Ca^{2+} channels influences the local $[Ca^{2+}]_i$, we wrote a computer program to simulate cytoplasmic diffusion of Ca^{2+} away from a tightly packed array of channels. The model assumed that 5% of the whole-cell Ca^{2+} current entered through channels scattered randomly within a 300-nm-diameter disk in a planar surface, and that Ca^{2+} then diffused freely, with a diffusion coefficient of 6×10^{-10} $m^2 \cdot s^{-1}$, into an infinite volume of water that initially contained no Ca^{2+}. The model did not take into account Ca^{2+} buffering in the cytoplasm or its removal by pumps. Although buffering and pumping are crucial to the overall Ca^{2+} economy of all cells, they probably had little influence over the extremely localized rise in $[Ca^{2+}]_i$ within the hair cell's active zones, for the reasons presented below.

Two types of Ca^{2+} buffers were present in the cells under our experimental conditions: a diffusible buffer introduced through the whole-cell pipette, and whatever immobile, endogenous buffers remained in the cytoplasm after diffusible buffers disappeared into the pipette. Immobile buffers can have no effect on steady-state Ca^{2+} concentrations because they are in equilibrium with the constant local $[Ca^{2+}]_i$ and therefore release one Ca^{2+} ion for every ion bound. Although diffusible buffers can, under some conditions, lower the local free Ca^{2+} concentration by binding an ion near the point of entry and carrying it some distance away before releasing it, two separate factors combined to make the diffusible buffer ineffective at active zones. The first was the time required for a Ca^{2+} ion to encounter and bind to a buffer molecule. Most of our experiments used 1 mM EGTA, which binds Ca^{2+} at a rate of only 10^4 s^{-1}.[37] This means that the average Ca^{2+} ion remained free in the cytoplasm for approximately 100 μs, long enough to diffuse about 500 nm. Because most Ca^{2+} ions diffused a substantial distance from their point of entry before binding to a buffer molecule, 1 mM EGTA had little effect at an active zone. A more rigorous mathematical treatment of this phenomenon was presented by Neher.[37] Note that this argument does not invoke saturation of the buffer and is therefore valid even for vanishingly small rates of Ca^{2+} influx. In some whole-cell recordings, we used high enough concentrations of rapid Ca^{2+} buffers to reduce the local rise in $[Ca^{2+}]_i$ produced by the Ca^{2+} currents. This effect is predicted by the theoretical treatment presented above; for the highest buffer concentration used, 50 mM BAPTA,[38] Ca^{2+} ions can diffuse less than 10 nm before being sequestered. Buffer concentrations below 1 mM were effective only during small Ca^{2+} currents, and appeared to saturate during whole-cell Ca^{2+} currents larger than 200 pA. The Ca^{2+} influx was then evidently fast enough to outpace the exchange of Ca^{2+}-BAPTA for free BAPTA. These two factors—the slowness of Ca^{2+} binding to buffer, and its rapid saturation—rendered diffusible Ca^{2+} buffers ineffective within a few hundred nanometers of an active zone under our experimental conditions.

During a hair cell's normal operation, the endogenous Ca^{2+} buffers are probably even less effective at lowering the local $[Ca^{2+}]_i$ at active zones. The precise concentrations and affinities of cytoplasmic Ca^{2+} buffers are unknown, but the total capacity of fast Ca^{2+} buffers is probably well below 1 mM.[9,39] At such a low concentration, both of the factors discussed above come into play. In addition, an intact cell would not have access to the vast reservoir of free buffer provided by the whole-cell pipette. Therefore, we think it unlikely that Ca^{2+} buffering has an important influence on electrical resonance or synaptic transmission in these hair cells.

We could also ignore active extrusion of Ca^{2+} in the model because the large number of pumps (or exchangers) needed to keep up with the Ca^{2+} influx at each active zone could not reasonably be located close enough to appreciably lower the local $[Ca^{2+}]_i$. In the model simulations, we found that even an instantaneous, unsaturable sink for Ca^{2+}, surrounding the entire active zone at a radius of 1 μm, had only a small effect on the $[Ca^{2+}]_i$ within the 300-nm-diameter disk at the center. Only pumps located within 1 μm of the active zone could perceptibly decrease the local $[Ca^{2+}]_i$. Within this region, there is scarcely room for enough pumps to keep pace with the steady Ca^{2+} influx associated with the resting whole-cell Ca^{2+} current of -20 pA. This current corresponds to an entry into the cytoplasm of about 6×10^7 Ca^{2+} ions per second. If the hair cell's Ca^{2+} pump resembles that in the sarcoplasmic reticulum, with a turnover rate of 200 s^{-1}, each hair cell requires more than 300,000 Ca^{2+} pumps operating at maximum capacity simply to maintain the resting $[Ca^{2+}]_i$. During a large, sustained stimulus, the average Ca^{2+} influx may be more than ten times as great. Even to lower the resting local $[Ca^{2+}]_i$ would therefore require packing some 15,000 pumps into the 1 μm^2 area around each active zone. This high a density of membrane proteins is possible, and has been observed for gap-junction channels, Na^+ channels at nodes of Ranvier, and acetylcholine receptors at neuromuscular synapses. In each of these cases a nearly close-packed array of intramembrane particles is evident in freeze-fracture electron micrographs.[40] Our freeze-fracture micrographs showed no increase in the density of large particles around active zones above the average density of about 1,100 μm^{-2} of basolateral surface. Given the average basolateral surface area near 1,000 μm^2, the cell's 300,000 or so hypothetical Ca^{2+} pumps could be spread evenly at a density exceeding 300 μm^{-2}. It therefore seems likely that a significant fraction, perhaps even the majority, of the particles on the basolateral membrane surface are Ca^{2+} pumps.

Although it is improbable that Ca^{2+} pumping could have much effect on local changes in $[Ca^{2+}]_i$ at active zones, the pumps are necessary to maintain a low average $[Ca^{2+}]_i$ throughout the cytoplasm. To justify modeling the dispersal of Ca^{2+} from active zones as diffusion into an infinite volume containing no free Ca^{2+}, we needed to assume an average cytoplasmic $[Ca^{2+}]_i$ below 1 μM. Based upon measurements of cytoplasmic $[Ca^{2+}]_i$ in other types of cells,[12] this is a reasonable assumption. Because 1 μM is less than 10% of the local $[Ca^{2+}]_i$ produced by the resting Ca^{2+} current, we could ignore this background $[Ca^{2+}]_i$ in the diffusion model. According to the model, there is a large, standing Ca^{2+} gradient around each active zone, even in an unstimulated hair cell.

The conclusions drawn from our model seem reliable because, once buffering and pumping are eliminated from the equations, there is only a minor uncertainty in the diffusion coefficient for Ca^{2+}. The Stokes-Einstein equation[41] predicts that diffusion coefficients in cytoplasm are half as large as in water because cytoplasm is about twice as viscous. Under the whole-cell recording conditions in these experiments, in which the cytoplasm had been partially replaced by the solution in the recording pipette, the intracellular viscosity was probably intermediate between those of cytoplasm and water. For simplicity, we therefore used the coefficient for

Ca^{2+} diffusion in water in the model calculations. It is important to keep in mind that many authors employ smaller diffusion coefficients that incorporate the effect of Ca^{2+} binding to fixed or slow-moving buffers in the cytoplasm. This apparent diffusion coefficient should not be confused with the coefficient for diffusion of free Ca^{2+}.[9,10,42] The coefficient of free diffusion applies at active zones because, as discussed above, buffering is not a factor this close to a site of Ca^{2+} influx. Because diffusion is not a saturable process, the model predicted a linear relationship between the rate of Ca^{2+} influx and the local $[Ca^{2+}]_i$, in agreement with the experimental findings.

The model contained no adjustable values or fitted parameters. We first computed the local Ca^{2+} current by dividing the whole-cell Ca^{2+} current by the number of active zones per cell, then assumed that this current entered through channels located in a membrane disk the size of the active zone's particle array. Because diffusion respects the principle of superposition, the $[Ca^{2+}]_i$ produced by many channels in a cluster was the sum of the channels' individual contributions, which were easily calculated from the equation for steady-state diffusion away from a point source in a planar boundary:

$$[Ca^{2+}]_i = \frac{-i}{4\pi FDr}.$$

Here i is the current entering at the point source, F is the Faraday constant, D is the diffusion coefficient, and r is the distance from the source. To calculate $[Ca^{2+}]_i$ at any point in space, it was necessary to determine the distance to each channel, apply the above equation to calculate each channel's contribution to $[Ca^{2+}]_i$, and add together the individual contributions. Although freeze-fracture micrographs revealed particles arrayed in several short bars within the active zone, we found the precise arrangement of channels within the disk to be of secondary importance in model calculations. Most calculations were accordingly carried out assuming the simplest possible arrangement: random scattering within a disk. In this case, the average $[Ca^{2+}]_i$ at the center of the disk was easily calculated to be -18 $\mu M/pA$ of whole-cell Ca^{2+} current. Digital simulation led to a slightly lower estimate, -15 $\mu M/pA$, for the average $[Ca^{2+}]_i$ throughout the disk.

It might be argued that these averages are not good representations of the $[Ca^{2+}]_i$ because of the variations that occur within the disk. In particular, $[Ca^{2+}]_i$ increases toward infinity at the point corresponding to each Ca^{2+} channel. A more reasonable average was obtained by prohibiting K^+ channels in the model from approaching within 10 nm of the mouth of a Ca^{2+} channel. When this region of excessively high $[Ca^{2+}]_i$ was excluded, however, the average local $[Ca^{2+}]_i$ declined only slightly, to -13 $\mu M/pA$. The two-dimensional spatial profile of $[Ca^{2+}]_i$ at the active zone's membrane can therefore be visualized as a smooth plateau supporting 90 tall spires, each centered on a Ca^{2+} channel. Because each spire is only a few nanometers in diameter, it contributes little to the average altitude.

Given the approximate nature of our calculations, the agreement between the calculated values and the measured value of -34 $\mu M/pA$ was remarkably good. There are, moreover, several reasons to expect that the model should slightly underestimate the local change in $[Ca^{2+}]_i$. As mentioned above, Ca^{2+} diffuses more slowly in cytoplasm than in water. In addition, the synaptic body that lies directly behind the active zone's membrane may retard diffusion into the cell's interior. Finally, active-zone particles are organized into several short bars in which channels are closer together than we assumed in our model. Our modeling studies showed that channel clustering is sufficient to explain the steep relationship between the Ca^{2+}

current and $[Ca^{2+}]_i$, and yielded a reasonable quantitative agreement with physiological measurements. They also demonstrated that some type of clustering is necessary to achieve the measured high concentrations of Ca^{2+}.

Our results also argued against a direct coupling between Ca^{2+} channels and Ca^{2+}-activated K^+ channels, in which Ca^{2+} is funneled from Ca^{2+} channels to binding sites on Ca^{2+}-activated K^+ channels without diffusing through the cytoplasm. In this case no amount of a buffer would suffice to block communication between the two. We found instead that highly concentrated buffers behaved as expected for a diffusion-mediated process. They were able to suppress the opening of K^+ channels during small Ca^{2+} currents, but were saturated by large ones. We conclude that the two types of channels occur together in clusters and communicate by cytoplasmic diffusion of Ca^{2+}.

CONCLUSION

Our results indicate that each of a hair cell's 20 or so active zones contains a cluster of Ca^{2+} channels that can pass up to -75 pA of current, producing a local concentration of free Ca^{2+} that can exceed 1 mM. This value, though high, squares with theoretical calculations based upon the rate of Ca^{2+} entry at each active zone, the diameter of the region of membrane containing Ca^{2+} channels, and the diffusion coefficient of Ca^{2+}. Because a large Ca^{2+} current flows through a small membrane area at each active zone, a modest depolarization can produce a sizable increase in presynaptic $[Ca^{2+}]_i$. Walrond and Reese[35] observed that presynaptic membranes at neuromuscular junctions on a lizard's tonic muscle fibers had only 13 intramembrane particles (and putative Ca^{2+} channels) per active zone, compared to 17 particles per active zone on twitch fibers, and suggested that this difference was related to the larger number of quanta released per action potential at twitch synapses. By similar reasoning, the much larger number of particles per active zone in hair cells is likely a functional adaptation related to the cells' nonspiking character. Clustering of ion channels at presynaptic active zones permits changes in membrane potential much smaller than an action potential to modulate both the exocytosis of synaptic vesicles and the activity of Ca^{2+}-activated K^+ channels.

ACKNOWLEDGMENT

The authors thank J. C. Weeks for comments on the manuscript.

REFERENCES

1. HOWARD, J., W. M. ROBERTS & A. J. HUDSPETH. 1988. Mechanoelectrical transduction by hair cells. Annu. Rev. Biophys. Biophys. Chem. **17:** 99–124.
2. ROBERTS, W. M., J. HOWARD & A. J. HUDSPETH. 1988. Hair cells: transduction, tuning, and transmission in the inner ear. Annu. Rev. Cell Biol. **4:** 63–92.
3. HUDSPETH, A. J. 1989. How the ear's works work. Nature **341:** 397–404.
4. FURUKAWA, T., Y. HAYASHIDA & S. MATSUURA. 1978. Quantal analysis of the size of excitatory post-synaptic potentials at synapses between hair cells and afferent nerve fibres in goldfish. J. Physiol. (Lond.) **276:** 211–226.
5. BLEDSOE, S. C., JR. 1986. Pharmacology and neurotransmission of sensory transduction in the inner ear. Semin. Hear. **7:** 117–137.

6. GLEISNER, L., Å. FLOCK & J. WERSÄLL. 1973. The ultrastructure of the afferent synapse on hair cells in the frog labyrinth. Acta Oto-laryngol. **76:** 199–207.
7. MILLER, M. R. & J. BECK. 1988. Auditory hair cell innervational patterns in lizards. J. Comp. Neurol. **271:** 604–628.
8. ROBERTS, W. M., R. A. JACOBS & A. J. HUDSPETH. 1990. Colocalization of ion channels involved in frequency selectivity and synaptic transmission at presynaptic active zones of hair cells. J. Neurosci. **10:** 3664–3684.
9. SIMON, S. M. & R. R. LLINÁS. 1985. Compartmentalization of the submembrane calcium activity during calcium influx and its significance in transmitter release. Biophys. J. **48:** 485–498.
10. AUGUSTINE, G. J., M. P. CHARLTON & S. J. SMITH. 1987. Calcium action in synaptic transmitter release. Annu. Rev. Neurosci. **10:** 633–693.
11. SMITH, S. J. & G. J. AUGUSTINE. 1988. Calcium ions, active zones and synaptic transmitter release. Trends Neurosci. **11:** 458–464.
12. HERNÁNDEZ-CRUZ, A., F. SALA & P. R. ADAMS. 1990. Subcellular calcium transients visualized by confocal microscopy in a voltage-clamped vertebrate neuron. Science **247:** 858–862.
13. FETTIPLACE, R. 1987. Electrical tuning of hair cells in the inner ear. Trends Neurosci. **10:** 421–425.
14. CHAY, T. R. 1986. On the effect of the intracellular calcium-sensitive K$^+$ channel in the bursting pancreatic β-cell. Biophys. J. **50:** 765–777.
15. WONG, R. K. S. & D. A. PRINCE. 1978. Participation of calcium spikes during intrinsic burst firing in hippocampal neurons. Brain Res. **159:** 385–390.
16. JAHNSEN, H. & R. LLINÁS. 1984. Ionic basis for the electroresponsiveness and oscillatory properties of guinea-pig thalamic neurones *in vitro.* J. Physiol. (Lond.) **349:** 227–247.
17. MEECH, R. W. 1978. Calcium-dependent potassium activation in nervous tissues. Annu. Rev. Biophys. Bioeng. **7:** 1–18.
18. LANDÒ, L. & R. S. ZUCKER. 1989. "Caged calcium" in *Aplysia* pacemaker neurons. Characterization of calcium-activated potassium and nonspecific cation currents. J. Gen. Physiol. **93:** 1017–1060.
19. LEWIS, R. S. & A. J. HUDSPETH. 1983. Voltage- and ion-dependent conductances in solitary vertebrate hair cells. Nature **304:** 538–541.
20. HUDSPETH, A. J. & R. S. LEWIS. 1988. Kinetic analysis of voltage- and ion-dependent conductances in saccular hair cells of the bull-frog, *Rana catesbeiana.* J. Physiol. (Lond.) **400:** 237–274.
21. LEWIS, R. S. & A. J. HUDSPETH. 1983. Frequency tuning and ionic conductances in hair cells of the bullfrog's sacculus. *In* Hearing—Physiological Bases and Psychophysics. R. KLINKE & R. HARTMANN, Eds.:17–22. Springer-Verlag. Berlin.
22. HUDSPETH, A. J. & R. S. LEWIS. 1988. A model for electrical resonance and frequency tuning in saccular hair cells of the bull-frog, *Rana catesbeiana.* J. Physiol. (Lond.) **400:** 275–297.
23. CRAWFORD, A. C. & R. FETTIPLACE. 1981. An electrical tuning mechanism in turtle cochlear hair cells. J. Physiol. (Lond.) **312:** 377–412.
24. KROESE, A. B. A., A. DAS & A. J. HUDSPETH. 1989. Blockage of the transduction channels of hair cells in the bullfrog's sacculus by aminoglycoside antibiotics. Hearing Res. **37:** 203–218.
25. MARTY, A. & E. NEHER. 1983. Tight-seal whole-cell recording. *In* Single-Channel Recording. B. SAKMANN & E. NEHER, Eds: 107–122. Plenum. New York.
26. STÜHMER, W., W. M. ROBERTS & W. ALMERS. 1983. The loose patch clamp. *In* Single-Channel Recording. B. SAKMANN & E. NEHER, Eds.: 123–132. Plenum. New York.
27. NOWYCKY, M. C., A. P. FOX & R. W. TSIEN. 1985. Three types of neuronal calcium channel with different calcium agonist sensitivity. Nature **316:** 440–443.
28. ROBERTS, W. M. 1987. Sodium channels near end-plates and nuclei of snake skeletal muscle. J. Physiol. (Lond.) **388:** 213–232.
29. THOMPSON, S. & J. COOMBS. 1988. Spatial distribution of Ca currents in molluscan neuron cell bodies and regional differences in strength of inactivation. J. Neurosci. **8:** 1929–1939.

30. JONES, O. T., D. L. KUNZE & K. J. ANGELIDES. 1989. Localization and mobility of ω-conotoxin-sensitive Ca^{2+} channels in hippocampal CA1 neurons. Science **244:** 1189–1193.

31. SILVER, R. A., A. G. LAMB & S. R. BOLSOVER. 1990. Calcium hotspots caused by *L*-channel clustering promote morphological changes in neuronal growth cones. Nature **343:** 751–754.

32. BARRETT, J. N., K. L. MAGLEBY & B. S. PALLOTTA. 1982. Properties of single calcium-activated potassium channels in cultured rat muscle. J. Physiol. (Lond.) **331:** 211–230.

33. HEUSER, J. E., T. S. REESE & D. M. D. LANDIS. 1974. Functional changes in frog neuromuscular junctions studied with freeze-fracture. J. Neurocytol. **3:** 109–131.

34. PUMPLIN, D. W., T. S. REESE & R. LLINÁS. 1981. Are the presynaptic membrane particles the calcium channels? Proc. Natl. Acad. Sci. USA **78:** 7210–7213.

35. WALROND, J. P. & T. S. REESE. 1985. Structure of axon terminals and active zones at synapses on lizard twitch and tonic muscle fibers. J. Neurosci. **5:** 1118–1131.

36. JACOBS, R. A. & A. J. HUDSPETH. 1990. Ultrastructural correlates of mechanoelectrical transduction in hair cells of the bullfrog's internal ear. Cold Spring Harbor Symp. Quant. Biol. **55:** 547–561.

37. NEHER, E. 1986. Concentration profiles of intracellular calcium in the presence of a diffusible chelator. *In* Experimental Brain Research, Series 14.: 80–96. Springer-Verlag. Berlin.

38. TSIEN, R. Y. 1980. New calcium indicators and buffers with high selectivity against magnesium and protons: design, synthesis, and properties of prototype structures. Biochemistry **19:** 2396–2404.

39. SALA, F. & A. HERNÁNDEZ-CRUZ. 1990. Calcium diffusion modeling in a spherical neuron. Relevance of buffering properties. Biophys. J. **57:** 313–324.

40. ALMERS, W. & C. STIRLING. 1984. Distribution of transport proteins over animal cell membranes. J. Membr. Biol. **77:** 169–186.

41. HILLE, B. 1984. Ionic Channels of Excitable Membranes. Sinauer Associates. Sunderland, Massachusetts.

42. HODGKIN, A. L. & R. D. KEYNES. 1957. Movements of labelled calcium in squid giant axons. J. Physiol. (Lond.) **138:** 253–281.

Membrane Fusion as Seen in Rapidly Frozen Secretory Cells[a]

DOUGLAS E. CHANDLER

Department of Zoology
Arizona State University
Tempe, Arizona 85287

INTRODUCTION

Since 1959, when Palade first reported electron microscopic evidence for secretion from the exocrine pancreas,[1] exocytosis has remained one of the best studied examples of biological membrane fusion. Early thin-sectioning studies revealed the presence of three fusion intermediates.[2-5] The membrane of the secretory granule and that of the plasma membrane first became apposed with elimination of all cytoplasm to form a pentalaminar structure. The pentalaminar structure was then thought to rearrange to form a single bilayer continuous with both the plasma membrane and secretory granule membrane—the so-called trilaminar structure. The trilaminar structure was considered to be unstable, breaking down to form a pore joining the granule interior with the extracellular space.

Subsequent freeze-fracture studies have visualized intermediates during exocytosis, which appear to substantiate the three-step sequence previously developed from thin sections. In freeze-fracture replicas, widespread contact between the plasma and secretory granule membranes appears as dome-shaped IMP free areas, which have been thought to be equivalent to the pentalaminar structures seen in thin sections.[6-8] Likewise, the trilaminar structure has been visualized in freeze fracture as a distinct single bilayer diaphragm that is continuous with both plasma and granule membranes.[9]

Many of the observations in glutaraldehyde-fixed tissues described above, however, have not been confirmed in tissues, which have been rapidly frozen without chemical fixation and then freeze-fractured. This has led to the conclusion that the character or extent of the proposed intermediates have been altered by chemical fixation. Indeed, there is good evidence that chemical fixation results in the formation of plasma membrane blebs exactly at the site of membrane fusion,[10] and that glycerination, which is required for normal freeze-fracture protocols, can actually induce artifactual membrane fusion.[11]

What has been seen in quick-frozen secretory cells, including the adrenal medulla,[12] amebocytes,[13] and mast cells,[14] is that fusion always begins with a single small pore ranging from 10 to 40 nm in diameter. Pore formation and growth is not accompanied by areas cleared of IMPs, and during growth the pore is circular in cross section, with its total length remaining very short, about 40 to 100 nm.

[a]The studies described above were supported by a Grant from the NSF (DCB-8810200).

234

RESULTS AND DISCUSSION

Formation of the pore and its subsequent enlargement in mast cells can be best seen in stereographic figures. In the rat mast cell the most peripheral layer of granules is generally separated from the plasma membrane by a 50 to 200 nm thick layer of cytoplasm (FIG. 1), although occasionally these two membranes approach each other to within 25 nanometers. In cells that have been stimulated with the polycation 48/80, the earliest sign of membrane interaction is dimpling of the plasma membrane towards the granule membrane (FIG. 2). These indentations bring the two membranes within 10 nm of each other and presumably lead to initial contact within a very small localized region. Dimples can be as great as 100 nm in depth.

The initial pore formed from such contacts, as judged by electrophysiological measurements could be as small as 2 to 8 nm in diameter and may not be visible in freeze fracture. Somewhat larger pores, from 8 to 20 nm in diameter, are visible, as shown in FIGURE 3. In this case, both membranes, that of a fused granule and that of an unfused granule, are distended toward each other, with a small 8 nm diameter pore joining the two. At higher magnification, the pore appears to include several IMPs at its edge (FIG. 4); the presence of IMPs, however, is not typical and is seen only occasionally. The structural rearrangements that produce a pore must therefore take place in a very small region, probably no greater than within a 30 nm diameter area.

Pore growth is accompanied by a variable morphology. Some granules appear to be pulled away from the plasma membrane as the pore grows to 70 nm in diameter (FIG. 5). Other granules are still spherical in shape, the granule membrane being well separated from the plasma membrane except where the pore joins the two (FIG. 6). Pore length remains variable during further enlargement of the pore. In some cases, although not common, pore length can be as large as 200 nm during the period in which pore diameter is about 100 to 200 nm (FIG. 7). By contrast, in its final stages of growth, the pore is usually surrounded by a thin lip of cytoplasm, and thus its effective length is quite short (FIG. 8).

Two areas in which electron microscopy has contributed to the mechanism of exocytosis is in characterizing the structural variability of pores during growth and in assessing the role of osmotic forces in promoting pore widening. Recently, electrophysiological studies have shown that the initial exocytic pore appears to be of variable conductance, suggesting that it is not a typical channel but rather one that is variable in structure (see papers by Zimmerberg and by Almers, this volume). Unfortunately, these smallest pores, assuming bulk aqueous conductivity throughout their interior, are probably 2 to 8 nm in diameter, too small to be easily observed in freeze-fractured samples. Despite this, electron microscopy does show that the smallest pores observed (8 to 20 nm in diameter) are variable in structure. Some pores are relatively short, having a length about equal to their diameter. Other pores are more elongated with lengths as much as three to four times their diameter. These observations, combined with electrophysiological evidence that pores can expand, contract, pause, and even reversibly open and reclose early in their life history, suggest that pores may comprise lipid and variable numbers of pore-forming protein subunits whose sequence of assembly can vary from one pore to the next.[15,16] Unfortunately, our freeze fracture studies have not consistently shown the presence of IMPs within the pore structure (although see FIG. 4). It is possible, however, that pore-forming proteins may fracture cleanly, leaving little trace of their presence.

For over fifteen years osmotic forces have been implicated in pore formation and

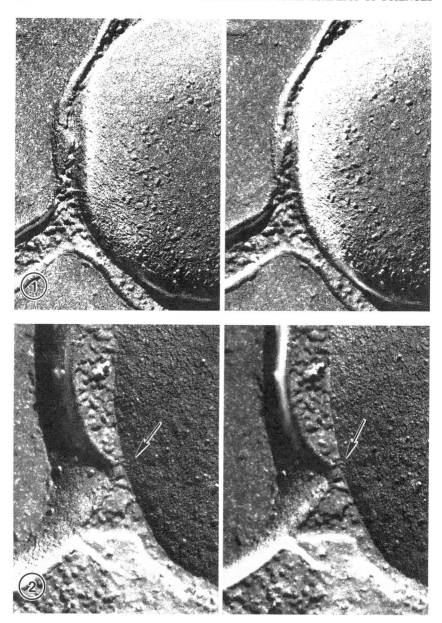

FIGURE 1. Freeze-fracture replica of a secretory granule in a rat mast cell prior to fusion with the plasma membrane. Note that a thin layer of cytoplasm separates the two membranes even at their closest approach. Sample was stimulated with 8 μg/mL 48/80, quick-frozen on a liquid helium-cooled copper block 15 s later, and freeze-fractured. Stereo pair; ×120,000, reduced by 10%.

FIGURE 2. A dimple in the plasma membrane approaches the granule membrane (arrow). Sample was stimulated and quick-frozen 15 s later as described in FIG. 1. Stereo pair; ×140,000, reduced by 10%.

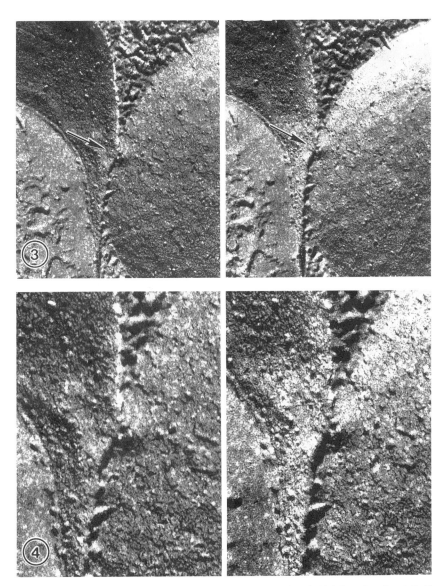

FIGURES 3 and 4. A small pore (arrow) forms between fused (right) and unfused (left) granule membranes. At high magnification (FIG. 4) the pore appears to be associated with IMPs. Sample was stimulated and quick-frozen 15 s later as described in FIG. 1. Stereo pairs; FIG. 3. ×110,000, reduced by 10%; FIG. 4 ×250,000, reduced by 10%.

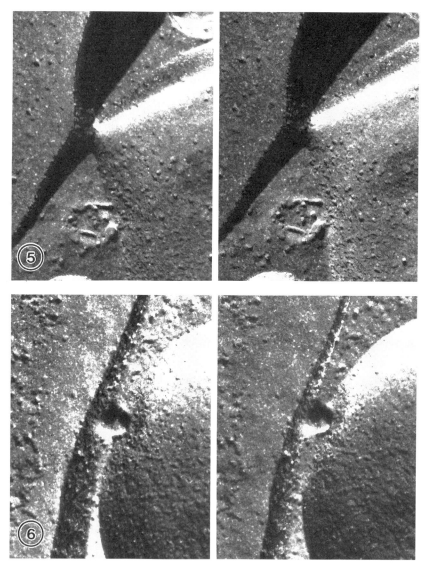

FIGURES 5 and 6. During pore growth the granule membrane surrounding the pore is well separated from the plasma membrane. Samples were stimulated and quick-frozen 17 s later as described in Fig. 1. Stereo pairs; Figures 5 and 6, ×170,000, reduced by 13%.

expansion. High medium osmolarity has been shown to inhibit exocytosis in a number of cells including sea urchin eggs,[17,18] adrenal chromaffin cells,[19,20] platelets,[21] and neutrophils.[22] This effect was originally interpreted to suggest that water flux into the secretory granule was critical for initiation of fusion between the granule and plasma membrane and that such flux was reduced in hyperosmotic media. This

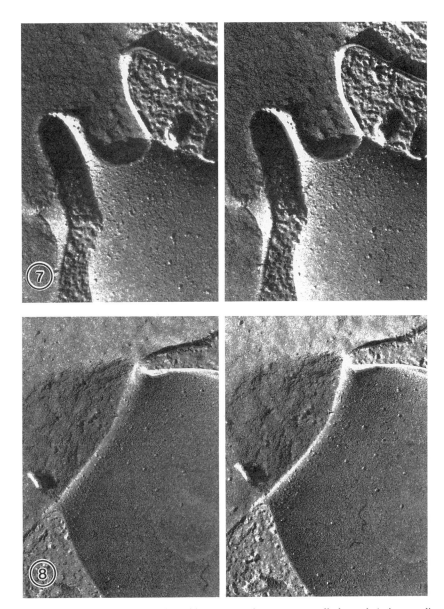

FIGURES 7 and 8. The pore further widens as granule contents are discharged. At intermediate stages of growth (FIG. 7), the pore can be several diameters in length, while at late stages (FIG. 8) the mouth of the pore is surrounded by a thin lip of cytoplasm probably due to compression by the expanding granule matrix. Samples were stimulated and quick-frozen 15 s later as described in FIG. 1. Stereo pairs; FIG. 7, ×90,000, reduced by 12%; FIG. 8, ×82,000, reduced by 12%.

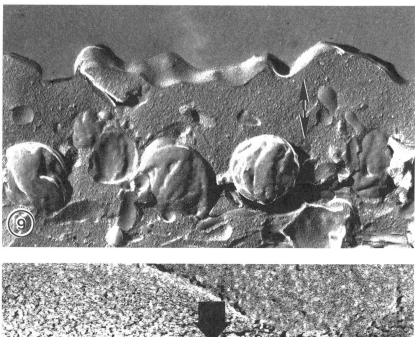

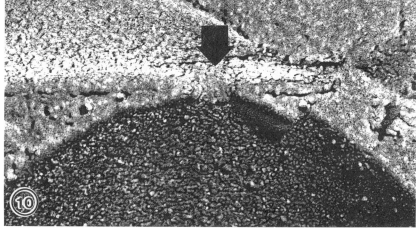

FIGURES 9 and 10. Treatment of sea urchin eggs (*L. pictus* or *S. purpuratus*) with hyperosmotic sea water containing 0.8 M stachyose (2.6 osM/Kg) leads to formation of a granule-free zone (arrows, FIG. 9) in the cell cortex and separation of 90% of cortical granules from the plasma membrane. The remainder of the granules fuse with the plasma membrane with the formation of small pores (arrow, FIG. 10), but pore widening is arrested. FIG. 9: Samples were treated with 0.8 M stachyose in sea water for 5 minutes, then quick-frozen; ×50,000, reduced by 10%. Fig. 10: Samples were treated with 0.8 M stachyose in sea water for five minutes, activated with 60 μM A23187, and quick-frozen 5 minutes later; ×300,000, reduced by 10%. (Chandler *et al.*[27] With permission from the Rockefeller University Press.)

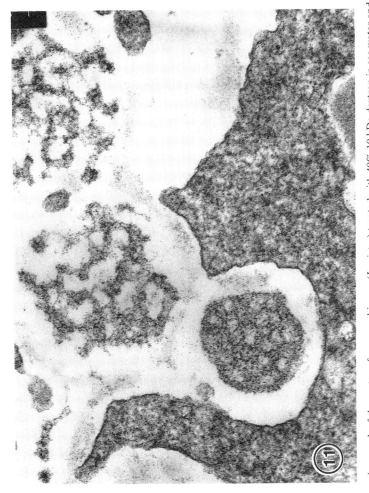

FIGURE 11. Electron micrograph of the cortex of a sea urchin egg (*L. pictus*) treated with 40% 10 kDa dextran in sea water and activated with 60 μM A23187. The egg exhibits numerous exocytic pockets containing intact granule cores. Sample was fixed with 2% glutaraldehyde 5 min after activation, postfixed with osmium tetroxide in seawater, stained en bloc with 1% uranyl acetate, dehydrated in ethanol, and embedded in Spurr's epoxy resin; ×60,000.

hypothesis was strengthened by the finding that fusion of unilammellar liposomes with planar bilayers was facilitated by an osmotic gradient[23] and that certain secretory granules, notably those in sea urchin eggs, were observed to swell before fusion with the plasma membrane.[24]

Both light- and electron-microscopic evidence now argue against such a scenario. Zimmerberg et al.[25] have shown in beige mouse mast cells, through simultaneous electrical recording of pore conductance and video/light microscopic imaging of granule diameter, that swelling of granules does not occur until after the fusion pore has formed and expanded to reach its full conductance. Even in hyperosmotic media these authors have found that granule fusion is not preceded by granule swelling. In fact, electron-microscopy studies show that exocytosis in hyperosmotic media is prevented by formation of an organelle-free zone in the cortex of the cell. In neutrophils, for example, both azurophil and specific granules are separated from the plasma membrane by a 0.2 μm thick layer of cytoskeletal filaments within seconds after incubation of the cells in hyperosmotic medium.[22]

In the sea urchin egg the cytoskeletal layer formed in response to hyperosmolality (0.6 M Na_2SO_4 in sea water, 2.25 osM/kg) is even thicker ($0.5 - 1$ μm; see FIG. 9) and appears to be composed of a dense meshwork of actin-containing filaments.[26] This layer forces 90% of the cortical granules away from the plasma membrane so that they are not even in position to undergo fusion. Upon activation with calcium ionophore, however, the 10% of granules remaining do fuse with the plasma membrane, demonstrating that fusion itself is not blocked by hyperosmolality.[18] Of those granules that fuse nearly all are arrested at early stages of pore growth. Pores as small as 33 nm are seen five minutes after calcium ionophore activation, long after initiation of exocytosis and at a time when all exocytic pockets should have been fully opened and flattened (see FIG. 10).

There is good reason to think that opening of the pore and flattening of the exocytic pocket are related to the ability of the granule matrix to absorb water and to disassemble. Exposure of eggs to sea water containing 30% dextran (10 kDa; Pharmacia, Piscataway, NJ) blocks granule matrix disassembly and at the same time inhibits the final stages of granule pocket opening[27] (see FIG. 11). It appears that the high molecular weight polysaccharide is able to bind enough water to its numerous hydroxyl groups that insufficient amounts of water are available to hydrate the cortical granule matrix. Whitaker and Zimmerberg have postulated that the dextran is unable to enter the granule matrix thus ensuring that the water activity is lowered outside the matrix.[28]

Recently, we have been able to distinguish between osmotic and ionic requirements at the moment of pore formation and during pore growth as opposed to requirements for granule matrix disassembly once the exocytic pocket is wide open. If sea urchin eggs are sperm-activated so as to initiate a wave of exocytosis, the wave can be stopped by addition of hyperosmotic sucrose to raise osmolality to 2.3 osM/kg or above.[29] Eggs fixed in glutaraldehyde after such a hyperosmotic block exhibit cortical granules at the front of the wave, which have undergone fusion but which have not undergone pore widening. Thus inhibition of pore widening can be achieved by either an ionic osmoticant, such as sodium sulfate (see above), or by a nonionic osmoticant, as in the case of sucrose. This supports our contention that it is high osmolality and not ionic composition that retards pore growth at this early stage.

By contrast, matrix disassembly after pore growth appears to be specifically sensitive to high concentrations of certain ions in the sea water. Because 30% 10-kDa dextran blocks granule matrix disassembly without inhibiting pore widening, we used eggs activated in dextran sea water as a model for matrix disassembly. As pointed out above, eggs activated in dextran exhibit numerous exocytic pockets that are filled with granule matrix cores. Exposure of these cores to hyperosmotic sucrose (after dextran has been washed out) has shown that granule matrices undergo complete disassembly.[29] Thus, hyperosmotic media without ions will not inhibit the later stages of granule matrix disassembly.

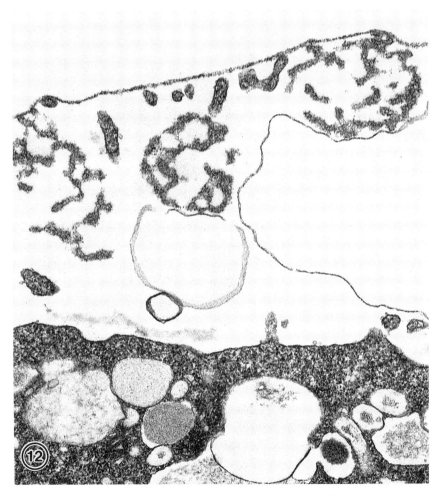

FIGURE 12. Cortex of a sea urchin egg (*L. pictus*) treated with 40% 10 kDa dextran in divalent cation-free sea water, then activated with A23187. Exocytic pockets have flattened, and cores have partially disassembled. Sample was fixed and prepared for electron-microscopy as described in FIG. 11; ×41,000, reduced by 10%.

These later stages, however, can be retarded by the presence of sodium, calcium, or magnesium. Although sodium does not inhibit at concentrations found in sea water, it does block matrix disassembly at high ionic strength. For example, either 0.5 M Na_2SO_4 or 0.5 M Na_2HPO_4 in sea water preserves the matrix core inasmuch as the ionic strength is well above that of sea water. The effects of calcium and magnesium, however, appear to be specific because they occur at much lower concentrations. If eggs are activated in sea water containing 30% dextran but no divalent cations, exocytic pockets flatten, and all but the final stages of granule matrix disassembly are observed (see FIG. 12). By contrast, if either calcium or magnesium is present in dextran solutions, the granule matrix remains intact.

In summary, the exocytotic process appears to be divided into at least four distinct phases: membrane adhesion, pore formation, pore widening, and granule matrix discharge.[27] Membrane adhesion is characterized by formation of a small indentation in the plasma membrane that serves to contact the granule membrane in a highly localized region. Pore formation within this region appears first as a reversible, variable conductance as detected in patch clamp recordings. The pore is thought to go through a phase of early growth before it reaches the 10 to 20 nm diameter range in which it is first detected by freeze-fracture electron-microscopy. Further pore widening requires inward movement of water and hydration of the granule contents. It is this stage that is sensitive to hyperosmotic inhibition of inward water flux. Finally, the last step, matrix dispersal, appears to depend on water availability, on a sufficiently low ionic strength, and on a sufficiently low concentration of divalent cations.

REFERENCES

1. PALADE, G. E. 1959. Functional changes in the structure of cell components. *In* Subcellular Particles. T. Hayashi, Ed.: 64–80. Ronald Press. New York.
2. PALADE, G. E. & R. R. BRUNS. 1969. Structural modulations of plasmalemmal vesicles. J. Cell Biol. **37:** 633–649.
3. PALADE, G. E. 1975. Intracellular aspects of the process of protein synthesis. Science **189:** 347–358.
4. PLATTNER, H. 1981. Membrane behaviour during exocytosis. Cell Biol. Int. Rep. **5:** 435–459.
5. CHANDLER, D. E. 1988. Exocytosis and endocytosis: membrane fusion events captured in rapidly frozen cells. Curr. Top. Membr. Trans. **32:** 169–202.
6. CHI, E. Y., D. LAGUNOFF & J. K. KOEHLER. 1976. Freeze fracture study of mast cell secretion. Proc. Natl. Acad. Sci. USA **73:** 2823–2827.
7. FRIEND, D. S., L. ORCI, A. PERRELET & R. YANAGIMACHI. 1977. Membrane particle changes attending the acrosome reaction in guinea pig sperm. J. Cell Biol. **74:** 561–577.
8. LAWSON, D., M. C. RAFF, B. D. GOMPERTS, C. FEWTRELL & N. B. GILULA. 1977. Molecular events during membrane fusion. A study of exocytosis in rat peritoneal mast cells. J. Cell Biol. **72:** 242–259.
9. PINTO DA SILVA, P. & M. L. NOGUEIRA. 1977. Membrane fusion during secretion. A hypothesis based on electron microscope observation of *Phytophthora palmivora* zoospores during encystment. J. Cell Biol. **73:** 161–181.
10. CHANDLER, D. E. 1984. Comparison of quick-frozen and chemically fixed sea urchin eggs: structural evidence that cortical granule exocytosis is preceded by a local increase in membrane mobility. J. Cell Sci. **72:** 23–36.
11. CHANDLER, D. E. & J. HEUSER. 1979. Membrane fusion during secretion. Cortical granule exocytosis in sea urchin eggs as studied by quick-freezing and freeze fracture. J. Cell Biol. **83:** 91–108.
12. SCHMIDT, W., A. PATZAK, G. LINGG, H. WINKLER & H. PLATTNER. 1983. Membrane events in adrenal chromaffin cells during exocytosis: a freeze-etching analysis after rapid cryofixation. Eur. J. Cell Biol. **32:** 31–37.
13. ORNBERG, R. L. & T. S. REESE. 1981. Beginning of exocytosis captured by rapid freezing of *Limulus* amebocytes. J. Cell Biol. **90:** 40–54.

14. CHANDLER, D. E., M. CURRAN, F. S. COHEN & J. ZIMMERBERG. 1989. Exocytosis in mast cells is accompanied by dimpling of the plasma membrane and formation of small (< 10 nm) pores. J. Cell Biol. **109:** 300a.

15. ALMERS, W. 1990. Exocytosis. Annu. Rev. Physiol. **52:** 607–624.

16. CURRAN, M., J. ZIMMERBERG & F. S. COHEN. 1988. Dynamics of pore formation in mast cells of the beige mouse. Biophys. J. **53:** 322a.

17. ZIMMERBERG, J., C. SARDET & D. EPEL. 1985. Exocytosis of sea urchin egg cortical vesicles *in vitro* is retarded by hyperosmotic sucrose: kinetics of fusion monitored by quantitative light-scattering microscopy. J. Cell Biol. **101:** 2398–2410.

18. MERKLE, C. & D. E. CHANDLER. 1989. Hyperosmolality inhibits exocytosis in sea urchin eggs by formation of a granule-free zone and arrest of pore widening. J. Membr. Biol. **112:** 223–232.

19. HAMPTON, R. Y. & R. W. HOLZ. 1983. Effects of changes in osmolality on the stability and function of cultured chromaffin cells and the possible role of osmotic forces in exocytosis. J. Cell Biol. **96:** 1082–1088.

20. POLLARD, H. B., C. J. PAZOLES, C. E. CREUTZ, J. H. SCOTT, O. ZINDER & A. HOTCHKISS. 1984. An osmotic mechanism for exocytosis from dissociated chromaffin cells. J. Biol. Chem. **259:** 114–1121.

21. POLLARD, H. B., K. TACK-GOLDMAN, C. J. PAZOLES, C. E. CREUTZ & N. R. SHULMAN. 1977. Evidence for control of serotonin secretion from human platelets by hydroxyl ion transport and osmotic lysis. Proc. Natl. Acad. Sci. USA **74:** 5295–5299.

22. KAZILEK, C. J., C. J. MERKLE & D. E. CHANDLER. 1988. Hyperosmotic inhibition of calcium signals and exocytosis in rabbit neutrophils. Am. J. Physiol. **254:** C709–C718.

23. FINKELSTEIN, A., J. ZIMMERBERG & F. COHEN. 1986. Osmotic swelling of vesicles: its role in the fusion of vesicles with planar phospholipid bilayer membranes and its possible role in exocytosis. Annu. Rev. Physiol. **48:** 163–174.

24. ZIMMERBERG, J. & M. WHITAKER. 1985. Irreversible swelling of secretory granules during exocytosis caused by calcium. Nature (Lond.) **315:** 581–584.

25. ZIMMERBERG, J., M. CURRAN, F. S. COHEN & M. BRODWICK. 1987. Simultaneous electrical and optical measurements show that membrane fusion precedes secretory granule swelling during exocytosis of beige mouse mast cells. Proc. Natl. Acad. Sci. USA **84:** 1585–1589.

26. MERKLE, C. J. & D. E. CHANDLER. 1989. Hyperosmolality induces intracellular alkalinization and formation of a filamentous network in the cortex of sea urchin eggs. J. Cell Biol. **109:** 127a.

27. CHANDLER, D. E., M. WHITAKER & J. ZIMMERBERG. 1989. High molecular weight polymers block cortical granule exocytosis in sea urchin eggs at the level of granule matrix disassembly. J. Cell Biol. **109:** 1269–1278.

28. WHITAKER, M. & J. ZIMMERBERG. 1987. Inhibition of secretory granule discharge during exocytosis in sea urchin eggs by polymer solutions. J. Physiol. (Lond.) **389:** 527–539.

29. MERKLE, C. J. & D. E. CHANDLER. 1990. Cortical granule matrix disassembly during exocytosis in sea urchin eggs. J. Cell Biol. **111:** 488a.

Review of Evidence for Loss of Motor Nerve Terminal Calcium Channels in Lambert-Eaton Myasthenic Syndrome[a]

ANDREW G. ENGEL

*Department of Neurology
and Muscle Research Laboratory
Mayo Clinic
Rochester, Minnesota 55905*

The Lambert-Eaton myasthenic syndrome (LEMS) is an autoimmune disease in which pathogenic antibodies deplete the voltage-sensitive calcium channels (VSCC) of the motor nerve terminal (MNT) by antigenic modulation. This communication reviews freeze-fracture and immunoelectron microscopic evidence for loss of VSCC from the MNT and that this is caused by pathogenic autoantibodies. The work summarized here was done between 1980 and 1988 in collaboration with E. H. Lambert,[1] M. Osame,[1,2] H. Fukunaga,[1-3] T. Fukuoka,[4-6] and S. Nagel[6] at the Mayo Clinic, and with John Newsom-Davis,[3-6] B. Lang,[3-6] A. Vincent,[3,5] C. Prior,[4] and D. Wray[4] at the Royal Free Hospital in London. I will begin with a brief review of our current understanding of LEMS.

The characteristic symptoms are weakness and abnormal fatigability of the trunkal and mostly of the proximal limb muscles. Cranial muscles tend to be spared. Strength facilitates at the start of contraction. Autonomic disturbances, such as decreased salivation, lacrimation, and sweating, orthostatism, impotence, and abnormal pupillary light reflexes occur in about 75% of the patients. Two-thirds of LEMS patients have carcinoma, and more than 80% of the neoplasms are small cell carcinomas of the lung (reviewed by Engel[7] and O'Neill *et al.*[8]). The electrophysiologic basis of LEMS is a decreased release of acetylcholine quanta from the MNT by nerve impulse.[9,10] The decreased quantal release is not due to reduced synthesis or storage of acetylcholine, because the acetylcholine content and choline acetyltransferase activity of LEMS muscle are normal.[11] Repetitive stimulation or raising the external calcium concentration, which increase the probability of quantal release, improve the transmission defect.[10]

A possible autoimmune origin of LEMS had been suggested by the response to immunosuppressants and plasma exchange, an association with other autoimmune disorders, HLA-B8 and DRw3 antigens, and organ-specific autoantibodies (reviewed by O'Neill *et al.*[8]). The conclusive evidence for an autoimmune etiology of LEMS, however, came from the passive transfer to mice with IgG of the electrophysiologic[12-14] and morphologic[3,4,6] features of the disease.

[a]Work in the author's laboratory was supported by Grant NS 6277 from the National Institutes of Health and by a Research Center Grant from the Muscular Dystrophy Association.

PAUCITY OF ACTIVE ZONE PARTICLES (AZP) ON THE MNT
IN HUMAN LEMS

In 1980, we postulated that the reduced quantal release from the MNT by nerve impulse in LEMS was caused by a depletion or disorganization of the AZP of the MNT. This hypothesis was based on the fact that opening of VSCC increases the probability of quantal release,[15–18] and the assumption that the AZP comprise the VSCC. At that time, there were three reasons to assume that the VSCC and AZP were identical structures: (1) In 1976, Llinás and his associates demonstrated that at the squid giant synapse the latency between the onset of the calcium current and transmitter release was only 0.2 ms, and during this time Ca^{2+} ions could diffuse only 150 nm from their site of entry into the MNT[19]; subsequent observations on the same synapse by Pumplin, Reese, and Llinás indicated that the maximum presynaptic calcium current is related to the number of AZP.[20] (2) In 1979, Heuser and co-workers found that synaptic vesicle exocytosis captured by quick freezing occurred near the AZP.[21] (3) Also in 1979, Ceccarelli et al. showed that the AZP can specify sites of exocytosis even when dispersed by exposure to a low-Ca^{2+} medium.[22]

Visualization of the AZP requires freeze-fracture electron-microscopy. Using this technique, the AZP are readily recognized as large particles, 10–12 nm in diameter, packed in double parallel arrays. Each array consists of two parallel rows, and each row contains a number of AZP (FIG. 1). Quantitative freeze-fracture analysis, however, presents a number of problems: the MNTs, which occupy only a small fraction of a muscle sample, are hard to find in freeze-fracture replicas; the AZP are best observed in face-on views of the protoplasmic (P) leaflet of the presynaptic membrane, but only one in four fractures traversing MNT yields this view. Further, the density (number per unit area) of AZP cannot be determined in a conventional electron-micrograph because the projection of a curving membrane surface on a two-dimensional micrograph reduces the membrane area. We resolved these problems by fracturing many muscle segments enriched in MNTs, stereo-imaging all MNTs found in the replicas, and estimating the presynaptic membrane area by a computer-assisted stereometric method.[1,2]

The freeze-fracture studies revealed several striking alterations in the LEMS MNTs: the density of the active zones and AZP was markedly reduced, the number of particles per active zone was also reduced, and a proportion of the remaining AZP was aggregated into clusters (FIGURES 2A, 2B, and 3). The AZP were selectively affected, for there was no change in the density or size distribution of those membrane particles that were not associated with either active zones or clusters.[1] From these results and the assumption that the AZP represent VSCC, the physiologic defect in LEMS could now be attributed to the loss of VSCC from the MNT.[1] This study was published in 1982 from the Muscle Research Laboratory at the Mayo Clinic. By this time, Lang and co-workers at the Royal Free Hospital had transferred the physiologic defect of LEMS to mice with IgG.[12] Therefore, we could infer that the AZP (i.e., the VSCC) were (1) targets of the LEMS autoantibodies, (2) aggregate because they were cross-linked by IgG, and (3) depleted by the mechanism of antigenic modulation.[1] Subsequent joint studies by the two laboratories obtained adequate evidence for each of these postulates.

THE AZP ARE TARGETS OF LEMS AUTOANTIBODIES[3]

The mediation of the membrane lesions in LEMS by IgG was established by freeze-fracture studies on diaphragm muscles of mice treated with 10 mg control or

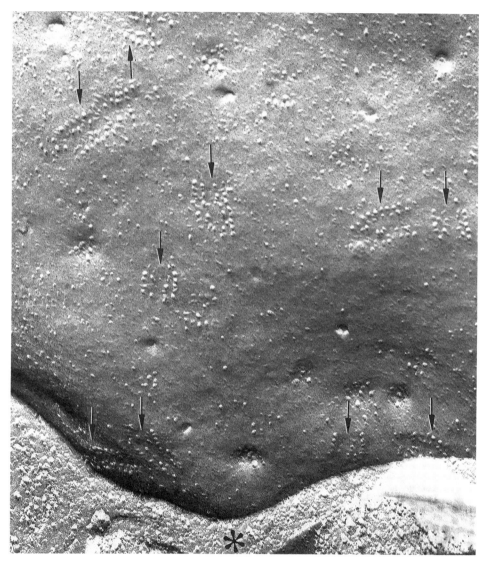

FIGURE 1. Freeze-fracture electron-micrograph of control presynaptic membrane P-face viewed face on. Ten active zones can be identified (arrows). Each zone contains two arrays; each array consists of two parallel rows of large particles. The active zones vary in length, and not all rows in a given zone have the same number of particles. Asterisk indicates primary synaptic cleft; ×100,000.

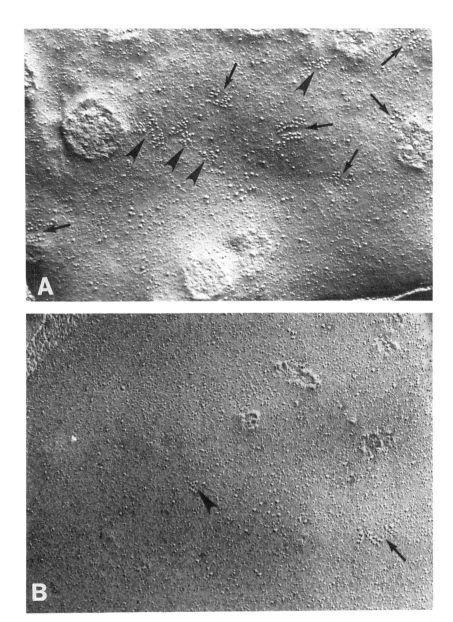

FIGURE 2. LEMS presynaptic membrane P-faces. In **A,** membrane leaflet shows 6 recogniz-able active zones (arrows) and 4 clusters of particles (arrowheads). In **B,** entire membrane contains only one short active zone and a single cluster of large particles (compare with FIG. 1). **A,** ×59,800; **B,** ×61,100. (Fukunaga *et al.*[1] With permission from *Muscle and Nerve.*)

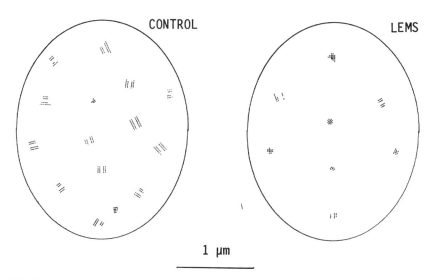

FIGURE 3. Stereometric reconstruction of control and LEMS presynaptic membranes, showing numbers, sizes, and configurations of active zones and numbers and sizes of particle clusters. The analysis is based on 83 control and 93 LEMS samples. A 5-μm^2 region is imaged in each case. Control membrane contains 13 active zones and 2 clusters. LEMS membrane contains 3 active zones and 5 clusters. The active zones are smaller, and the clusters are larger in LEMS than in control membrane. (Fukunaga et al.[1] With permission from *Muscle and Nerve.*)

LEMS IgG per day for 27–75 days. The LEMS IgG was from three patients. IgG from patients 1 and 2 transferred the electrophysiologic defect to mice, but IgG from patient 3 did not. The morphologic study, which was done blindly, demonstrated clustering and depletion of AZP only in those mice that received IgG from patients 1 and 2 (FIG. 4).

THE AZP ARE SUFFICIENTLY CLOSE TOGETHER TO BE CROSS-LINKED BY THE TWO ANTIGEN-BINDING SITES OF IgG[4]

The spacing of AZP in normal mouse diaphragm MNTs was determined by freeze-fracture analysis. To obviate the foreshortening of distances in two-dimensional images of three-dimensional membranes, a computer program was written for measuring interparticle distances in stereo-pair electron-micrographs using the x, y, and z coordinates of each point. This study established that the shortest distance between AZP in an outer row (7.3 nm), inner row (4.6 nm), or in two adjacent rows (9.6 nm) of an array was less than the 14 nm distance between the two antigen-binding sites of IgG (FIGURES 5A and 6A). Therefore, the AZP of a given array were sufficiently close together to be cross-linked by IgG. The shortest distance, however, between particles in two adjacent arrays of an active zone (27.8 nm) could not be spanned by IgG as long as the rectilinear and parallel orientation of the inner rows of the arrays was maintained.

AGGREGATION OF AZP IS AN EARLY EFFECT OF LEMS IgG[4]

In mice treated with 120–180 mg pathogenic LEMS IgG over 2 days, the initial alteration in the active zone was a decrease in the distance between particles in a given row and between adjacent rows of an array; the distance between the two arrays of the active zone remained unaltered (FIGURES 5B and 6B). In more affected active zones, the parallel orientation of the rows was disturbed (FIGURES 5B and 6C), and the arrays became clusters (FIGURES 5B and 6D). After two days of treatment there was also a significant (31%) decrease in the density of large membrane particles found in active zones and clusters. The end-plate potential quantal content in the same diaphragm muscles was reduced by 45–58% below the control mean.

DIVALENCY OF LEMS IgG IS AN ESSENTIAL REQUIREMENT FOR THE AGGREGATION AND DEPLETION OF AZP[6]

All the above morphologic data were consistent with modulation of AZP cross-linked by LEMS IgG. If this were the case, then only divalent LEMS IgG and $F(ab')_2$ should aggregate and deplete the AZP and monovalent LEMS Fab should be without effect. To test this hypothesis, mouse diaphragms were exposed to control and LEMS IgG and IgG fragments in organ culture for 24 hours and then studied by quantitative freeze-fracture electron-microscopy (FIG. 7). Divalent LEMS IgG (FIG. 7B) and $F(ab')_2$ (FIG. 7C) aggregated and depleted the active zone particles, whereas monovalent Fab was without effect (FIG. 7D). The findings reconfirmed that LEMS IgG binds to the AZP and gave direct evidence for modulation of the AZP by LEMS IgG. The findings were also in harmony with parallel electrophysiologic studies of the

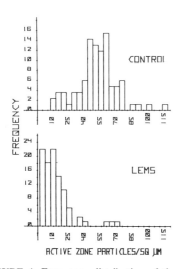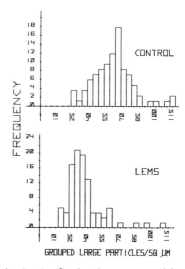

FIGURE 4. Frequency distribution of the density (no./μm^2) of active zones particles (left panel) and of large membrane particles in active zones and clusters (right panel) in control mice (83 membrane samples) and mice treated with pathogenic LEMS IgG (77 membrane samples).

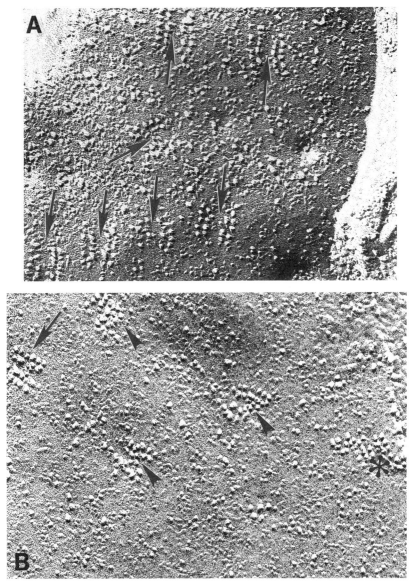

FIGURE 5. Presynaptic membrane P-faces from diaphragm muscles of mice treated for two days with 120 mg control IgG (**A**) and pathogenic LEMS IgG (**B**). Numerous normal active zones are present in **A** (arrows). **B** contains one normal-appearing active zone (arrow) and several abnormal active zones (arrowheads). In the abnormal zones the particles in individual rows are aggregated, but the two arrays remain distinct. A particle cluster, in which the space between the arrays is obliterated, is also imaged (asterisk); ×117,000. (Fukuoka et al.[4] With permission from the *Annals of Neurology.*)

effects of LEMS IgG fragments on transmitter release in the same diaphragm muscles.[23]

IMMUNOELECTRON MICROSCOPY LOCALIZATION OF LEMS IgG AT THE MOTOR END-PLATE[5]

The freeze-fracture studies gave evidence that LEMS IgG binds to the AZP and reduces their density by antigenic modulation. This notion was further substantiated by the immunolocalization of LEMS IgG to the active zones. The mouse passive

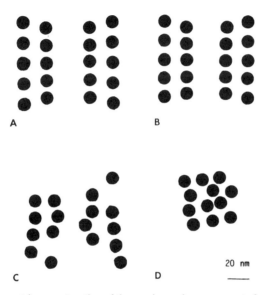

FIGURE 6. Stereometric reconstruction of the spacing and arrangement of particles in normal active zones of control mice (**A**) and in mice treated with LEMS IgG (**B, C,** and **D**). **B** shows reconstruction of active zones judged to be normal by simple inspection. Exact measurements, however, reveal a slight reduction of particle spacing within the two arrays. **C** is reconstruction of active zones with more pronounced particle aggregation. **D** represents a cluster. Calibration mark at the lower right indicates 20 nm. (Fukuoka *et al.*[4] With permission from the *Annals of Neurology.*)

transfer model was used. Special problems in this study were the paucity of AZP (about $50/\mu m^2$ normally and still lower in LEMS) and diffusion artifacts in the immunoperoxidase method. These difficulties were obviated by the use of (1) sensitive avidin-biotin detection systems, (2) both peroxidase and ferritin labels, and (3) quantitative immunoelectron microscopy and end-plate morphometry. Mice treated with LEMS IgG, control IgG, and no IgG were compared. In all mice, nonspecific background staining was found in the basal lamina covering the muscle fibers and Schwann cells. When a single dose of 10 mg IgG was injected intravenously, IgG samples from 12 patients (FIG. 8 A–C) produced significant immunostaining of the mouse active zones; IgG samples from 7 patients did not produce

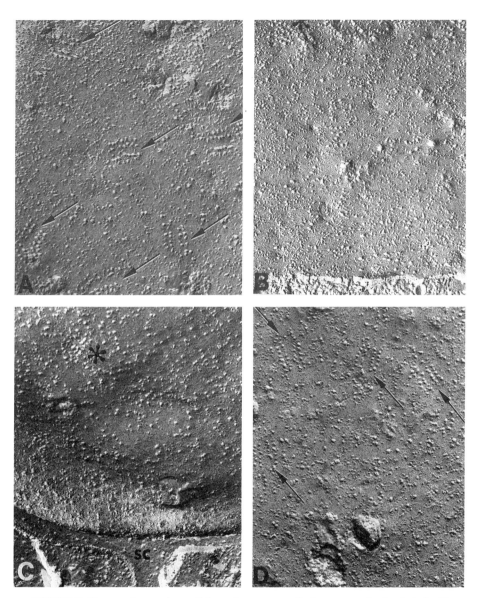

FIGURE 7. Presynaptic membrane P-faces from mouse diaphragm muscles incubated with normal IgG (**A**), LEMS IgG (**B**), LEMS F(ab')$_2$ (**C**), and LEMS Fab (**D**). Numerous normal active zones (arrows) are present in **A** and **D**. Normal active zones are absent from the imaged regions in **B** and **C**; asterisks in **B** and **C** indicate large membrane particles aggregated into clusters. sc = synaptic cleft; ×75,000. (Nagel *et al.*[6] With permission from the *Annals of Neurology.*)

significant immunostaining. Higher doses of IgG injected intraperitoneally (20 mg three times a day for 2 days, or 10 mg a day for 15 days) from each of four patients caused significant immunostaining of mouse active zones (FIG. 8D): (1) the mean density (no./μm presynaptic membrane length) of positive active zones was 0.72 in the immunoperoxidase and 0.91 in the immunoferritin study (control values: 0.12

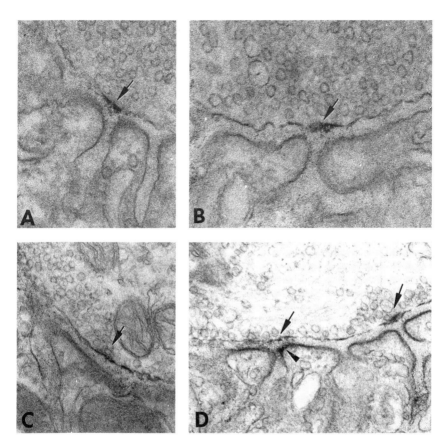

FIGURE 8. Immunoperoxidase localization of human IgG in mice treated with single intravenous (**A, B,** and **C**) or multiple intraperitoneal (**D**) injections of LEMS IgG. Arrows indicate immunostained active zones. Postsynaptic staining vis-a-vis positive active zones (arrowhead in **D**) is attributed to diffusion artifact. **A,** ×50,300; **B** ×58,200; (**C**) ×44,00; (**D**) ×43,800. (Fukuoka et al.[5] With permission from the *Annals of Neurology*.)

and 0.02) (FIG. 9); (2) 43% of the ferritin particles in the primary synaptic cleft were concentrated at the active zones, and the rest were scattered randomly (control value: 5.3%). These findings clearly established that LEMS IgG binds to presynaptic membrane active zones.[5]

THE AZP AND VSCC OF THE MNT ARE IDENTICAL STRUCTURES

Recent electrophysiological studies also suggest that LEMS IgG causes a loss of VSCC from the MNTs. When mice are treated with LEMS IgG, spontaneous quantal release from MNTs depolarized by high K^+ concentrations is significantly reduced over a range of Ca^{2+} concentrations.[24] Further, LEMS IgG has now been shown to reduce functional VSCC in small-cell carcinoma,[25,26] rat pheochromocy-toma (PC12),[25] anterior pituitary,[27] adrenal chromaffin,[28] and neuroblastoma-glioma hybrid cells.[29] Finally, IgG from some LEMS patients immunoprecipitates ^{125}I-ω-conotoxin-labeled VSCC extracted from human neuroblastoma[30,31] and small cell carcinoma[32] cells. Observations on the adrenal chromaffin, anterior pituitary, and

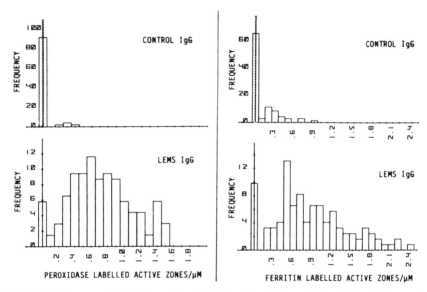

FIGURE 9. Frequency distribution of the density (no./μm^2) of peroxidase-labeled (left panel) and ferritin-labeled (right panel) active zones in mice treated with multiple doses of control IgG (49 and 70 end-plate regions) and LEMS IgG (138 and 122 end-plate regions). Each end-plate region contains one primary synaptic cleft. (Fukuoka et al.[5] With permission from the *Annals of Neurology.*)

neuroblastoma-glioma hybrid cells suggest that LEMS IgG has a selective effect on L Ca^{2+} channels, whereas immunoprecipitation by some LEMS IgG of ^{125}I-ω-conotoxin-labeled VSCC implies binding to N and a subtype of L Ca^{2+} channels. These observations, however, do not mean that the MNT VSCC is either L or N in type, because LEMS IgG might recognize homologous and antigenically similar domains in different types of Ca^{2+} channels. Although the kinetic properties and molecular structure of the MNT VSCC are still undefined, the freeze-fracture data, indicating that LEMS IgG depletes the AZP,[1,3,4,6] in conjunction with the early studies suggesting that AZP comprise the VSCC of the MNT[19-22] and with studies on effects of LEMS IgG on the VSCC of different cell lines,[25-32] are sufficient evidence to assume that the AZP and the VSCC of the MNT are identical structures. Immunocytochemical localization of fluorescent ω-conotoxin at the frog motor nerve terminal, reported in this volume, is also consistent with this assumption.[33]

REFERENCES

1. FUKUNAGA, H., A. G. ENGEL, M. OSAME & E. H. LAMBERT. 1982. Paucity and disorganization of presynaptic membrane active zones in the Lambert-Eaton myasthenic syndrome. Muscle & Nerve **5:** 686–697.
2. ENGEL, A. G., H. FUKUNAGA & M. OSAME. 1982. Stereometric estimation of the area of the freeze-fractured membrane. Muscle & Nerve **5:** 682–685.
3. FUKUNAGA, H., A. G. ENGEL, B. LANG, J. NEWSOM-DAVIS & A. VINCENT. 1983. Passive transfer of Lambert-Eaton myasthenic syndrome IgG from man to mouse depletes the presynaptic membrane active zones. Proc. Natl. Acad. Sci. USA **80:** 7636–7640.
4. FUKUOKA, T., A. G. ENGEL, B. LANG, J. NEWSOM-DAVIS, C. PRIOR & D. W.-WRAY. 1987. Lambert-Eaton myasthenic syndrome: I. Early morphologic effects of IgG on the presynaptic membrane active zones. Ann. Neurol. **22:** 193–199.
5. FUKUOKA, T., A. G. ENGEL, B. LANG, J. NEWSOM-DAVIS & A. VINCENT. 1987. Lambert-Eaton myasthenic syndrome: II. Immunoelectron microscopy localization of IgG at the mouse motor end-plate. Ann. Neurol. **22:** 200–211.
6. NAGEL, A., A. G. ENGEL, B. LANG, J. NEWSOM-DAVIS & T. FUKUOKA. 1988. Lambert-Eaton syndrome IgG depletes presynaptic membrane active zone particles by antigenic modulation. Ann. Neurol. **24:** 552–558.
7. ENGEL, A. G. 1986. Myasthenic syndromes. *In* Myology. A. G. Engel & Banker, Eds.: 1955–1990. McGraw-Hill. New York.
8. O'NEILL, J. H., N. M. F. MURRAY & J. NEWSOM-DAVIS. 1988. The Lambert-Eaton myasthenic syndrome. A review of 50 cases. Brain **111:** 577–596.
9. ELMQVIST, D. & E. H. LAMBERT. 1968. Detailed analysis of neuromuscular transmission in a patient with the myasthenic syndrome sometimes associated with bronchogenic carcinoma. Mayo Clin. Proc. **43:** 689–713.
10. LAMBERT, E. H. & D. ELMQVIST. 1971. Quantal components of end-plate potentials in the myasthenic syndrome. Ann. N.Y. Acad. Sci. **183:** 183–199.
11. MOLENAAR, P. C., J. NEWSOM-DAVIS, R. L. POLAK & A. VINCENT. 1982. Eaton-Lambert syndrome: acetylcholine and choline acetyltransferase in skeletal muscle. Neurology **32:** 1061–1065.
12. LANG, B., J. NEWSOM-DAVIS, D. W. WRAY, A. VINCENT & N. MURRAY. 1981. Autoimmune aetiology for myasthenic (Lambert-Eaton) syndrome. Lancet **ii:** 224–226.
13. LANG, B., J. NEWSOM-DAVIS, C. PRIOR & D. W.-WRAY. 1983. Antibodies to motor nerve terminals: an electrophysiological study of a human myasthenic syndrome transferred to mouse. J. Physiol. (London) **344:** 335–345.
14. KIM, Y. I. 1985. Passive transfer of the Lambert-Eaton myasthenic syndrome: neuromuscular transmission in mice injected with plasma. Muscle & Nerve **8:** 162–172.
15. KATZ, B. & R. MILEDI. 1967. The timing of calcium action during neuromuscular transmission. J. Physiol. (London) **189:** 535–544.
16. KATZ, B. & R. MILEDI. 1967. The release of acetylcholine from nerve endings by graded electrical pulses. Proc. R. Soc. Lond. Biol. Sci. **167:** 23–28.
17. LLINÁS, R. & C. NICKELSON. 1975. Calcium in depolarization secretion coupling: An aequorin study in squid giant synapse. Proc. Natl. Acad. Sci. USA **72:** 187–190.
18. CHARLTON, M. P., S. J. SMITH & R. ZUCKER. 1982. Role of presynaptic calcium ions and channels in synaptic facilitation and depression at the squid giant synapse. J. Physiol. (London) **323:** 173–193.
19. LLINÁS, R., I. Z. STEINBERG & K. WALTON. 1976. Presynaptic calcium currents and their relation to synaptic transmission: Voltage clamp study in squid giant synapse and theoretical model for the calcium gate. Proc. Natl. Acad. Sci. USA **73:** 2918–2922.
20. PUMPLIN, D. W., T. S. REESE & R. LLINÁS. 1981. Are the presynaptic membrane particles calcium channels? Proc. Natl. Acad. Sci. USA **78:** 7210–7213.
21. HEUSER, J. E., T. S. REESE, M. J. DENNIS, Y. JAN, L. YAN & L. EVANS. 1979. Synaptic

vesicle exocytosis captured by quick freezing and correlated with quantal transmitter release. J. Cell Biol. **81:** 275–300.

22. CECCARELLI, B., F. GROHAVAZ & W. P. HURLBUT. 1979. Freeze-fracture studies of frog neuromuscular junctions during intense release of neurotransmitter. I. Effects of black widow spider venom and Ca^{2+} free solutions on the structure of the active zones. J. Cell Biol. **81:** 163–177.

23. LANG, B., J. NEWSOM-DAVIS, C. PEERS & D. W.-WRAY. 1987. The action of myasthenic syndrome antibody fragments on transmitter release in the mouse. J. Physiol. (London) **390:** 173P.

24. LANG, B., J. NEWSOM-DAVIS, C. PEERS, C. PRIOR & D. W.-WRAY. 1987. The effect of myasthenic syndrome antibody on presynaptic calcium channels in mouse. J. Physiol. (London) **390:** 257–270.

25. LANG, B., A. VINCENT, N. M. F. MURRAY & J. NEWSOM-DAVIS. 1989. Lambert-Eaton myasthenic syndrome: Immunoglobulin G inhibition of Ca^{2+} flux in tumor cells correlates with disease severity. Ann. Neurol. **25:** 265–271.

26. DE AIZAPURA, H. J., E. H. LAMBERT, G. E. GRIESMANN, B. M. OLIVERA & V. A. LENNON. 1988. Antagonism of voltage-gated calcium channels in small cell carcinomas of patients with and without Lambert-Eaton myasthenic syndrome by autoantibodies, ω-conotoxin and adenosine. Cancer Res. **48:** 4719–4724.

27. LOGIN, I. S., Y. I. KIM, A. M. JUDD, B. L. SPANGELO & R. M. MACLEOD. 1987. Immunglobulins of Lambert-Eaton myasthenic syndrome inhibit rat pituitary hormone release. Ann. Neurol. **22:** 610–614.

28. KIM, Y. I. & E. NEHER. 1988. IgG from patients with Lambert-Eaton syndrome blocks voltage-dependent calcium channels. Science **239:** 405–408.

29. PEERS, C., B. LANG, J. NEWSOM-DAVIS & D. W.-WRAY. 1987. Selective action of Lambert-Eaton myasthenic syndrome antibodies on calcium channels in a rodent neuroblastoma × glioma hybrid cell line. J. Physiol. (London). **421:** 293–308.

30. SHER, E., C. GOTTI, N. CANAL, C. SCOPETTA, G. PICCOLO, A. EVOLI & F. CLEMENTI. 1989. Specificity of calcium channel autoantibodies in Lambert-Eaton myasthenic syndrome. Lancet **ii:** 640–643.

31. LEYS, K., B. LANG, A. VINCENT & J. NEWSOM-DAVIS. 1989. Calcium channel autoantibodies in Lambert-Eaton myasthenic syndrome. Lancet **ii:** 1107.

32. LENNON, V. A. & E. H. LAMBERT. 1989. Autoantibodies bind solubilized calcium channel-ω-conotoxin complexes from small cell lung carcinoma: a diagnostic aid for Lambert-Eaton myasthenic syndrome. Mayo Clin Proc. **64:** 1498–1504.

33. ROBITAILLE, R. & M. P. CHARLTON. Unpublished observations from the conference.

Role of Specific Lipids and Annexins in Calcium-Dependent Membrane Fusion[a]

PAUL MEERS,[b] KEELUNG HONG,[c]

AND DEMETRIOS PAPAPHADJOPOULOS[c]

[b]Department of Pathology
William B. Castle Hematology Laboratory
Boston University School of Medicine
Boston, Massachusetts 02118-2394

[c]Cancer Research Institute
University of California
San Francisco, California

INTRODUCTION

The concentration of intracellular Ca^{2+} is highly regulated during cellular secretion and other membrane fusion events. Therefore, it is thought that Ca^{2+} may play some role, direct or indirect, in these processes. One early indication of a direct role in membrane fusion was the observation that Ca^{2+} could induce aggregation and leakage of contents from model membrane vesicles composed of the most abundant naturally occurring acidic phospholipid, phosphatidylserine (PS).[1] Later these phenomena were shown to be associated with fusion of the vesicles.[2] Subsequently, the ability to produce large unilamellar vesicles (LUV)[3–5] and the development of fluorescent fusion assays[5,6] has allowed detailed studies of the factors that mediate Ca^{2+}-dependent membrane fusion, particularly fusion of PS vesicles.[5] A simple mass action model for the kinetics of membrane fusion that could describe or predict the results of fusion assays under certain conditions resulted from such studies.[7,8] A prominent feature of this model was that the overall fusion process was treated as a two-step reaction involving first aggregation of vesicles followed by actual fusion. Using this rational framework, the factors explicitly involved at each step can be discussed separately.

CALCIUM-INDUCED FUSION OF PHOSPHOLIPID VESICLES

Application of these methods to the fusion of PS vesicles has helped delineate the ways in which Ca^{2+} acts in the overall fusion process. For instance, Ca^{2+} can accelerate aggregation of PS vesicles through charge neutralization,[9,10] but a major factor that makes Ca^{2+} fusogenic is the formation of an anhydrous "trans" intermembrane complex[11–14] where Ca^{2+} actually may bind between the headgroups of PS molecules from separate apposed bilayers. The affinity for Ca^{2+} in this complex is much higher than in single bilayer ("cis") complexes.[11,13] The ability of Ca^{2+} to form

[a]This investigation was supported by research Grant 1570 C-1 from the Massachusetts Chapter of the American Cancer Society (P. Meers), a postdoctoral fellowship (P. Meers) from the Arthritis Foundation, and partially by Grant GM-28117 (K. Hong and D. Papahadjopoulos) and Grant GM-41790-01A1 (P. Meers) from the National Institutes of Health.

259

an anhydrous intermembrane complex is crucial to membrane fusion, as dehydration of the phospholipid headgroups is the major energy barrier to the close approach necessary for fusion and mixing of lipids from each interacting bilayer.[15] Because Mg^{2+} does not form such a complex with PS,[11] fusion of LUV is absolutely specific for Ca^{2+}, although both cations can cause aggregation of these vesicles. The dissociation constant for the Ca^{2+}-PS intermembrane complex has been measured and ranges from 0.1 to 3 μM depending on the species of PS.[14] These results suggest that this type of complex could participate in intracellular membrane fusion at physiologically relevant Ca^{2+} concentrations.

In contrast to LUV, a number of ions are able to induce fusion of small unilamellar vesicles (SUV), probably due to the relatively less stable nature of these highly curved membranes.[16] The amount of bound ion on the surface of these vesicles was found to be critical in determining the rate of fusion.[9,17] For equal amounts bound, the sequence of effectiveness for divalent cations was $Ba^{2+} > Ca^{2+} > Sr^{2+} > Mg^{2+}$ under conditions where aggregation of the vesicles was rate-limiting. When the actual fusion of the vesicles was rate-limiting, Ca^{2+} was shown to be more effective than Ba^{2+} at equal bound cation concentrations.

Fusion is also observed with some other phospholipid compositions but with

TABLE 1. Threshold Concentrations of Ca^{2+} and Mg^{2+} (mM) for Fusion of LUV Composed of Pure Phospholipids[a]

Phospholipid	Aggregation		Fusion	
	Ca^{2+}	Mg^{2+}	Ca^{2+}	Mg^{2+}
Phosphatidylinositol	3	6	[b]	—
Phosphatidylglycerol[c]	5	20	15	—
Phosphatidylserine	2	5	2	—
Phosphatidate	0.2	0.4	0.2	0.4

[a]All experiments were performed at 25°C at pH 7.4.
[b]Indicates no fusion.
[c]Data from Sundler,[76] Rosenberg et al,[77] and N. Düzgünes, unpublished.

different cation specificities and threshold concentrations. The Ca^{2+} and Mg^{2+} concentration thresholds for aggregation and fusion of various acidic phospholipids is shown in TABLE 1. Phosphatidate (PA) is the most sensitive to Ca^{2+}, with a submillimolar Ca^{2+} dependence, followed by PS and phosphatidylglycerol (PG). Much of the Ca^{2+} required for fusion of the acidic vesicles results from the necessity for charge neutralization. Phosphatidylinositol (PI), however, does not show fusion even at cation concentrations that induce aggregation. Phosphatidylcholine, one of the most hydrated of these phospholipids, does not allow fusion even though it has a net neutral charge. The resistance of PC toward Ca^{2+}-mediated fusion prevails even in liposomes in which the major bilayer components are fusion-susceptible.[18,19] When PS is mixed with large percentages of phosphatidylethanolamine (PE), Mg^{2+} is also able to cause fusion. This is presumably due to the instability and low hydration of pure PE bilayers. Apposition of the PS/PE bilayers by any cation capable of charge neutralization of the acidic component is sufficient to allow fusion. In a sense, this situation is similar to that with SUV of PS, where Mg^{2+} can also cause fusion despite lack of evidence for a dehydrated complex. The propensity of PE to form nonbilayer structures may be an important factor making such membranes fusogenic. The mechanism of this fusion may be significantly different from fusion of PS vesicles induced by Ca^{2+}.[20]

Besides the dehydration of the headgroups that allows critically close apposition of interacting bilayers, rearrangements of the acyl chains of the phospholipids are also important in the membrane fusion process. Düzgünes *et al.*[21] and Bentz *et al.*[22] showed that increased molecular motion induced by increased temperatures enhanced the rate of membrane fusion. The same studies showed that phase transitions of the phospholipid bilayers were not necessary for fusion.

Conformational rearrangements of the acyl chains from bilayer packing to some other phase is also important in the membrane fusion process. The ability of phospholipids to form the inverted hexagonal II phase has been correlated with fusogenicity.[23–26] It has been suggested that hexagonal II phase or lipidic particles, which have been associated with hexagonal II phase, may be general intermediates in membrane fusion. This is probably not the case with phospholipids, however, that do not form inverted phases, such as PS in the presence of Ca^{2+}. Rapid-freeze electron-microscopy studies have clearly shown that lipidic particles and hexagonal II phase are not observed during fusion of liposomes, even those that contain phospholipids with a tendency to form hexagonal II phase.[27] It seems likely that Ca^{2+}-dependent membrane fusion of acidic phospholipid vesicles involves a relatively small and transient perturbation in bilayer structure at the point of interbilayer contact. This may involve a small defect or some other means of exposing the hydrophobic acyl chains of interacting bilayers.[28–30] It could be related to inverted phases or could be a different type of structure. Recent data suggest that fusion involving phospholipids that readily form inverted phases could include formation of interlamellar attachments (ILA) that are related to the cubic phase.[20]

These studies of Ca^{2+}-dependent fusion have elucidated three major steps in the fusion process. First, long-range electrostatic repulsive forces must be overcome by double layer screening and binding of cations to neutralize charge. Then water of hydration at the surface of the bilayer must be stripped off to allow very close approach of membrane surfaces. Finally a perturbation in the bilayer packing of the phospholipids that may involve some small transient intermediate structure may be necessary to promote fusion of the bilayers. The importance of each step in any given system may vary or they may even exist as one concerted step.

PROTEIN-MEDIATED MEMBRANE FUSION: ROLE OF ANNEXINS

Despite the advances in elucidation of the mechanisms of Ca^{2+}-dependent fusion of liposomes, the mechanisms of intracellular membrane fusion remain unclear. Several facts suggest that protein factors may help modulate Ca^{2+}-dependent membrane fusion. One important fact is that the Ca^{2+} requirement for liposome fusion (TABLE 1) is several orders of magnitude higher than the maximal Ca^{2+} concentration attained in the cytoplasm in stimulated cells (near 1 μM).[55] This difference is probably due to the necessity to screen the surface charge of acidic liposomes and the low concentration of liposomes that must be used in fusion assays. Factors that can overcome the charge repulsion and enhance the rate of vesicle aggregation potentially decrease the Ca^{2+} requirement. Indeed, acidic liposomes containing glycolipid can fuse at significantly lower Ca^{2+} concentrations when preaggregated by specific lectins.[31,32] A second, more compelling argument for the existence of fusion-mediating proteins is the problem of regulation and specificity. Simply regulating Ca^{2+} levels does not confer specificity on the site of fusion and does not allow fine-tuning of fusion through regulatory cascades. It is also likely that movement of vesicles through structurally complex cytoskeletal barriers requires protein mediation. Although Ca^{2+}-phospholipid intermediates may ultimately define the final step in intracellular fusion, it is likely that proteins exist to mediate and enhance specific interactions, thus imposing temporal and spatial control.

The annexins are a group of Ca^{2+}-dependent membrane-binding proteins with a variety of putative intracellular and extracellular functions. These include Ca^{2+}-dependent membrane fusion[33-38] as well as membrane-cytoskeletal interactions,[39-41] intracellular signaling as kinase substrates,[42-45] control of cell growth,[42,46] inhibition of blood coagulation,[47] and anchoring of cells to collagen.[48] Most of these putative functions depend on the common ability of annexins to bind to membrane phospholipids at Ca^{2+} concentrations in the range of 0.7 to several hundred μM. In addition, some annexins are able to cause the aggregation of model and biological vesicles in a Ca^{2+}-dependent manner. Structurally, there is a striking homology between the various members of the human family (40–50% identity) in the C-terminal 80–90% of the proteins.[49] This portion of the sequence consists of a repeated 60–80 amino acid segment that shows high intrapolypeptide homology. A short N-terminal sequence is unique in composition and length in each annexin, suggesting that it may confer functional specificity. Modification of the N terminus affects the Ca^{2+} sensitivity of several of the annexins.[37,50,51] The annexin sequences do not contain a classical

TABLE 2. Effect of Synexin on Calcium-Dependent Aggregation and Fusion of Various Phospholipid Vesicles[54]

Phospholipid Composition	Aggregation	Fusion
PS, PS/PE, PA/PE[a]	enhanced	enhanced
PS/PC	enhanced	no effect
PI/PE	enhanced	inhibited

[a]PA, phosphatidate prepared from egg phosphatidylcholine; PC, egg phosphatidylcholine; PE, phosphatidylethanolamine transesterified from egg phosphatidylcholine; PI, bovine phosphatidylinositol; PS, bovine brain phosphatidylserine.

EF-hand Ca^{2+}-binding site.[52] Though some proposals have been made for the structure of Ca^{2+} and phospholipid binding domains,[53] determination of the structure of membrane bound annexins awaits further investigation.

The first indication that annexins could mediate membrane fusion came from one of the earliest isolated members of this class, a protein called synexin (annexin VII).[33] Early investigations showed that synexin was capable of aggregating chromaffin granules in a Ca^{2+}-dependent manner. Hong et al.[18,34,54] showed that synexin could enhance fusion of phospholipid vesicles composed of acidic phospholipids (TABLE 2), whereas other Ca^{2+}-binding proteins had no effect. Synexin reduces the Ca^{2+}-concentration dependence for fusion of PA/PE vesicles by two orders of magnitude from the millimolar range to approximately 10 μM. This is higher than the free Ca^{2+} concentration that produces 50% activation of catecholamine release in electropermeabilized chromaffin cells.[55] A later study on depolarized chromaffin cells, however, estimates that the Ca^{2+} entry into the cytosolic space can reach up to 170–340 μM in one second during a short depolarization.[56]

In the presence of Ca^{2+}, synexin binds to isolated secretory vesicles and also self-associates to form extended rods in the absence of vesicles.[57] The threshold concentration of Ca^{2+} required for self-association (> 100 μM) is higher than that for binding to vesicles (6 μM). At 10–50 μM Ca^{2+} and sufficient protein and vesicle concentrations, most ($> 70\%$) synexin added is found associated with liposomes under conditions where fusion occurs.[18,54] Self-association of synexin prior to addition of vesicles for fusion inhibits the synexin effect.[36] These facts suggest that extended rods of synexin are probably not involved in the fusion of liposomes. There is some evidence, however, for significant activity of polymerized synexin.[36]

In order to determine whether synexin enhances aggregation of vesicles, actual fusion of vesicles or both, studies were initiated to isolate these kinetic steps by making one or the other the rate-limiting step in the overall process. This was done by varying phospholipid concentration, ionic composition, or phospholipid composition.[36] In all cases synexin exerted positive effects on the overall rate of fusion only under aggregation rate-limiting kinetics. When the actual fusion step was rate-limiting, synexin was either inhibitory or had no effect. Synexin-mediated fusion required a phospholipid composition itself susceptible to fusion at some Ca^{2+} concentration. It is likely that most annexins assist in membrane fusion of liposomes solely by enhancing the rate of aggregation and that the rate of fusion itself is dependent on other membrane components.

Synexin, as a Ca^{2+}-dependent "aggregator," acts synergistically with promoters of the actual fusion step. Free fatty acids are generated upon stimulation of many secretory cells (*e.g.* ref. 58–60). They have also been shown to enhance fusion of small unilamellar vesicles.[61,62] Fatty acids enhance the rate of the fusion step but not the aggregation step for a number of lipid vesicle systems.[63] Because of this kinetic specificity, they act synergistically with synexin. It is important to note that this synergy is a result of action at different kinetic steps and does not imply direct interaction between fatty acids and synexin. In fact all data thus far suggest that fatty acids (fusion promoters) and synexin (aggregation promoter) act at spatially separate sites. This distinction is quite important for determining the detailed mechanism by which a promoter of the overall fusion process acts in the cell.

Evidence for the possible importance of synexin in degranulation of human neutrophils was found using specific granules and cytosolic proteins isolated from this system.[35] Antibodies against bovine liver synexin showed that human neutrophils contain this protein. When cytosol from human neutrophils is exposed to a liposome affinity column, a group of three major proteins, including the putative synexin, bind in a Ca^{2+}-dependent manner. Bovine synexin and these neutrophil cytosol proteins mediate Ca^{2+}-dependent aggregation of specific granules. Synexin also mediates Ca^{2+}-dependent fusion of specific granules with liposomes. These data suggest that synexin or a synexin-like protein may be involved in human neutrophil degranulation. It is to be noted, however, that fusion is not observed below approximately 100 μM Ca^{2+} under the conditions of the experiments, a concentration that is much higher than that observed after stimulation of the neutrophil. One possible resolution is that transiently higher Ca^{2+} concentrations occur locally in the cell, but quantitative evidence for this phenomenon has been difficult to obtain in this cell.

Recently, fusion has been observed in the concentration range of 1 μM Ca^{2+} using annexin II. This protein, referred to as calpactin, exists as a heterotetramer with two annexin subunits and two 10 kDa subunits. It allows aggregation of chromaffin granules at 0.7 μM Ca^{2+} [37] and mediates exocytosis of permeabilized chromaffin cells at 1–3 μM Ca^{2+}.[38] Thus annexins are implicated in membrane fusion at physiological Ca^{2+} levels, and calpactin specifically in the chromaffin cell system. There have also been indications that lipocortin I (annexin I) can interact with membranes at micromolar levels of Ca^{2+} [64] and can mediate fusion of neutrophil-derived plasma membranes with phospholipid vesicles at 10 μM Ca^{2+} or less (P. Meers, unpublished data).

INTERACTIONS OF ANNEXINS WITH PHOSPHOLIPID VESICLES

The structure of the membrane-bound annexin is of particular interest in that it may help to elucidate the mechanism of annexin-mediated aggregation and fusion of vesicles. Because of the difficulty of crystallization of a membrane-bound protein to a form suitable for detailed X-ray diffraction analysis, it is desirable to use other approaches to study this form as well. One method has been to use the intrinsic tryptophan fluorescence of the annexins.[65] Most human annexins contain a single tryptophan, providing an ideal site-specific marker. For example, human lipocortin V (annexin V) contains a single tryptophan in the third consensus sequence. When this protein binds to vesicles composed of 50% phosphatidylserine and 50% phosphatidyl-choline in the presence of 100 μM Ca^{2+}, a marked increase in fluorescence intensity is observed, accompanied by a red shift indicating a conformational change upon binding.[65] The tryptophan fluorescence of the bound lipocortin V is quenched strongly when phosphatidylcholine (PC) is replaced by a derivative with a nitroxide moiety at the 5 position of the acyl chain (FIG. 1). This indicates that the third consensus sequence probably makes close contact with the phospholipids of the membrane. Quenching by derivatives with the nitroxide more deeply localized in the membrane is weaker, suggesting an interfacial location for the tryptophan. The single tryptophan in lipocortin I (annexin I), located in the N-terminal region, shows little interaction with the phospholipid quenchers, suggesting that this tryptophan does not make close contact with the phospholipids. Subsequently it was shown that the tryptophan in the third consensus sequence of calpactin (annexin II) is in close proximity to a Tb^{3+} binding site.[66] Taken together, these results suggest the possibility that the third consensus sequence in annexins participates in a ternary annexin-Ca^{2+}-phospholipid complex, where the Ca^{2+} ion has both protein and phospholipid ligands.

A simple sensitive assay is desirable to determine the factors responsible for

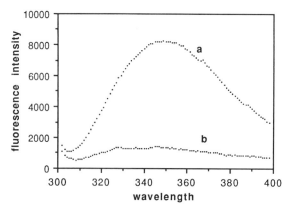

FIGURE 1. Tryptophan emission spectrum of lipocortin bound to phospholipid vesicles. All samples consisted of 10 μg/mL lipocortin V and 50 μM total phospholipid in 100 μM free Ca^{2+}, 100 μM EDTA, 100 mM NaCl, 5 mM N-[tris(hydroxymethyl)methyl]-2-aminoethanesulfonic acid (TES), pH 7.4, at 25°C. The phospholipid compositions were (a) PS/PC (1/1) and (b) PS/5-PC (1/1). 5-PC = 1-palmitoyl-2-(5-doxyl)stearoyl-sn-glycero-3-phosphocholine. Lipocortin V was generously supplied in purified form by R. Blake Pepinsky.

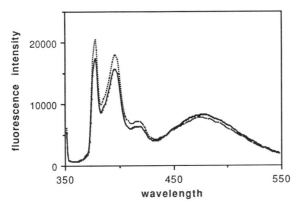

FIGURE 2. Emission spectrum of 5 mol% pyrene-PC incorporated into phosphatidylserine vesicles at a total phospholipid concentration of 0.25 μM. Each sample contained 156 nM endonexin and was in a total volume of 2 mL of 100 mM NaCl, 5 mM TES, 0.1 mM EDTA at pH 7.4 and 25°C. The solid curve is in buffer alone. The broken curve contains 100 μM free Ca^{2+}. Endonexin was purified by the method of Südhof *et al.*[74,75] with small modifications.

annexin binding to membranes. We have found various fluorescent phospholipid probes useful to characterize this binding.[67,68] Binding of annexins to phospholipid vesicles causes dequenching of membrane-incorporated fluorophors quenched in a concentration-dependent manner. For instance, when synexin binds to vesicles containing 0.75 mol% each of *N*-(7-nitrobenz-2-oxa-1,3-diazol-4-yl)dipalmitoyl-L-α-phosphatidylethanolamine (NBD-PE) and *N*-(lissamine rhodamine B sulfonyl)dipalmitoyl-L-α-phosphatidylethanolamine (Rh-PE), an increase in the NBD fluorescence is observed.[69] NBD-PE is the donor of this resonance energy transfer pair and is partially quenched by the presence of the acceptor Rh-PE. When NBD-PE alone is incorporated into vesicles at 5 mol% of the total phospholipid, it is partially selfquenched. Binding of annexins to this type of vesicle also increases the NBD fluorescence. In both cases the fluorescence change observed is dependent on the simultaneous presence of both an annexin and Ca^{2+}. It is also dependent on a fluorescent phospholipid derivative that is quenched in a concentration-dependent manner.

Because the NBD group is interfacially localized and potentially susceptible to artifactual effects,[70–72] a hydrophobic acyl chain probe was also tested. 3-Palmitoyl-2-[1-pyrenedecanoyl]-L-α-phosphatidylcholine (pyrene-PC) forms excited state complexes called excimers at a sufficiently high proportion of the probe in the membrane. When annexins bind to PS vesicles with this probe, a decrease in the excimer-to-monomer ratio is observed. In FIGURE 2, the effect of binding of endonexin (annexin IV) is shown. Peaks from monomers at 377 and 396 nm increase in intensity, and the broad peak at 480 nm from excimers decreases in intensity when endonexin binds in the presence of Ca^{2+}. The increase in intensity of the 377 nm peak can be followed as a function of time, as in FIGURE 3. From this FIGURE it is clear that the response is dependent on the protein concentration within this range. Other nonannexin proteins do not cause the observed effect. Based on the lack of probe specificity and results indicating no change in fluorescence lifetimes, the most likely cause of this effect is a decrease in the effective bulk lateral mobility of membrane phospholipids upon annexin binding.

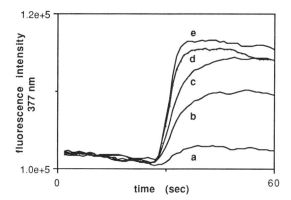

FIGURE 3. Dependence of probe response on protein concentration. Endonexin at a final concentration of 7.8 nM (a), 15.6 nM (b), 31.2 nM (c), 62.5 nM (d), or 125 nM (e) was added to vesicles composed of 5 mol% pyrene-PC in PS at a total phospholipid concentration of 1 μM in 100 mM NaCl, 5 mM TES, 0.1 mM EDTA, pH 7.4, at 25°C. At approximately 30 seconds a final concentration of 100 μM Ca^{2+} was added to the sample, and fluorescence at 377 nm was monitored. The excitation wavelength was 344 nm.

The reversibility of endonexin binding was also assessed using the pyrene response. When EDTA is added to bound endonexin a complete and rapid reversal of the fluorescence increase is observed. The polycation spermine is also able to reverse the annexin-mediated fluorescence increase (FIG. 4). The presence of spermine before Ca^{2+} addition also inhibits the fluorescence increase. These results indicate that ionic interactions may dominate the binding of endonexin under the chosen conditions.

Pyrene-PC fluorescence could also be used to measure competition of unlabeled vesicles with labeled PS vesicles. In FIGURE 5 is shown the effect of competing vesicles on the fluorescence increase induced by binding of the 67 kDa calelectrin (annexin VI). Clearly there is significant competition by unlabeled PS vesicles. By binding the protein first to the labeled vesicles and then adding the unlabeled vesicles the rate of exchange between vesicles could also be monitored. In this case the exchange is very slow on the time scale of minutes. Endonexin binding to vesicles of varying percentages of PS in PC was also measured by competition and is shown in TABLE 3. The effect of phospholipid composition was observed both in directly labeled vesicles and by competition of unlabeled vesicles with labeled vesicles. There is an apparent cutoff in the binding of endonexin when the PS composition drops below approximately 25–50 percent. This is probably related to the necessity for the protein to access a minimum number of PS molecules within the surface area covered by the protein. Binding to phosphatidate is also observed using this probe.

By varying the protein or phospholipid concentration it was possible to generate binding isotherms at 100 μM Ca^{2+}. These binding isotherms have been modeled in terms of monomers of annexin binding to n phospholipids. Reasonable agreement with the data can be obtained by assuming the n phospholipids are perturbed in such a way as to decrease the excimer-to-monomer ratio of the pyrene probe by a certain percentage. In FIGURE 6, the binding of endonexin is shown. A reasonable fit to the data can be obtained by taking n = 25. This number represents the space occupied by the protein on the membrane surface, not the actual number of phospholipid binding sites on the protein. If 25–50% of the phospholipids must be PS, 6–12 PS binding sites may exist in the protein in agreement with Junker and Creutz.[73]

The still emerging picture is that annexins bind to phospholipids by mainly ionic interactions and do not normally insert deeply into the membrane under the conditions of our experiments. This interaction does, however, perturb the lateral mobility of a number of the phospholipids. At least one consensus sequence, the third, makes close contact with phospholipids and may form a protein-Ca^{2+}-

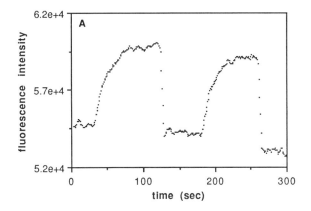

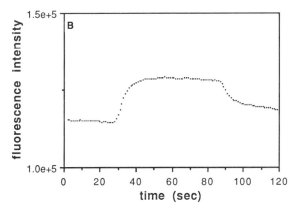

FIGURE 4. Reversibility of annexin binding. **A:** Sample contained 0.25 μM total phospholipid of 5 mol% pyrene-PC in PS and 15 nM endonexin. Additions were 100 μM Ca^{2+} at 30 s (first arrow), 110 μM EDTA at 120 s (second arrow), 110 μM Ca^{2+} at 180 s (third arrow), and 110 μM EDTA at 250 s (fourth arrow). Experimental conditions were as in FIG. 3. **B:** 31 nM endonexin and 1 μM total phospholipid composed of 5 mol% pyrene-PC in PS. 100 μM Ca^{2+} was added at the first arrow and 100 μM spermine at the second arrow. Spermine alone had no effect but inhibited the Ca^{2+} response.

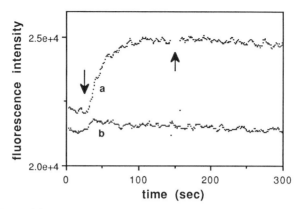

FIGURE 5. Competition of vesicles for annexin binding. Initial preparations contained 7.5 nM of the 67 kDa calelectrin and either 0.25 μM of 5 mol% pyrene-PC in PS (a) or 0.25 μM of 5 mol% pPC in PS along with 5 μM PS (b). In a and b 100 μM Ca^{2+} was added at the first arrow. In a 5 μM PS was added at the second arrow. Other experimental conditions were as in FIG. 3. The 67 kDa calelectrin was prepared by the method of Südhof *et al.*[74,75] with modifications.

TABLE 3. Effect of Phospholipid Composition on the Change in Pyrene-PC Fluorescence due to Endonexin (annexin IV) Binding

Phospholipid Composition	Percent Fluorescence Increase[a]	Competition Index[b]
PS	13.0	0.95
PS/PC (3/1)	—	0.95
PS/PC (1/1)	3.2	0.84
PS/PC (1/3)	0.4	0.01
PC	0	—
PA	8.5	—

[a]Percentage increase in pyrene-PC fluorescence at 377 nm upon addition of 100 μM Ca^{2+} to 1 μM total phospholipid with no competing unlabeled vesicles. Vesicles were of the noted composition and contained 5 mol% pyrene-PC. Final endonexin concentration was 31 nM. Experiments were performed in 100 mM NaCl, 5 mM TES, 0.1 mM EDTA, pH 7.4, at 25°C. Endonexin was purified by the method of Südhof *et al.*[74,75] with small modifications.

[b]Samples contained 47 nM endonexin and 2 μM total phospholipid of vesicles composed of PS with 5 mol% pyrene-PC. Also included was 2 μM total phospholipid of competing unlabeled vesicles of composition indicated in the first column. The competition index was defined as

$$\frac{I_{max} - I_{obs}}{I_{max} - I_{1/2}}$$

where I_{max} is the maximal percentage increase without competing vesicles, I_{obs} is the observed percent increase in fluorescence, and $I_{1/2}$ is the percent increase for half of the original amount of protein (10 nM), *i.e.* $I_{1/2}$ is the percent increase expected if endonexin bound equally well to the competing vesicles. An index of 1.0 denotes equal binding to the labeled and competing vesicles, whereas 0 indicates no binding to the competing vesicles. Experiments were performed in 100 mM NaCl, 5 mM TES, 0.1 mM EDTA, pH 7.4, at 25°C.

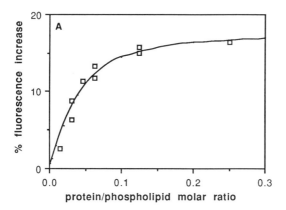

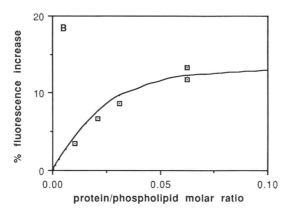

FIGURE 6. Binding isotherms for endonexin. **A:** Samples contained vesicles of 5 mol% pyrene-PC in PS at a total phospholipid concentration of 1 μM and varying concentrations of endonexin. Molar ratios of protein/phospholipid are based on one-half of the total phospholipid concentration. Solid lines represent curves fit to the data using an apparent binding constant (K) of $1.2 \times (10^8)$ M^{-1} and an apparent lipid/protein stoichiometry (n) of 25. Other experimental conditions were as in Fig. 3. **B:** Samples contained vesicles of 5 mol% pyrene-PC in PS at a varying phospholipid concentration and an endonexin concentration of 31 nM.

phospholipid ternary complex. Further structural characterization will help define the mechanism of annexin binding and its effects on fusion of membranes.

CONCLUDING REMARKS

Because membrane fusion, as we have defined it, may be a critical step in exocytosis, we have attempted to understand the mechanism at the molecular level. Our approach has been the establishment of a relatively simple experimental model system amenable to a detailed study of the role of individual components of this complex reaction. This system is the vesicle fusion system, starting with phospholipid vesicles (liposomes) and proceeding to isolated secretory granules and plasma membrane vesicles. The relative advantages of this cell-free system are as follows: simplicity of starting material, with incremental complexity; accessibility of detailed kinetic studies by the use of sensitive fluorescence assays; independent assessment of the specificity of various lipids, proteins, metal ions, and other "effectors;" and possible study of structure-function relationships of the individual components.

The kinetic analysis of fusion has proved to be extremely important in defining the role of specific components. This is because the overall fusion reaction involves two in-series reactions: one, the aggregation of the vesicles, and the other, the actual fusion of their membranes. Thus, it is essential to define whether a particular reactant is active in promoting the aggregation (recognition, close contact) or fusion (mixing of membranes and vesicle contents) step. The overall fusion rate could be affected by participation in either step, depending on which is the rate-limiting reaction. Our results with synexin indicate that its ability to enhance the overall vesicle fusion reaction is due to increasing the aggregation rate and not the rate of fusion per se. Polyamines such as spermine and spermidine seem to have a similar effect by the same criteria. On the contrary, long chain fatty acids, such as arachidonate, seem to have an effect in enhancing the rate of fusion itself, rather than the rate of aggregation.

Concerning the mechanism of interaction of some of the annexins with the phospholipid bilayer, our recent results indicate that these proteins (annexins I, IV, V, and VI, which are known to bind to negatively charged bilayer vesicles in the presence of Ca^{2+}) bind only to the surface of the bilayer in a reversible manner with only a small degree of penetration into the bilayer interior. Further detailed studies, however, of the role of various cytoplasmic and membrane proteins are needed for a thorough understanding of the mechanism of membrane fusion during exocytosis. The vesicle fusion system we have reviewed here has proven to be a valuable tool in that pursuit.

REFERENCES

1. PAPAHADJOPOULOS, D. & A. D. BANGHAM. 1966. Biochim. Biophys. Acta 126: 185–188.
2. PAPAHADJOPOULOS, D., G. POSTE, B. E. SCHAEFFER & W. J. VAIL. 1974. Biochim. Biophys. Acta 352: 10–28.
3. SZOKA, F. & D. PAPAHADJOPOULOS. 1978. Proc. Natl. Acad. Sci. USA 75: 4194–4198.
4. SZOKA, F., F. OLSON, T. HEATH, W. VAIL, E. MAYHEW & D. PAPAHADJOPOULOS. 1980. Biochim. Biophys. Acta 601: 559–571.
5. WILSCHUT, J., N. DÜZGÜNES, R. FRALEY & D. PAPAHADJOPOULOS. 1980. Biochemistry 19: 6011–6021.
6. ELLENS, H., J. BENTZ & F. C. SZOKA. 1985. Biochemistry 24: 3099–3106.
7. NIR, S., J. BENTZ & J. WILSCHUT. 1980a. Biochemistry 19: 6030–6036.
8. BENTZ, J., S. NIR & J. WILSCHUT. 1983. Colloids Surf. 6: 333–363.
9. NIR, S., J. BENTZ & A. R. PORTIS, JR. 1980b. Adv. Chem. Ser. 188: 75–106.
10. MCLAUGHLIN, S. 1989. Annu. Rev. Biophys. Biophys. Chem. 18: 113–136.
11. PORTIS, A., C. NEWTON, W. PANGBORN & D. PAPAHADJOPOULOS. 1979. Biochemistry 18: 780–790.
12. REHFELD, S. J., N. DÜZGÜNES, C. NEWTON, D. PAPAHADJOPOULOS & D. J. EATOUGH. 1981. FEBS Lett. 123: 249–251.
13. EKERDT, R. & D. PAPAHADJOPOULOS. 1982. Proc. Natl. Acad. Sci. USA 79: 2273–2277.
14. FEIGENSON, G. W. 1986. Biochemistry 25: 5819–5825.
15. RAND, R. P. 1981. Annu. Rev. Biophys. Bioeng. 10: 277–314.

16. BENTZ, J. & N. DÜZGÜNES. 1985. Biochemistry **24:** 5436–5443.
17. DÜZGÜNES, N., S. NIR, J. WILSCHUT, J. BENTZ, C. NEWTON, A. PORTIS & D. PAPAHADJO-POULOS. 1981a. J. Memb. Biol. **59:** 115–125.
18. HONG, K., N. DÜZGÜNES, R. EKERDT & D. PAPAHADJOPOULOS. 1982b. Proc. Natl. Acad. Sci. USA **79:** 4642–4644.
19. DÜZGÜNES, N., J. WILSCHUT, R. FRALEY & D. PAPAHADJOPOULOS. 1981b. Biochim. Biophys. Acta **642:** 182–195.
20. ELLENS, H., D. P. SIEGEL, D. ALFORD, P. L. YEAGLE, L. BONI, L. J. LIS, P. J. QUINN & J. BENTZ. 1989. Biochemistry **28:** 3692–3703.
21. DÜZGÜNES, N., J. PAIEMENT, K. FREEMAN, N. G. LOPEZ, J. WILSCHUT & D. PAPAHADJO-POULOS. 1984a. Biochemistry **23:** 3486–3494.
22. BENTZ, J., N. DÜZGÜNES & S. NIR. 1985. Biochemistry **24:** 1064–1072.
23. CULLIS, P. R. & M. J. HOPE. 1978. Nature **271:** 672–674.
24. VERKLEIJ, A. J., C. MOMBERS, W. J. GERRITSEN, L. LEUNISSEN-BIJVELT & P. R. CULLIS. 1979. Biochim. Biophys. Acta **555:** 358–361.
25. VERKLEIJ, A. J., C. J. A. VAN ECHTELD, W. J. GERRITSEN, P. R. CULLIS & B. DE KRUIFF. 1980. Biochim. Biophys. Acta **600:** 620–624.
26. SIEGEL, D. 1984. Biophys. J. **45:** 399–420.
27. BEARER, E. L., N. DÜZGÜNES, D. S. FRIEND & D. PAPAHADJOPOULOS. 1982. Biochim. Biophys. Acta **693:** 93–98.
28. HUI, S. W., T. P. STEWART, L. T. BONI & P. L. YEAGLE. 1981. Science **212:** 921–923.
29. HORN, R. G. 1984. Biochim. Biophys. Acta **778:** 224–228.
30. MARRA, J. & J. ISRAELACHVILI. 1985. Biochemistry **24:** 4608–4618.
31. SUNDLER, R. & J. WIJKANDER. 1983. Biochim. Biophys. Acta **730:** 391–394.
32. DÜZGÜNES, N., D. HOEKSTRA, K. HONG & D. PAPAHADJOPOULOS. 1984b. FEBS Lett. **173:** 80–84.
33. CREUTZ, C. E., C. J. PAZOLES & H. B. POLLARD. 1978. J. Biol. Chem. **253:** 2858–2866.
34. HONG, K., N. DÜZGÜNES & D. PAPAHADJOPOULOS. 1981. J. Biol. Chem. **256:** 3641–3644.
35. MEERS, P., J. D. ERNST, K. HONG, N. DÜZGÜNES, J. FEDOR, I. M. GOLDSTEIN & D. PAPAHADJOPOULOS. 1987a. J. Biol. Chem. **262:** 7850–7858.
36. MEERS, P., J. BENTZ, D. ALFORD, S. NIR, D. PAPAHADJOPOULOS & K. HONG. 1988a. Biochemistry **27:** 4430–4439.
37. DRUST, D. S. & C. E. CREUTZ. 1988. Nature **331:** 88–91.
38. ALI, S. M., M. J. GEISOW & R. D. BURGOYNE. 1989. Nature **340:** 313–315.
39. GERKE, V. & K. WEBER. 1984. EMBO J. **3:** 227–233.
40. GLENNEY, J. 1986. Proc. Natl. Acad. Sci. USA **83:** 4258–4262.
41. IKEBUCHI, N. W. & D. M. WAISMAN. 1990. J. Biol. Chem. **265:** 3392–3400.
42. FAVA, R. A. & S. COHEN. 1984. J. Biol. Chem. **259:** 2636–2645.
43. GLENNEY, J. R. & B. F. TACK. 1985. Proc. Natl. Acad. Sci. USA **82:** 7884–7888.
44. ISACKE, C. M., I. S. TROWBRIDGE & T. HUNTER. 1986. Mol. Cell Biol. **6:** 2745–2751.
45. CREUTZ, C. E., W. J. ZAKS, H. C. HAMMAN, S. CRANE, W. H. MARTIN, K. L. GOULD, K. M. ODDIE & S. J. PARSONS. 1987. J. Biol. Chem. **262:** 1860–1868.
46. PEPINSKY, R. B. & L. K. SINCLAIR. 1986. Nature **321:** 81–84.
47. FUNAKOSHI, T., R. L. HEIMARK, L. E. HENDRICKSON, B. A. MC MULLEN & K. FUJIKAWA. 1987. Biochemistry **26:** 5572–5578.
48. PFÄFFLE, M., F. RUGGIERO, H. HOFMANN, M. P. FERNÁNDEZ, O. SELMIN, Y. YAMADA, R. GARRONE & K. VON DER MARK. 1988. EMBO J. **7:** 2335–2342.
49. PEPINSKY, R. B., R. TIZARD, R. J. MATTALIANO, L. K. SINCLAIR, G. T. MILLER, J. L. BROWNING, E. P. CHOW, C. BURNE, K.-S. HUANG, D. PRATT, L. WACHTER, C. HESSION, A. Z. FREY & B. P. WALLNER. 1988. J. Biol. Chem. **263:** 10799–10811.
50. SCHLAEPFER, D. & H. T. HAIGLER. 1987. J. Biol. Chem. **262:** 6931–6937.
51. ANDO, Y., S. IMAMURA, Y.-M. HONG, M. K. OWADA, T. KAKUNAGA & R. KANNAG. 1989. J. Biol. Chem. **264:** 6948–6955.
52. KRETSINGER, H. & C. E. CREUTZ. 1986. Nature (Lond.) **320:** 573.
53. GEISOW, M. J., J. H. WALKER, C. BOUSTEAD & W. TAYLOR. 1987. Biosci. Rep. **7:** 289–298.
54. HONG, K., N. DÜZGÜNES & D. PAPAHADJOPOULOS. 1982a. Biophys. J. **37:** 297–305.
55. BAKER, P. F. & D. E. KNIGHT. 1978. Nature **276:** 620–622.

56. ARTALEJO, C. R., A. G. GARCIA & D. AUNIS. 1987. J. Biol. Chem. **262:** 915–926.
57. CREUTZ, C. E., C. J. PAZOLES & H. B. POLLARD. 1979. J. Biol Chem. **254:** 553–558.
58. STENSON, W. F. & C. W. PARKER. 1979. J. Clin. Invest. **64:** 1457–1465.
59. WAITE, M., L. R. DeCHATELET, L. KING & P. S. SHIRLEY. 1979. Biochem. Biophys. Res. Commun. **90:** 984–992.
60. WALSH, C. E., B. M. WAITE, M. J. THOMAS & L. R. DeCHATELET. 1981. J. Biol. Chem. **256:** 7228–7234.
61. KANTOR, H. L. & J. H. PRESTEGARD. 1975. Biochemistry **14:** 1790–1795.
62. KANTOR, H. L. & J. H. PRESTEGARD. 1978. Biochemistry **17:** 3592–3597.
63. MEERS, P., K. HONG & D. PAPAHADJOPOULOS. 1988b. Biochemistry **27:** 6784–6794.
64. BLACKWOOD, R. A. & J. D. ERNST. 1990. Biochem. J. **266:** 195–200.
65. MEERS, P. 1990. Biochemistry **29:** 3325–3330.
66. MARRIOTT, G., W. R. KIRK, N. JOHNSSON & K. WEBER. 1990. Biochemistry **29:** 7004–7011.
67. MEERS, P., D. PAPAHADJOPOULOS & K. HONG. 1987b. Biophys. J. **51:** 169a.
68. MEERS, P., D. PAPAHADJOPOULOS & K. HONG. 1988c. Biophys. J. **53:** 319a.
69. MEERS, P., K. HONG & D. PAPAHADJOPOULOS. 1990b. Submitted to Biochem. Biophys. Res. Commun.
70. SILVIUS, J. R., R. LEVENTIS, P. M. BROWN & M. ZUCKERMANN. 1987. Biochemistry **26:** 4279–4287.
71. SILVIUS, J. R., R. LEVENTIS & P. M. BROWN. 1988. In Molecular Mechanisms of Membrane Fusion. S. Ohki, D. Doyle, T. D. Flanagan, S. W. Hui & E. Mayhew, Eds.: 531–542. Plenum Press. New York.
72. DÜZGÜNES, N., T. M. ALLEN, J. FEDOR & D. PAPAHADJOPOULOS. 1988. In Molecular Mechanisms of Membrane Fusion. S. Ohki, D. Doyle, T. D. Flanagan, S. W. Hui & E. Mayhew, Eds.: 543–555. Plenum Press. New York.
73. JUNKER, M. & C. E. CREUTZ. 1990. Biophys. J. **57:** 461a.
74. SÜDHOF, T. C. & D. K. STONE. 1987. Methods Enzymol. **139:** 30–35.
75. SÜDHOF, T. C., M. EBBECKE, J. H. WALKER, U. FRITSCHE & C. BOUSTEAD. 1984. Biochemistry **23:** 1103–1109.
76. SUNDLER, R. 1984. In Biomembranes M. Kates & L. A. Manson, Eds. **12:** 563–583. Plenum Press. New York.
77. ROSENBERG, J., N. DÜZGÜNES & C. KAYALAR. 1983. Biochim. Biophys. Acta **735:** 173–180.

Video Microscopy Studies of Vesicle-Planar Membrane Adhesion and Fusion[a]

WALTER D. NILES AND FREDRIC S. COHEN

Department of Physiology
Rush Medical College
Chicago, Illinois 60612

Membrane fusion, the melding of two phospholipid bilayers into a single lamella with the discharge of the vesicular contents to external medium, is the fundamental event underlying the quantal release of neurotransmitter. This report is divided into two parts. In the body of the text, we describe a model system of synaptic vesicle exocytosis, in which phospholipid vesicles fuse with a planar lipid membrane. In the model system, calcium promotes the tight adhesion of negatively charged phospholipid bilayers, the initial step in membrane fusion. This indicates that calcium is capable of regulating quantal transmitter release through physical processes at an early stage in the exocytotic process. In the Appendix, the extent to which this early calcium-dependent step in membrane fusion accounts for features of the presynaptic kinetics of quantal transmitter release is examined.

THE ROLE OF CALCIUM IN A MODEL SYSTEM OF EXOCYTOSIS

At the synapse, neurotransmitter is released by the incorporation of the synaptic vesicle membrane into the axolemma at a release site and the discharge of the vesicle contents into the synaptic cleft.[1,2] The process is termed synaptic vesicle exocytosis, and it results in the release of a quantal packet of transmitter. The rate of release depends on the calcium concentration in the axoplasm just under the axolemma, which is increased when voltage-dependent calcium channels spanning the axolemma adjacent to the release sites are opened.[3] Calcium may regulate exocytosis through a potentially large set of proteins and enzyme cascades. For example, the cytosolic domain of p65, an integral membrane protein of synaptic vesicles, exhibits about 40% homology with the C2 region identified in some types of protein kinase C and binds anionic phospholipids and sphingolipids.[4] p65 could regulate membrane fusion directly through disruption of the lamellar arrangement of lipid membranes in a calcium-dependent process, bypassing or supplementing enzyme cascades such as kinases and other effectors regulated by GTP-binding proteins. The biochemical processes that regulate synaptic vesicle exocytosis, however, ultimately converge to a single series of physical events. The synaptic vesicle membrane adheres to a small region of the plasmalemma, and the two phospholipid bilayer membranes subsequently meld into a single lamella within this contact zone, resulting in the intermixing of the vesicular contents with external medium.

We have turned to a model system of exocytosis, the fusion of a phospholipid vesicle with a planar phospholipid membrane,[5,6] to study membrane fusion at a

[a] This work was supported by NIH Grant GM 27367.

fundamental level and to understand how membrane fusion determines or limits the rate of quantal transmitter release. Calcium promotes the adhesion but not the fusion between anionic phospholipid membranes,[7] so that the vesicle is held in a "prefusion" state. To overcome the physical barriers to fusion, additional stress must be supplied to the region of vesicle-planar membrane contact, and this is readily achieved by osmotic swelling of the vesicle.[6,8,9]

VIDEO MICROSCOPY OF VESICLE-PLANAR MEMBRANE ADHESION AND FUSION

To study the physical chemistry of adhesion and fusion, we use a fluorescence microscope to view in video single phospholipid vesicles interacting with a planar phospholipid membrane separating two buffer-filled compartments. Large unilamellar vesicles, 1–10 μm in diameter, are made containing 200 mM calcein, a water-soluble, membrane-impermeant fluorescent dye. At this concentration, the fluorescence of the dye is self-quenched, so that when a vesicle's membrane is ruptured, either through fusion with the planar membrane or simple lysis, an easily detectable, localized emission of fluorescence is observed. We have termed this brief light emission a "flash." By placing cobalt, a quencher of calcein fluorescence, on either the *cis* (vesicle-containing) or *trans* side of the planar membrane, we can determine whether the flash is due to dye release to the *trans* compartment by fusion or release to the *cis* compartment by lysis.[10] The vesicles are delivered directly to the surface of the planar membrane by pressure-ejection from an L-shaped pipette. Vesicles adhering to the planar membrane are observed as discrete fluorescent spots, situated within a single plane of focus. The bound vesicles drift slowly in the direction of the convection currents of the stirred chamber buffer and provide a direct, observable event for determining the parameters of the adhesion step of the fusion process.

The bound vesicles are induced to fuse with the planar membrane by osmotic swelling.[5-7] The intravesicular hydrostatic pressure that is generated can be calculated from the equations describing solute and water fluxes.[11] The hydrostatic pressure stresses the vesicle membrane and the region of the planar membrane adhering to the vesicle. The stress drives the molecular rearrangements in the contact zone, resulting in the formation of a single membrane. The hydrostatic pressures that result in fusion are in the range of those necessary to elastically rupture phospholipid membranes.[12]

CALCIUM AND THE ADHESION OF VESICLES TO THE PLANAR MEMBRANE

Adhesion of vesicles to the planar membrane requires calcium (or other divalent cations) when the membranes contain anionic lipids.[6,7] We usually use asolectin to form membranes, a lipid mix with 20% negatively charged phospholipids.[13] These anionic lipids include phosphatidylinositol, phosphatidic acid, and small amounts of phosphatidylserine. The remaining phospholipids are the zwitterions phosphatidylcholine and phosphatidylethanolamine. We have measured the calcium dependence of the binding of asolectin vesicles with asolectin planar membranes by ejecting vesicles at planar membranes bathed by buffers of varying calcium concentration. When observed in the video fluorescence microscope, some of the ejected vesicles adhere to the planar membrane; the unadherent vesicles are swept away by the continual stirring of the *cis* compartment. The bound vesicles all lie within a single plane of focus and drift very slowly, about 1–10 μm/s, in the direction of the stirring. This indicates that the vesicles are strongly attached to the planar membrane, because they are not torn away by the continual stirring. The slowly drifting bound vesicles have a terminal velocity determined by the force of the stirred buffer near the surface of the planar membrane, which, as shown below, is primarily opposed by the viscosity of the two-dimensional fluid planar membrane.

We measure binding as the fraction of vesicles that remain bound after a brief period of exposure of the vesicles to the planar membrane. After the vesicles are ejected, we count the total number of vesicles in focus at the planar membrane, and, then, after the unbound vesicles move away, we count the remaining adherent, in-focus vesicles. The fraction bound is the ratio of the number of bound vesicles to the total number of vesicles encountering the planar membrane. We consider the vesicles that were in-focus initially but were swept away by the end of the counting interval to be those that had an opportunity to bind, but did not do so. The dependence of the fraction bound on the calcium concentration is shown in FIGURE 1. At zero calcium, no vesicles are bound. Binding increases over the millimolar range of calcium concentration, with about 2 to 3 mM required to obtain a fraction significantly greater than zero. Half-maximal binding is obtained at 15 mM, whereas binding is saturated by 30 mM. At calcium concentrations sufficient to saturate the fraction bound, about 70% of the vesicles encountering the planar membrane adhere, indicating that the membranes are very sticky in the presence of calcium. The vesicles remain adherent despite convection.

VELOCITY OF VESICLE MOVEMENT AND THE STRENGTH OF ADHESION

We can estimate the strength of the binding interaction from the terminal velocity of the bound vesicles when the *cis* compartment is stirred (see FIG. 2). The bound vesicles are moved by frictional coupling to the convective flow of the aqueous solution. As the viscosity of water, 0.01 poise, is only about 1% that of lipid bilayer,[14] the planar membrane remains relatively stationary in spite of vigorous stirring, resulting in the classical unstirred layer adjacent to the planar membrane. We treat the vesicular and planar membranes as effectively "spot-welded" together by calcium in the region of contact. Any force imparted to the vesicle by the stirring is fully transmitted to the planar membrane in the region of contact by the binding interaction (*i.e.,* the region of planar membrane adhering to the vesicle in the contact zone moves with it). While the fluid near the planar membrane travels at a high velocity (1 cm/s), the terminal velocity of the bound vesicle typically reaches only 10 μm/s. This reflects the small viscosity of water (compared to lipid bilayer), which results in small frictional coupling to the vesicle. For the vesicle to remain attached through the contact zone, the calcium-mediated binding interaction must equal or exceed the force exerted by stirring. As the vesicle moves at a constant terminal velocity, this stirring force equals the viscous force, which must be overcome to translate the contact zone laterally within the plane of the planar membrane. Treating the contact zone as a circular disk of radius r that moves at velocity v in a two-dimensional fluid of viscosity n, the frictional force is given by the Stokes-Einstein relation in two dimensions,[15] $F = 4\pi nrv$. For a vesicle 1 μm in radius with 20% of its surface area in the contact zone moving at velocity $v = 10$ μm/s, $F = 1.26 \times 10^{-6}$ dyne. Therefore, the binding force, distributed over an area of about 3×10^{-8} cm², must be at least 21 dyne/cm². Equivalently, the binding energy is at least -21

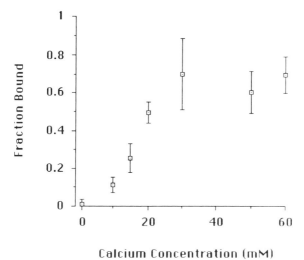

FIGURE 1. Calcium dependence of the fraction of asolectin vesicles bound to planar asolectin membranes. See text for details.

erg/cm^2 or -10 erg/cm^2 for each membrane (the sign is negative because binding is favored).

If the adhesive energy were greater than the cohesive energy of lipid bilayers, then binding, per se, would lead to bilayer destabilization. But as the estimated adhesive energy is less than the cohesive energy of phospholipid bilayers,[12] about 70 erg/cm^2, vesicles bind to the planar membrane and attain equilibrium without creating stress in the vesicle membrane. Also leading to stability upon adhesion is that the planar bilayer is supported by a torus of bulk phospholipid molecules. The adhesion zone of the bound membranes increases in area, due to the favorable binding interaction, as new phospholipid molecules from the bulk phase are pulled into the planar membrane.[7] In the region of contact with the vesicle membrane, the otherwise flat planar membrane curves locally when wrapping around a fraction of the vesicle's surface area and the tension of planar membrane is increased. The adherent vesicle, however, need not have its membrane stressed. Thus, the vesicle bound to the planar membrane reaches a stable equilibrium, and additional stress must be applied to the vesicle membrane in the region of contact (by osmotic swelling) to cause membrane fusion. This can be contrasted with the case when two vesicles adhere to one another. Again, the adhesion zone increases in area, due to the favorable binding interaction, by pulling more and more membrane into the contact zone. But in this case, because each vesicle has a fixed number of lipid molecules, an expansion stress is generated in each vesicle's membrane. The expansion stress may rupture the vesicles or cause fusion, particularly when lipids forming nonlamellar phases are used.[16] Hence, whereas calcium alone only produces adhesion between the vesicle and the planar membrane, it can produce fusion between vesicles.

THE SPACE BETWEEN THE VESICULAR AND PLANAR MEMBRANES

The vesicular and planar bilayer membranes remain separate and distinct within the region of contact. The binding interaction mediated by calcium does not involve the melding of the outer monolayer of the vesicle with the vesicle-facing monolayer of the planar membrane.[10,17] The water-filled gap remaining between the vesicular and planar membranes in the region of contact is small: swelling can be induced by imposing an osmotic gradient across the planar membrane;[6,7,11] only those vesicles very close to planar membrane imbibe water and swell.[7] Any separation or gap between the vesicular and planar membranes in the region of contact allows a portion of the water that flows across the planar membrane to be shunted around, rather than into, the vesicle. This produces a smaller hydrostatic pressure than would occur if there were no gap.

The fraction of water that enters the vesicle, f, is determined from the ratio of the osmotic gradient needed to lyse the membranes if none of the water were shunted around the vesicle to the osmotic gradient experimentally needed to produce fusion, as described quantitatively.[7] The theoretical gradient is that needed to produce an intravesicular hydrostatic pressure sufficient to lyse a phospholipid bilayer membrane. This pressure is given by Laplace's law, pressure $P = 2T/r$, where r is the radius and T is the tension at lysis (3 dyne/cm). The transbilayer osmotic gradient needed for fusion is usually at least 0.2 osmole/kg.[6,18,19] The hydrostatic pressure resulting from a transbilayer gradient is calculated using known equations.[11] For a gradient of 0.2 osmol/kg, the hydrostatic pressure is 5×10^6 dyne/cm^2 or about 5 atm. The separation between membranes, modeled as two square parallel plates of length l separated by a distance d, is easily obtained from equation 3 of appendix I of Akabas et al:[7] $f = 1.7 \times 10^{-13}(l^2/d^3)/(1 + 1.7 \times 10^{-13} \times l^2/d^3)$, where the water permeability coefficient of the vesicular membrane is 2×10^{-3} cm/s. For a 1 μm

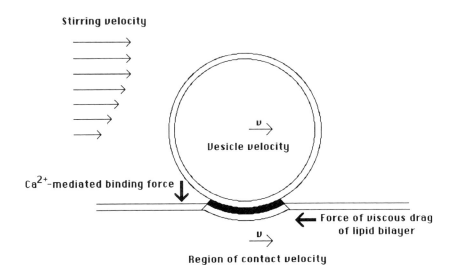

FIGURE 2. Diagram of a vesicle bound to a planar membrane swept along by stirring. The velocity of the stirred aqueous buffer is depicted by the arrows from the left. The stirred buffer exerts a force on the vesicle that pushes the vesicle in the direction parallel to the planar membrane. The vesicle adheres to the planar membrane by way of the calcium-mediated binding force. Movement of the vesicle together with the adherent region of planar membrane is opposed by the viscous drag of the large expanse of planar membrane outside the adhesion zone. The vesicle remains attached to the planar membrane as long as the binding force is greater than the force required to overcome the viscous drag.

radius vesicle (theoretical lysis pressure = 0.06 atm) with 20% of the vesicular surface area in contact with the planar membrane, (l = 0.9 μm), the ratio of the experimentally needed pressure to the theoretical hydrostatic pressure is 1.2 percent. Thus, d is 4.8 nm. With a 100 nm radius vesicle, l is 90 nm, the lysis pressure is 0.6 atm, f is 12%, and d is only 0.48 nanometers. The larger separation predicted for the 1 μm vesicle results from the longer path length for water flow, which increases the hydrodynamic resistance for exiting the gap.[7] Nevertheless, the separation remaining between the vesicular and planar membranes is narrow and is within the ranges predicted for the electrostatic and hydration barriers to membrane apposition.[20] The larger distance is consistent with the location of the primary minimum in the electrostatic energy between zwitterionic membranes.[21] The smaller distance corresponds to the length of 2–3 water molecules, consistent with the large energy required to fully dehydrate the phospholipid headgroups.[22] This simplified model suggests that the phospholipid headgroups are partially, but not completely, dehydrated within the adhesion zone and that the hydration barrier remains the primary force limiting membrane adhesion and direct molecular contact of the membranes.

The interaction between membranes mediated by calcium may weaken the region of contact. A surprisingly large fraction of the vesicles that release dye due to swelling fuse with the planar membrane.[10] In 20 mM calcium, a concentration at which the fraction of vesicles bound is saturated, about half of the vesicles that swell and release dye fuse with the planar membrane. Calcium may exert additional effects within the region of contact that promote membrane fusion. In 100 mM calcium, a concentration at which the same fraction of vesicles bind as at 20 mM, nearly 70% of the swelling vesicles fuse.[10] It is presently unresolved whether the higher calcium concentration leads to a larger area of contact, and/or further dehydration of the headgroups, thus reducing the size of the interposing gap.

HOW DOES CALCIUM PROMOTE TIGHT ADHESION OF THE MEMBRANES?

The close approach of two phospholipid membranes is opposed by electrostatic forces between like surface charges on the two membranes[21,23] and repulsive forces due to hydration of the headgroups.[22] The electrostatic surface potentials between anionic membranes are well-recognized as governing the long-range interactions between lipid membranes.[24] The more recently discovered hydration barrier, however, ultimately limits the closest approach of the membranes, whether or not they possess a net charge. Within a distance of about 3 nm, depending on the headgroup, the hydration force is the primary barrier limiting the close approach of phospholipid membranes.

Calcium overcomes both the electrostatic and hydration barriers to membrane adhesion. The divalent cation binds anionic headgroups in the apposing monolayers, neutralizes both surface charges, and lowers the repulsive surface potential. In addition, calcium binding dehydrates the anionic headgroups,[25] generates an adhesive bond between two apposed phospholipid molecules, one from each facing monolayer, and spans the gap by local sites of adhesion. The intrinsic dissociation constant for the binding of calcium to a single anionic phospholipid (*e.g.,* phosphatidylserine) in isolated membranes is around 100 mM.[26] Calcium binding between membranes can be much more avid, however. When phosphatidylserine is allowed to complex freely with calcium in the presence of excess water,[27] the neutral $Ca(PS)_2$ forms with an equilibrium constant of only 4 μM Ca. It may be noteworthy that this is a concentration attained in the axoplasm near the active zones of synaptic sites.[28,29]

Our kinetic measure for the calcium concentration of half-maximal binding of vesicles to the planar membrane is about 15 mM. This higher value may occur because the vesicle-planar membrane adhesion zone is far from equilibrium or because the formation of $Ca(PS)_2$ bridges between the two membranes is sterically hindered. In coordination complexes of calcium, such as $Ca(PS)_2$, the interatomic distance between the calcium atom and the charged atom is on the order of 0.24 nm.[30] Thus, we expect that the minimum separation between adherent membranes is about 0.48 nm, when the interaction is mediated by calcium cross-bridge formation. This distance is consistent with our calculation of the separation. We envision that lipids in apposing monolayers that are cross-bridged by calcium are in very close proximity, whereas the lipids in the adhesion zone that remain unliganded retain their bound water.

Membranes composed entirely of zwitterionic phospholipids are able to adhere and fuse in the absence of calcium.[7,18] The binding interaction between these macroscopically neutral membranes is weaker than the interaction mediated by calcium between anionic membranes.[31] We have explored the adhesion and fusion properties of oppositely charged membranes and compared this electrostatically mediated interaction to the calcium-mediated one. Positively charged planar membranes were made containing different amounts of the cationic pseudophospholipid, dioleyltrimethylammonium propane (DOTAP), which was synthesized and graciously supplied to us by Dr. John Silvius of the Department of Biochemistry, McGill University, Montreal, Quebec.[32] The fraction of anionic asolectin vesicles bound is shown plotted against the mole fraction of DOTAP in the planar membrane in FIGURE 3. Half-maximal binding was obtained with 20 to 25% DOTAP, and binding was saturated with 40% cationic lipid. As with calcium-mediated binding (FIG. 1), 70% of the vesicles contacting the planar membrane adhered at maximum binding. Because the mole fraction of anionic lipids in the asolectin vesicles was 20% and because the range of DOTAP surface densities over which vesicle binding increased bracketed this percentage, we conclude that the binding was mediated by electrostatic interactions between the oppositely charged membranes. When the vesicles were osmotically swollen with a *trans*-to-*cis* flow of water, however, less than 5% of the vesicles were observed to release dye (as opposed to more than 12% with calcium-mediated binding[10]). This indicates that the binding mediated by the electrostatic interaction left a relatively large gap between the vesicular and planar membranes in the contact zone; the water flux was shunted around the vesicle so that the resulting hydrostatic pressure was insufficient to cause fusion. Therefore, the calcium-mediated binding between anionic membranes dehydrates the headgroups more than the electrostatically induced binding (which may involve the formation of salt bridges).

In summary, calcium mediates the close approach of phospholipid membranes, most likely by dehydration and cross-bridging. Adhesion of membranes does not lead to membrane fusion. The stresses imparted to the lipid bilayers by interactions with calcium are insufficient to destabilize the bilayers, even though calcium binding is known to increase the surface tension of anionic lipid monolayers.[33] The physical chemistry of membrane adhesion mediated by calcium in the model system may or may not extrapolate to biological systems. Nevertheless, the results garnered in the model system provide a framework for determining the stages of the quantal release of neurotransmitters where calcium may work at a purely physical level and where intervention by proteins is necessary. We offer the hypothesis that calcium serves to weld the vesicle to the axolemma in tight association as a first stage in the release process and that proteins, perhaps calcium-activated, generate stresses that cause the molecular rearrangements of fusion.

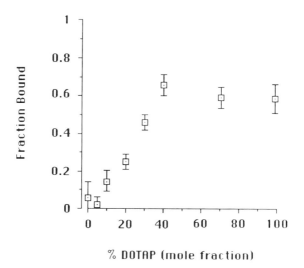

% DOTAP (mole fraction)

FIGURE 3. Vesicle binding mediated by electrostatic interaction. The fraction of negatively charged asolectin vesicles bound to planar membranes containing various amounts of the cationic lipid dioleyltrimethylammonium propane (DOTAP) is shown. The remainder of the planar membrane is diphytanoylphosphatidylcholine.

APPENDIX: THE PRESYNAPTIC RELEASE PROCESS AND CALCIUM[b]

Calcium action at an early stage in synaptic vesicle exocytosis, perhaps by causing the adhesion of the vesicular membrane and the axolemma, is suggested by the rapid rate of quantal release following a nerve impulse. Transmitter release at the squid giant synapse can be as fast as 200 μs following depolarization of the presynaptic membrane at 15°C.[3] Even at temperatures as low as 0.5 to 4°C at the crayfish walking leg excitatory neuromuscular junction, the minimum synaptic delay between the focally recorded nerve terminal potential and the postsynaptic quantal potential is less than 10 ms.[34-39] The readily apparent steep temperature dependence reveals that the presynaptic process underlying quantal release comprises a series of reaction steps. The nerve impulse regulates the process by controlling calcium entry. The time-course of calcium entry, limited by the activation kinetics of voltage-dependent calcium channels and the buildup of axoplasmic calcium by permeation through the channels, determines the time-course of transmitter release.[40] Indeed, the temperature-dependence of the synaptic delay probably manifests the channel activation kinetics.[37] The series of reactions that is interposed between the entry of calcium and the release of the quantal unit of transmitter, therefore, probably occurs on a relatively fast time-scale. This is indicated by the ability of calcium to rapidly diffuse into the axoplasm through calcium channels and the fast time-course of the molecular reorientations underlying membrane fusion. For example, the time required for lipid bilayers to develop localized intermediate thermodynamic phases is less than 1 μs,[41] and, once an opening or "fusion pore" has been created,[42,43] the collapse of the vesicle membrane into the planar membrane is limited by viscosity on a time scale of 100 nanoseconds. Thus, the role of calcium is to load synaptic vesicles into a very

[b]This section was written by Walter D. Niles.

rapid queue of final reaction steps that culminate in release. An early, calcium-dependent stage of quantal release has been proposed to account for the time-course of nerve-evoked release.[44,45]

The kinetics of quantal release are measured with a focal recording electrode judiciously placed over one or very few active sites of quantal release from the nerve terminal.[39] The field potentials arising from the depolarization of the presynaptic membrane directly under the electrode and the depolarization of the postsynaptic membrane due to the action of the locally released quanta of neurotransmitter are recorded. The gap in time between the nerve terminal potential and the subsequent quantal potential is the synaptic delay[35] or quantal latency,[46] which occurs with a characteristic temporal distribution.[35,38,39,44,47] Crayfish neuromuscular junctions in the distal regions of the walking leg dacyl opener excitatory axon have active zones spaced as much as 20 μm apart,[48] and quantal release from a single synaptic site can be recorded. The number of quanta evoked per nerve impulse (quantal content) for a single site is often less than one so that single quantal potentials can be timed. Multiple quantal potentials evoked at low temperature, probably from two adjacent release sites under the electrode, are temporally separated, and their individual latencies can be measured. In FIGURE 4, some focally recorded quantal potentials evoked by nerve stimulation at 1 Hz (1°C) are shown together with the frequency distribution of quantal latencies.

The presynaptic process underlying quantal release can be described as a series of configurational states of presynaptic membrane or reactions involving transitions between these states. No spatial restriction is placed on the sites, which may be discrete and localized or continuous and spread out over a large region of axolemma. The sites are created by the action of calcium on phospholipids (or, perhaps,

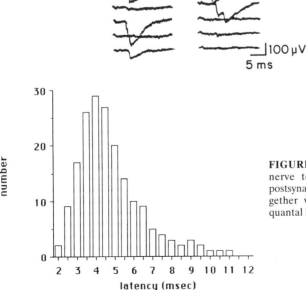

FIGURE 4. Focally recorded nerve terminal potentials and postsynaptic quantal potentials together with the distribution of quantal latencies.

proteins), but many cellular reactions mediated by proteins and initiated by calcium may be needed to move a vesicle to the presynaptic membrane. Once the vesicle has achieved contact, the series of reactions ensues as a stochastic process so that the amount of time spent by the site in a particular state is a random variable, and the time required for any vesicle to complete the series successfully and fuse with the axolemma is also a random variable. We assume each successful quantal release occurs independently of other nearby sites in various steps of the reaction, but that the same physical process occurs at all sites. If there are k states and the transition rate (v) to exit each state to the next is the same for each step, then the synaptic delay is distributed as a gamma-function, where the probability density for the first release at time t after a nerve impulse is $g(t)dt = (1/(k-1)!)v^k t^{k-1}e^{vt}dt$. The probability density for any quantal release at time t, $\alpha(t)dt$, is $\alpha(t)dt = g(t)dt/\int_t^\infty g(u)du$. $\alpha(t)$ is the likelihood that any vesicle-bound site completes the series of reactions culminating in fusion by time t. With $\alpha(t)$ as the fundamental rate, the master equation for quantal release as a function of time can be derived and solved for the time-course of the average number of releases following a nerve impulse (unpublished derivation). This treatment is similar to previous interpretations of the time-course of quantal release.[35,36,46,47] It yields a nonuniform, nonstationary binomial distribution of quantal content, the probability that m quanta have been released by time t after the nerve impulse given that n sites with vesicles were present at time t = 0.[49]

Several features of the delay and latency distributions reveal the role of calcium in quantal release from synaptic sites. When extracellular calcium is varied, only the magnitude of the release probability $\alpha(t)$ is changed, but not its time-course.[36,44,45] The time-course of $\alpha(t)$ is resistant to pharmacological manipulations.[47] When extracellular calcium is substituted with strontium, a divalent cation that permeates calcium channels, $\alpha(t)$ is unchanged.[50] Thus, the time-course is unaffected by the equilibrium binding constant between the divalent cation and the intracellular receptor that triggers release. Even 5-hydroxytryptamine at the crayfish neuromuscular junction, which increases the quantal content by an order of magnitude, has no effect on the time-course of impulse-evoked quantal release.[39] This indicates that the presynaptic process is initiated by calcium, but that once it is started, calcium has no effect on the intrinsic transition rates. In summary, we view the cellular reactions of synaptic vesicle exocytosis from the perspective of the presynaptic axolemma. Calcium, by lowering the energy barrier of adhesion, favors the entry of the vesicle into the series of reactions leading to fusion. An increase in the amount of calcium simply increases the number of vesicles that enter the first reaction step of the queue. Although more vesicles enter the first stage in the presence of increased calcium, the subsequent transitions leading to exocytosis occur at a rate independent of the calcium concentration. Calcium thus switches or gates this process, and the time-course of quantal release is independent of the magnitude of the calcium concentration. This is consistent with the role of calcium discerned in the model system of causing vesicle-planar membrane adhesion. The adhesion serves to prepare the vesicle for fusion with the planar membrane, but does not directly act to cause the membrane rearrangements inherent in fusion. In neurosecretion, a synaptic vesicle might, for example, be loaded onto the reaction queue by the action of a calcium-triggered enzyme cascade that frees the vesicle from attachment to a cytoskeletal element and allows calcium-mediated membrane adhesion between vesicle and axolemma. Subsequent stages correspond to intermediate axolemmal structures, possibly intermediate phases of phospholipid membranes.[41]

REFERENCES

1. KATZ, B. 1969. The Release of Neural Transmitter Substances. Liverpool University Press. New York.
2. HEUSER, J. E. & T. S. REESE. 1973. J. Cell Biol. **57:** 315–344.
3. LLINÁS, R., I. Z. STEINBERG & K. WALTON. 1981. Biophys. J. **33:** 323–351.
4. PERIN, M. S., V. A. FRIED, G. A. MIGNERY, R. JAHN & T. C. SUDHOF. 1990. Nature **345:** 260–263.
5. ZIMMERBERG, J., F. S. COHEN & A. FINKELSTEIN. 1980. J. Gen. Physiol. **75:** 241–250.
6. COHEN, F. S., J. ZIMMERBERG & A. FINKELSTEIN. 1980. J. Gen. Physiol. **75:** 251–270.
7. AKABAS, M. H., F. S. COHEN & A. FINKELSTEIN. 1984. J. Cell Biol. **98:** 1063–1071.
8. COHEN, F. S., M. H. AKABAS & A. FINKELSTEIN. 1982. Science **217:** 458–460.
9. ZIMMERBERG, J., F. S. COHEN & A. FINKELSTEIN. 1980. Science **210:** 906–908.
10. NILES, W. D. & F. S. COHEN. 1987. J. Gen. Physiol. **90:** 703–735.
11. NILES, W. D., F. S. COHEN & A. FINKELSTEIN. 1989. J. Gen. Physiol. **93:** 211–244.
12. EVANS, E. A. & R. SKALAK. 1983. Mechanics and Thermodynamics of Biomembranes. CRC Press. Boca Raton, FL.
13. ERDAHL, W. T., A. STOLYHWO & O. S. PRIVETT. 1973. J. Am. Oil Chem. Soc. **50:** 513–515.
14. SHINITZKY, M., A.-C. DIANOUX, C. GITLER & G. WEBER. 1971. Biochemistry **10:** 2106–2111.
15. BATCHELOR, G. K. 1983. Introduction to Fluid Dynamics. Cambridge University Press. New York.
16. KACHAR, B., N. FULLER & R. P. RAND. 1986. Biophys. J. **50:** 779–788.
17. PERIN, M. S. & R. C. MACDONALD. 1989. J. Membr. Biol. **109:** 221–232.
18. COHEN, F. S., M. H. AKABAS, J. ZIMMERBERG & A. FINKELSTEIN. 1984. J. Cell Biol. **98:** 1054–1063.
19. COHEN, F. S., W. D. NILES & M. H. AKABAS. 1989. J. Gen. Physiol. **93:** 201–210.
20. BLUMENTHAL, R. 1987. Curr. Top. Membr. Trans. **29:** 203–254.
21. MCLAUGHLIN, S. 1989. Annu. Rev. Biophys. Biophys. Chem. **18:** 113–136.
22. RAND, R. P. & V. A. PARSEGIAN. 1989. Biochim. Biophys. Acta **988:** 351–376.
23. NIR, S. & J. BENTZ. 1978. J. Colloid Interface Sci. **65:** 399–414.
24. VERWEY, E. J. W. & J. T. G. OVERBEEK. 1948. Theory of the Stability of Lyophobic Colloids. Elsevier North Holland. New York.
25. PORTIS, A., C. NEWTON, W. PANGBORN & D. PAPAHADJOPOULOS. 1979. Biochemistry **18:** 780–790.
26. MCLAUGHLIN, S., N. MULRINE, T. GRESALFI, G. VAIO & A. MCLAUGHLIN. 1981. J. Gen. Physiol. **77:** 445–473.
27. FEIGENSON, G. W. 1986. Biochemistry **25:** 5819–5825.
28. SIMON, S. M. & R. R. LLINÁS. 1985. Biophys. J. **48:** 485–498.
29. ZUCKER, R. S. & A. L. FOGELSON. 1986. Proc. Natl. Acad. Sci. USA **83:** 3032–3036.
30. WILLIAMS, R. J. P. 1980. *In* Calcium-binding Proteins: Structure and Function. F. L. Siegel, E. Carafoli, R. H. Kretsinger, D. H. MacLennan & R. H. Wasserman, Eds. Elsevier North Holland, Inc. New York.
31. NILES, W. D. & M. E. EISENBERG. 1985. Biophys. J. **48:** 321–326.
32. STAMATATOS, L., R. LEVENTIS, M. J. ZUCKERMANN & J. R. SILVIUS. 1988. Biochemistry **27:** 3917–3925.
33. OHKI, S. 1984. J. Membr. Biol. **77:** 265–275.
34. DUDEL, J. & S. W. KUFFLER. 1961. J. Physiol. **155:** 514–525.
35. KATZ, B. & R. MILEDI. 1965a. Proc. R. Soc. Lond. B Biol. Sci. **161:** 483–495.
36. KATZ, B. & R. MILEDI. 1965b. Proc. R. Soc. Lond. B Biol. Sci. **161:** 496–503.
37. KATZ, B. & R. MILEDI. 1965c. J. Physiol. **181:** 656–670.
38. ZUCKER, R. S. 1973. J. Physiol. **229:** 787–810.
39. NILES, W. D. & D. O. SMITH. 1982. J. Physiol. **329:** 185–202.
40. AUGUSTINE, G. J., M. P. CHARLTON & S. J. SMITH. 1985. J. Physiol. **367:** 143–162.
41. SIEGEL, D. P. 1984. Biophys. J. **45:** 399–420.

42. ZIMMERBERG, J., M. CURRAN, F. S. COHEN & M. BRODWICK. 1987. Proc. Natl. Acad. Sci. USA **84:** 1585–1589.
43. BRECKENRIDGE, L. J. & W. ALMERS. 1987. Proc. Natl. Acad. Sci. USA **84:** 1945–1949.
44. PARNAS, H., G. HOVAV & I. PARNAS. 1989. Biophys. J. **55:** 859–874.
45. BENNETT, M. R. & J. ROBINSON. 1990. Proc. R. Soc. Lond. B Biol. Sci. **239:** 329–358.
46. BARRETT, E. F. & C. F. STEVENS. 1972. J. Physiol. **227:** 665–689.
47. DATYNER, N. B. & P. W. GAGE. 1980. J. Physiol. **303:** 299–314.
48. JAHROMI, S. S. & H. L. ATWOOD. 1974. J. Cell Biol. **63:** 599–613.
49. HATT, H. & D. O. SMITH. 1976. J. Physiol. **259:** 367–393.
50. MILEDI, R. 1966. Nature **212:** 1233–1234.

A Dissection of Steps Leading to Viral Envelope Protein-Mediated Membrane Fusion

ROBERT BLUMENTHAL, CHRISTIAN SCHOCH,
ANU PURI, AND MICHAEL J. CLAGUE

Section on Membrane Structure and Function
LMMB
National Cancer Institute
National Institutes of Health
Bldg 10, Rm 4B56
Bethesda, Maryland 20892

INTRODUCTION

An increase in $[Ca^{2+}]$ at the presynaptic nerve terminal sets a complex set of biochemical events in motion that finally terminates in the specific fusion of the membrane of the secretory vesicle with the plasma membrane.[1] In studying the action of Ca^{2+} at the presynaptic terminal a distinction has to be made between processes that occur in the cytosol that result in the triggering of the fusion event, and the final membrane fusion event itself. Although specific fusogenic proteins have been postulated to mediate exocytotic membrane fusion, the molecular components of exocytotic membrane fusion machinery remain to be identified.

Our own studies have focused on pH-regulated viral fusion for which the participatory proteins have been identified.[2] The first steps in infection of animal cells by enveloped virus are binding and fusion of the cell and viral membranes.[3] Those events are mediated by viral envelope glycoproteins. Some virus strains infect cells by acid-activated fusion following endocytosis (*e.g.* influenza and vesicular stomatitis virus (VSV)), whereas others fuse directly with the plasma membrane at neutral pH (*e.g.* human immunodeficiency virus (HIV) and Sendai virus). Fusion of the acid-triggered viruses with the plasma membrane can be induced by lowering the external pH following binding. The threshold pH for fusion varies between 6.5 and 5.2 for different virus strains, independent of the nature of the target membrane or method of assay. The pH-dependence of fusion is related to the pH dependence of the conformational changes of the viral fusion protein.[2]

FIGURE 1 summarizes a series of events that presumably take place upon binding of virus to their cell surface receptors on target membrane. They include (1) triggering of a conformational change by receptor binding, or by lowering the pH; (2) approach of membranes; (3) formation of intermediates; and (4) the final fusion event itself. Using a variety of biochemical, cell biological, and biophysical techniques, we have been able to analyze the various conformational and kinetic components of the overall fusion process.[4-7] In this chapter we will describe these components. The data are mainly derived from work with influenza hemagglutinin (HA) whose structure is best characterized among the viral envelope proteins.[8,9]

pH-INDUCED CHANGES IN HA STRUCTURE

The membrane of influenza virus has two major spike glycoproteins, a neuramini-dase, and the hemagglutinin (HA), which contains both the capacity to bind to cell surface sialic acid residues and to catalyze fusion.[9] HA consists of two disulfide-linked glycopolypeptide chains, HA1 and HA2, which are arranged as a trimeric rod consisting of an α-helical stem extending some 10 nm from the virus membrane, surmounted by a globular top portion rich in β structure, as determined by X-ray crystallography to 0.3 nm resolution.[8] The C terminal of HA2 contains the viral membrane–spanning region, and the N terminal contains the relatively hydrophobic fusion peptide. The sialic acid–binding site is on a portion of HA1 that is at the top of the stalk. Beyond the threshold pH of fusion, the stalks open up, resulting in exposure of the hydrophobic amino terminus of HA2, which plays a critical role in

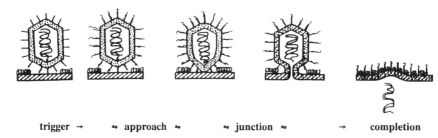

trigger →   ⇌ approach ⇌   ⇌ junction ⇌   →   completion

FIGURE 1. Schematic drawing of hypothetical steps in viral fusion. Five stages going from left to right are shown. (1) Viral envelope proteins (spikes) mediate association of the virus with binding sites on the target membrane. (2) The viral envelope proteins undergo a conforma-tional change (indicated by the squiggly appearance of the spikes). (3) Movement brings the two membranes into close apposition (prefusion state). (4) Fusion results in merging of membranes and contiguity of aqueous compartments. (5) In the final stage the membrane components and aqueous components are completely mixed. The membranes of the virions are stippled, and the plasma membrane is cross-hatched to indicate separate membrane compo-nents (lipids, proteins). After fusion they are intermixed. The cytoskeletal components are not shown. The nucleocapsid of the virion is drawn as two wavy lines and is seen in the cytoplasm after fusion. The spikes on the virion represent viral spike glycoproteins, and the fuzzy "broccoli" on the plasma membrane represents cell surface carbohydrates (glycoproteins, glycolipids).

fusion.[10] Extensive studies have been performed on the acid-triggered conforma-tional change that is related to the fusogenic activity of influenza virus HA. Electron-microscopy of negatively stained as well as unstained, frozen, hydrated influenza virus has revealed that the HA spikes in the intact virion at neutral pH are regular rectangular projections about 13 nm in length.[6,11] Acid treatment of influenza from the X31 strain results in a disordered appearance consistent with the tops coming apart (FIG. 2D). This drastic structural change does not happen with all strains of influenza virus. For instance, acid treatment induces conformational changes in the HA of the Japan strain, as indicated by sensitivity to proteolytic digestion and release of the fusion peptide, but the regular projections are still intact (FIG. 2B). Models have been proposed in which the heads of HA come apart but remain globular, the stem region remains trimeric, and there is no major change in overall secondary structure.[2] White and Wilson have probed the details of the

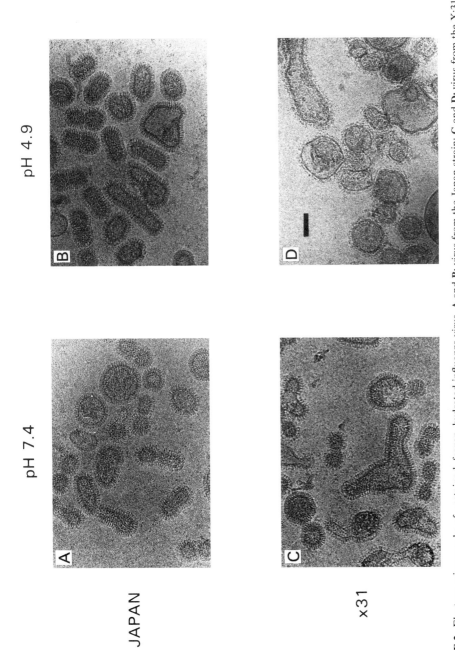

FIGURE 2. Electron micrographs of unstained, frozen, hydrated influenza virus. **A** and **B**: virus from the Japan strain; **C** and **D**: virus from the X:31 strain. **A** and **C**, virus at pH 7.4 and 37°C; **B** and **D**, virus incubated for 15 min at pH 4.9 and 37°C, and subsequently neutralized.[6]

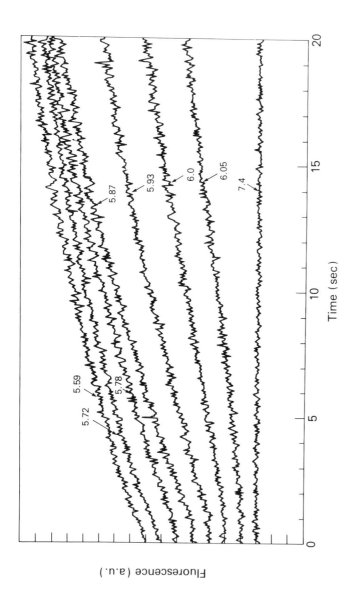

$$D_m \leftarrow \cdots D_1 \leftrightarrow T_0 \leftrightarrow R_0 \leftrightarrow R_1 \cdots \rightarrow R_n$$

FIGURE 3

pH-dependent conformational changes in the X:31 HA using a panel of anti–HA-peptide antibodies.[12] The results of the study indicate that the acid-triggered conformational change of isolated HA occurs in at least two steps: the fusion peptide comes out of the trimer interface ("intermediate state") followed by dissociation of the globular heads. A key question in the field is, Which of the states is associated with membrane fusion?

RAPID KINETIC STUDIES WITH INTACT VIRUS

To examine details about the initial stages of viral fusion, we have measured the kinetics and extent of fusion of intact virions with a variety of targets using an assay for continuous monitoring of fluorescence changes.[13] The assay uses the lipophilic fluorescent dye octadecylrhodamine B (R18), which is incorporated into intact virions under self-quenching conditions without redistribution of the probe into the target membrane under conditions where no fusion occurs.[14] Once fusion has occurred, the fluorophore diffuses into the larger target resulting in relief of selfquenching. Consequently an increase in the fluorescence signal is observed. Control experiments show that R18 dequenching is specific for the fusion reaction. In our studies the fusion event is dominated by virus associated with binding sites on the target membrane at the time of mixing. Thus, we can neglect consideration of diffusion-limited virus-cell association in our analysis.

To obtain a high-time resolution for the initial rates, we performed stopped flow kinetic measurements of viral fusion at 50 ms intervals.[7] The curves in FIGURE 3 show the kinetics of fusion of VSV with erythrocyte ghosts at different pH values. Similar results were seen with influenza virus.[15] The kinetics indicate that fusion does not follow a simple exponential behavior as would be expected from an instantaneous establishment of lipid continuity. The kinetics show a rather complex structure reminiscent of ion gating kinetics. At pH values close to threshold a lag time of about two seconds was followed by a relatively slow rise. The lag time decreased, and the rise time increased as the pH came closer to optimum. We interpret the lag time as reflecting the relative rates of rearrangements into the fusogenic state where membrane mixing takes place.

The final extents of fusion are also pH-dependent. A scheme with pH-dependent rate constants for the various activation steps would lead to the same extent of fusion irrespective of pH. To account for the pH-dependence of extents of fusion, we invoke a "desensitization" pathway.[7] According to that model, pH-dependent viral fusion occurs when the envelope proteins undergo pH-activated conformational changes while the virus is appropriately bound to the target membrane. pH-dependent conformational transitions, occurring while the virus is not in the proper apposition

---

FIGURE 3. Rapid kinetics of fluorescence changes upon fusion of R18-labeled VSV with erythrocyte ghosts. The reaction was triggered by rapid mixing of equal volumes of an R18VSV-ghost suspension and a low pH buffer solution at 37°C. Ten data sets were averaged for each pH indicated in the figure. Fluorescence at zero time, when suspension was mixed, was the same for all pH values, but offset for clarity. The scheme shown at the bottom of the figure represents a model of minimal complexity that gives an adequate fit to the complete set of kinetic data. The T_0 and R_0 to R_{n-1} states represent "prefusion" states, the D states desensitized states, whereas the R_n state represents the "fusion junction" that allows mixing of lipids. The T and R states might represent different degrees of apposition with the target membrane, of which only the most advanced can enter into a fusogenic state.[7]

with respect to the target membrane, will result in a failure to fuse, or desensitization. If the rates of activation reactions leading to fusion are slow relative to those of the desensitization pathway, suboptimal extents will be reached, whereas rapid activation rates will yield optimal extents. All the data were fit to a multiple state model indicated in FIG. 3.[7]

The complex features of the kinetics indicate that the fusion process undergoes a cascade of activation steps before the lipid-mixing event occurs. The next challenge is to identify molecular processes underlying that complex cascade. To do so we have studied the fusion activity of the influenza virus HA expressed on surfaces of cells. This system allows us to modify important parameters that may play a role in the fusion kinetics, such as surface density. Moreover the system offers the possibility to examine variants of viral envelope proteins constructed by site-directed mutagenesis.

CELL FUSION MEDIATED BY INFLUENZA HEMAGGLUTININ

Cells expressing HA have been shown by light microscopy to fuse with erythrocytes (bearing the appropriate sialoglycolipid/sialoglycoprotein receptors) if the cells are placed in a low pH medium for 30–60 s followed by incubation at neutral pH for >30 min.[16] We developed assays for continuously monitoring the fusion between membranes of HA cells and erythrocytes by two fluorescent events: cytoplasmic continuity and lipid mixing.[4,5] For these studies we have used a line of 3T3 fibroblasts (GP4F cells), which constitutively express large amounts of HA from the Japan strain at the cell surface.[17] Using spectrofluorometric and video microscopic techniques, fluorescence changes were monitored before and during the fusion on single cells as well as on cell populations. The time lag for the onset of fusion HA-expressing cells with erythrocytes is in the order of tens of seconds, which is about an order of magnitude longer than the time lag for the onset of intact virus-cell fusion. The maximal extent is reached within minutes. A correspondence of the kinetics of small aqueous and lipid fluorophores indicates that the cytoplasmic connections form as rapidly as the outer bilayers mix. Movement of aqueous fluorophores between effector and target, however, is restricted during the initial events in fusion, consistent with the opening of small junctional pore(s). The properties of those fusion pores are discussed in more detail by Zimmerberg and Almers in other chapters of this volume.

By taking advantage of the longer lag time of fusion with HA-expressing cells we could distinguish between the triggering process and subsequent activation steps. To do this we monitored the kinetics of lipid mixing after switching the pH back and forth at various times before onset of fusion.[4] In the experiment shown in FIGURE 4, fusion was triggered by lowering the pH to 5.0. Bringing the pH back to 7.4 after 4 s resulted in about the same initial rate, but a 45% lower amplitude than the no-neutralization control. Neutralization after 10 s yielded 77% fluorescence-dequenching. When the pH was neutralized beyond 15 s the reaction was 100% complete. Fusion that was partially arrested after 4 s, could be reactivated by reacidification after 100 s (FIG. 4). These results indicate that only a brief treatment (<15 s) at low pH is required to trigger HA-mediated fusion. Following that, fusion can proceed at neutral pH. This is consistent with the notion that low pH triggering of HA leads to an irreversible commitment to the fusogenic state. This observation has recently been confirmed for single cell fusion events.[18]

Studies with variants of HA with single amino acid mutations in the fusion peptide indicate that only the relatively rapid components (commitment time) in the overall fusion reaction depend on the structure of the fusion peptide, whereas the slower processes are governed by other factors.[19]

MOLECULAR INTERPRETATION FOR THE LAG TIME

The difference in lag time between intact virus-cell fusion and HA-induced cell fusion could be interpreted in terms of the surface density of HA on the GP4F cells, which is about 1/10 that found in a virion.[17] Moreover, cells that express HA at double

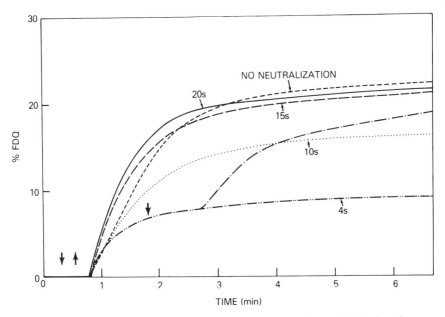

FIGURE 4. Effect of pH neutralization on HA-induced cell fusion. R18-labeled erythrocytes bound to GP4F cells were suspended in 2 mL PBS, pH 7.4, at 37°C in a spectrofluorometer cuvette. Fusion was triggered by lowering the pH to 5.0 using 0.5 M citrate (arrow down). The pH was switched back to neutral by adding 3.3 M Tris after various times (arrow up). - - -, no neutralization; -··, neutralization after 4 s; ···, neutralization after 10 s; — —, neutralization after 15 s; —, neutralization after 20 s; –·–, neutralization after 4 s, followed by reacidification to pH 5.0 after 100 s.[4]

density increase their fusion efficiency with liposomes bearing glycophorin 4–5-fold.[17] Those results indicate that more than one trimer is needed for HA-mediated fusion. According to the model shown in FIGURE 5 formation of a fusion junction occurs by the lateral association of several HA trimers. Assuming that the rate-limiting step of fusion is the formation of the higher order HA complex, the number (n) of HA trimers required to form the complex can be estimated from the dependence of the lag time on surface density. As shown in the appendix, n is the slope of a log-log plot of delay as a function of surface density.[17]

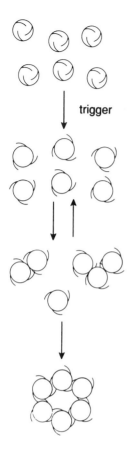

FIGURE 5. A model for cooperative assembly of a fusion complex. The HA trimers are viewed in cross-section parallel to the plane of the membrane. Initially they are randomly dispersed throughout the membrane with their fusion peptides tucked in. Triggering results in exposure of the fusion peptide, association of HA trimers into higher order complexes, and finally a structure that could resemble a fusion pore. Lipids are not depicted.

To examine the role of surface density, we studied the kinetics of HA-mediated cell fusion as a function of surface density of HA.[15] We modulated surface density in two ways: (1) HA expressed on the cell surface requires proteolytic cleavage with trypsin from an inactive HA0 form. We have limited the extent of proteolysis. (2) We have infected CV-1 cells with a recombinant SV40 virus bearing the influenza HA gene. The surface expression of HA is a function of time postinfection. For low pH–induced fusion of both types of cells with erythrocytes, the lag time decreases with increasing HA density, with a slope of 0.2 on a log-log plot.[15] This indicates that the fusion process is not positively cooperative at the level of the rate-determining step. Positive cooperativity, however, could still occur at early (*e.g.* commitment) steps.

The slope of 0.2 would predict a threefold decrease in delay for a tenfold increase in surface density. The decrease in delay between GP4F cells and intact virus, however, is about tenfold (20 s versus 2 s). This indicates that, normalized to surface density, fusion of intact virus is about three times more rapid than cell-cell fusion. The physical basis for those differences are still being studied.

CONCLUSIONS

Triggering of viral fusion sets a complex set of events in motion that finally terminates in the coalescence of membranes and aqueous spaces. TABLE 1 shows a timetable for the different events in fusion of HA-expressing cells with erythrocytes that have been resolved kinetically. Our goal is to find a molecular basis for those different events. We had surmised that the first (5–10 s) period was required to bring a critical number of viral envelope proteins to a fusogenic conformation. Our more recent data suggest that also the initial interaction of the fusion peptide with the target membrane, and perhaps lateral association, are part of that commitment process. What happens during the second (20–30 s) pH-independent time period is at present unclear. That delay has been suggested to represent the time required for movement of membranes into an apposition appropriate for fusion.[20] Other possibilities (*e.g.* removal of hydration repulsion barriers) also need to be considered. The observation of a two-step fusion process, the latter of which is not dependent on the regulatory cation, has also been reported in studies of exocytosis in a cell-free system.[21] In that system the Ca^{2+}-dependent step is considered to be required for activation of phospholipase and liberation of unsaturated fatty acids, and the Ca^{2+}-independent step is interpreted as the time required for modification of the membrane microenvironment that readies the plasma membrane to fuse with the secretory granule. The concepts and techniques used to dissect steps leading to viral protein–mediated membrane fusion may be applied to the resolution of the more complex exocytotic membrane fusion machinery.

APPENDIX

We have proposed the following model:

$$R_0 \overset{\text{trigger}}{\longrightarrow} R_1 \overset{k}{\to} \cdots R_f. \tag{1}$$

The viral envelope proteins complexes (in the case of HA, trimers) are originally in the inactive R_0 state. Triggering induces conformational changes. Subsequently, a

TABLE 1. A Dissection of Steps Leading the Fusion of HA-Expressing Cells with Erythrocytes

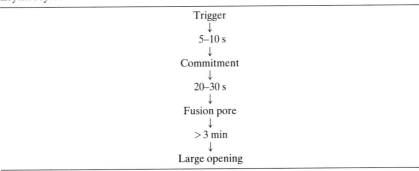

Trigger
↓
5–10 s
↓
Commitment
↓
20–30 s
↓
Fusion pore
↓
> 3 min
↓
Large opening

number of activation steps occur that then result in the formation of the fusogenic form, R_f. Fluorescence dequenching occurs after a critical concentration of R_f (R_f(crit)) has been reached:[22]

$$F(t) = F_0, \qquad 0 < t < t_1$$

$$F(t) = F_\infty(1 - e^{-\gamma(t-t_1)}), \qquad t > t_1, \tag{2}$$

where F_0 is the background fluorescence, $F(t)$ the fluorescence at time t, F_∞ the fluorescence after complete redistribution of dye, t_1 the time required to reach R_f(crit), and γ the redistribution rate of fluorophores from a single erythrocyte to a cell. In a model where fusion protein aggregation is the rate-limiting step, a number (n) of viral envelope proteins are needed to form a fusogenic complex. The scheme in equation 1 can be written in the form of a differential equation assuming that the triggering is instantaneous, that is, at t = 0 the maximal surface concentration (a) of units in the R_1 state has been produced:

$$\frac{d[R_f]}{dt} = k[R_1]^n. \tag{3}$$

By solving equation 3 for different values of n, we can get an estimate of the number of units needed to form a junction. Let us define $[R_1]$ at t = 0 as a and $[R_f]$ at any given time t as x. For single units (n = 1) the differential equation becomes

$$\frac{dx}{dt} = k(a - x). \tag{4}$$

Integrating equation 4 yields

$$\ln\left(1 - \frac{x}{a}\right) = kt. \tag{5}$$

At t = t_1 the critical concentration (x = x_1) of R_f is reached, where $F(t) > F_0$ (onset of fluorescence dequenching). Assuming that the number of such complexes is small compared to the total number of units ($x_1 \ll a$), we can rearrange equation 5 to

$$\frac{x_1}{a} \approx kt_1. \tag{6}$$

According to equation 6, the delay time should be inversely proportional to surface density if the rate-limiting step for onset of fluorescence dequenching is activation of single viral envelope protein units.

If two units (n = 2) are involved in the fusion complex, equation 3 becomes

$$\frac{dx}{dt} = k(a - 2x)^2. \tag{7}$$

Integrating equation 7 yields

$$\frac{x}{a(a - 2x)} = kt. \tag{8}$$

As above, we define the delay (t_1) when a threshold level, x_1, has been reached. For $x_1 \ll a$, equation 8 can be rearranged to

$$\frac{1}{t_1} = \left(\frac{k}{x_1}\right) a^2. \tag{9}$$

Thus, for two units, a logarithmic plot of $1/t_1$ versus a (total surface density) should yield a slope of 2.

It can be shown that an approximate solution for n units is

$$\frac{1}{t_1} = \left(\frac{k}{x_1}\right) a^n. \tag{10}$$

Thus, a logarithmic plot of $1/t_1$ versus **a** should yield as a slope the number of units required for a fusion junction.

REFERENCES

1. ALMERS, W. 1990. Exocytosis. Annu. Rev. Physiol. **52:** 607–624.
2. WHITE, J. M. 1990. Viral and cellular fusion proteins. Annu. Rev. Physiol. **52:** 675–697.
3. COMPANS, R. W., A. HELENIUS & M. OLDSTONE. 1989. Cell Biology of Virus Entry, Replication and Pathogenesis. Alan R. Liss. New York.
4. MORRIS, S. J., D. P. SARKAR, J. M. WHITE & R. BLUMENTHAL. 1989. Kinetics of pH-dependent fusion between 3T3 fibroblasts expressing influenza hemagglutinin and red blood cells. J. Biol. Chem. **264:** 3972–3978.
5. SARKAR, D. P., S. J. MORRIS, O. EIDELMAN, J. ZIMMERBERG & R. BLUMENTHAL. 1989. Initial stages of influenza hemagglutinin-induced cell fusion monitored simultaneously by two fluorescent events: cytoplasmic continuity and lipid mixing. J. Cell Biol. **109:** 113–122.
6. PURI, A., F. BOOY, R. W. DOMS, J. M. WHITE & R. BLUMENTHAL. 1990. Conformational changes and fusion activity of influenza hemagglutinin of the H2 and H3 subtypes: effects of acid pretreatment. J. Virol. **64:** 3824–3832.
7. CLAGUE, M. J., C. SCHOCH, L. ZECH & R. BLUMENTHAL. 1990. Gating kinetics of pH-activated membrane fusion of vesicular stomatitis virus with cells: stopped flow measurements by dequenching of octadecylrhodamine fluorescence. Biochemistry **29:** 1303–1308.
8. WILSON, I. A., J. J. SKEHEL & D. C. WILEY. 1981. Structure of the hemagglutinin membrane glycoprotein of influenza virus at 3 A resolution. Nature **289:** 366–373.
9. WILEY, D. C. & J. J. SKEHEL. 1987. The structure and function of the hemagglutinin membrane glycoprotein of influenza virus. Annu. Rev. Biochem. **56:** 365–394.
10. GETHING, M-J., R. W. DOMS, D. YORK & J. WHITE. 1986. Studies on the mechanism of membrane fusion: Site-specific mutagenesis of the hemagglutinin of influenza virus. J. Cell Biol. **102:** 11–23.
11. BOOY, F. P., R. W. RUIGROK & E. F. VAN BRUGGEN. 1985. Electron microscopy of influenza virus. A comparison of negatively stained and ice-embedded particles. J. Mol. Biol. **184:** 667–676.
12. WHITE, J. M. & I. A. WILSON. 1987. Anti-peptide antibodies detect steps in a protein conformational change:low-pH activation of the influenza virus hemagglutinin. J. Cell Biol. **56:** 365–394.
13. PURI, A., M. J. CLAGUE, C. SCHOCH & R. BLUMENTHAL. 1991. Kinetics of fusion of enveloped viruses with cells. Methods Enzymol. In press.
14. HOEKSTRA, D., T. DE BOER, K. KLAPPE & J. WILSCHUT. 1984. Fluorescence method for measuring the kinetics of fusion between biological membranes. Biochemistry **23:** 5675–5681.

15. CLAGUE, M. J., C. SCHOCH & R. BLUMENTHAL. 1991. The delay time for influenza hemagglutinin-induced membrane fusion depends on the haemagglutinin surface density. J. Virol. **65:** 2402–2407.

16. DOXSEY, S. J., J. SAMBROOK, A. HELENIUS & J. WHITE. 1985. An efficient method for introducing macromolecules into living cells. J. Cell Biol. **101:** 12–27.

17. ELLENS, H., J. BENTZ, D. MASON, F. ZHANG & J. M. WHITE. 1990. Fusion of influenza hemagglutinin-expressing fibroblasts with glycophorin-bearing liposomes:role of hemagglutinin surface density. Biochemistry. **29:** 9697–9707.

18. KAPLAN, D., J. ZIMMERBERG, A. PURI, D. P. SARKAR & R. BLUMENTHAL. 1991. Single cell fusion events induced by influenza hemagglutinin: studies with rapid-flow, quantitative fluorescence microscopy. Exp. Cell Res. **195:** 137–144.

19. SCHOCH, C. & R. BLUMENTHAL. 1991. Kinetics of pH-dependent fusion induced by influenza hemagglutinin and mutants in the fusion peptide. Biophys. J. **59:** 133a (Abstract)

20. DIMITROV, D. S. & A. E. SOWERS. 1990. A delay in membrane fusion: Lag times observed by fluorescence microscopy of individual fusion events induced by an electric field pulse. Biochemistry **29:** 8337–8344.

21. KARLI, U. O., T. SCHAFER & M. M. BURGER. 1990. Fusion of neurotransmitter vesicles with target membrane is calcium independent in a cell-free system. Proc. Natl. Acad. Sci. USA **87:** 5912–5915.

22. CHEN, Y. & R. BLUMENTHAL. 1989. Use of self-quenching fluorophores in the study of membrane fusion: Effect of slow probe redistribution. Biophys. Chem. **34:** 283–292.

Evidence for a Model of Exocytosis That Involves Calcium-Activated Channels

GERALD EHRENSTEIN, ELIS F. STANLEY,
SUSAN L. POCOTTE, MIN JIA, KUNI H. IWASA,
AND KEITH E. KREBS

Laboratory of Biophysics
National Institute of Neurological Disorders and Stroke
Building 9, Room 1E124
National Institutes of Health
Bethesda, Maryland 20892

INTRODUCTION

Experiments on secretory cells suggested that fusion of secretory vesicles with the plasma membrane requires an osmotic gradient that can cause vesicle lysis.[1] Subsequent experiments on model systems composed of lipid vesicles and planar lipid bilayers demonstrated directly that fusion in these model systems requires an osmotic gradient in the direction that causes water to enter the vesicles.[2-5] It was concluded that the role of this water flow was to cause vesicle lysis. Experiments on sea urchin eggs[6] and chromaffin cells[7] demonstrated that the fusion of vesicles with the plasma membrane requires micromolar concentrations of cytoplasmic calcium. In order to link the calcium requirement with the putative osmotic requirement, Akabas *et al.*[8] suggested that the role of cytoplasmic calcium might be to increase the osmolarity of secretory vesicles by opening calcium-activated ion channels located in the vesicle membranes. Stanley and Ehrenstein[9] considered this possibility in detail and concluded that the opening of calcium-activated ion channels located in vesicle membranes is a feasible mechanism for the osmotic lysis of vesicles.

The hypothesis that osmotic swelling of secretory vesicles leads to vesicle fusion was tested in the mast cells of beige mice by comparing the time-course of vesicle fusion, as monitored by the capacitance of the plasma membrane, with the time-course of vesicle swelling.[10,11] Because of the large size of the secretory vesicles in these cells, vesicle swelling could be monitored by video microscopy. It was found that the capacitance increase always preceded vesicle swelling, indicating that vesicle swelling is not the cause of vesicle fusion in these cells. Furthermore, even flaccid vesicles were found to fuse,[10] demonstrating that mechanical stress on vesicle membranes is not required.

Although the hypothesis that calcium-activated ion channels play an important role in vesicle fusion was first considered together with the vesicle-swelling hypothesis, the negative results regarding the latter do not necessarily rule out the former. In fact, the results of several types of experiments were found to be consistent with an important role for calcium-activated ion channels. One of the purposes of this paper is to summarize these results.

The experimental support for the calcium-activated-channel hypothesis led us to search for an overall model of exocytosis that combines a role for calcium-activated channels with a physical process for fusion that does not depend on vesicle swelling. The physical process we chose for further consideration is that described in the experiments of Fisher and Parker,[12] wherein fusion results from the removal of water from the space between two apposed lipid bilayers.

WATER REMOVAL FROM INTERMEMBRANE SPACE

In the experimental setup used by Fisher and Parker, two large hemispheric lipid bilayer vesicles were forced together, and the capacitance between the vesicles and between each vesicle and the bath was measured, as shown in FIGURE 1. After an osmotic difference between the vesicles and the bath was established in the direction to withdraw water from the space between the bilayers, a single central bilayer formed spontaneously, as indicated by the change in capacitance shown in FIGURE 2. The time between the establishment of the osmotic difference and the change in capacitance depended systematically on the magnitude of the osmotic difference and the area of contact. For an osmotic difference of 200 mM, a typical time delay was 20 seconds. The area of the central bilayer determined by direct measurement of the contact area was in agreement with the area determined from the observed capacitance change. After its formation, the central bilayer sometimes ruptured spontaneously, the topological equivalent of exocytosis.

The results on fusion of hemispheric lipid bilayer vesicles suggested that water removal from the intermembrane space between a secretory vesicle and a plasma membrane could lead to exocytosis. There are three important differences, however, between fusion in the model system and exocytosis in biological systems. Exocytosis does not involve perfusion with a low-osmolarity solution; exocytosis usually requires calcium, and exocytosis can occur in less than a millisecond. As indicated in the model description below, these differences can be resolved if a secretory vesicle membrane contains a calcium-activated cation channel and an anion channel in the region of the intermembrane space.

DESCRIPTION OF MODEL

The steps of the model, leading from opening of a calcium channel in the plasma membrane to fusion of a secretory vesicle with the plasma membrane, are shown schematically in FIGURE 3.

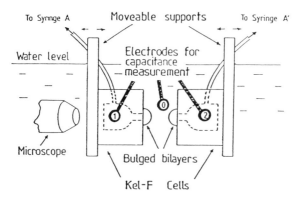

FIGURE 1. Schematic diagram of apparatus used to detect fusion between bilayers. After bulged bilayers are formed, they are moved together by a micrometer-driven stage. Capacitance is measured between electrodes placed at points labeled 0, 1, and 2. (Fisher & Parker.[12] With permission from the *Biophysical Journal.*)

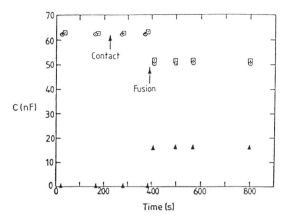

FIGURE 2. Capacitances of the bilayers before and after fusion. Circles show capacitance between points 0 and 1 of FIG. 1, squares show capacitance between points 0 and 2, and triangles show capacitance between points 1 and 2. (Fisher & Parker.[12] With permission from the *Biophysical Journal.*)

FIGURE 3A shows a secretory vesicle, whose membrane contains a calcium-activated cation channel and an anion channel, closely apposed to a plasma membrane containing a calcium channel. The three channels all face the intermembrane space. As the result of an appropriate stimulus, such as depolarization of the plasma membrane, the calcium channel opens.

FIGURE 3B indicates that calcium ions move through the calcium channel into the cytoplasm, resulting in the opening of the calcium-activated cation channel. If the impermeable transmitter or hormone in the vesicle is cationic, there will be a much higher concentration of sodium and potassium ions in the cytoplasm than in the vesicle. Therefore, when the calcium-activated cation channel opens, these cations will tend to enter the vesicle, as shown in FIGURE 3C. (If the impermeable species is anionic, a slight variation of the model would be required, with the secretory vesicle membrane containing a calcium-activated anion channel and a cation channel.)

The movement of cations into the vesicle causes the inside of the vesicle to become more positive relative to the cytoplasm, and this change in the potential of the vesicle causes anions to enter the vesicle. The combined movement of cations and anions into the vesicle results in an osmolarity difference between vesicle and cytoplasm, causing water to move from the intermembrane space into the vesicle. Both ions and water enter the vesicle through the vesicle channels, as also shown in FIGURE 3C. Because this water movement is primarily through ion channels, it is much more rapid than water movement through hemispheric lipid bilayers. This can explain why exocytosis can occur much more rapidly than osmotically induced fusion of hemispheric bilayers.

Because of the high viscosity of the thin layer of water in the intermembrane space, the movement of water from the cytoplasm to replace the water from the intermembrane space will be relatively slow. As a result, there will be a net removal of water from the intermembrane space, thus allowing the hydrophobic force between the two membranes to draw them closer together. When the two membranes become close enough, they spontaneously form a single central bilayer (not shown). The central bilayer then ruptures, resulting in fusion of the vesicle with the plasma membrane (FIG. 3D).

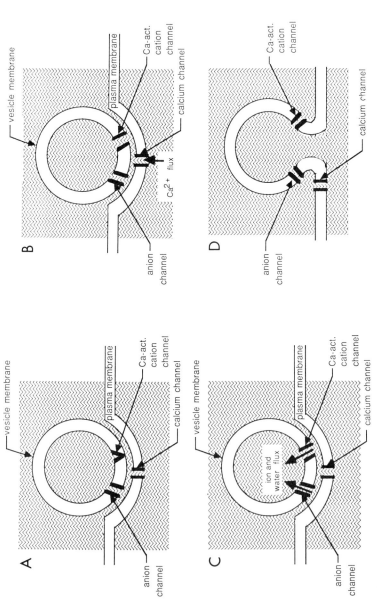

FIGURE 3. Schematic diagram of steps leading to fusion of vesicle membrane and plasma membrane. Vesicle membrane contains a calcium-activated cation channel and an anion channel. Plasma membrane contains a calcium channel. **A:** Calcium channel in plasma membrane opens. **B:** Calcium-activated cation channel in vesicle membrane opens. **C:** Ions and water move from the intermembrane space into the vesicle through the vesicle channels. As a result of water loss from the intermembrane space, the two membranes move closer together and spontaneously form a single central bilayer (not shown). **D:** The central bilayer ruptures, resulting in fusion.

EXPERIMENTAL EVIDENCE REGARDING CALCIUM-ACTIVATED CHANNELS

When the calcium-activated-channel hypothesis was first considered,[8,9] there was no experimental evidence that such channels are present in the membranes of secretory vesicles. Since that time, however, calcium-activated cation channels have been reported to be present in vesicles of the bovine neurohypophysis,[13] the rat neurohypophysis,[14] and the *Torpedo* electric organ,[15] and calcium-activated anion channels have been reported to be present in neurosecretory granules of the bovine neurohypophysis.[16] In addition, anion channels have been reported to be present in vesicles of the bovine neurohypophysis[17] and the rat neurohypophysis.[14] Thus, the channels required for the model are present in at least some secretory cells.

Does the opening of calcium-activated channels in secretory vesicles play an important role in secretion? If so, a correlation would be expected between the calcium dose-response curve for the opening of these channels and the calcium dose-response curve for secretion. For a wide range of secretory cells, the dose-response curve for secretion is sigmoidal, with half-maximum at a cytosolic calcium concentration of about 1 μM. Representative dose-response relations summarized by Knight and Scrutton[18] are shown in FIGURE 4. Although dose-response curves for the opening of calcium-activated channels in secretory vesicles have not yet been reported, preliminary information on calcium-activated channels in secretory vesicles of the rat neurohypophysis[14] is consistent with a calcium dose-response relation for channel opening similar to the curves in FIGURE 4.

A more definitive test for the correlation of dose-response curves is afforded by the parathyroid cell. The dependence of parathyroid hormone (PTH) secretion on extracellular calcium is anomalous; secretion decreases when the calcium concentration increases.[19] In order to determine whether this is related to the properties of calcium-activated channels in these cells, we have measured dose-response curves for secretion[20] and for the calcium-activated-channel open probability[21] in bovine parathyroid cells. The independent variable for both measurements was cytosolic calcium concentration. Nygren *et al.*[22] independently measured the dose-response curve for PTH secretion by a completely different method. As shown in FIGURE 5, both secretion measurements indicate that the dose-response curve is biphasic, with a peak at about 200 nM. The right-hand limb of FIGURE 5, which corresponds to the physiological range of cytosolic calcium, indicates that the dependence of secretion on intracellular calcium, as well as its dependence on extracellular calcium, is anomalous. This is consistent with the view that the intracellular calcium concentration is proportional to the extracellular calcium concentration.

A direct test of the role of calcium-activated channels in vesicles during exocytosis requires comparison of the curves in FIGURE 5 with the dose-response curve for the open-channel probability of calcium-activated channels in the vesicles of parathyroid cells, but these data are not yet available. As a first step, however, we have measured the dose-response curve for the open probability of these channels in the plasma membrane of parathyroid cells, and this curve is shown in FIGURE 6. Because vesicle channels are incorporated into the plasma membrane during fusion, some of the channels in the plasma membrane may have originated in the vesicles, and comparison of the curves in FIGURES 5 and 6 provides an indirect test of the role of these channels in exocytosis. Both secretion and open-channel probability curves are biphasic, and the peaks for both curves occur at a cytosolic calcium concentration of about 200 nM. The agreement between these curves is consistent with a role in exocytosis for calcium-activated channels in secretory vesicles. The agreement also suggests that the explanation for the anomalous secretion of parathyroid cells lies in the unusual properties of calcium-activated channels in these cells.

DELAY TIME FOR TRANSMITTER RELEASE

The time duration between the entrance of calcium and the release of transmitter in the squid giant synapse is not more than 200 microseconds.[23] This very rapid

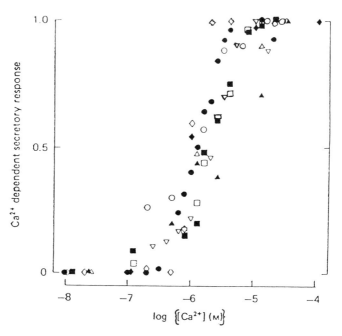

FIGURE 4. Calcium-dependent secretory responses from various electropermeabilized cell preparations summarized in ref. 18. Filled circles relate to catecholamine secretion from bovine adrenal medullary cells; open diamonds relate to Met-enkephalin secretion from bovine adrenal medullary cells; open circles relate to cortical granule discharge from sea urchin eggs; filled diamonds relate to insulin secretion from pancreatic beta cells; filled squares relate to 5-hydroxyl[14C]tryptamine secretion from human platelets; open squares relate to β-N-acetylglucosaminidase secretion from human platelets; downward-pointing open triangles relate to amylase secretion from pancreatic acinar cells; upward-pointing open triangles relate to acetylcholine secretion from *Torpedo* synaptosomes; and upward-pointing closed triangles relate to ATP secretion from *Torpedo* synaptosomes. (Knight & Scrutton.[18] With permission from the *Biochemical Journal*.)

response time provides an important constraint on models of exocytosis. In terms of the present model, this constraint requires that the entire process, including opening of calcium-activated ion channels, movement of ions into vesicles, and movement of water into vesicles, can occur within 200 microseconds. It may appear that channel opening would not be fast enough, because a typical time constant for opening

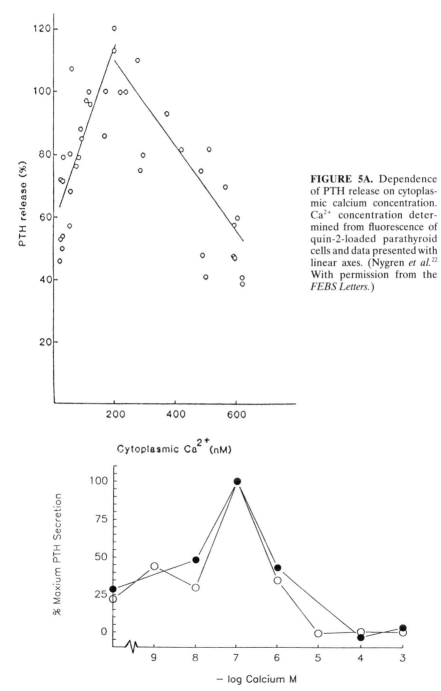

FIGURE 5A. Dependence of PTH release on cytoplasmic calcium concentration. Ca^{2+} concentration determined from fluorescence of quin-2-loaded parathyroid cells and data presented with linear axes. (Nygren *et al.*[22] With permission from the *FEBS Letters.*)

FIGURE 5B. Ca^{2+} concentration established by electropermeabilizing parathyroid cells and data presented with semilogarithmic axes. (Pocotte & Ehrenstein.[20] With permission from *Endocrinology.*)

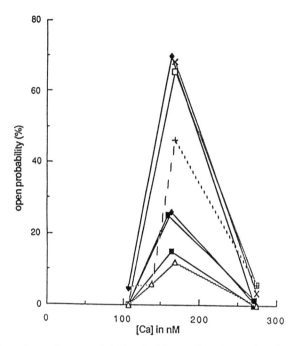

FIGURE 6. Dependence of open probability of calcium-activated potassium channel in parathyroid cell on cytoplasmic calcium concentration. Experiment was performed by patch-clamping inside-out patches from bovine parathyroid cells and varying the Ca^{2+} concentration of the bath. Membrane potentials were -30 mV (solid lines), 0 mV (lines with horizontal dashes), and -50 mV (line with vertical dashes). Each point is based on a 23-second observation. (Jia *et al.*[21] With permission from the *Proceedings of the National Academy of Sciences USA.*)

calcium-activated channels is about 2 milliseconds.[24] It has been shown, however, that only about 3% of available vesicles fuse during transmitter release.[25] Thus, with a 2 msec time constant, only 60 μsec would be required for the requisite number of channels to open.

We can also estimate the time for water to leave the corridor after a calcium-activated channel opens. Although the thickness of the corridor has not been measured, the spacing between lipid bilayers in a lamellar lipid-water system has been reported to be between 0.5 and 2 nm,[26,27] suggesting that the corridor thickness is approximately one nanometer. Assuming that the area of fusion is several times larger than the cross-sectional area of a fusion pore,[10] the total volume of water to be removed is about 30 nm,[3] corresponding to about 1,000 water molecules. Assuming that the ion current through a calcium-activated channel is at least 1 picoamp and that each ion carries at least two water molecules, the water would be removed by electro-osmosis in less than 80 microseconds. Thus, both the channel-opening and water-removal steps of the model can occur fast enough to meet the experimental constraint on delay time.

REFERENCES

1. POLLARD, H. B., C. J. PAZOLES, C. E. CREUTZ & O. ZINDER. 1979. The chromaffin granule and possible mechanisms of exocytosis. Int. Rev. Cytol. **58:** 159–197.
2. MILLER, C. & E. RACKER. 1976. Ca^{++}-induced fusion of fragmented sarcoplasmic reticulum with artificial planar bilayers. Cell **9:** 283–300.
3. COHEN, F. S., J. ZIMMERBERG & A. FINKELSTEIN. 1980. Fusion of phospholipid vesicles with planar phospholipid bilayer membranes. II. Incorporation of a vesicular membrane marker into the planar membrane. J. Gen. Physiol. **75:** 251–270.
4. ZIMMERBERG, J., F. S. COHEN & A. FINKELSTEIN. 1980. Micromolar Ca^{2+} stimulates fusion of lipid vesicles with planar bilayers containing a calcium-binding protein. Science **210:** 906–908.
5. COHEN, F. S., M. H. AKABAS & A. FINKELSTEIN. 1982. Osmotic swelling of phospholipid vesicles causes them to fuse with a planar phospholipid bilayer membrane. Science **217:** 458–460.
6. BAKER, P. F. & M. J. WHITAKER. 1978. Influence of ATP and calcium on the cortical reaction in sea urchin eggs. Nature **276:** 513–515.
7. BAKER, P. F. & D. E. KNIGHT. 1978. Calcium-dependent exocytosis in bovine adrenal medullary cells with leaky plasma membranes. Nature **276:** 620–622.
8. AKABAS, M. H., F. S. COHEN & A. FINKELSTEIN. 1984. Separation of the osmotically driven fusion event from vesicle-planar membrane attachment in a model system for exocytosis. J. Cell Biol. **98:** 1063–1071.
9. STANLEY, E. F. & G. EHRENSTEIN. 1985. A model for exocytosis based on the opening of calcium-activated potassium channels in vesicles. Life Sci. **37:** 1985–1995.
10. ZIMMERBERG, J., M. CURRAN, F. S. COHEN & M. BRODWICK. 1987. Simultaneous electrical and optical measurements show that membrane fusion precedes secretory granule swelling during exocytosis of beige mouse mast cells. Proc. Natl. Acad. Sci. USA **84:** 1585–1589.
11. BRECKENRIDGE, L. J. & W. ALMERS. 1987. Final steps in exocytosis observed in a cell with giant secretory granules. Proc. Natl. Acad. Sci. USA **84:** 1945–1949.
12. FISHER, L. R. & N. S. PARKER. 1984. Osmotic control of bilayer fusion. Biophys. J. **46:** 253–258.
13. STANLEY, E. F., G. EHRENSTEIN & J. T. RUSSELL. 1988. Evidence for cation and anion permeable channels in secretory vesicle membranes. Biophys. J. **51:** 46a.
14. LEMOS, J. R., K. A. OCORR & J. J. NORDMAN. 1989. Possible role for ionic channels in neurosecretory granules of the rat neurohypophysis. Soc. Gen. Physiol. Ser. **44:** 333–347.
15. RAHAMIMOFF, R., S. A. DERIEMER, B. SAKMANN, H. STADLER & N. YAKIR. 1988. Ion channels in synaptic vesicles from Torpedo electric organ. Proc. Natl. Acad. Sci. USA **85:** 5310–5314.
16. KREBS, K. E. & G. EHRENSTEIN. 1991. Secretory-vesicle-specific ion permeable channels from the neurohypophysis. Biophys. J. **59:** 373a.
17. STANLEY, E. F., G. EHRENSTEIN & J. T. RUSSELL. 1988. Evidence for anion channels in secretory vesicles. Neurosci. **25:** 1035–1039.
18. KNIGHT, D. E. & M. C. SCRUTTON. 1986. Gaining access to the cytosol: the technique and some applications of electropermeabilization. Biochem. J. **234:** 497–506.
19. SHERWOOD, L. M., G. P. MAYER, C. F. RAMBERG, JR., D. S. KRONFELD, G. D. AURBACH & J. T. POTTS, JR. 1968. Regulation of parathyroid hormone secretion: proportional control by calcium, lack of effect of phosphate. Endocrinology **83:** 1043–1051.
20. POCOTTE, S. L. & G. EHRENSTEIN. 1989. The biphasic calcium dose-response curve for parathyroid hormone secretion in electropermeabilized adult bovine parathyroid cells. Endocrinology **125:** 1587–1592.
21. JIA, M., G. EHRENSTEIN & K. IWASA. 1988. Unusual calcium-activated potassium channels of bovine parathyroid cells. Proc. Natl. Acad. Sci. USA **85:** 7236–7239.
22. NYGREN, P., R. LARSSON, E. LINDH, S. LJUNGHALL, J. RASTAD, G. AKERSTROM & E.

GYLFE. 1987. Bimodal regulation of secretion by cytoplasmic Ca^{+2} as demonstrated by the parathyroid. FEBS Lett. **213:** 195–198.

23. LLINÁS, R., I. Z. STEINBERG & K. WALTON. 1981. Relationship between presynaptic calcium current and postsynaptic potential in squid giant synapse. Biophys. J. **33:** 323–352.

24. MOCZYDLOWSKI, E. & R. LATORRE. 1983. Gating kinetics of Ca^{2+}-activated K^+ channels from rat muscle incorporated into planar lipid bilayers. J. Gen. Physiol. **82:** 511–542.

25. KUSANO, K. & E. M. LANDAU. 1975. Depression and recovery of transmission at the squid giant synapse. J. Physiol. **245:** 13–22.

26. LIS, L. J., M. MCALISTER, N. FULLER, R. P. RAND & V. A. PARSEGIAN. 1982. Interactions between neutral phospholipid bilayer membranes. Biophys. J. **37:** 657–665.

27. MCINTOSH, T. J. & S. A. SIMON. 1986. Area per molecule and distribution of water in fully hydrated dilauroylphosphatidylethanolamine bilayers. Biochemistry **25:** 4948–4952.

A Lipid/Protein Complex Hypothesis for Exocytotic Fusion Pore Formation[a]

JOSHUA ZIMMERBERG,[b,d] MICHAEL CURRAN,[b,d] AND
FREDRIC S. COHEN[c]

[b]*Laboratory of Theoretical and Physical Biology*
National Institute of Child Health and Human Development
National Institutes of Health
Bethesda, Maryland 20892

[c]*Department of Physiology*
Rush Medical College
Chicago, Illinois 60612

INTRODUCTION

It has long been appreciated that exocytotic secretion results in the formation of a fusion pore connecting the interior of a secretory granule with the extracellular space.[1] In the early 1980s, however, structures seen in the electron-microscope were identified as small fusion pores.[2-5] Recently, large increases in electrical cell capacitance, resulting from the addition of membrane inserted by fusion during exocytosis, were observed in mast cells with large granules.[6,6A] These large increases in capacitance coupled with the greater time resolution than previously employed showed that the capacitance changes were not instantaneous. A method predicting the growth of pore size from the measured time-course of the capacitance increase was described.[6] Finally, it was shown that the conductance of the initial fusion pore could be determined by measuring the discharge of granule potential that results from fusion.[7] The formation of the initial pore and its growth are being vigorously investigated.[8,9] Based on these electrical measurements, predominantly on mast cells from beige mice, models of the initial fusion pore have been considered wherein preformed protein pores, analogous to gap junctions, span the two membranes, allowing vesicular discharge.[10,11] Lipids participate in pore-widening only after the lumen of the granule is in contact with the extracellular space. In this paper we present an alternate model wherein lipids participate in the formation of the initial pore. We contrast the two competing models.

When conceiving molecular models for membrane fusion, one strives to integrate biophysical data on fusion in its various biological settings. This parsimonious view is taxed when the molecular events must occur within a short time. At the giant synapse in squid, exocytosis can occur as fast as 200 μs after calcium entry into the presynaptic terminal,[12,13] and at the frog neuromuscular junction, as fast as 400 μs at 20°C.[14] This short time has led to models in which fusion proteins are preassembled in membranes, and when triggered by calcium, exhibit rapid conformational changes leading to the opening of a fusion pore.[11] Thus, in this model the initial pore is totally

[a]This work was supported by National Institutes of Health Grant GM 27367.
[d]Address for correspondence: Bldg. 10, Room 6C101, National Institutes of Health, Bethesda, MD 20892.

proteinacious, and when the pore is initially detected, fusion has not occurred as lipid does not intercalate between protein subunits until the pore begins to enlarge.

POSSIBLE ROLE OF LIPIDS IN FUSION PORE

Lipid Movement

Lipids can diffuse over molecularly significant distances in short times. In 100 μs, a lipid with a diffusion constant of 10^{-8} cm^2/s will diffuse 200 Å. As lipids occupy 60 Å^2, 25 lipid molecules lie within 200 Å. Further, phospholipids in model systems can adopt nonlamellar configurations.[15] In the presence of proteins this ability of lipids is undoubtedly increased. Thus, there is little *a priori* reason to exclude lipids as a structural component of the initial pore. There is also direct experimental evidence indicating that lipids move before fusion is complete.[16]

Exocytotic fusion is usually thought to be irreversible. Endocytotic retrieval of membrane is considered a fundamentally different process. In mast cells, however, a reversible structural intermediate of fusion has been detected electrically. In addition to the usual cases where irreversible increases in capacitance are observed, occasionally reversible capacitance "flicker" is seen wherein the capacitance increases only to quickly decrease.[17] This flicker is readily explained as due to a fusion pore transiently opening and closing.[6,7,18] Lipid continuity between granules and plasma membrane is established during flicker.[9] As fusion is still reversible and not fully committed during flicker, models should allow for lipid flux through the fusion pore early in the fusion process.

Fusion Proteins

Packing considerations of fusion proteins and candidate fusion proteins also suggest that lipid is involved in the structure of the fusion pore. Only in the case of virus are the fusion proteins unambiguously identified.[19,20] For viruses the fusion proteins consist of a single transmembrane alpha helix and a large extraviral ectodomain. In the case of influenza, the crystal structure of the fusion protein has been obtained to 3 Å resolution.[21] This fusion protein is trimeric with each monomer approximately 74 kilodaltons. The ectodomain is about 135 Å long and 40 Å in diameter. Simple considerations of packing show that when these proteins touch in the aqueous extraviral domain, significant distances exist between the membrane-spanning helices of separate trimers. In this system, it is difficult to imagine how preformed pores composed solely of protein could expand. It is easy to envision that the membrane-spanning regions of trimers are separated from each other by lipids. Further, more than one fusion trimer is needed for fusion competence.[22] Although it is possible that the membrane-spanning alpha helices of the fusion protein could form a water-filled pore in the viral envelope as part of the fusion pore, there are *a priori* conceptual difficulties with this notion. These membrane-spanning alpha helices are composed solely of nonpolar and hydrophobic amino acids, making it unlikely that they form a pore. As channels can be formed from nonpolar amino acids, however,[23] this possibility cannot be ruled out. A specific, detailed model considering the role of lipids in viral fusion has been presented.[24]

If the polar headgroups of lipids were to form part of the lining of the pore, then a space for ionic milieu would result. A pore composed of lipid and protein would also mean that fusion was essentially complete when the pore was formed. This would be consistent with the demonstration of lipid flow early in the virus fusion process.[16] In nerve cells, the candidate fusion proteins have the bulk of their mass on the cytoplasmic side. With these proteins the packing problem is not as severe as with the viral fusion proteins; but again if lipid is a component of the pore, all such constraints are removed.

Pore Conductance

The data indicate that the fusion pore is not a static, stable structure. The size distribution of the initial pore is broad.[8] The decay of granule potential through a

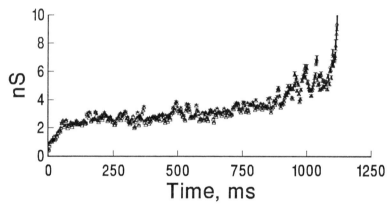

FIGURE 1. Experimentally derived exocytotic fusion-pore conductances. The pore conductance during a single exocytotic event was obtained from the room temperature measurement of capacitance of a beige mouse mast cell, using the whole-cell patch-clamp technique.[6,50] The cell was stimulated with GTP-γ -S and a sine wave of 800 Hz. Pore conductance, in nanosiemens (nS), is shown as a function of time. The zero time is chosen as the first detectable change in capacitance above noise.

fusion pore of fixed conductance would follow a single exponential. It seldom does,[7] establishing that the pore varies its conductance on the submillisecond time-scale. Direct time measurements show that the conductance of the fusion pore varies dramatically on the millisecond time-scale.[6,8] FIGURE 1 shows an example of the time-course of the growth of the pore. In this record, three phases are apparent. In the first phase, the conductance rapidly increases, and in the second phase, the conductance transiently plateaus to a semistable value. The third phase is characterized by a rapid enlargement to immeasurably large conductance values. Although there is large variation in the time-course of conductance among fusion pores, most exhibit these three phases.

With the possible exception of gap junctions, fusion pores are clearly different from other known pores. As the gap junction does span two membranes, analogies of the fusion pore to gap junctions have been reasonably and repeatedly made.[7,11,25] Because gap junctions exhibit broad distributions of sizes[26] and time-varying single channel conductances,[27] this analogy could well have physical reality. Even if fusion proteins should prove to have some sequence or functional homology to gap junctions, however, the essential difference between fusion pores and gap junctions is their role in fusion. Gap junctions allow communication between connecting cells, but they do not cause fusion. Similarly, if proteins of plasma and vesicular membranes (unrelated to the gap junction/connexin proteins) dock with each other to form fusion pores, as several groups have suggested,[28,29] lipid continuity must be established for fusion to have occurred. The melding of two bilayers into one is a key characteristic of fusion. We suggest that the lipid movement needed to complete fusion occurs early in the process; by the time the fusion pore is detected, lipid rearrangements have already occurred.

Pure Lipid Fusion Pores

The exocytotic pore enlarges gradually with varied time-course, unlike the pore that occurs when phospholipid vesicles fuse to planar membranes. In phospholipid bilayers the pore conductance is greater than 100 nS within 200 μs.[30] In addition, the smallest phospholipid vesicles have external diameters of 21 nm and internal diameters of 10 nm,[31] considerably larger than the diameter of initial exocytotic pores, which are less than one nanometer. It is unlikely, therefore, that the earliest detectable pore is composed totally of lipids.

PROTEIN AND LIPID IN PORE FORMATION AND ENLARGEMENT

Fusion involves three major components: protein, lipid, and water. We present a model that explicitly considers the possible roles of each of these components. We hypothesize a fusion pore composed of lipid and protein. Water, using both hydrophobic and hydration forces, drives fusion. For a model to be viable, the movements of the constituent molecules must be continuous—the incremental steps must be infinitesimal. We present the model in sequential steps to emphasize that the transitions between the panels represent small and physically reasonable conformational and structural changes. We point out biophysical motifs that may be important for pore formation and growth. We then mathematically describe each of the key transitions to illustrate the predictive power of the model. Different models for pore formation have been proposed. There are many proteins that may be involved in fusion. In exocytosis, the vesicular integral membrane proteins VAMP-1,[32] synaptobrevin,[33] and synaptophysin, alternatively known as p38,[34,35] are leading candidates. Peripheral membrane and cytoplasmic proteins such as NSF,[36] other NEM-sensitive proteins,[37] SNAP,[38] synapsin I,[39] and annexins[40] have also been implicated in fusion in both exocytosis and intracellular trafficking. For convenience we refer to the fusion-inducing proteins as "fusins." We imagine that upon stimulation of secretion, complementary polar surfaces are generated between fusins of the opposing membranes. Short-range attractive forces between fusins (possibly attractive hydration forces[41]) cause them to dehydrate and bind across the extracellular space (FIG. 2B) and bind transversely (FIG. 2C). Alternatively, a fusin in one membrane might undergo a conformational change and insert into or attach to the apposing membrane, thereby causing the intimate contact of FIGURE 2C. Lipid headgroups, however, remain hydrated and separated.[42]

As a consequence of these multiple associations, which resemble spot weldings between the membranes,[3] the vesicular and plasma membranes are brought close together. Because hydration forces repel at distances less than 2 nm,[43] we envision that a pressure develops in this region of apposition (shown by double arrow in FIG. 2D). A strain on the lipids in the region of contact ensues and a blister-like structure forms. Conformational changes of the fusins, due to binding, pressure, or other motifs, lead to exposure of hydrophobic surfaces.[44] The acyl chains of the lipids in the region of strain flip from the bilayer to a more energetically favorable position on the newly exposed hydrophobic surfaces of the fusins (FIG. 2E). As some water is associated with the polar head groups of the lipids, the lipids and fusins line a hydrated lumen. Thus a pore has formed (FIG. 2E), as suggested previously.[45] As in the fusion of phospholipid membranes,[30,46,47] we suggest that pressure plays a role in providing the force responsible for molecular rearrangements. In biological fusion, however, this pressure is not a result of osmotic swelling of the vesicle but rather is a result of protein conformational changes that restrict the pressures and the resulting tensions and strains to within the region of contact. Granule contents are completely secreted, with no leakage into the cytoplasm, because the rearranging lipids are constrained to the associated fusin complexes.

This fusin model predicts many of the experimental observations. The initial pore conductance is variable because it depends on the number of fusin complexes, the number of lipids, and the electrostatic structure of the headgroups of the lipids that happen to constitute part of the polar lining of the pore. The movement of lipid between bilayer and fusin structures, and variation in the number of fusin complexes in the pore, cause pore conductance fluctuations. Lateral dissociations and associations of complexes cause closures and reformations of the pore lumen, seen as flickering. The hydration force between the lipid headgroups lining the pore provides a repulsive force that widens the pore. Formation and accretion of additional fusin complexes and associated lipid rearrangements also leads to growth of the pore. The small radius of curvature of the inner pore lipids will also tend to widen the pore and increase the pore length, resulting in an hourglass shape (FIG. 2F) as observed experimentally.[48] The initial rapid growth of the pore, however, will decelerate and stabilize, because the number of fusin complexes is finite, as discussed below. In addition, fusin complexes may stabilize the pore as they constrain the opposing bilayers in the manner of spot welds. Finally, concomitant with the overall growth due to these processes, the neck stretches, and the omega figure flattens. At this point fusin complexes dissociate transversely (FIG. 2G), which removes constraints on the pore, allowing for its rapid enlargement.

When fusion is very fast, as in nerve, fusin complexation may be complete in the opposing membranes before the initiation of fusion. Diffusion of additional fusin molecules ($D \approx 10^{-10}$ cm^2/s) to the site of membrane fusion is relatively slow. Within the context of the model, lipid arrangements occur before the fusion pore is detected.

A key feature of our model is the exposure of hydrophobic surfaces, to promote the movement of lipid from a bilayer configuration to the newly exposed hydrophobic surfaces. For some viral fusion proteins, it is known that conditions that lead to fusion also lead to exposure of hydrophobic sequences. A similar mechanism, movement of lipid onto new surface, can also account for viral-induced membrane fusion.[24]

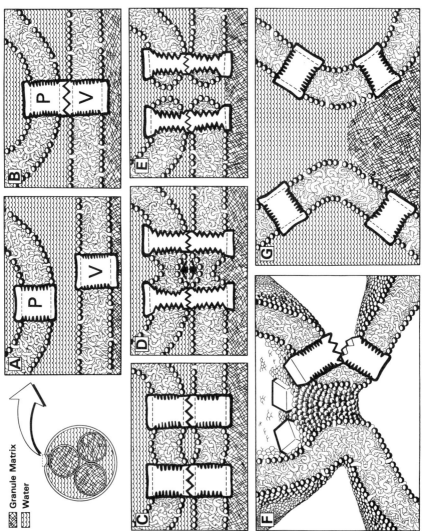

FIGURE 2.

THE MODEL'S QUANTITATIVE PREDICTIONS FOR THE KINETICS OF PORE GROWTH

We describe the steps of the model of FIGURE 2 in kinetic terms to demonstrate that our hypothesis could quantitatively account for the experimental observations. We depict the formation of fusin complexes by equations 1 and 2. The consequent lipid movement that results in pore formation is given by equations 3–6. We show that the model predicts semistable pore conductances as seen experimentally (FIG. 1) and that whereas fusin complexation leads to formation and gradual growth of a pore conductance, an additional process is necessary to account for the rapid increase in pore conductance (the third phase).

We denote the fusins in the vesicular and plasma membranes of FIGURE 2A by V and P, respectively. The association reaction forming the complex of fusins, VP, shown in FIGURE 2B is given by

$$V + P \overset{k}{\rightarrow} VP.$$

The rate is given by

$$\frac{d}{dt}[VP] = k([V]_0 - [VP])([P]_0 - [VP]), \tag{1}$$

where [VP] is the concentration of VP at time t. The general solution for [VP] with time is given by

$$[VP] = \frac{[V]_0 \left\{ e^{([V]_0 - [P]_0)kt} - 1 \right\}}{\left\{ \dfrac{[V]_0}{[P]_0} e^{([V]_0 - [P]_0)kt} \right\} - 1}. \tag{2a}$$

Note that [VP] increases without a time-lag and saturates with time (because $[V]_0$ and $[P]_0$ are finite). An algebraically convenient form is obtained if the fusins in either membrane are in large excess, which we take to be P for concreteness. Then

$$[VP] = [V]_0 \left(1 - e^{-k[P]_0 t} \right). \tag{2b}$$

Equation 2b yields the same features for VP as the general solution. VP increases monotonically with no time delay and reaches saturation. Equation 3b can therefore be used to illustrate the general quantitative consequences of the model in FIGURE 3.

As illustrated by FIGURE 2D, the formation of VP complexes results in the

---

FIGURE 2. Model for pore formation and enlargement during exocytosis, illustrating some hypothetical sequential steps of membrane contact and fusion. **A** and **B:** As the plasma membrane (top) and vesicle membrane (bottom) approach one another (the inward dimpling of the plasma membrane toward a vesicle membrane[49]), the fusins of opposing membranes undergo conformational changes and bind. **C:** Due to multiple associations of opposing fusins, the bilayers are brought into close proximity. Consequently, repulsive forces between the bilayers produce "blisters." **D:** The acyl chains move into the newly created hydrophobic portions of the fusins. **E:** A hydrated lipid-lined protein pore forms that connects the vesicle interior to the extracellular space. **F:** As more fusin complexes form, the pore widens, and the plasma and vesicular membranes mix. **G:** The fusins dissociate, and the pore formation becomes irreversible.

exposure of binding sites for lipids. The nature and number of binding sites will vary with time. In the absence of any information about these sites, we assume the simplest model: there are B independent and identical binding sites on each fusin complex and at any time t, L(t) of these sites are occupied by bound lipid (*i.e.* the fusin complex is a Langmuir adsorption surface for lipids). Then,

$$\frac{d}{dt}(B - L) = -k'(1 - L/B), \tag{3}$$

where k' is a proportionality constant. Solving equation 3 yields

$$L(t) = L_\infty (1 - e^{-k't}), \tag{4}$$

where L_∞ is the steady-state number of bound lipids per VP complex.

The exocytotic pore of FIGURE 2 is an assembly of lipids and fusin complexes. The experimentally measured quantity, the conductance of the pore, is a function of

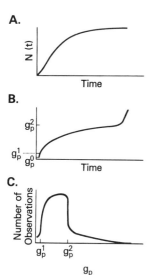

FIGURE 3. Kinetic model of fusion. **A:** The number of lipids within a pore assembly, N, as a function of time. **B:** The pore conductance as a function of time, where g_p^0 is the initial pore conductance; g_p^1 and g_p^2 are two sequential pore conductances. The conductance increases relatively slowly between g_p^1 and g_p^2. **C:** Theoretical histogram of pore conductances.

the number of VP complexes and the number of bound lipids. Because the quantitative relation between pore conductance and these numbers cannot be stated *a priori*, we can only assume that the conductance increases as the number of bound lipids increases. Hence, we calculate the number of bound lipids. When a VP complex forms at time τ, the binding of lipids to this complex is initiated. Therefore, at any time t ($t > \tau$) the lipids have been binding to this complex for duration $[t - \tau]$. In a time interval $\delta\tau$, the increment in the number of lipids that bind to the fusins is proportional to the number of fusin complexes times the rate of lipid binding times $\delta\tau$. Hence, the number of lipids within a pore assembly, N(t), at time t is given by

$$N(t) = \beta \int_0^t [VP](\tau)\, d/dt\, [L(t - \tau)]\, d\tau \tag{5}$$

where β is a proportionality constant. Note that $N(t)$ is simply a convolution of VP with dL/dt. For ease of illustration, we use equation 2b to describe the time course of VP. This yields

$$N(t) = \beta[V]_0 L_\infty (1 - e^{-k't})(1 - e^{-k[P]_0 t}). \tag{6}$$

When an individual exocytotic pore is detected (FIG. 2F) its initial conductance, g_p^0, is variable. It depends on the number of lipids and VP complexes and on the particular phospholipids (*e.g.* acidic vs. zwitterionic) that constitute the lining of the water-filled pore. The conductance increases as more VP complexes and lipids contribute to the macromolecular assembly of the exocytotic pore. In the simplified treatment, $g_p(t)$ is a monotonic function of $N(t)$. FIGURE 3A shows $N(t)$ as a function of time. Because $N(t)$ saturates with time, so would $g_p(t)$ if only association of fusion were involved. Therefore, once the pore forms and fusion is complete, additional processes must be contributing to the accelerated enlargement of the pore. Our model predicts that $g_p(t)$, therefore, has the overall shape indicated by the curve of FIGURE 3B.

The pore conductance increases relatively slowly between values denoted by g_p^1 and g_p^2. Conductances between these values should therefore be observed relatively frequently. The shape of the expected histogram for the frequency of observed pore sizes, FIGURE 3C, is similar to experimentally derived histograms. Note that adding complexities to the quantitative treatment of the model, such as assuming the number of lipid-binding sites (equation 5) varies with time or that sites are not identical, can confer additional characteristics to the shape of FIGURE 3C. Discrete additions of VP complexes to the multimacromolecular complexes would result in discrete increases in g_p. The basic shape of FIGURE 3C follows from FIGURE 2 and is independent of the purposely simplified treatment. Because even this simplest of treatments has many free parameters (*e.g.* k', β, precise relationship between $N(t)$ and $g(t)$), we do not attempt to curve-fit the model to experimental data. If the lipid-protein complex of the exocytotic pore is formed by sequential stages of molecular rearrangements, the time evolution of the pore is conveniently described by convolving the time functions of these stages (equation 5).

CONCLUSION

In exocytosis the first recordable event is a fusion pore. We propose a molecular model where the fusion pore is composed of lipid and protein, rather than solely of protein. The model predicts variable pore sizes and flicker, as is experimentally observed, and can account for the expected time-courses and frequency-distributions of pore conductance. This model proposes that the hydration barrier to membrane fusion is overcome by intermembrane protein adhesion, leaving pockets of trapped water between strained lipids. The lipids rearrange and coat the membrane fusion proteins; a pore forms. This initial pore subsequently widens by accretion of proteins and lipids.

ACKNOWLEDGMENT

We thank Bob Polaski for his artistic contributions to this paper.

REFERENCES

1. COLE, K. S. 1968. Membranes, Ions, and Impulses. University of California Press. 35–36. Berkeley, CA.
2. CHANDLER, D. E. & J. E. HEUSER. 1980. J. Cell Biol. **86:** 666–674.
3. ORNBERG, R. L. & T. S. REESE. 1981. J. Cell Biol. **90:** 40–54.
4. SCHMIDT, W., W. PATZAK, G. LINGG & H. WINKLER. 1983. Eur. J. Cell Biol. **32:** 31–37.
5. OLBRICHT, K., H. PLATTNER & H. MATT. 1984. Exp. Cell Res. **151:** 14–20.
6. ZIMMERBERG, J., M. CURRAN, F. S. COHEN & M. BRODWICK. 1987. Proc. Natl. Acad. Sci. USA **84:** 1585–1589.
6A. Breckenridge, L. J. & W. Almers. 1987. Proc. Natl. Acad. Sci. USA **84:** 1945–1949.
7. BRECKENRIDGE, L. J. & W. ALMERS. 1987. Nature (Lond.) **328:** 814–817.
8. SPRUCE, A. E., L. J. BRECKENRIDGE, A. K. LEE & W. ALMERS. 1990. Neuron **4:** 643–654.
9. MONCK, J. R., G. A. DETOLEDO & J. M. FERNANDEZ. 1990. Proc. Natl. Acad. Sci. USA **87:** 7804–7808.
10. ZIMMERBERG, J. 1988. In Molecular Mechanism of Membrane Fusion. S. Ohki, D. Doyle, T. D. Flanagan, S. W. Hui & E. Mayhew, Ed.: 181–195. Plenum Press. New York.
11. ALMERS, W. & F. W. TSE. 1990. Neuron **4:** 813–818.
12. LLINÁS R., I. Z. STEINBERG & K. WALTON. 1981. Biophys. J. **33:** 323–351.
13. DELANEY, K. R. & R. S. ZUCKER. 1990. J. Physiol. (Lond.). **426:** 473–498.
14. KATZ, B. & R. MILEDI. 1965. Proc. R. Soc. Lond. B. Biol. Sci. **161:** 483–495.
15. CULLIS, R. P., M. J. HOPE, R. NAYAR & C. P. S. TILCOCK. 1985. In Phosholipids in the Nervous System. L. A. Horrocks, Ed.: 71–86. Raven Press. New York.
16. SARKAR, D. P., S. J. MORRIS, O. EIDELMAN, J. ZIMMERBERG & R. BLUMENTHAL. 1989. J. Cell Biol. **109:** 113–122.
17. FERNANDEZ, J. M., E. NEHER & B. D. GOMPERTS. 1984. Nature (Lond.) **312:** 453–455.
18. DE TOLEDO, G. A. & J. M. FERNANDEZ. 1988. Cell Physiology of Blood. R. B. Gunn & J. C. Parker, Ed.: 233–243. Rockefeller University Press. New York.
19. WHITE, J., M. KIELIAN & A. HELENIUS. 1983. Q. Rev. Biophys. **16:** 151–195.
20. WILEY, D. C. & J. J. SKEHEL. 1987. Annu. Rev. Biochem. **56:** 365–394.
21. WILSON, I. A., J. J. SKEHEL & D. C. WILEY. 1981. Nature **289:** 368–373.
22. ELLENS, H., J. BENTZ, D. MASON, F. ZHANG & J. M. WHITE. 1990. Biochemistry **29:** 9697–9707.
23. LEAR, J. D., Z. R. WASSERMAN & W. F. DEGRADO. 1988. Science **240:** 1177–1181.
24. BENTZ, J., H. ELLENS & D. ALFORD. 1990. FEBS Lett. **276:** 1–5.
25. ALMERS, W. 1990. Annu. Rev. Physiol. **52:** 607–624.
26. SOMOGYI, R. & H. A. KOLB. 1988. Pfluegers Arch. **412:** 54–65.
27. VEENSTRA, R. D. & R. L. DeHAAN. 1988. Am. J. Physiol. **255:** H170–H180.
28. THOMAS, L., K. HARTUNG, D. LANGOSCH, H. REHM, E. BAMBERG, W. W. FRANKE & H. BETZ. 1988. Science **242:** 1050–1053.
29. BIRMAN, S., F. M. MEUNIER, B. LESBATS, J. R. LeCAER, J. ROSSIER & M. ISRAEL. 1990. FEBS Lett. **261:** 303–306.
30. COHEN, F. S., J. ZIMMERBERG & A. FINKELSTEIN. 1980. J. Gen. Physiol. **75:** 251–270.
31. HUANG, C. & J. T. MASON. 1978. Proc. Natl. Acad. Sci. USA **75:** 308–310.
32. TRIMBLE, W. S., D. M. COWAN & R. H. SCHELLER. 1988. Proc. Natl. Acad. Sci. USA **85:** 4538–4542.
33. BAUMERT, M., P. R. MAYCOX, F. NAVONE, P. DE CAMILLI & R. JAHN. 1989. EMBO J. **8:** 379–384.
34. JOHNSTON, P. A., R. JAHN & T. C. SUDHOF. 1989. J. Biol. Chem. **264:** 1268–1273.
35. NAVONE, F., R. JAHN, G. DI GIOIA, H. STUKENBROK, P. GREENGARD & P. DE CAMILLI. 1986. J. Cell Biol. **103:** 2511–2527.
36. MALHOTRA, V., L. ORCI, B. S. GLICK, M. R. BLOCK & J. E. ROTHMAN. 1988. Cell **54:** 221–227.
37. JACKSON, R. C., K. K. WARD & J. G. HAGGERTY. 1985. J. Cell Biol. **101:** 6–11 (Erratum:101: 1167).
38. CLARY, D. O., I. C. GRIFF & J. E. ROTHMAN. 1990. Cell **61:** 709–721.
39. DE CAMILLI, P. & P. GREENGARD. 1986. Biochem. Pharmacol. **35:** 4349–4357.

40. ZAKS, W. J. & C. E. CREUTZ. 1990. J. Bioenerg. Biomembr. **22:** 97–120.
41. RAND, R. P., N. FULLER, V. A. PARSEGIAN & D. C. RAU. 1988. Biochemistry **27:** 7711–7722.
42. RAND, R. P. & V. A. PARSEGIAN. 1989. Biochim. Biophys. Acta. **988:** 351–376.
43. RAND, R. P. & V. A. PARSEGIAN. 1986. Annu. Rev. Physiol. **48:** 201–212.
44. POLLARD, H. B., E. ROJAS, A. L. BURNS & C. PARRA. 1988. *In* Molecular Mechanisms of Membrane Fusion. S. Ohki, D. Doyle, T. D. Flanagan, S. W. Hui & E. Mayhew, Eds.: 341–345. Plenum Press. New York.
45. NILES, W. D. 1981. Ph.D. Thesis. University of Wisconsin. Madison, Wisconsin.
46. NILES, W. D., F. S. COHEN & A. FINKELSTEIN. 1989. J. Gen. Physiol. **93:** 211–244.
47. WOODBURY, D. J. & J. E. HALL. 1988. Biophys. J. **54:** 1053–1063.
48. CURRAN, M., D. E. CHANDLER, F. S. COHEN & J. ZIMMERBERG. In preparation.
49. CHANDLER, D. E., M. CURRAN, F. S. COHEN & J. ZIMMERBERG. 1989. J. Cell Biol. **109:** 300A.
50. NEHER, E. & A. MARTY. 1982. Proc. Natl. Acad. Sci. USA **79:** 6712–6716.

Millisecond Studies of Single Membrane Fusion Events[a]

W. ALMERS, L. J. BRECKENRIDGE,[b] A. IWATA,

A. K. LEE, A. E. SPRUCE,[c] AND F. W. TSE

Department of Physiology and Biophysics
University of Washington
Seattle, Washington 98195

One of the major challenges in transmitter release is to understand how it can happen so quickly. When an action potential invades the presynaptic terminal of a frog neuromuscular junction, the terminal releases acetylcholine after a median delay of only 1 ms at 19°C.[1] Within this short time, Ca channels must open, Ca must bind to receptors (so far unknown) that trigger exocytosis, the receptors must change their conformation, and finally, the vesicles must undergo exocytosis and release their contents into the synaptic cleft. Moreover, quantal analysis of transmitter release has shown that, at any one moment, only a small portion of the synaptic vesicles in a terminal can respond to an action potential by exocytosis. It is not known in detail what distinguishes this select group of vesicles from all the others in a nerve terminal. In response to an action potential, however, they perform exocytosis with high probability (for a review, see ref. 2). The synaptic delay gives us, therefore, a lower limit on the rate constant of the exocytic reaction. In motor neurons at 19°C, this rate constant would be > 1000/second.[1] In the squid giant synapse, the shorter synaptic delay of 0.2 ms[3] suggests even higher rate constants. In synapses, nature has gone to great lengths to ensure that the cytosolic messenger (Ca^{2+}) is supplied quickly. Synapses may be the only biological system where one of the rate-limiting steps in secretion is exocytosis itself, rather than the supply of messenger that regulates exocytosis. Hence they teach a unique lesson: membrane fusion can be triggered and executed with rate constants of thousands per second.

All other membrane fusion reactions studied so far are at least 1000-fold slower. At 20°C, rate constants for the fusion of aggregated cardiolipin vesicles are of the order of 1/s; rate constants for the fusion of viral envelopes with cell membranes at 20°C are even slower (< 0.1/s, for a review, see ref. 4). On thermodynamic grounds, the fusion of viral envelopes is expected to be slow because it takes time for the viral fusion protein to insinuate itself into the lipid bilayer of the host cell membrane. In pure lipid vesicles, it will similarly take time to form the nonbilayer lipid fusion intermediates that are thought to be required before two bilayers can become one. In both cases, the common denominator is that fusion requires, at least locally, the disruption of the lipid bilayer. The lipid bilayer is a very stable structure, hence it is unlikely that major disruptions can be generated with rate constants of thousands per second.

Transmitter release also requires the fusion of bilayers, namely those of the synaptic vesicle and plasma membrane. To explain why it happens so quickly, we

[a]This work was supported by NIH Grants AR-17803 and GM-39520.
[b]Present address: Department of Cell Biology, University of Glasgow, Glasgow G12 8QQ, Scotland, U.K.
[c]Present address: Department of Zoology, University of Washington, Seattle, WA 98195.

have suggested[4,5] that a macromolecule, bridging both the vesicle and the plasma membrane, is already in place before the action potential arrives. When the action potential causes an increase in cytosolic Ca^{2+}, the macromolecule binds Ca^{2+} and, within fractions of a millisecond, forms a pore connecting the inside of the vesicle to the outside of the cell. Through this "fusion pore," transmitter can escape. Under this hypothesis, the Ca-induced opening of the pore is the only event in transmitter release that needs to be fast. Putting the macromolecule in place can be slow and, once the transmitter has escaped, the actual collapse of the vesicle into the plasma membrane can also be slow. Inasmuch as there are many precedents for the rapid, ligand-induced opening of ion channels, it is tempting to think that the fusion pore is in some ways similar to an ion channel that spans both the vesicle membrane and the plasma membrane. A structural hypothesis on how an ion channel–like structure could cause membrane fusion has been described.[4,5] Because transmitter release is so rapid, and because of possible similarities between fusion pores and ion channels, we have tried to study single biological fusion events with the patch clamp, much as others have used this technique to study ion channels. An assay sensitive enough to detect single fusion events exists at the neuromuscular junction, where the miniature endplate potential (MEPP) reports the exocytosis of single vesicles.[6] Although MEPPs do report exocytosis at millisecond time resolution, they provide little detail about the exocytic event itself.

PLASMA MEMBRANE CAPACITANCE AS AN ASSAY FOR EXOCYTOSIS AND ENDOCYTOSIS

Every exocytic event increases, and every endocytic event decreases, the cell surface area. Because all biological membranes have a uniform capacitance of 1 $\mu F/cm^2$, the cell surface area, and hence exo- and endocytosis, can be monitored by time-resolved measurement of the membrane capacitance.[7,8] This method has now been applied to a wide variety of secretory cells, among them chromaffin cells,[9] synaptic terminals,[10,11] and endocrine pituitary cells.[12,13] In cells with large (> 0.3 μm diameter) vesicles, single exocytic events can be detected as step increases in membrane capacitance.[9,14] Unfortunately, synaptic vesicles are much too small for this approach; therefore we performed our experiments on mast cells, in particular on mast cells from a murine mutant, the beige mouse. Although in normal rats or mice, a mast cell contains some 1000 vesicles of 0.8 μm average diameter,[15] mast cells from beige mice contain 10–20 giant vesicles of up to 5 μm diameter. Exocytosis of single vesicles results in large (0.1–1 pF) and stepwise increases in capacitance. The following pieces of evidence indicate that the capacitance changes represent exocytosis and secretion. (1) In rat mast cells, the histogram of capacitance step amplitudes agrees well with the histogram of morphologically observed vesicle surface areas.[14] (2) In mast cells of normal and beige mice, secretion of vesicle contents was monitored as the loss of a fluorescent dye, quinacrine, that accumulates in the acidic environment usually found in vesicles. The time-course of fluorescence loss closely paralleled that of capacitance increase. Furthermore, in mast cells of beige mice, the loss of fluorescence is often episodic, and each episode begins with a large capacitance step.[16] (3) In mast cells of beige mice, vesicles swell during exocytosis.[17] Simultaneous capacitance and video microscopy measurements have shown that the swelling of each vesicle is preceded by a step increase in capacitance.[16,18] The amplitude of the step is proportional to the surface area calculated from the diameter of the vesicle immediately before it swelled, the proportionality constant

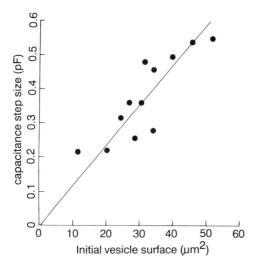

FIGURE 1. Relationships between vesicle surface area and the capacitance step in mast cells of beige mice. The surface area of a secretory vesicle was calculated from video micrographs recorded immediately before the vesicle performed exocytosis and swelled. The amplitude of the capacitance step recorded immediately before the vesicles swelled (ΔC) is plotted against the surface area. The line is the best least-square fit, constrained to go through the origin. It has a slope of 1.17 μF/cm^2 of vesicle surface. From Almers & Breckenridge;[20] data first reported by Breckenridge & Almers.[16]

being 1.17 μF/cm^2 (FIG. 1, see ref. 16) or 0.57 μF/cm^2,[18] in fair agreement with the specific capacitance of about 1 μF/cm^2 measured on other biological membranes (for a review, see ref. 19). Combined video microscopy and capacitance measurements have also shown that even in vesicles shrunk by hypertonic solutions, the capacitance step (and, hence, membrane fusion) preceded swelling. This result suggests that exocytosis can occur even if the vesicle's membrane is slack,[16,18,20] and argues against a central role of osmotic swelling and/or mechanical stress in the initiation of fusion.

HOW LARGE IS THE FUSION PORE IN MAST CELLS?

Vesicles quickly frozen in early stages of exocytosis show fusion pores of diameters down to 10–20 nm connecting the inside of vesicles with the cell exterior.[21-23] Because this is close to the limit of resolution in quick-freeze electron-micrographs, we asked whether the fusion pore seen in electron-micrographs has smaller precursors. Our approach was to measure the conductance of a single fusion pore and to infer from it the pore diameter.

Time-resolved measurements of the pore conductance can be made by analyzing the electrical admittance contributed by a fusing vesicle. FIGURE 2 shows a brief episode during secretion by a beige mouse mast cell; during this episode, a single vesicle performed exocytosis. The cell was under whole-cell voltage clamp,[24] and the plasma membrane potential was forced to undergo sinusoidal oscillations. The sinusoidal current needed to do this was decomposed with a lock-in amplifier[9] into its "real" (in phase with the voltage, G_{ac}) and "imaginary" components (90° out-of-phase, capacitance (C) in FIG. 2). The final change in C is proportional to the C of the vesicle, whereas the transient change in G_{ac} results from the increasing conductance of the fusion pore. Using circuit analysis (equations 1 and 2), this conductance can be calculated independently either from the C or the G_{ac} trace. The conductance (trace g in FIGURE 2) is seen to increase gradually until it is too large to measure. On the right-hand side of FIGURE 2, the pore conductance is converted to pore diameter, using an equation given by Hille[25] and assuming the pore to have the length of a gap junction channel (15 nm) and to be filled with electrolyte of 100 Ωcm resistivity, slightly larger than that of our external bathing solution. For most of the trace, the pore diameter remains well below that measured in electron-micrographs. Hence the experiment suggests that the "fusion pores" seen, for example, by Chandler and Heuser[26] arise from much smaller, short-lived precursors. The method used here, however, provides only one measurement every sinusoidal cycle (800 Hz), and hence

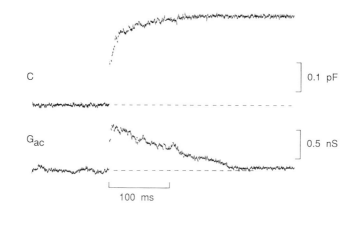

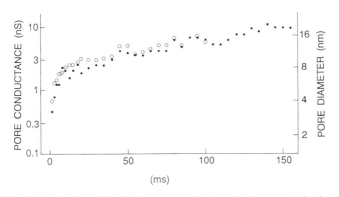

FIGURE 2. Determination of the fusion pore conductance during exocytosis of a single vesicle in a beige mouse mast cell. Capacitance (C), in-phase component of sinusoidal admittance (G_{ac}) and pore conductance (g) of a mast cell secretory vesicle during exocytosis. The gradual rise of capacitance to a final value reflects the gradual dilation of the fusion pore, as does the transient increase in G_{ac}. The pore conductance was calculated from C (circles) or G_{ac} (dots) by

$$g = \frac{2\pi f C_v}{\sqrt{C_v/C - 1}} \tag{1}$$

$$g = \frac{2G_{ac}}{1 + n\sqrt{1 - (G_{ac}/\pi f C_v)^2}} \tag{2}$$

where C_v is the final amplitude of the capacitance change and f the frequency of the sinusoid (800 Hz); $n = 1$, while $C < C_v/2$ and -1 otherwise. The righthand ordinate of the g versus time plot converts pore conductance into pore diameter, as explained in the text.

cannot resolve events happening in less than 2.5 milliseconds. FIG. 2 does not exclude, for instance, that the pore conductance increases gradually from zero to very large values.

To address this question, we took advantage of the finding that the admittance changes shown in FIGURE 2 are preceded by a brief current transient flowing through the fusion pore as the pore first opens. This current is generated as the vesicle membrane discharges its large (inside positive) potential through the nascent fusion pore. One such transient is shown in FIGURE 3A. FIGURE 3B shows the time integral

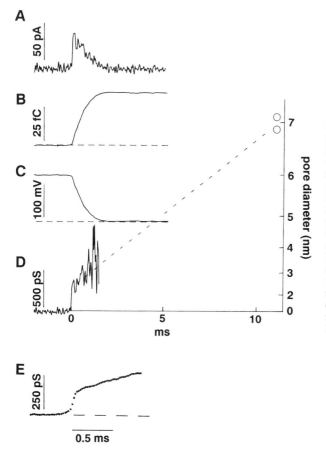

FIGURE 3. The fusion pore conductance during the first millisecond of exocytosis in a beige mouse mast cell. Analysis of the current transient flowing through the nascent fusion pore was performed as described in the text.[29] E is the average of 219 traces as in D. g_i, the initial pore conductance, was obtained by fitting a straight line to trace D over the interval 0 to 1.5 ms and extrapolating the line to zero time.

of the current, and FIGURE 3C the potential across the fusion pore, calculated by subtracting trace B from its final value and dividing the result by the final amplitude of the capacitance step that followed (not shown). Because the potential in trace C drives the current in trace A, the pore conductance can be obtained simply by dividing trace C by trace A. The result is shown in FIGURE 3D. The trace suggests that the pore opened abruptly to an initial conductance, g_i (see legend of FIG. 3). The conductance then increased more gradually, as if the pore dilated.

Unlike ion channels, g_i varies over a broad range, with median values of 285 pS at 23°C and 190 pS at 14°C. Nonetheless, it is clear that g_i is in the range observed for large ligand-gated ion channels. Of special interest is the gap junction channel, because it is the only channel that spans two membranes and whose conductance has been measured. This analogy is consistent with our suggested model of exocytosis at synapses.[4,5] The conductance of a fully open single gap junction channel is 120 pS[27] to 240 pS,[28] not much less than g_i. The comparison suggests that the fusion pore initially has a diameter of 2–3 nm, only slightly larger than that of a single gap junction channel.[29]

Unfortunately, synaptic vesicles are too small to allow similar measurements with existing technology, and the initial pore conductance for synaptic vesicles is unknown. The escape of acetylcholine (ACh) through a 280 pS pore, however, would be rapid. If concentration gradients within the small volume of a synaptic vesicle (vol. = 27,000 nm³),[30] are ignored, ACh would escape exponentially (equation 3):

$$[ACh]_{vesicle} = C_o \exp - (t/\tau), \tag{3}$$

where C_o is the initial ACh concentration in the vesicle and

$$\tau = V/\rho\, Dg. \tag{4}$$

Equation (4)[31] was derived by combining equations (8-1) and (8-6) in Hille;[25] g is the pore conductance, ρ the resistivity of the pore lumen (assumed 100 Ωcm), and D is the diffusion coefficient of ACh. If ACh existed as a complex with 4 ATP molecules, its diffusion coefficient would probably be around 3.5×10^{-6} cm²/s,[4] and a vesicle would lose its ACh with a time constant of only 260 microseconds. Clearly, the synaptic delay would allow sufficient time for a synaptic vesicle to discharge most of its contents through a 280 nm pore. The pore may not even have to dilate. Indeed, it is conceivable that a fusion pore could open, discharge its transmitter and then close again a millisecond later. Such a vesicle could be refilled with cytoplasmic transmitter and would then be once more available for synaptic transmission without the time-consuming cycle of complete exocytosis followed by endocytosis. Admittedly, the membrane of many vesicles clearly does fuse with the nerve terminal membrane, and is retrieved by endocytosis.[32,33] In addition, there is no evidence that fusion pores in synaptic vesicles close again, or that synaptic vesicles can be readied for a second round of release having bypassed the exocytosis-endocytosis cycle; however, there is also no evidence to rule out this possibility. Mast cell fusion pores have been observed to close again,[14,16,18,34,35] even after they have dilated severalfold[29] and, possibly, have allowed the exchange of lipid between plasma and vesicle membranes.[36]

In conclusion, the rapid opening of the fusion pore predicted for a synapse can be observed in mast cells. It is tempting to consider that the final steps in exocytic fusion occurs similarly in both cells, and that only the control mechanisms differ.

PROPERTIES OF THE FUSION PORE FORMED BY A WELL-CHARACTERIZED FUSION PROTEIN

So far, the only known fusion proteins are those found in the envelopes of animal viruses (see refs. 37 and 38, and Blumenthal *et al.,* this volume). Among them, the hemagglutinin (HA) of the influenza virus is the best characterized, and we were interested in using the patch clamp to study fusion mediated by HA. Virions are too small to be patch-clamped; therefore we used fibroblasts transfected to express the fusion protein on their cell surface.[39] For our purposes, these cells may be thought of as giant viruses that can be patch-clamped while they fuse to erythrocytes.[40]

FIGURE 4 shows an experiment similar to FIGURE 2, plotting the C and conductance components (G_{ac}) of the sinusoidal admittance of a fibroblast. A single erythrocyte (RBC) had bound to the fibroblast. When the fibroblast's HA was activated by the application of H^+, C increased, ultimately by about 1 pF, while G_{ac} rose and fell. The following findings indicate that the events in FIGURE 4 are due to the HA-mediated fusion of fibroblast and RBC.[40] (1) The final value of the increase in C is identical to the capacitance of a single RBC. (2) The events are not observed when no RBC is bound to the fibroblast, and never occur without acidification. (3) The HA must be subjected to proteolytic cleavage before it can cause fusion;[37] correspondingly, the events in FIGURE 4 occur only with fibroblasts that had previously been treated with trypsin.

As in FIGURE 2, the C and G_{ac} signals can each be used to calculate the conductance (g) developing between the two cells. The resulting trace resembles that in FIGURE 2, except that the conductance changes occur more than 1000-fold more slowly. When the initial portions of g traces are plotted on an extended time scale, they often resemble recordings from single ion channels in that the conductance rapidly fluctuates around a constant value that can be maintained for more than 10 s.[41] These experiments suggest that the HA-mediated fusion pore can dilate only slowly.

To measure the initial conductance of the HA-mediated fusion pore, we proceeded as in FIGURE 3. Measuring capacitance and G_{ac} only intermittently, we looked for current transients immediately preceding the increase in C and G_{ac}.[41] Unlike in mast cells, the current transients recorded were inward because we held the

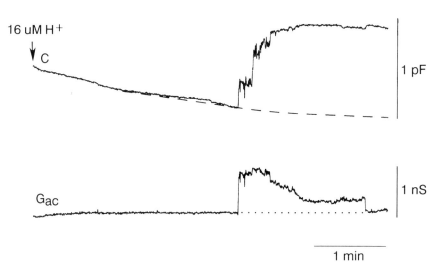

FIGURE 4. Cell fusion mediated by the influenza HA. Capacitance and G_{ac} changes recorded from a fibroblast expressing the fusion protein (HA) of the influenza virus envelope are plotted against time. The fibroblast had been mildly trypsinized to make the HA fusion competent. A single RBC had bound to it, and fusion with this RBC caused the C and G_{ac} changes observed here. These changes were triggered by acidifying the external solution to pH 4.8. Experimental conditions as in ref. 41.

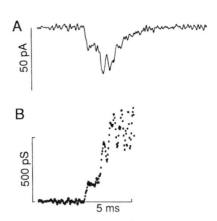

FIGURE 5. The first milliseconds of fusion mediated by the influenza fusion protein. **A:** Current transient through the nascent fusion pore formed by the influenza HA during fusion of a fibroblast with an RBC. **B:** conductance (g) calculated from **A** as in FIG. 3. Experimental conditions similar to FIG. 4.[41]

fibroblasts at around −40 mV, and because at the low pH required to activate fusion, RBCs had a slightly positive internal potential. FIGURE 5 shows one such current transient, and beneath it is shown the conductance trace calculated from the current transient, as in FIGURE 3. During the first 1–2 ms, the pore conductance remained at only about 130 pS in FIGURE 3; the mean value in other, similar experiments was 150 pS. At first, the conductance increases rapidly, as in mast cells. Soon, however, the increase is temporarily arrested at a conductance of 0.4–1 nanoseconds. Occasionally, the pore closes again completely, and a second opening generates a second current transient.[41] Why the conductance becomes arrested at 0.4–1.0 nS is unknown. It is hard to imagine how a 1 nS pore could allow the viral genome to pass into the host cell. Conceivably, the arrest of pore dilation could be a consequence of the rigid cytoskeleton of the RBC, or it could mean that rapid dilation requires factors that are lacking in the fibroblast/RBC assay system.

Experiments as in FIGURE 4 were carried out also with RBCs whose lipid bilayers were loaded with fluorescent phosphatidylethanolamine.[42] Following fusion, fluorescent lipid was lost from the RBC membrane as it was distributed over the membrane of the fibroblast, and this process was monitored by digital image analysis. The fusion pore opened long (sometimes minutes) before lipid transfer could be observed. While the pore conductance remained < 6 nS, lipid transfer was less than 20,000–40,000 lipid molecules/s, the limit of our detection. Clearly, the opening of the fusion pore is the earliest event in fusion observed with the methods currently available (see also Zimmerberg *et al.*, this volume).

In summary, exocytic fusion and the fusion mediated by the influenza HA both begin with the abrupt formation of an aqueous pore with the conductance of a large ion channel. Initially, the estimated pore diameters are much too small to be visible in quick-freeze electron-micrographs. The pore conductance, however, increases with time as if the pores dilated (as, indeed, they must). Most likely, dilation represents incorporation of membrane lipid into the pore.

Despite an abundance of speculative models, the molecular details of pore formation and pore dilation are likely to remain a mystery for some time. Nonetheless, it may be hoped that the first eukaryotic fusion proteins will be identified within the next few years. The experiments described here suggest that the patch clamp will be a useful tool for studying their function at millisecond time resolution.

REFERENCES

1. KATZ, B. & R. MILEDI. 1965. The measurement of synaptic delay and the time course of acetylcholine release at the neuromuscular junction. Proc. R. Soc. Lond. Biol. Sci. **161:** 483–495.
2. MCLACHLAN, E. M. 1978. The statistics of transmitter release at chemical synapses. *In* International Review in Physiology, Neurophysiology III. R. Porter, Ed. **17:** 49–117. University Park. Baltimore, MD.
3. LLINÁS, R., I. Z. STEINBERG & K. WALTON. 1981. Relationship between presynaptic calcium current and postsynaptic potential in squid giant synapse. Biophys. J. **33:** 323–351.
4. ALMERS, W. & F. W. TSE. 1990. Transmitter release from synapses: does a preassembled fusion pore initiate exocytosis? Neuron **4:** 813–818.
5. ALMERS, W. 1990. Exocytosis. Annu. Rev. Physiol. **52:** 607–624.
6. DEL CASTILLO, J. & B. KATZ. 1954. The effect of magnesium on the activity of motor nerve endings. J. Physiol. **124:** 553–559.
7. PENNER, R. & E. NEHER. 1989. The patch-clamp technique in the study of secretion. Trends Neurosci. **12:** 159–163.
8. LINDAU, M. 1991. Time-resolved capacitance measurements: monitoring exocytosis in single cells. Quart. Rev. Biophys. **24:** 75–101.
9. NEHER, E. & A. MARTY. 1982. Discrete changes of cell membrane capacitance observed under conditions of enhanced secretion in bovine adrenal chromaffin cells. Proc. Natl. Acad. Sci. USA **79:** 6712–6716.
10. GILLESPIE, J. I. 1979. The effect of repetitive stimulation on the passive electrical properties of the presynaptic terminal of the squid giant synapse. Proc. R. Soc. Lond. Biol. Sci. **206:** 293–306.
11. LIM, N. F., M. C. NOWYCKY & R. J. BOOKMAN. 1990. Direct measurement of exocytosis and calcium currents in single vertebrate nerve terminals. Nature **344:** 449–451.
12. SIKDAR, S. K., R. ZOREC, D. BROWN & W. T. MASON. 1989. Dual effects of G-protein activation on Ca-dependent exocytosis in bovine lactotrophs. FEBS Lett. **253:** 88–92.
13. THOMAS, P., A. SURPRENANT & W. ALMERS. 1990. Cytosolic Ca^{2+}, exocytosis, and endocytosis in single melanotrophs of the rat pituitary. Neuron **5:** 723–733.
14. FERNANDEZ, J. M., E. NEHER & B. D. GOMPERTS. 1984. Capacitance measurements reveal stepwise fusion events in degranulating mast cells. Nature **312:** 453–455.
15. HELANDER, H. F. & D. BLOOM. 1973. Quantitative analysis of mast cell structure. J. Microsc. (Oxf.) **100** (Part B): 315–321.
16. BRECKENRIDGE, L. J. & W. ALMERS. 1987a. Final steps in exocytosis observed in a cell with giant secretory granules. Proc. Natl. Acad. Sci. USA **84:** 1945–1949.
17. CURRAN, M. J., M. S. BRODWICK & C. EDWARDS. 1984. Direct visualization of exocytosis in mast cells. Biophys. J. **45:** 170a.
18. ZIMMERBERG, J., M. CURRAN, S. COHEN & M. BRODWICK. 1987. Simultaneous electrical and optical measurements show that membrane fusion precedes secretory granule swelling during exocytosis of beige mouse mast cells. Proc. Natl. Acad. Sci. USA **84:** 1585–1589.
19. ALMERS, W. 1978. Gating currents and charge movements in excitable membranes. Rev. Physiol. Biochem. Pharmacol. **82:** 96–190.
20. ALMERS, W. & L. J. BRECKENRIDGE. 1988. Early steps in the exocytosis of secretory vesicles in mast cells. *In* Molecular Mechanisms of Membrane Fusion. S. Ohki, D. Doyle, T. D. Flanagan, S. W. Hui & E. Mayhew, Eds.: 197–208. Plenum Publishing Corp. New York.
21. HEUSER, J. E. & T. S. REESE. 1981. Structural changes after transmitter release at the frog neuromuscular junction. J. Cell Biol. **88:** 564–580.
22. ORNBERG, R. L. & T. S. REESE. 1981. Beginning of exocytosis captured by rapid-freezing of Limulus amebocytes. J. Cell Biol. **90:** 40–54.
23. CHANDLER, D. E., M. WHITAKER & J. ZIMMERBERG. 1989. High molecular weight polymers block cortical granule exocytosis in sea urchin eggs at the level of granule matrix disassembly. J. Cell Biol. **109:** 1269–1278.

24. HAMILL, O. P., A. MARTY, E. NEHER, B. SAKMANN & F. J. SIGWORTH. 1981. Improved patch-clamp techniques for high resolution current recording from cells and cell-free patches. Pflügers Arch. **391:** 85–100.

25. HILLE, B. 1984. Ionic Channels in Excitable Membranes. 186–188. Sinauer Associates. Sunderland, MA.

26. CHANDLER, D. E. & J. E. HEUSER. 1980. Arrest of membrane fusion events in mast cells by quick-freezing. J. Cell Biol. **86:** 666–674.

27. NEYTON, J. & A. TRAUTMANN. 1985. Single channel currents of an intercellular junction. Nature **317:** 331–335.

28. VEENSTRA, R. D. & R. L. DEHAAN. 1988. Cardiac gap junction channel activity in embryonic chick ventricle cells. Am. J. Physiol. **254:** H170–H180.

29. SPRUCE, A. E., L. J. BRECKENRIDGE, A. K. LEE & W. ALMERS. 1990. Properties of the fusion pore that forms during exocytosis of a mast cell secretory vesicle. Neuron **4:** 643–654.

30. STEINBACH, J. H. & C. F. STEVENS. 1976. Neuromuscular transmission. *In* Frog Neurobiology. R. Llinás & W. Precht, Eds.: 33–92. Springer-Verlag. New York.

31. ALMERS, W., L. J. BRECKENRIDGE & A. E. SPRUCE. 1989. The mechanism of exocytosis during secretion in mast cells. *In* Secretion and Its Control. Society of General Physiologists 42nd Annual Symposium. G. S. Oxford & C. M. Armstrong, Eds.: 269–282. Rockefeller University Press. New York.

32. VON WEDEL, R. J., S. S. CARLSON & P. A. LARSSON. 1981. Transfer of synaptic vesicle antigens to the presynaptic plasma membrane during exocytosis. Proc. Natl. Acad. Sci. USA **78:** 1014–1018.

33. MILLER, T. M. & J. E. HEUSER. 1984. Endocytosis of synaptic vesicle membrane at the frog neuromuscular junction. J. Cell Biol. **98:** 685–698.

34. BRECKENRIDGE, L. J. & W. ALMERS. 1987b. Currents through the fusion pore that forms during exocytosis of a secretory vesicle. Nature **328:** 814–817.

35. ALVAREZ DE TOLEDO, G. & J. M. FERNANDEZ. 1988. The events leading to secretory granule fusion. *In* Cell Physiology of Blood. R. B. Gunn & J. C. Parker, Eds.: 333–344. Rockefeller University Press. New York.

36. MONCK, J. R., G. ALVAREZ DE TOLEDO & J. M. FERNANDEZ. 1990. Tension in secretory granule membranes causes extensive membrane transfer during exocytotic fusion. Proc. Natl. Acad. Sci. USA **87:** 7804–7808.

37. STEGMANN, T., R. W. DOMS & A. HELENIUS. 1989. Protein-mediated membrane fusion. Annu. Rev. Biophys. Biophys. Chem. **18:** 187–211.

38. WHITE, J. M. 1990. Viral and cellular membrane fusion proteins. Annu. Rev. Physiol. **52:** 675 697.

39. DOXSEY, S. J., J. SAMBROOK, A. HELENIUS & J. M. WHITE. 1985. An efficient method for introducing macromolecules into living cells. J. Cell Biol. **101:** 19–27.

40. SPRUCE, A. E., A. IWATA, J. M. WHITE & W. ALMERS. 1989. Patch clamp studies of single cell-fusion events mediated by a viral fusion protein. Nature **342:** 555–558.

41. SPRUCE, A. E., A. IWATA & W. ALMERS. 1991. The first milliseconds of the pore formed by a fusogenic viral envelope protein during membrane fusion. Proc. Natl. Acad. Sci. USA **88:** 3623–3627.

42. TSE, F. A., A. IWATA & W. ALMERS. 1991. The fusion pore opens before membrane lipids mix when a viral fusion protein mediates cell fusion. Soc. Neurosci. Abstr. In press.

Synexin: Molecular Mechanism of Calcium-Dependent Membrane Fusion and Voltage-Dependent Calcium-Channel Activity

Evidence in Support of the "Hydrophobic Bridge Hypothesis" for Exocytotic Membrane Fusion

HARVEY B. POLLARD, EDUARDO ROJAS,
RICHARD W. PASTOR,[a] EDUARDO M. ROJAS,
H. ROBERT GUY,[b] AND A. LEE BURNS

Laboratory of Cell Biology and Genetics
National Institute of Diabetes, and Digestive and Kidney Diseases
National Institutes of Health
Bethesda, Maryland 20892

[a]Biophysics Laboratory
Center for Biologics Evaluation and Research
Food and Drug Administration
Bethesda, Maryland 20892

[b]Laboratory of Mathematical Biology
National Cancer Institute
National Institutes of Health
Bethesda, Maryland 20892

INTRODUCTION TO THE PROBLEM OF MEMBRANE FUSION DURING EXOCYTOSIS

Membrane fusion is a process of central importance in cell biology, being necessary for such diverse events as exocytotic and apocrine secretion, endocytosis, vesicle trafficking, viral invasion and release, sperm-egg fusion, cell division, and other related events (see reference 1 for a recent general review). Nonetheless, the precise mechanism for this critical process in any of the above events presently remains unknown. Our own experimental work over the past few years has focused on the process of exocytosis from chromaffin cells, where our specific aims have been to understand the energetics and specificity of the fusion event, which occurs between the chromaffin granule and the plasma membrane. The critical problem in this, and other instances of fusion between membranes, is the requirement for overcoming the profound electrostatic repulsion forces apparently preventing the two membrane bilayers from coming close enough to fuse.[2]

With regard to the energetics of fusion, biochemical studies on chromaffin granules initially led to the explicit hypothesis that the chemiosmotic properties of the organelle might provide a motive force for the secretion process.[3-6] A variant of this hypothesis featuring K^+ rather than H^+ has also been proposed.[7] In particular, the hypothesis envisioned that granule swelling might expand the enclosed bilayer to the point where interaction of the lipids with those of another bilayer might be favored. A more biophysical set of applications of this principle were later introduced for fusion of liposomes with bilayers,[8] and these studies then expanded to more biological systems (*e.g.* refs. 9 and 10). Recently, however, enthusiasm for the osmotic hypothesis has been tempered by experimental ambiguities,[5,6] and the tactical approach to this impass has been to direct more attention to the fundamental question of mechanism and specificity of the processes inducing the membrane contact event occurring before fusion.

The specificity of the fusion reaction during secretion has been approached most frequently through concerns for the apparent primacy of calcium in regulating the process. Indeed, chromaffin cells are dependent on the influx of extracellular calcium to drive the secretion process.[11] Historically, the direct cross-linking of the target membranes by calcium was considered as a plausible mechanism for inducing fusion. The concentrations of calcium needed, however, in model membrane fusion reactions appeared to be too high and too nonselective with respect to magnesium. Thus calcium appeared to require an intermediary factor. The first possibility was tubulin, inasmuch as calcium was known to cause depolymerization of microtubules. Although interactions between tubulin and plasma and chromaffin granule membranes certainly occur, however,[12,13] the role of tubulin in chromaffin cells presently appears to be that of regulating intracellular transport of organelles.

Historically, contractile proteins have also been considered for a role in fusion. The conceptual basis has been that parallels might exist between the processes of stimulus/contraction coupling and stimulus/secretion coupling. Indeed, F-actin cross-links chromaffin granules to each other in a reversible and calcium-dependent manner.[14,15] F-actin, however, did not cause fusion between cross-linked granules or granule ghosts. Presently, interactions between F-actin and chromaffin granules remain understood as illustrative of reversible cytoskeletal interactions with organelles in the cytosol or subcortical web. In this situation $[Ca^{2+}]_{free}$ is low but can fluctuate upwards in response to secretory signals, thereby permitting granules the freedom to diffuse towards the membrane for subsequent fusion.[4,15]

This still leaves unresolved, however, the question of how calcium might directly mediate fusion. In contractile tissues, the direct calcium signal to actomyosin is mediated by troponin C; and based on a homology argument, calmodulin has therefore been widely considered for a role in regulating calcium-dependent secretion. In fact, calmodulin occurs in large amounts in chromaffin cells, and anticalmodulin antibodies interfere to some extent with secretion.[16] Calmodulin, however, is not presently viewed as a direct participant in the fusion process because the protein does not cause membrane contact or fusion in granule or model systems. Furthermore, whereas the phenothiazine drug trifluoperazine (TFP) inhibits both calmodulin activity and secretion from chromaffin cells, promethazine (PMTHZ), a phenothiazine drug with poor potency for calmodulin, is nearly as potent as TFP as an inhibitor of secretion from cells.[17] Similar results were obtained with glucose-activated insulin secretion from islets of Langerhans.[18]

More recently, we have turned our attention to the protein synexin as a possible mediator of calcium-dependent membrane fusion. Synexin is a calcium-binding protein with membrane fusion and calcium channel properties,[19] which we initially isolated from adrenal medullary tissue.[20,21] We now know it to be widely distributed throughout both the body and phylogeny, and to be equally sensitive to low concentrations of both phenothiazine drugs, TFP and PMTHZ. In the remainder of this chapter we will first review some of the results of a kinetic analysis of synexin-driven membrane fusion and provide some information regarding the biophysical basis for the interaction of synexin with membranes. We will then present a model, based on our recent studies, of the molecular biology of the synexin gene, for the three-dimensional structure of synexin when within the membrane. Finally, we will describe a possible mechanism by which synexin promotes membrane fusion. This mechanism involves the formation of a hydrophobic bridge of synexin molecules between fusing membrane partners. In this context, we will also provide a rationale for this "hydrophobic bridge hypothesis" for membrane fusion, which is consistent with the physical properties of phospholipid bilayers as determined by experiment and computer simulation.

KINETIC ANALYSIS SHOWS THAT SYNEXIN DIRECTLY AFFECTS THE RATES OF MEMBRANE CONTACT AND MEMBRANE FUSION

In the presence of calcium, synexin causes the fusion of both acidic phospholipid liposomes[22] and chromaffin granule ghosts.[23] In addition, the earliest studies had shown that synexin could fuse together intact chromaffin granules with the further aid of arachidonic acid.[24,25] The kinetic mechanism by which synexin fuses membranes has been studied in the most detail by Nir et al.,[26] for the case of chromaffin granule ghosts. In that study, the fusion process was modeled in terms of aggregation of two ghosts to form a dimer, and then higher order aggregates, followed by subsequent fusion of the closely apposed membranes to form a larger vesicle with a shared volume. As summarized in TABLE 1, different contributions of synexin to each of these two rates could be discerned at different weight ratios of synexin/ghost. For example, at a low ratio of synexin/ghost (e.g., 0.13), the aggregation rate constant was 4×10^8 $M^{-1}sec^{-1}$, whereas the rate constant for fusion was 1 sec^{-1}. Nir et al.[26] commented that this fusion rate constant was "among the largest reported for vesicle fusion . . . or for virus-liposome fusion."

Moreover, as shown in TABLE 1, an increase in the ratio of synexin/ghost to 0.41 caused an eightfold elevation in the aggregation rate constant to 3.2×10^9 $M^{-1}sec^{-1}$ while increasing the fusion rate constant by ca. 30 percent. Under these conditions Nir et al.[26] observed that the rate constant for aggregation was already close to the diffusion limit, that is, approximately ca. 5×10^9 $M^{-1}sec^{-1}$ (ref. 27; and see footnote c for details on this calculation). Thus, the contributions that synexin makes to the fusion process are not only that it affects the fusion rate, per se, but perhaps more importantly, that it also eliminates the potential energy barrier, otherwise theoretically preventing the close approach of ghost membranes that are destined to fuse. Thus, in this biologically based fusion process there appears to be no need for additional energy to surmount the barrier. We view this phenomenon as reminiscent of the contributions other types of proteins (e.g., enzymes) make to catalysis of reactions that are otherwise kinetically unfavorable.

At an even higher synexin/ghost ratio (e.g., 1.15), Nir et al.[26] observed that the aggregation rate constant was not further elevated, but that the fusion rate constant

---

[c]The first approximation for a diffusion-limited bimolecular rate constant is given by the Smoluchowski equation: $k_s = 4\pi \ Dr_0N_0 \times 10^{-3}$, where D and r_0 are the sum of the diffusion constants and radii of the reacting species, respectively, and N_0 is Avogadro's number. The factor 10^{-3} serves to convert k_s to units of $M^{-1}s^{-1}$ when cgs units are used for D and r_0. If we assume that the ghosts are spheres of equal radii a, and that the friction constant is given by Stokes law, then $D = 2kT/6\pi\eta a$ and $k_s = (8kT/3\eta) \ N_0 \times 10^{-3}$, where k is Boltzmann constant, T is temperature, and η is viscosity of the solvent. Inserting the value $\eta = 0.0069$ p for water at 307K leads to $k_s = 9.9 \times 10^9 M^{-1}sec^{-1}$. This is an upper limit, as we have assumed that the particles are hard spheres and that all collisions are reactive.

was decreased 5–10-fold. While no mechanism for this effect is yet apparent, the data indicate that synexin appears to be able either to increase or to decrease the fusion rate constant, somewhat independently of how it affects the aggregation rate constant.

Finally, the experiments by Nir *et al.*[26] with synexin and granule ghosts clearly distinguished the more rapid process of membrane mixing from that of the slower process of volume mixing, which marks authentic fusion. As shown in TABLE 1, the fusion rate constant deduced by measuring membrane mixing by octadecyl-rhodamine dequenching was ≥ 10-fold greater (≥ 10 sec^{-1}) than that measured by volume mixing (1 sec^{-1}) at the same synexin/ghost ratio. Nir *et al.*[26] cautioned that at least two synexin-mediated processes could be responsible for the higher membrane-mixing rate, including not only hemifusion, but also exchange of the probe between otherwise closely apposed membranes. It is therefore our contention that a complete explanation for synexin action in the membrane fusion process should also address the mechanism and meaning of the more rapid and apparently coincident membrane-mixing event.

TABLE 1. Rate Constants Describing Aggregation and Fusion of Chromaffin Granule Ghosts by Synexin[26]

Fusion Assay	Synexin/Ghost Ratio (W/W)	Aggregation Rate Constant ($M^{-1}sec^{-1}$)	Fusion Rate Constant (sec^{-1})
Volume-mixing	0.13	4×10^8	1.0
	0.41	3.2×10^9	1.3
	1.15	$2-4 \times 10^9$	0.1–0.3
Membrane-mixing	0.41	5×10^9	≥ 10

BIOPHYSICAL EVIDENCE THAT SYNEXIN ENTERS AND SPANS TARGET MEMBRANES

Most informative from a mechanistic viewpoint has been our observation that calcium-activated synexin can raise the capacitance of phospholipid bilayers and natural membranes and therein exhibit capacitative transients.[28] This result indicates that synexin dipoles can be inserted into the bilayer interior. Consistently, calcium-activated synexin was found to raise the surface pressure of phosphatidylserine (PS) monolayers, as calculated here from surface tension data in reference 29. In addition, calcium-activated synexin preferentially adhered to the air/PS interface, as determined from measurements of 45-[Ca] recruited to the interface in synexin-bound form.[29] Moreover, we subsequently observed that synexin could also support specific and selective calcium channel activity across the same membranes in which we had detected the capacitance transients.[30] It would thus appear that these capacitative transients could well be "gating currents" for the synexin channels, by analogy with equivalent results from studies on sodium channels.[31,32]

We have previously interpreted these data to mean that in the presence of calcium, synexin not only enters the membrane, but also spans the membrane. Furthermore, once within the membrane, synexin molecules can also move within the membrane in response to the electric field. Our conclusion from these studies has

```
      S: MSYFGYPPTGYPPPFGYPPAGQESSFPPSGQYPYPSGFPPHGGGAYPQVPSSGYPGAGGYP
         APGGYPAPGGYPGAPQPGGAPSYPGVPPGQGFGVPPGGAGFSGYPQPPSQSYGGGPAQVP
                                         *
         LPGGFPGGQMPSQYPGGQPTYPSQPATVTQVTQGTIRPAANFDAIR
 E2:                                 KAQVLRGTVTDFFGFDERA
 L1: MAMVSEFLKQAWFIENEEQEYVQTVKSSKGGPGSAVSPYPTFNPSS
 C1:     MSTVHEILCKLSLEGDHSTPPSAYGSVKAYINFDAER
 P2:                               AAKGGVKAASGFNAAE
  c:                            MAKPAQGAKYRGSIHDFFGFDPNQ
```

AMINO TERMINAL DOMAIN

```
      *    *    * * *   *      *    ***        *  **   *
   S: DAEILRKAMKGFGTDEQAIVDVVANRSNDQRQKIKAAFKTSYGKDLIKDLKSELSGNMEELILALFMPPTYY
 E2:    T      L   ES LTLLTS   A   E S    LF R LD    T KF K   V  MK SRL
 L1: VAA H   IMVK V  AD I LLTK N A    Q      LQET   P LET  KA T HL  VV    LKT AQF
 C1: LNIET I TK V  VD  NLLT    A   D AF YQRRTK E ASA   A   HL TV  G LKT AQ
 P2: QT      L    D IS L Y   TA    E RT Y STI R  LD         F QV  GMMT TVL
 c1:   A YT      S KE  L IITS   R   EVCQSY SL    A     Y T KF R  VG MR  A C
 c5: KA         L   DT I IITH    V    Q RQT  SHF R  MT       I  DLAR   G M   AH
```

FIRST REPEAT

```
      *       * *** *  *  *  **     **        *     *        ***       *
   S: DAWSLRKAMQGAGTQERVLIEILCTRTNQEIREIVRCYQSEFGRDLEKDIRSGTSGHFERLLVSMCQGNRDENQSINHQMAQE
 E2: YE KH LK    N K T  IAS   PE L A KQV EE Y SS  D VVG    YYQ M  VLL A   PDAG DEAQVEQ
 L1: DE  A  KL  D DT      AS   K  D N V RE LK   A  T     D RNA L LAK D S  DFGV  EDL DS
 C1: SE KAS K L  D DS     I S     LQ  N V KEMYKT       I      D RK M ALAK R A  DG VIDYELIDQ
 P2: VQE  R       D GC     S  PE   R NQT  LQY  S  D       FM Q V   LSA G   GNYLDDALVRQ
 c2: KEIKD IS I  D KC     AS    EQMHQL AA KDAYE    A  IG      QKM  VLL  T E  DDVVSEDLV Q
 c6: KQ K  E     D KA     A    A  NEA KEDYHKS   DALS         R I I LAT H E  GGENLD AREDAQVAA
```

SECOND REPEAT

```
                                  *       *                *  *
   S: DAQRLYQAGEGRLGTDESCFNMILATRSFPQLRATMEAYSRMANRDLLSSVSREFSGYVESGLKTILQCALNRPAFF
 E2:   A F    LKW     EK IT FG    VSH  KVFDK MTISGFQIEETID  T  NL QL LAVVKSIRS I   YL
 L1: RA  E    R K    VNV T  T    Y     RVFQK TKYSKH MNKVLDL LK DI KC TA VK  TSK A
 C1: RD  D  VK K     VPKWIS MTE  V H QKVFDR KSYSPY M E IRK VK DL NAFLNLV  IQ K LY
 P2:   D E    KKW    VK LTV CS NRNH   HVFDE K ISQK IEQ IKS T  SF DA LA VKCMR KS Y
 c3: V D  E   LKW     AQ IY  GN  KQH   LVFDE LKTTGKPMKA IRG L  DF KLMLAVVK IRST EY
 c7: EILELADTPS DKTSL TR MT   C  TY H   RVFQEFIK T Y VEHTIKK M  D RDAFVA V SVK K L
```

THIRD REPEAT

```
      *  *   *** ** *    *                          *  *
   S: AERLYYAMKGAGTDDSTLVRIVVTRSEIDLVQIKQMFAQMYQKTLGTMIAGUTSGDYRRLLLAIVGQ
 E2:    T         H I VM S      FN RKE RKNFATS YS  K      KKA  LLC EDD
 L1:   K HQ     V  RHKA I  M S    MND  AFYQK  GIS CQA LDE K    EKI V LC GN
 C1:  D   DS    K  R KV I  M S    V MLK RSE KRK G S YYY QQ  K   QKA  YLC GDD
 P2:    KS     L  N I VM S A    MMD RAN KRL G S YSF K        KV  ILC GDD
 c4:    FK     L  R N  I  M S    L MLD REI RTK E S YS  KN    E  KKT  KLS GDD
 c8: DK  KS       EK  T  M S     LN RRE IEK D S HQA E       FLKA  LC GED
```

FOURTH REPEAT

FIGURE 1. Comparison of the amino acid sequence of human synexin with homologous annexins. S is synexin (annexin VII); E2 is endonexin II (annexin V); L1 is lipocortin 1 (annexin I); C1 is calpactin 1, heavy chain (annexin II); and C is calelectrin 67K (annexin VI).[34] Horizontal lines show regions of high homology. Asterisk marks highly conserved residues. Spaces denote sequence identity with synexin.

been that the fusion activity intrinsic to synexin might be mediated by these physical properties. As a specific example, we have recently advanced the hypothesis that synexin might initiate fusion by forming a hydrophobic bridge between fusing membranes, across which phospholipids could cross and mix.[33] Further evidence supporting this hypothesis has been accumulated in the interim, as will be made evident in succeeding parts of this chapter.

SYNEXIN IS A MEMBER OF THE ANNEXIN GENE FAMILY

Our understanding of the structural basis for both channel and membrane fusion activity has been greatly illuminated by recent studies on the molecular biology of synexin.[34] As shown in FIGURE 1, cloning and sequencing studies revealed that synexin was homologous with a family of calcium/phospholipid binding proteins, presently termed the "annexins." Each of these proteins has a unique N-terminal domain, but all share a homologous C-terminal tetrad (or octad in one case) repeat. The C-terminal tetrad is composed of four segments of *ca.* 70 amino acids each, comprising about 32,000 kDa in mass. The N-terminal of synexin is an unusually large (16,700 kDa) and highly hydrophobic sequence composed primarily of proline and glycine, (which are common in beta turns and coils); phenylalanine, tyrosine, and alanine (all hydrophobic); and glutamine. By contrast, the other annexins have much smaller N-terminal domains, one of the smallest being endonexin II, with only 19, mostly hydrophilic, residues. In endonexin II, 30% (6 of 19 amino acids) are in fact identical to those shared with synexin in this proximal 19-residue segment.

One step in understanding the structural basis of the channel activity was our realization that a low resolution, two-dimensional model of the channel could be constructed directly from the hydrophobicity plot. For this purpose we created a box of the four segments of the horizontal axis of the hydrophobicity plot corresponding to the four repeats, respectively. We then placed contiguous hydrophobic sequences on the outer edge of the box and continguous hydrophilic sequences on the inside. Indeed, the structure of the hydrophobicity plot made this a simple maneuver. This view "down the mouth" of the channel proved useful in constructing site-directed mutants and in predicting the results of new experiments. One of these new experiments is described in the next section.

EVIDENCE THAT THE C-TERMINAL DOMAIN OF SYNEXIN IS THE LOCUS OF THE CHANNEL

An important assumption in the preceding analysis was that the C-terminal domain was the locus of the channel activity. In principle, it was just as possible that the hydrophobic N-terminal domain could have been responsible for the channel activity. When we subjected native and recombinant forms of the annexin homologue endonexin II to the same studies as those described above for synexin, however, we found similar calcium channel activity.[35] An example is shown in FIGURE 2. In distinction to synexin, endonexin II channels were somewhat less selective, much like the calcium-release channels from the sarcoplasmic reticulum. By way of further contrast to synexin, endonexin II was incapable of inducing aggregation or fusion of chromaffin granule or phosphatidylserine liposomes. Thus the conclusion is inescapable that the C-terminal domain is likely to be the material basis of the channel.

In FIGURE 3 we show a two-dimensional hydrophobic plot for endonexin II, which is equivalent to that for synexin in FIGURE 4. From FIGURE 3 we note that many charged residues are conserved, especially in the mouth of the channel, and

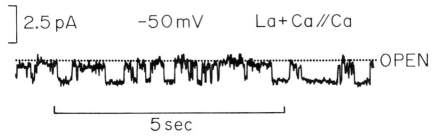

FIGURE 2. Single endonexin II channel currents. The membrane was formed at the tip of a patch pipet from a phosphatidylinositol monolayer. The chamber and pipet contained 50 mM $CaCl_2$ and 10 mM Cs-Hepes, pH 7.4. $LaCl_3$ (0.6 mM) was added to the bath (chamber) to block some of the channels. The pipet voltage was −50 mV, and the positive current is flowing into the pipet.[35]

that, in common with synexin, each repeat has four or five "loops" of residues that cross or touch the axis. Consistently, we also found that endonexin II, like synexin, could increase the surface pressure of a PS monolayer (see FIG. 5). Taken together, the channel and surface-tension data appear to indicate that the C-terminal domains in both synexin and endonexin II can penetrate the bilayer and displace phospholipids.

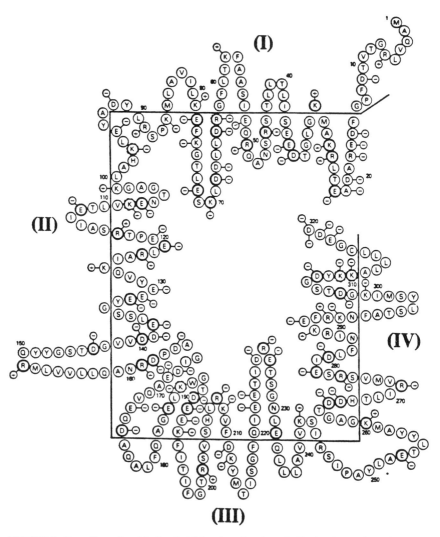

FIGURE 3. Two-dimensional hydrophobicity plot of endonexin II, showing a view "down the mouth" of the channel. Details of the construction and properties are as described for synexin in FIG. 4. Heavily marked circles represent conserved, charged residues. Intermittent, heavily marked circles represent residues in which arginine (R) is replaced by lysine (K), or vice-versa. This only occurs six times, and only one anionic residue exchange (*e.g.,* E for D) occurs in Repeat III.[35]

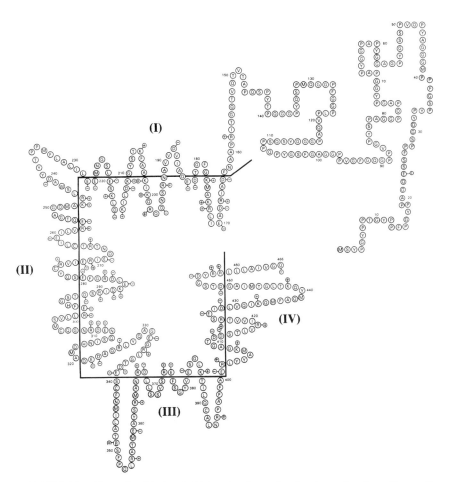

FIGURE 4. Two-dimensional hydrophobicity plot of synexin, showing a view down the mouth of the channel. The "exterior" of the box is exposed to the lipid domain, parallel to the plane of the paper. The numerals, **I–IV**, represent the tetrad repeats. The lengthy hydrophobic N-terminal domain is represented by the segment outside the box. The charged amino acids are clustered in the center with a negative net charge, suitable for attracting cations and repelling anions.[34]

A "TIM BARREL" MODEL FOR SYNEXIN CHANNELS

Our initial examination of the predicted secondary structure of synexin had failed to delineate the hydrophobic transmembrane alpha helices characteristic of membrane-resident channels.[34] A similar problem presented itself when we attempted such an analysis on endonexin II.[35] Indeed, this problem had led us to the temporary expedient of the two-dimensional plots in FIGURES 3 and 4. Using a homology-based search for potential alpha-helical regions, however, and justifying the choices with the Delphi program, we were able to define five segments (A–E) in each repeat that could form alpha helices.[36] The same secondary-structure prediction had been made previously by Taylor and Geisow[37] using similar methods. Furthermore, these predictions have been confirmed only recently in X-ray crystallographic studies of annexin V (endonexin II), on what we believe to be the water-soluble form.[38] In our own studies we noted that the segments between A and B (S_1) and between D and E (S_2) were highly conserved and contained negatively charged residues.

Recent work by Guy and Conti,[39] in an analysis of the activation mechanism and ion selectivity of voltage-gated channels, had proposed a characteristic motif for these processes involving a transmembrane cylinder of hydrophobic alpha helices surrounding an eight-stranded beta barrel. These enclosed beta strands had negative charges. An ensuing comparison revealed similarities between putative structures defining selectivity in these bona fide membrane resident channels and those available in synexin.

The model we favor presently is shown in FIGURE 6, in which S_1 and S_2 are beta strands, assembled to form an eight-stranded beta barrel that is surrounded by the more hydrophobic B and E helices. Such a structure is termed a TIM barrel, after the prototypic structure found in the glycolytic enzyme *tri*osephosphate *isom*erase. The view is from the *cis* or cytosolic face of the inserted synexin, down the center of the barrel, into the patch pipet. The N-terminal and C-terminal residues are oriented towards the aqueous phase, but the N-terminal domain of synexin is not included in the model. Macroscopically, the structure of the C-terminal channel domain is that of a "hollow screw," in which the head of the screw, formed by the A, C, and D helices of each of the four covalently linked repeats, is deeply buried in the *cis* monolayer. The TIM barrel spans the *trans* monolayer of the membrane.

The critical elements of this model include hydrophobic external domains for interaction with lipids in the membrane; a highly conserved, negatively charged interior channel for conduction of cations; an asymmetric orientation in the membrane, consistent with the voltage-dependent character of the channel activity; and structural characteristics to be discussed below that suit our present understanding of how synexin (or other structural homologues) might promote fusion processes.

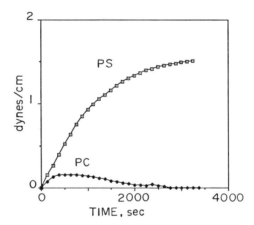

FIGURE 5. Endonexin II decreases the surface tension (makes the surface pressure less negative) of a phosphatidylserine (PS) monolayer in the presence of calcium. Endonexin II (18 μg in a 5 μL aliquot) was diluted into 20 mL of equilibrated hypophase buffer and observed to cause a reduction in the surface tension, as estimated by the Wilhelmy plate method. The total decrease was *ca.* 2 dyne/cm. Virtually no change was observed when a phosphatidylcholine (PC) monolayer was used as the target monolayer instead of PS.

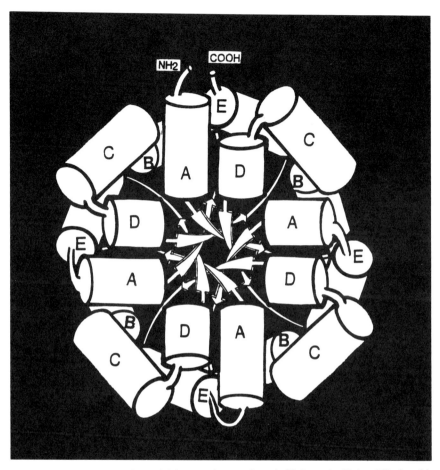

FIGURE 6. A "TIM barrel" model for synexin or endonexin II channels. Hydrophilic (amphipathic) A, C, and D helices displace lipids in the *cis* monolayer. The segments S1 (between A and B helices) and S2 (between D and E helices) form beta strands that assemble to form an 8-stranded beta barrel. The barrel is surrounded by the hydrophobic B and E helices, and the entire barrel structure penetrates the *trans* leaflet. In general, the view is down the shaft of a "hollow screw," in which the head is made up of the A, C, and D helices and the shaft is made up of the TIM barrel.

CALCIUM CAUSES A CONFORMATIONAL CHANGE IN SYNEXIN, WHICH PERMITS SUBSEQUENT INSERTION OF THE PROTEIN INTO THE TARGET MEMBRANE

As an approach to understanding how synexin promotes membrane fusion, we first consider how synexin might approach, contact, and insert into one membrane. We know this occurs because of our experiments with channel formation in bilayers at the tip of a patch pipet. A substantial body of experiments on both synexin and other annexins[40] indicates that upon binding calcium the proteins undergo a confor-

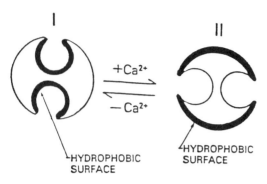

FIGURE 7. A two-dimensional model for a conformational transition in synexin mediated by calcium. In the presence of calcium, hydrophobic surfaces, previously cryptic, become exposed. This allows more facile interactions between protein and membrane. The solid lines represent hydrophobic regions, whereas the thin lines represent hydrophilic regions.[33]

mational transition. For the case of synexin this transition changes the protein from a water-soluble conformation state to a more hydrophobic, less water-soluble conformation.[21]

To help us in our analysis of the ramifications of this process we have characterized this transition in the simplified two-dimensional diagram shown in FIGURE 7. The heavily shaded surfaces represent hydrophobic regions, shielded from water in the absence of calcium (I), or exposed to water in the presence of calcium (II). We presume that the hydrophobic regions eventually allow synexin to reside within the low dielectric interior of the bilayer. The thinly lined surfaces represent hydrophilic regions, perhaps responsible for solubility in water at low ambient calcium levels, recognition of acidic phospholipid headgroups, or involvement in channel function. We have not included any surface area proportional to the N-terminal domain, because the C-terminal tetrad repeat (ca. 32 kDa) is apparently sufficient for contact and insertion. Furthermore, although we now believe the structure of synexin to be highly asymmetric within the membrane, as defined by the preceding TIM barrel model, this structural distinction is not necessary for the more general purposes of the forthcoming analysis.

In brief, we presume that inasmuch as synexin (and other annexins) are highly selective for acidic phospholipids, the initial interactive step must include specific contact between the calcium-activated synexin and the phospholipid headgroup. The next step must involve insertion of the activated synexin molecule(s) into the membrane. The mechanism and anticipated kinetics of this process, however, must depend on the state and disposition of the lipids. For example, the phospholipids could be arrayed in a rigidly ordered structure, with minimum allowed deviation from the orientation perpendicular to the bilayer normal. In that case, induced changes in such a structure might indeed be energetically costly (*e.g.,* see concerns in reference 41). Although more rigidly ordered phospholipid bilayers can occur, however, as in the L_β form occurring at low temperature and low water content,[42] the situation under biologically relevant conditions is quite different. It is this more fluid L_α form that we shall use for the development of our model, and upon which we shall briefly dwell before proceding to a further consideration of the synexin insertion process.

AN ANALYSIS OF EXPERIMENT AND COMPUTER SIMULATION SHOWS THAT THE MEMBRANE INTERIOR IS HIGHLY DISORDERED

Since the introduction of the fluid mosaic model for membranes by Singer and Nicholson in 1972, it has been widely understood that phospholipids in bilayers are engaged in a variety of high frequency changes in state. These states are summarized in TABLE 2, along with their associated parameters. Here we discuss some of the equilibrium properties of the bilayer, and in the following sections consider dynamical details.

Perhaps one of the best views of the average structure of a phospholipid bilayer can be derived from a consideration of the deuterium order parameter, S_{CD} (TABLE 2 and reference 43). This parameter is a measure of the average orientation of the methylene groups within the bilayer. The value of the deuterium order parameter is given by the equation, $S_{CD} = \frac{1}{2} \langle 3\cos^2\theta - 1 \rangle$, where θ is the angle between the vector along the C-D bond and the bilayer normal. The importance of this equation is that if the average vector described by the hydrocarbon chains were exclusively perpendicular to the bilayer normal, the value of $\cos\theta$ would be 0 and the value of S_{CD} would therefore be -0.5. By contrast, if the chains were randomly oriented, S_{CD} would be 0. Experimentally, the value of S_{CD} falls between -0.1 and -0.2 for both purified phospholipids and a variety of biological membranes.[44] The physical basis for such a result is that although the hydrocarbon chains are rapidly isomerizing, the phospholipid molecules are both rotating in the plane of the membrane and processing, "as if wobbling in a cone."[45]

The length distributions of the chains in the membrane, as measured by neutron diffraction,[42] are consistent with the high degree of freedom manifested by the deuterium order parameter. For example, consider the distance between carbonyl carbons of the acyl chains on opposite sides of the bilayer; this distance, denoted $d(C_1 - C'_1)$, is basically the width of the "pure hydrophobic" membrane interior. If the chains of a dipalmitylphosphatidylcholine (DPPC) molecule were fully extended (*i.e.*, all *trans*) and parallel to the bilayer normal (as in the L_β phase), then $d(C_1 - C'_1)$ would be approximately 40 Å. An analysis of simulation[45-47] and experiment,[42] however, indicates this distance is 28–30 Å. The surface area per lipid is also 65–70 Å^2,[46,48] which is consistent with the notion that the density of the membrane interior is comparable to neat hexadecane.

Unfortunately, the development of a more detailed physical picture of the bilayer interior has been hampered by the significant model dependence associated with the interpretation of most experiments. Certainly, molecular dynamics simulations[49,50] can provide a valuable compliment to experimental data. The application of computer simulations to phospholipid bilayers, however, is a relatively new enterprise, and many of the results are best considered preliminary. Essentially, multinanosecond trajectories are required to simulate the relevant motions (cf. TABLE 2), whereas even on supercomputers, trajectories of only several hundred picoseconds are possible using the traditional deterministic equations. Of course, this is not suitable for consideration of possible mechanisms of membrane fusion, because in what may be the most rapidly known system, the squid giant synapse, fusion may occur in *ca.* 200 microseconds.[51] Even longer times are required in other fusion systems (ms-s). In

TABLE 2. Equilibrium and Dynamic Properties of Phospholipids in Bilayers

Property	Value	Reference
Gauche-to-*trans* isomerization	2×10^{10}/s	47
Trans-to-*gauche* isomerization	4×10^9/s	47
Rotational diffusion constant	10^8-10^{10}/s	57–59
Translational diffusion constant	10^{-8} cm^2/s	60
Collective motions	10^3-10^0/s	59
Deuterium NMR order parameter	*ca.* $-$ 0.2	42,52

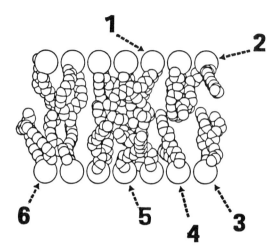

FIGURE 8. A space-filling simulation of a phospholipid bilayer composed of 14 phospholipids. Individual conformations are randomly chosen from among 30,000 structures generated over a 160 nanosecond time interval at 37°C. Some phospholipids are numbered to indicate those that appear to deviate particularly from the orientation perpendicular to the bilayer normal.

fact, detailed dynamic information is needed over these longer time scales to help decide whether possible models have kinetic or steric validity.

Recently, Pastor et al.[45–47] have developed a simulation strategy based on stochastic methods. Only a small part of the complete system is explicitly simulated, and the effect of the remainder is parametrized by random forces (with distributions related to the solvent viscosity) and an average orienting potential (similar to ones used in the theory of liquid crystals). With this approach, simulations can be carried out to the required 100 nanosecond time scale. The most attractive aspect of these studies is that they give an excellent fit when compared with the experimental results on DPPC as discussed above. Specifically, the simulations are consistent with the deuterium order parameters obtained by Seelig and Seelig,[44,52] with the T_1 spin lattice relaxation times of Brown and co-workers,[53] and the length distributions from Zaccai et al.[42]

An analysis of the simulations, both in Pastor et al.[45–47] and in DeLoof et al.,[54] reveals the liquid-like nature of the bilayer interior, as well as details that would be impossible to discern from experiment alone. For example, the terminal methylene groups are found to spend a significant time close to the aqueous interface, either because the entire chain moves close to the surface, or because the distal methyl group looks back to the headgroup. To illustrate these concepts we refer to FIGURE 8, which shows a space-filling representation of a section (or slice) of bilayer composed of 14 phospholipids. Each conformation pictured was randomly chosen from the 30,000 different conformations generated in a 160 ns time interval at 37°C and was packed into an 84 lipid assembly in a manner consistent with experiment. In the FIGURE, a few lipids are marked with numbers to indicate conformations in which the hydrocarbon chains deviate particularly from the orientation perpendicular to the bilayer. In short, biological membranes have a "high degree of chain disorder and entanglement."[45]

SYNEXIN INSERTION INTO MEMBRANES MAY TAKE ADVANTAGE OF NATURALLY OCCURRING MEMBRANE DISORDER IN THE SUBMICROSECOND TIME RANGE

As indicated in the preceding section, an enormous array of conformations is available to phospholipids in the subnanosecond to submicrosecond time domains.

Such rapid processes are of interest because of our ultimate goal of understanding the fusion process. Accordingly, in the short term, our approach to the problem of how synexin might further interact with membranes has been to place mechanistic significance on the frequent excursions of hydrocarbon chains to the vicinity of the bilayer surface.

Specifically, our strategy has been to presume that the calcium-activated synexin molecule (FIG. 7, state II) first finds an acidic phospholipid headgroup on a target membrane of choice. This is shown in FIGURE 9, panel I. From this model it is apparent that mere adherence of the synexin molecule to a charged phospholipid headgroup may also bring hydrophobic domains of synexin into close association with the membrane surface. Thus for association to occur between the protein and some hydrocarbon chains, the protein need not force itself into the membrane, nor need the protein extract a phospholipid from the membrane interior. These would presumably be energetically unfavorable processes. Instead, the protein merely waits over the submicrosecond time domain for an appropriately oriented hydrocarbon chain to diffuse to the protein surface.

The next step in movement of the protein into the membrane is depicted in panel II of FIGURE 9. In this case, some phospholipids, with orientations essentially exactly

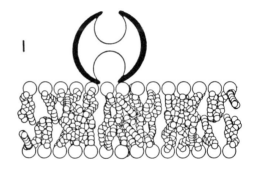

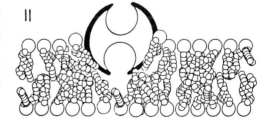

FIGURE 9. Penetration of a calcium-activated synexin molecule into a bilayer. **I.** Synexin molecule binds to an acidic phospholipid headgroup on the membrane. **II.** Synexin waits over a subnanosecond time period for phospholipid hydrocarbon chains on the *cis* leaflet to occur in an appropriate conformation for interaction. **III.** Synexin waits for appropriate conformations to occur on the *trans* leaflet, thereby completing its transfer into a transmembrane state.

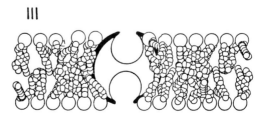

as occurring in the model bilayer, become juxtaposed to hydrophobic surfaces of the synexin molecule. The result is that the synexin molecule sinks into the bilayer, driven by the entropic hydrophobic forces and moving other phospholipids to peripheral positions. Indeed, both synexin and endonexin II (see FIG. 5) experimentally increase the surface pressure of acidic phospholipid monolayers, as predicted by this mechanism. Finally, the synexin molecule completes passage into the membrane, using naturally occurring nanosecond conformations of phospholipids on the *trans* leaflet as the steric pathway to its destined transmembrane state (panel III, FIG. 9). Thus, entry of a synexin molecule into a single membrane, as might occur during a channel experiment, would be very fast, compared with the relatively slow pace of known fusion processes. Perhaps relevant to this conclusion is the observation by Nir *et al.*,[26] described in an earlier section, in which under optimal conditions, membrane aggregation mediated by synexin was found to be an essentially diffusion limited process.

SYNEXIN-DRIVEN MEMBRANE FUSION MAY OCCUR BY SIMULTANEOUS PENETRATION INTO TWO MEMBRANES AND THE FORMATION OF A HYDROPHOBIC BRIDGE BETWEEN FUSION PARTNERS

At first glance, one possibility for driving fusion might be to let a synexin monomer bind to and penetrate two adjacent membranes, using the same mechanisms described for penetration into one membrane. An example of this possibility is shown in FIGURE 10. From the figure, however, it is apparent that the only result might be membrane mixing. Furthermore, if the asymmetric TIM barrel model of synexin were correct, in the sense that synexin interacts with membranes in an asymmetric manner, such an interaction might not even be possible. Indeed, endonexin II, although forming channels in bilayers, does not provoke membrane aggregation or fusion in either chromaffin granules or LUV PS liposomes. Perhaps coincidentally, endonexin II is not reported to form polymers when exposed to calcium.

Once calcium is added to synexin, however, the molecule polymerizes into cigar-shaped structures, 100 Å long by 50 Å wide, with cylindrical cross-sections.[21] The structure is likely to be a dimer and corresponds to state III in FIGURE 11. Immediately thereafter, the dimers form side-by-side associations, much like cigars in a cigar box. The negatively stained image obtained by electron-microscopy[21] is illustrated in FIGURE 11 (part IV). The driving force for formation of these structures is hydrophobic, because they depolymerize when the dielectric constant of the medium is lowered.

A single dimer could indeed simultaneously penetrate into two bilayers, and membrane mixing might ensue. An example of this process is shown in FIGURE 12. True fusion (*i.e.,* volume mixing), however, would be difficult to accomplish using the strategy described above. In passing we might note that recent work from our laboratory (Lee, de la Fuente, and Pollard, this volume and ref. 55) shows that a calcium-binding protein from bovine lung, sharing homology with lipocortin I (G 36), promotes only hemifusion of PS liposomes.

A synexin polymer, however, with at least four subunits, could promote a true fusion event, by a mechanism that we have previously called the hydrophobic bridge hypothesis.[29,33] The present version of this hypothesis is depicted in FIGURE 13. Briefly, we envision that synexin tetramers bind to phospholipids on two juxtaposed membranes (FIG. 13, stage 1) and that phospholipids cross over the hydrophobic bridge provided by the synexin polymer, using conformations naturally available over the submicrosecond time domain. This membrane-mixing step involving the *cis* leaflets may correspond to the rapid membrane-mixing rate constant described in TABLE 2. Synexin molecules are now surrounded by phospholipids and, in the absence of a hydrophobic driving force, dissociate. This exposes hydrophobic surfaces in the synexin molecules, which then provide an armature for expansion of the

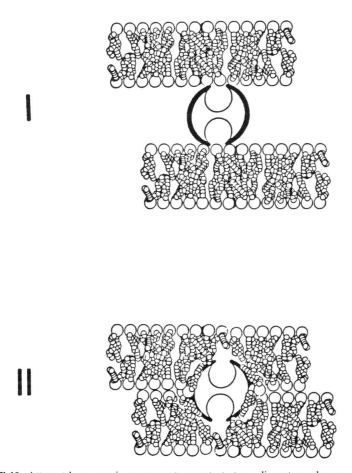

FIGURE 10. Attempt by a synexin monomer to penetrate two adjacent membranes simultaneously. As shown, this does not lead to fusion. Furthermore, if the TIM barrel model is correct, and insertion is asymmetric, this may be impossible.

phospholipids on the *trans* leaflets and complete fusion. This volume-mixing step, involving contact between the *trans* leaflets, very likely corresponds to the event described by the relatively slower fusion rate constant in TABLE 1, obtained from volume-mixing experiments. From experimental observations we know this last step occurs; but whether it occurs exactly in the manner shown is yet to be learned. For example, the process clearly occurs in three dimensions, and more than two synexin dimers may be required.

THE APPROXIMATE TIME TAKEN FOR FUSION TO OCCUR BY THE HYDROPHOBIC BRIDGE HYPOTHESIS IS FOUR MICROSECONDS

We have previously noted how some of the equilibrium properties of lipid bilayers are consistent with the proposed model for membrane fusion. It is now useful to estimate the molecular time scales involved, using the results of both simulation and experiment. In this way we may learn what event is rate-limiting, or even exclude certain models because they require unphysically slow transitions.

Isomerizations are rapid even on the nanosecond time scale (see TABLE 2). In the following estimate it is assumed that isomerizations of neighboring dihedrals and

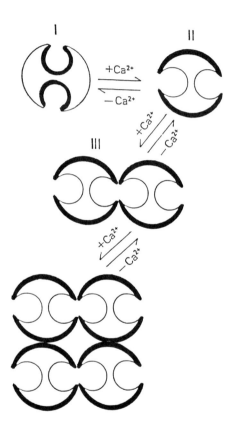

FIGURE 11. Synexin forms polymers when exposed to calcium. Upon exposure to calcium, the synexin molecules expose their hydrophobic regions and form dimers (state **II**). The dimers then polymerize into tetramers and subsequent three-dimensional arrays of such dimers.

chains are independent. We first define an average rate, k_{ave}, for an individual dihedral as

$$k_{\text{ave}} = 2\,k_{\text{gt}}p_{\text{g}} + k_{\text{tg}}p_{\text{t}},$$

where $p_{\text{g}} = \frac{1}{4}$ and $p_{\text{t}} = \frac{3}{4}$ are the approximate probabilities of *gauche* and *trans* conformations, respectively. (The factor of 2 in the *gauche*-to-*trans* rate, k_{gt}, takes $g_+ \to t$ and $g_- \to t$ into account.) From TABLE 1, then, we find that $k_{\text{ave}} = 13 \times 10^9$ ns^{-1}. The "waiting time" for a transition in a chain with 15 dihedral angles is $(15 \times k_{\text{ave}})^{-1}$

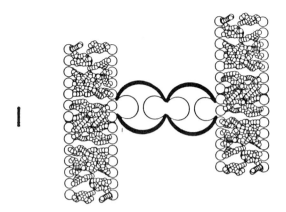

I

FIGURE 12. Attempt by synexin dimer to penetrate two adjacent membranes simultaneously and cause fusion. Membrane mixing can occur, as shown. Fusion involving volume mixing, however, is not evident.

II

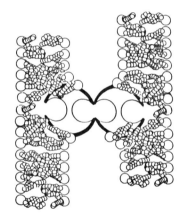

III

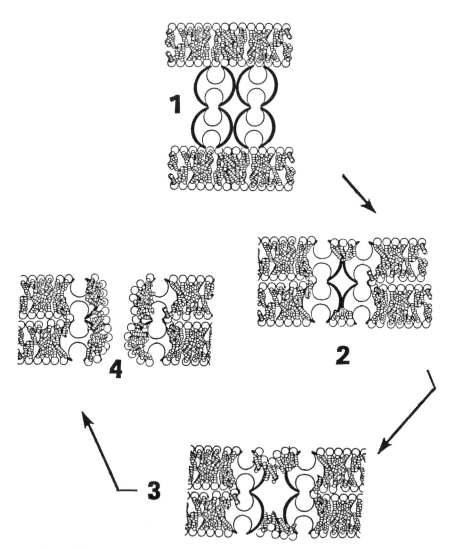

FIGURE 13. Hydrophobic bridge hypothesis for membrane fusion by synexin polymers. (**1**) Synexin tetramer binds to phospholipid headgroups on two adjacent membranes. (**2**) Phospholipids cross over the hydrophobic bridge using conformations available over the subnanosecond time domain. (**3**) Synexin polymer dissociates as hydrophobic forces driving polymerization disappear in the membrane interior. (**4**) Phospholipids migrate over the newly exposed hydrophobic synexin surface to complete the fusion process. The total distance traveled by phospholipids from the *trans* faces of the target membranes is *ca.* 40 Å, and occurs in *ca.* 4 microseconds. Details of the calculation are given in the text.

or *ca.* 5 picoseconds. Hence, in one nanosecond an average of 200 conformations are sampled for each chain. The time scale for "wobble" is several nanoseconds. This implies that a statistical distribution will result in the 100 ns to 1 μs time scale, at which point the chains are completely randomized.

With this information in hand we can now ask how long it might take for fusion to occur by the hydrophobic bridge hypothesis defined in FIGURE 13. From TABLE 2 we are reminded that translational diffusion is the slowest of the single molecule motions, and when we measure the longest distances over which phospholipids must move in this model, we find that lipids from the *trans* leaflet must diffuse a distance of approximately 40 Å. The time, Δt, required can be estimated from

$$\langle X^2 \rangle = 4 D \Delta t,$$

where D is the translational diffusion constant of the lipid. Letting $D = 10^{-8}$ cm²/s and $X = 40 \times 10^{-8}$ cm, $\Delta t = 4$ μs. Hence, all "single molecule" (as opposed to collective) events take place significantly faster than 100 microseconds. Inasmuch as the fastest known secretion process occurs in *ca.* 200 microseconds,[51] we can therefore conclude that the fusion event per se, taking only 4 microseconds, will not be a rate-limiting step.

SUMMARY AND CONCLUSIONS REGARDING THE ADVANTAGES OF THE HYDROPHOBIC BRIDGE HYPOTHESIS FOR MEMBRANE FUSION

The hydrophobic bridge hypothesis for the mechanism of synexin-driven membrane fusion has many advantages as an explanation for calcium-driven exocytotic fusion processes. First, there is the specificity for calcium, which was the basis for the discovery of synexin in the first place. To initiate secretion by a process depending on synexin, the cell need only allow calcium entry at the plasma membrane. Synexin molecules, soluble in the low calcium milieu of the resting cell, will then be available to bind calcium and form polymers with other activated synexin molecules. These activated synexin polymers are now able to bind to acidic phospholipids on either plasma membranes or chromaffin granule membranes, or both. According to this scenario, the location of a fusion event depends at the very least on a local increase in calcium concentration, availability of synexin molecules, and proximity of specific phospholipids.

The specificity of the synexin reaction for acidic phospholipids is also an advantage from the perspective of the biochemical asymmetry of phospholipids in most cells. In most cells, including chromaffin cells,[56] these phospholipids are localized to the cytosolic leaflets of plasma membranes. In chromaffin cells, specifically, the acidic phospholipids are also localized to the cytosolic leaflets of the chromaffin granule membranes. Thus, the specificity of synexin (and other annexins) for these specific lipids ensures that contacts could be generated either between granules and plasma membranes during simple exocytosis or between granules and other granule membranes during compound exocytosis.

A further advantage of the synexin mechanism for promoting membrane fusion is the favorable energetic considerations. In the resting cell, membranes seldom fuse. The reasons have been considered to include not only the repulsion forces between charged membrane surfaces, but also the space-occupying water molecules, which must be removed from between the membrane surfaces to permit close approach. In the case of synexin, however, these problems are circumvented. At least one profound contribution of the synexin molecule is to let contact between fusing membranes occur at a rate that is close to the diffusion limit.

We can best understand how synexin can circumvent the energetic barriers otherwise blocking membrane fusion in resting cells by appreciating that the hydrophobic bridge mechanism is consistent with the physical properties of membranes. In biological membranes under physiological conditions, the acyl chains are highly disoriented with respect to the bilayer plane. In fact, nonpolar CH_2 and distal CH_3 groups spend appreciable fractions of time close to the aqueous interface. These groups thereby provide local hydrophobic surfaces to which hydrophobic domains of calcium-activated synexin can adhere. Because the frequency of changes in conformation of phospholipids is well within the submicrosecond time domain, the synexin molecule need only wait over this time scale for adjacent phospholipids to present a favorable aspect for association.

Finally, an additional advantage of the hydrophobic bridge hypothesis is the time scale over which it permits synexin to engineer the fusion process. As calculated above, the model permits fusion to be accomplished in approximately four microseconds. The process is so rapid because the model allows smaller membrane lipids the opportunity to rapidly "lipidate" the larger protein molecule. This means that time is available for other regulatory processes to occur in the apparently minimum time interval of 200 μs, deduced from studies on the squid giant synapse.[51] Such processes might include calcium entry, binding of calcium to synexin (or other proteins), polymerization of synexin, and diffusion of activated synexin to target membranes. In this time interval other enzymatic or biophysical processes could also occur, such as those involving changes in cytoskeleton or activation of kinases.

In conclusion, it is our contention that the principle advantages of the synexin mechanism for exocytotic fusion include specificity with respect to regulating ligands, selectivity with respect to relevant phospholipids, favorable energetic considerations, consistency with the physical properties of biological membranes, and an appropriate time scale for catalyzing biological fusion processes. We can also point out at this juncture that although the synexin model has been constructed to explain the exocytotic fusion event, the principle behind the hydrophobic bridge hypothesis may be applicable to other types of membrane-fusion processes.

ACKNOWLEDGMENTS

The authors wish to thank Dr. Shlomo Nir and Dr. Ofer Eidelman for critical reviews of the manuscript, and Dr. Harry Haigler for the sample of endonexin II used to generate FIGURE 5.

REFERENCES

1. BLUMENTHAL, R. 1987. Membrane fusion. Curr. Top. Membr. Trans. **29:** 203–254.
2. WILSCHUT, J. 1988. Membrane interactions and fusion, *In* Energetics of the Secretion Response. J. W. N. Akkerman, Ed.: 63–80. CRC Press. Boca Raton, FL.
3. POLLARD, H. B., C. J. PAZOLES, C. E. CREUTZ & O. ZINDER. 1979. The chromaffin cell and possible mechanisms of exocytosis. Int. Rev. Cytol. **58:** 159–197.
4. POLLARD, H. B., C. E. CREUTZ, V. M. FOWLER, J. H. SCOTT & C. J. PAZOLES. 1982. Calcium-dependent regulation of chromaffin granule movement, membrane contact, and fusion during exocytosis. Cold Spring Harbor Symp. Quant. Biol. **46:** 819–834.
5. BROCKLEHURST, K. W. & H. B. POLLARD. 1988. Osmotic effects in membrane fusion during exocytosis. Curr. Top. Membr. Trans. **32:** 203–225.

6. POLLARD, H. B., C. J. PAZOLES, O. ZINDER & C. E. CREUTZ. 1984. An osmotic mechanism for exocytosis from dissociated chromaffin cells. J. Biol. Chem. **259:** 1114–1121.

7. STANLEY, E. F. & G. EHRENSTEIN. 1985. A model for exocytosis based on the opening of calcium-activated potassium channels in vesicles. Life Sci. **37:** 1985–1995.

8. FINKELSTEIN, A., J. ZIMMERBERG & F. S. COHEN. 1986. Osmotic swelling in vesicles: Its role in the fusion of vesicles with planar phospholipid bilayer membranes and its possible role in exocytosis. Annu. Rev. Physiol. **48:** 163–174.

9. KACHADORIAN, W. A., J. MULLER & A. FINKELSTEIN. 1981. Role of osmotic forces in exocytosis: Studies of ADH-induced fusion in toad urinary bladder. J. Cell Biol. **91:** 584–588.

10. PACE, C. S. & J. S. SMITH. 1983. The role of chemiosmotic lysis in the exocytotic release of insulin. Endocrinology **113:** 964–969.

11. ROSARIO, L. M., B. SORIA, G. FEUERSTEIN & H. B. POLLARD. 1989. Voltage-sensitive calcium flux into bovine chromaffin cells occurs through dihydropyridine-sensitive and dihydropyridine- and w-conotoxin-insensitive pathways. Neuroscience **29:** 735–747.

12. ZINDER, O., P. G. HOFFMAN, W. M. BONNER & H. B. POLLARD. 1978. Comparison of chemical properties of purified plasma membranes and secretory vesicle membranes from bovine adrenal medulla. Cell Tissue Res. **188:** 153–170.

13. BERNIER-VALENTIN, F., D. AUNIS & B. ROUSSET. 1983. Evidence for tubulin binding sites on cellular membranes: Plasma membranes, mitochondrial membranes and secretory granule membranes. J. Cell Biol. **97:** 209–216.

14. FOWLER, V. M. & H. B. POLLARD. 1982. Chromaffin granule membrane-F-actin interactions are calcium sensitive. Nature **295:** 336–339.

15. AUNIS, D. & D. PERRIN. 1984. Chromaffin granule membrane-F-actin interaction and spectrin-like protein of subcellular granules: a possible relationship. J. Neurochem. **42:** 1558–1569.

16. TRIFARO, J. M. & R. L. KOENIGSBERG. 1987. Chromaffin cell calmodulin. *In* Stimulus-Secretion Coupling in Chromaffin Cells. K. Rosenheck & P. I. Lelkes, Eds. CRC Press. Boca Raton, FL.

17. POLLARD, H. B., J. H. SCOTT & C. E. CREUTZ. 1983. Inhibition of synexin activity and exocytosis from chromaffin cells by phenothiazine drugs. Biochem. Biophys. Res. Commun. **113:** 908–915.

18. SUSSMAN, K. E., H. B. POLLARD, J. W. LIETNER, R. NESHER, J. ADLER & E. CERASI. 1983. Differential control of insulin secretion and somatostatin receptor recruitment in isolated islets. Biochem. J. **214:** 225–230.

19. POLLARD, H. B., A. L. BURNS & F. ROJAS. 1990. Synexin (annexin VII): a cytosolic calcium-binding protein which promotes membrane fusion and forms calcium channels in artificial bilayer and natural membranes. J. Membr. Biol. **117:** 101–112.

20. CREUTZ, C. E., C. J. PAZOLES & H. B. POLLARD. 1978. Identification and purification of an adrenal medullary protein (synexin) that causes calcium-dependent aggregation of chromaffin granules. J. Biol. Chem. **253:** 2858–2866.

21. CREUTZ, C. E., C. J. PAZOLES & H. B. POLLARD. 1979. Self-association of synexin in the presence of calcium: Correlation with synexin-induced membrane fusion and examination of the structure of synexin aggregates. J. Biol. Chem. **254:** 553–558.

22. PAPAHADJOPOULOS, D., S. NIR & N. DUZGUNES. 1990. Molecular mechanisms of calcium-induced membrane fusion. J. Bioenerg. Biomembr. **22:** 157–179.

23. STUTZIN, A. 1986. A fluorescence assay for monitoring and analyzing fusion of biological membranes *in vitro*. FEBS Lett. **197:** 274–280.

24. CREUTZ, C. E. 1981. Cis-unsaturated fatty acids induce the fusion of chromaffin granules aggregated by synexin. J. Cell Biol. **91:** 247–256.

25. CREUTZ, C. E. & H. B. POLLARD. 1982. A model for protein-lipid interactions during exocytosis: Aggregation and fusion of chromaffin granules in the presence of synexin and cis-unsaturated fatty acids. Biophys. J. **37:** 119–120.

26. NIR, S., A. STUTZIN, & H. B. POLLARD. 1987. Effect of synexin on aggregation and fusion of chromaffin granule ghosts at pH 6. Biochim. Biophys. Acta **903:** 309–318.

27. CANTOR, C. R. & P. R. SCHIMMEL. Biophysical Chemistry. Part III: The Behavior of Biological Macromolecules. WH Freeman and Co. San Francisco.

28. ROJAS, E. & H. B. POLLARD. 1987. Membrane capacity measurements suggest a calcium-dependent insertion of synexin into phosphatidylserine bilayers. FEBS Lett. **217:** 25–31.

29. POLLARD, H. B., E. ROJAS, A. L. BURNS & C. PARRA. 1988. Synexin, calcium and the hydrophobic bridge hypothesis for membrane fusion. *In* Molecular Mechanisms of Membrane Fusion. S. Ohki, D. Doyle, T. Flanagan, S. W. Hui & E. Mayhew, Eds.: 341–355. Plenum Press. New York.

30. POLLARD, H. B. & E. ROJAS. 1988. Calcium-activated synexin forms highly selective, voltage-gated channels in phosphatidylserine bilayer membranes. Proc. Natl. Acad. Sci. USA **85:** 2974–2978.

31. ROJAS, E. 1976. Gating mechanism for activation of the sodium conductance in nerve membranes. Cold Spring Harbor Symp. Quant. Biol. **XL:** 305–320.

32. ARMSTRONG, C. M. & F. BEZANILLA. 1976. Properties of the sodium channel gating current. Cold Spring Harbor Symp. Quant. Biol. **XL:** 297–304.

33. POLLARD, H. B., E. ROJAS & A. L. BURNS. 1987. Synexin and chromaffin granule membrane fusion: A novel "hydrophobic bridge" hypothesis for the driving and directing of the fusion process. Ann. N.Y. Acad. Sci. **493:** 524–541.

34. BURNS, A. L., K. MAGENDZO, A. SHIRVAN, M. ALIJANI, E. ROJAS & H. B. POLLARD. 1989. Calcium channel activity of purified human synexin and structure of the human synexin gene. Proc. Natl. Acad. Sci. USA **86:** 3798–3802.

35. ROJAS, E., H. B. POLLARD, H. HAIGLER, C. PARRA & A. L. BURNS. 1990. Calcium-activated endonexin II forms calcium channels across acidic phospholipid bilayer membranes. J. Biol. Chem. **265:** 21207–21215.

36. GUY, H. R., E. M. ROJAS, A. L. BURNS, E. ROJAS & H. B. POLLARD. 1991. A TIM barrel model of synexin channels. Biophys. J. **59:** 372a.

37. TAYLOR, W. R. & M. J. GEISOW. 1987. Predicted structure for the calcium-dependent membrane binding proteins, p35, p36 and p32. Protein Eng. **1:** 183–187.

38. HUBER, R., J. ROMISCH & E-P. PAQUES. 1990. The crystal and molecular structure of human annexin V, an anticoagulant protein that binds to calcium and membranes. EMBO J. **9:** 3867–3874.

39. GUY, H. R. & F. CONTI. 1990. Pursuing the structure and function of voltage-gated channels. Trends Neurosci. **13:** 201–206.

40. SMITH, V. L., M. A. KAETZEL & J. R. DEDMAN. 1990. Stimulus-response coupling: the search for intracellular calcium mediator proteins. Cell Regul. **1:** 165–172.

41. ALMERS, W. & F. W. TSE. 1990. Transmitter release from synapses: Does a preassembled fusion pore initiate exocytosis? Neuron **4:** 813–818.

42. ZACCAI, G., G. BULDT, A. SEELIG & J. SEELIG. 1979. Neutron diffraction studies on phosphatidylcholine model membranes. J. Mol. Biol. **134:** 693–706.

43. SEELIG, J. & P. M. MACDONALD. 1987. Phospholipids and proteins in biological membranes. ^{2}H-NMR as a method to study structure, dynamics and interactions. Acc. Chem. Res. **20:** 221–228.

44. SEELIG, J. & A. SEELIG. 1980. Lipid conformations in model membranes and biological membranes. Q. Rev. Biophys. **13:** 19–61.

45. PASTOR, R. W., R. M. VENABLE, M. KARPLUS & A. SZABO. 1988. A simulation based model of NMR T_1 relaxation in lipid bilayer vesicles. J. Chem. Phys. **89**(2): 1128–1140.

46. PASTOR, R. W., R. M. VENABLE & M. KARPLUS. 1990. A model for the structure of the lipid bilayer. Proc. Natl. Acad. Sci. USA. **88:** 892–896.

47. PASTOR, R. W. & R. M. VENABLE. 1988. Brownian dynamics simulation of a lipid chain in a membrane bilayer. J. Chem. Phys. **89**(2): 1112–1127.

48. RAND, R. P. & V. A. PARSEGIAN. 1989. Hydration forces between phospholipid bilayers. Biochem. Biophys. Acta. **998:** 351–376.

49. BROOKS, C. L., M. KARPLUS & B. M. PETTITT. 1988. Proteins: A Theoretical Perspective of Dynamics, Structure and Thermodynamics. Vol. LXXI. Wiley Series in Advances in Chemical Physics. I. Prigogine & S. Rice, Eds., Wiley Interscience. John Wiley and Sons. New York.

50. ALLEN, M. P. & D. J. TILDESLEY. 1987. Computer Simulation of Liquids. Clarendon Press. Oxford.

51. LLINÁS, R., I. Z. STEINBERG & K. WALTON. 1981. Relationship between presynaptic calcium current and postsynaptic potential in squid giant synapse. Biophys. J. **33:** 323–351.

52. SEELIG, A. & J. SEELIG. 1974. The dynamic structure of fatty acyl chains in a phospholipid bilayer measured by deuterium magnetic resonance. Biochemistry **23:** 4839–4845.

53. BROWN, M. F., A. A. RIBEIRO & G. D. WILLIAMS. 1983. New view of lipid bilayer dynamics from ^{2}H and ^{13}C NMR relaxation time measurements. Proc. Natl. Acad. Sci. USA **80:** 4325–4329.

54. DELOOF, H., S. C. HARVEY, J. P. SEGREST & R. W. PASTER. 1991. Mean field stochastic boundary molecular dynamics simulation of a phospholipid in a membrane. Biochemistry **30:** 2099–2113.

55. DE LA FUENTE, M., G. LEE & H. B. POLLARD. 1991. Induction of aggregation and hemifusion of acidic liposomes by a calcium or barium-dependent protein from bovine tissues. Biophys. J. **59:** 130a.

56. SCOTT, J. H., C. E. CREUTZ, H. B. POLLARD & R. O. ORNBERG. 1985. Synexin binds in a calcium dependent manner to oriented chromaffin cell plasma membranes. FEBS Lett. **180:** 17–23.

57. PETERSON, N. O. & S. I. CHAN. 1977. More on the motional state of lipid bilayer membranes: Interpretation of order parameters obtained from nuclear magnetic resonance experiments. Biochemistry **16:** 2657–2667.

58. SPEYER, J., R. WEBER, S. DAS GUPTA & R. GRIFFIN. 1989. Anisotropic ^{2}H NMR spin-lattice relaxation in L-(alpha) phase cerebroside bilayers. Biochemistry **28:** 9569–9574.

59. ROMMEL, E., F. NOACK, P. MEIER & G. KOTHE. 1988. Proton spin relaxation dispersion studies of phospholipid membranes. J. Phys. Chem. **92:** 2981–2987.

60. KIMMICH, R., G. SCHNUR & A. SCHEUERMANN. 1983. Spin-lattice relaxation and line shape parameters in nuclear magnetic resonance of lamellar lipid systems: fluctuation and spectroscopy of disordering mechanisms. Chem. Phys. Lipids **32:** 271–322.

Single Cell Assays of Excitation-Secretion Coupling[a]

RICHARD J. BOOKMAN,[b,f] NANCY FIDLER LIM,[c]
FELIX E. SCHWEIZER,[d] AND MARTHA NOWYCKY[e]

[b]Departments of Physiology and [c]Biophysics
University of Pennsylvania School of Medicine
Philadelphia, Pennsylvania

[d]Department of Molecular and Cellular Physiology
Stanford University
Stanford, California

[e]Department of Anatomy
Medical College of Pennsylvania
Philadelphia, Pennsylvania

INTRODUCTION

This report discusses some of our results on the problem of excitation-secretion coupling from two model systems: peptide-secreting nerve endings from the posterior pituitary and isolated adrenal chromaffin cells. By studying and comparing the mechanisms of transmitter and hormone release from these neuroendocrine cells, we are hoping to achieve two aims. On the one hand, we view these preparations as good model systems in which to study the mechanisms that couple membrane depolarization to the exocytotic release of hormones and neurotransmitters. In addition, we recognize that each endocrine system is likely to have unique properties that need to be understood in the context of its physiological role. For example, the timing requirements are likely to differ dramatically between a neuromuscular junction and a vascular delivery system like that in the posterior pituitary. The submillisecond delays observed at the neuromuscular junction and the differences in the cytoplasmic arrangement of the secretory granules may mean that the molecular solution is entirely different than that in neuroendocrine cells. An important reason why these preparations are of interest is due to their size and shape. Small spherical cells or secretosomes are amenable to patch clamp techniques and thereby permit the investigation of release mechanisms on individual cells. Central to our efforts in this regard is the utilization of small changes in membrane capacitance as an indicator of cell surface area changes and therefore of exocytosis.

Gillespie[1] demonstrated how to exploit the measurement of passive cell electrical properties in order to make inferences about the release of neurotransmitters. With the advent of patch-clamp techniques, Neher and Marty[2] were able to extend these observations to small cells (~ 10–20 μm diameter) and provide a new level of resolution of the exocytotic process. The measurement of capacitance has now been clearly demonstrated to provide significant information about the molecular and

[a]Support from the HHMI (R. J. Bookman), the NSF (R. J. Bookman), and the NIH (M. Nowycky) is gratefully acknowledged.
[f]Address for correspondence: Department of Molecular and Cellular Pharmacology, University of Miami School of Medicine, P.O. Box 016189, Miami, FL 33101.

kinetic details of excitation-secretion coupling in a number of model systems. These single cell assays for "release" offer the possibility of determining the kinetic relationships among membrane depolarization, Ca^{2+} entry, intracellular Ca^{2+} levels, membrane-membrane fusion, and exocytosis.

It seems clear that excitation-secretion coupling is a multistep process. Capacitance measurements offer us the possibility of making informed inferences about both the nature and number of these steps. In this way, we are using electrical events at the cell surface as a window through which to view cytoplasmic processes.

These approaches, however, have numerous limitations. For example, by measuring changes in cell surface area, we have no direct information about the actual release of transmitters or other compounds such as proteins and ATP. It is hard to resolve the rising phase of a capacitance increase that was triggered by membrane depolarization. One useful bit of information from such a measurement would be the length of the delay before the first fusion, because this could indicate something about the number and speed of any preliminary priming reactions. Also, with our present instrumentation, signal-to-noise considerations limit the ability to resolve individual fusion events. Thus it seems unlikely that we will soon have parallel information about the fusion pore that has been obtained from studies of mast cell exocytosis. The even smaller size of synaptic vesicles at the neuromuscular junction precludes for the moment the resolution of the presumptive quantal event in terms of a capacitance change.

METHODS FOR SINGLE CELL ASSAYS

The investigation of excitation-secretion coupling by means of measurement of small changes in membrane capacitance requires an understanding of some amount of circuit theory.[3,4] A number of papers have discussed the particulars with regard to patch-clamp techniques.[2,5-7] Here we want to add some comments that may help the nonpractitioners to understand both the challenges and limitations.

FIGURE 1 shows a schematic diagram of the recording situation showing a small cell being voltage-clamped using standard whole-cell patch-clamp techniques. For the purposes of this discussion and some of the analysis, we will neglect the additional capacitance that is on the input of the current-to-voltage converter arising from the electrode and electrode holder. These contributions to the admittance (the reciprocal of the impedance) usually can be successfully cancelled with the electrode compensation circuitry of the patch-clamp amplifier if the electrodes are Sylgarded. In the case of either chromaffin cells or isolated secretory terminals, there is 3–12 pF of whole-cell capacitance. In order to resolve the fusion of a small number of secretory granules with the plasma membrane, it is necessary to work at a fairly high gain (10–50 mV/pA). If our capacitance measurement method had sufficient dynamic range, we might be able to track the changes that occur as C_m increases from 4.5 pF to 4.55 pF. Unfortunately, neither the lock-in amplifier nor the computer-based approach have such dynamic range. Therefore, this initial, resting capacitance must be "cancelled" with the compensation circuitry of the amplifier.

It is interesting to contrast these methodological requirements with those used to study degranulation in mast cells. First of all, the stimulus for secretion in excitable cells is a brief depolarization, which, in and of itself, causes a change in the value of the circuit parameters by activating voltage-dependent ion channels. Second, we are trying to measure relatively small changes as 1–20 secretory granules fuse with the plasma membrane. In the case of mast cells or even more so with the mutant beige mouse mast cells, an individual secretory granule can contribute as much as 500 fF to the cell capacitance. The presumed unit event in our preparations is on the order of 1–4 fF. Third, we are interested in changes that occur fairly rapidly (ms) and usually find ourselves band-limited more than we would like.

The capacitance measurement method assumes that two models are valid. First we assume that we can represent the combination of the pipette and the cell as a three-element equivalent circuit as shown in FIGURE 1. Second, we assume that the admittance of the "whole cell" compensation network designed into the patch amplifier is the same as the unknown admittance of the pipette and cell combination. Sinusoidal excitation of a linear circuit such as this three-element model will produce a resulting current that will have the same frequency as the command voltage, but

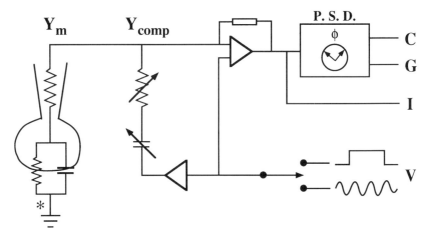

FIGURE 1. Schematic representation of the capacitance recording electronics. The cell and patch-pipette combination, drawn at left, is modeled as a three-element equivalent circuit, with an admittance function, $Y_m(\omega)$. The compensation network of the patch amplifier is designed to have the same transfer function (Y_{comp}) and is tuned so that the circuit elements match the values of the cell. The voltage command (V) can be switched between a pulse or sinusoid. The output of the patch-clamp amplifier, shown here only as an I-V converter, can either provide the membrane current signal (I) or can be fed to a phase-sensitive detector (PSD). We use either an analog lock-in amplifier or a computer-based PSD for this purpose. When the phase angle of this measurement, ϕ, is set properly the two orthogonal output signals are proportional to membrane capacitance (C) and a lumped conductance parameter (G). The phase angle is most easily set by switching a fixed resistor to ground (not shown, but located at * below the cell) in and out of the circuit.[7]

will differ with respect to its amplitude and phase. It is this amplitude and phase of the current that we can measure. These are usually transformed into magnitude measurements at two orthogonal phase angles analagous to a polar-to-rectangular coordinate transformation. This leaves us with two measured quantities in order to estimate the values of three circuit parameters. Clearly, the problem is underdetermined.

Assumption of the validity of these two models raises three questions regarding sources of error in the measurement of membrane capacitance. (1) Is the cell and pipette combination really behaving as a three-element equivalent circuit? In those cases where it has been more explicitly tested by using a wider band of excitation frequencies (*i.e.,* mast cells[8]), the equivalent circuit seems to be an adequate basis for these measurements. Providing that the cell is small and roughly spherical, the fit of the model parameters to the data obtained from stimulation between 100–1000 Hz is very good. Unfortunately, it is not presently very convenient to provide this assurance for every cell. (2) Is the whole-cell compensation network implementing the correct admittance function? Again, for these high resolution measurements we find it necessary to use the compensation circuitry. In most commercial patch-clamp amplifiers, the transfer admittance of the compensation network is based on the assumed three-element equivalent circuit of pipette and cell of FIGURE 1. Each has its own nuances, but they all seem adequate for the chromaffin cells and nerve terminals that we have studied. (3) Is the cancellation circuitry properly tuned? Judging by the quality of the cancellation using either small-step depolarizations or a sinusoid, the compensation networks adequately represent the equivalent circuit provided that the electrodes are carefully Sylgarded. This is also important for calibration of the signals because it is convenient to calibrate the signal through dithering the compensation potentiometers by a fixed and known amount.

Faced with an underdetermined problem, it is possible to estimate with good accuracy the value of the capacitance parameter by studying the properties of the admittance function and recognizing that the values of the circuit elements only change by very small amounts as a result of any one membrane depolarization. FIGURE 2A shows a family of curves in the complex admittance plane. Each one reflects the computation of the value for $Y_m(\omega)$, the admittance function, at a constant value of the frequency, f, the membrane resistance, R_m, and the series resistance, R_s, while C_m increases from 2 pF to 17 pF (equation 1).

$$Y_m(\omega) = \frac{j\omega C_m + \dfrac{1}{R_m}}{j\omega R_s C_m + \dfrac{R_s}{R_m} + 1} \qquad (1)$$

With only the C_m parameter increasing, each can be thought of as a secretory trajectory that the admittance travels along as the cell exocytotically releases hormones or neurotransmitters. In order to better understand the influence of the series resistance, different trajectories were computed using different values for the R_s parameter, as indicated in the FIGURE . Considering the four trajectories shown, the following points are worthy of mention. Notice that although all the trajectories are the same length in terms of capacitance units, their length in admittance units is different. It is as though you need a different ruler for with which to measure the capacitance for each value of series resistance. This reflects the fact that the change in the magnitude of the complex admittance for a given ΔC depends on the other circuit parameters and is particularly sensitive to R_s. Thus the trick is to figure out on which trajectory you are travelling, and how to measure small movements along it. In more proper terminology, these problems amount to setting the phase angle of the PSD and determining the calibration for capacitance measurement, respectively.

When you expand the scale for high-resolution measurements, the linearization discussed by Neher and Marty[2] and by Joshi and Fernandez[6] and the importance of the phase angle becomes easier to understand. The secretory trajectory helps us to define a new coordinate system in which to analyze the changes in the admittance function. If you imagine that there is a short line segment tangent to the secretory trajectory, then this can serve as the capacitance axis. Along the trajectory, or axis, the only quantity that is changing is C_m for small changes in C_m. Thus if we can

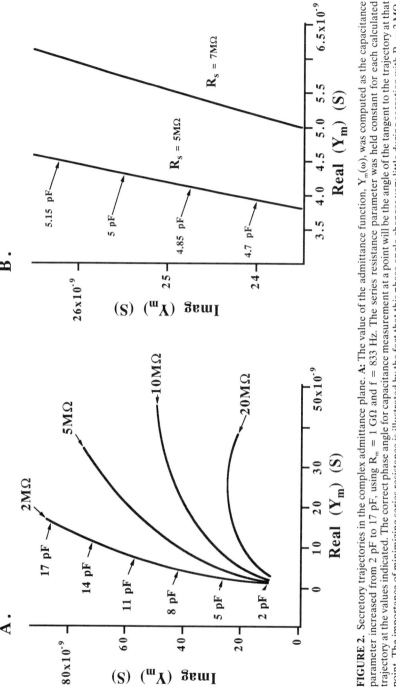

FIGURE 2. Secretory trajectories in the complex admittance plane. **A:** The value of the admittance function, $Y_m(\omega)$, was computed as the capacitance parameter increased from 2 pF to 17 pF, using $R_m = 1$ GΩ and $f = 833$ Hz. The series resistance parameter was held constant for each calculated trajectory at the values indicated. The correct phase angle for capacitance measurement at a point will be the angle of the tangent to the trajectory at that point. The importance of minimizing series resistance is illustrated by the fact that this phase angle changes very little during secretion with $R_s = 2$ MΩ. In fact, the imaginary part of the admittance is a reasonable approximation. With $R_s = 20$ MΩ, the phase angle can change a lot, and the capacitance signal can be seen to project mostly on the real Y axis. **B:** This detail of **A** illustrates the approximate linearity of the trajectory when working at high gain to observe small numbers of secretory vesicle fusions. Although the difference in phase angle for the two illustrated values of R_s is not great, incorrect settings will lead to errors in the estimate of the capacitance jump size.

measure the magnitude of the complex current at exactly that phase angle, then we will measure a change in C_m. The magnitude of the current is measured with a phase-sensitive detector that could be an analog lock-in amplifier or a computer-based implementation of the PSD algorithm.[6]

The phase angle of the analyzer is adjusted until one of the outputs of the PSD is aligned with this capacitance axis. In the case of the phase-tracking method,[7] this is done by switching a 500 kΩ resistor in and out of the circuit in series with the R_s-C_m branch and computing the value of the phase angle. With an analog lock-in amplifier, we can dither the value of the C_{slow} and G_{series} potentiometers while adjusting the phase angle on the lock-in until the C_{slow} dithers no longer project onto the G trace.

If the initial capacitance has been cancelled by the compensation circuitry prior to depolarization, then the origin in this coordinate system is the starting point for the measurement. After the pulse, the admittance will have a new value if the capacitance has increased. The magnitude of this change can be most easily estimated by calibrating the signal through the same dithering modifications to the patch-clamp amplifier. In this way, a calibrated 50 fF deflection can be inserted into the record.

CAPACITANCE JUMPS: FAST RESPONSES TO MEMBRANE DEPOLARIZATION

In our experiments, the most common stimulus protocol is a transient depolarization of the membrane potential for 5–200 ms in order to activate voltage-dependent calcium channels. We can then measure the amount by which the capacitance has increased as a result of the pulse. FIGURE 3 shows some sample records of the capacitance response to a single depolarizing pulse in an isolated nerve terminal (FIG. 3A) and an adrenal chromaffin cell (FIG. 3B). The cells are usually held at −80 mV, and the sinusoid (800–1000 Hz, 15 mV root mean square) is added to this holding potential. At the beginning of the traces in FIGURE 3A, there are large fluctuations in the C and G traces as the phase-tracking resistor is switched in and out of the circuit. Following three such changes, the proper phase angle is computed and then set in software.[7] The phase-tracking resistor is then switched in and out three more times. In each position, a new value of C and G is computed. Notice that for these last three computed values, there is no significant change in the C value. The lack of projection of these G dithers on the C trace is verification that the phase angle has been properly set. Baseline points are then collected.

During the depolarizing pulse, we must chose between more accurate measurement of the Ca^{2+} current (by turning off the sinusoid during the pulse) and more continuous measurement of C_m. Our present methods, however, do not enable us to track accurately the capacitance signal during the pulse. Two problems are limiting: first, large transients obscure the C_m signal at the beginning and end of the pulse. This can be minimized by aligning the rising and falling edges of the pulse with zero-crossings of the sine wave. Second, the activation of voltage-dependent Ca^{2+} channels changes the value of R_m, and therefore the C signal may no longer represent a pure measure of ΔC_m. In either case, we have little or no information about the capacitance changes during the pulse, and therefore we have no information about the rising phase of exocytotic release. We can record the Ca^{2+} current during the pulse, however, and thus have a measure of the amount of Ca^{2+} that entered the cell.

As soon as we can recover the signals (FIG. 3A or B), note that C_m has increased, whereas the G signal remains essentially constant. In both of these neuroendocrine preparations, the fusion of a single hormone-containing vesicle is expected to add

1–4 fF of capacitance to the membrane. Thus we could interpret the C_m increase in terms of some number of fused vesicles. The G signal is more complicated, and upward deflections represent the sum of R_s increases and G_m increases. Note that G_m is more accurately thought of as the parallel combination of the membrane conductance and the seal conductance. What can signals like these tell us about the process of excitation-secretion coupling?

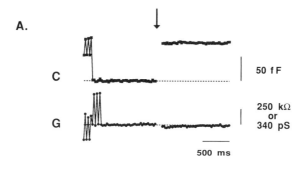

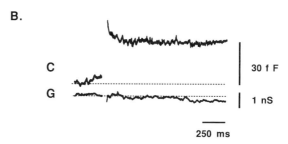

FIGURE 3. Rapid capacitance jumps elicited by transient membrane depolarization in two neuroendocrine cell types. **A:** This recording from an isolated posterior pituitary secretory ending illustrates the stability of the capacitance and conductance signals after setting the phase angle by switching the phase tracking resistor. In the middle of the trace, the sinusoidal stimulation was stopped and the membrane was depolarized to +30 mV from a holding potential of −90 mV for 76 ms. The first capacitance value after the pulses indicates an increase of ∼80 fF or 20–80 secretory vesicles. Thereafter, the C trace is stable. No significant change occurs in the conductance trace. **B:** The same features are observed in this recording from a bovine adrenal chromaffin cell. Here the cell was depolarized to +20 mV for 50 ms. The membrane current was analyzed with an analog lock-in amplifier that is responsible for the small initial transient after the pulse seen on the C trace. For both cell types, note the stability of the C traces after depolarization. This is consistent with a little endocytosis occurring over this time scale. (**A** modified from Lim et al.[17]; **B** modified from Bookman and Schweizer.[15])

Several points must be kept in mind when interpreting these records. First of all, the step-like appearance of these records should not be confused with the similar patterns in unambiguous records of single granule fusions from mast cells. Mast cell secretory granules, particularly those from beige mice, are considerably larger than neuroendocrine secretory granules. The increases we observe are too large to be accounted for by a single fusion event from a single secretory granule. We assume that the unit event in stimulated exocytosis is the fusion of a single granule and believe that the capacitance jumps reflect the fusions of numerous individual granules. It remains possible that numerous granules fuse together prior to the formation of a single fusion pore through the plasma membrane. Second, the C_m signal is a measurement of the net change in membrane capacitance. We think of the increase as reflecting exocytotic activity. Inasmuch as we have little control over endocytosis, the measured C_m increase only provides us with a lower bound of the amount of exocytosis. In addition, we are blind during the pulse so we have no information about the rising phase. Therefore, it is possible that the "true" time-course and extent of exocytosis is not reflected in our C signal. We think this is not likely. Preliminary modeling studies indicate that either endocytosis is absent or it is at least as fast as the exocytotic process and does not proceed to the same extent. We have analyzed the three cases that differ with respect to the relative rates of exo- and endocytosis (faster, same, and slower). At least qualitatively, we are unlikely to be missing an early peak in the C_m signal inasmuch as shortening the pulse always leads to a decrease in the size of the capacitance jump. Third, the capacitance signal does not tell us how much, if any, hormone is released, nor the identity of the released material.

Nevertheless, our observations indicate that depolarization-triggered release from two neuroendocrine preparations can approach the speed that has been demonstrated, for example, in squid giant synapse.[9,10] Depolarizations as brief as 5 ms can produce measurable increases in capacitance. What sort of molecular mechanisms might underlie these rapid neuroendocrine release systems?

EVIDENCE FOR A RELEASABLE POOL AND A DOCKING PROTEIN

One mechanism that might account for the speed of stimulated exocytosis centers on the idea of a releasable pool of secretory vesicles. As experiments by Schäfer *et al.*[11] suggest, these vesicles can be viewed as having already been primed and have only one or a few reactions required for fusion to occur. Palade[12] suggested that there might be an intracellular receptor for secretory vesicles that could act to keep the vesicles docked to the membrane, thereby shortening the latency to fusion after a stimulus. A candidate for such a putative docking protein is a 51 kDa plasma membrane protein isolated on the basis of its binding to purified chromaffin granules. This 51 kDa chromaffin granule binding protein (CGBP) was isolated using an affinity column constructed from purified secretory granules. Using two different assays in two different cell types, we have found evidence that functional obstruction of this docking protein with antibodies from either polyclonal sera or Fab fragments can block exocytosis.[13]

FIGURE 4 illustrates the results obtained using capacitance measurements as the assay for release. The patch pipette contained not only the Fab fragment against CGBP, but also a fluorescently tagged nonspecific antibody in order to control for the diffusion of the antibody (Ab) into the cell. Following break-in, many minutes are required for a high molecular weight Ab to diffuse into the cell.[14] This delay in Ab action is actually useful as it permits us to use each cell as its own control. Prior to Ab equilibration, we are able to depolarize the cell and measure the calcium current and the capacitance response (FIG. 4A). Some 15 minutes later, after establishing that the fluorescent label was uniformly distributed in cytoplasm, the cell was no longer able to secrete as indicated by the flat capacitance trace (FIG. 4B). This was not the

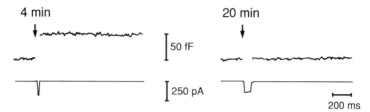

FIGURE 4. Rapid capacitance jumps are blocked by a specific antibody. Antibodies raised against CGBP, a candidate "docking protein," were included in the patch pipette and allowed to diffuse into the cell. The large size of the Ab molecules means that long times are required for diffusion. Thus 4 minutes after breaking into the cell (left), a 20 ms pulse produced an inward Ca^{2+} current (lower record) and a ~50 fF capacitance jump. After 20 minutes (right), the Ca^{2+} current (lower record) was relatively unaffected. The capacitance response was blocked despite the fact that total calcium entry was greater due to the use of a longer pulse. (Modified from Schweizer *et al.*[13])

result of blockade of the calcium channels because the current trace shows that even more Ca^{2+} entered the pulse due to the longer duration of the stimulating pulse.

CALCIUM DEPENDENCE OF CAPACITANCE JUMPS

The simultaneous measurement of calcium current and changes in membrane capacitance can provide new information about the calcium dependence of hormone and transmitter release. It is clear that the capacitance increase depends on calcium current, but not simply on the transmembrane flux of calcium because high concentrations of EGTA can greatly diminish the magnitude of the capacitance increase. FIGURE 5 shows a plot of the voltage-dependence of both the peak macroscopic

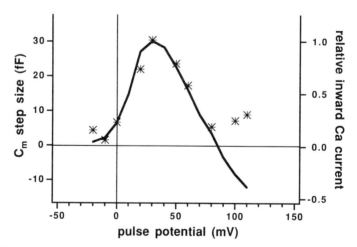

FIGURE 5. Calcium dependence of capacitance jumps observed in an isolated secretosome. The capacitance jump sizes (*, left axis) are plotted as a function of the amplitude of the depolarization. The relative peak inward current is plotted as a solid line.

current as well as ΔC_m from an isolated pituitary secretosome. Both show a bell-shaped dependence on voltage, peaking near a pulse potential of +30 mV (given a ~15 mV junction potential). As the voltage increases further, the secretory response is suppressed, reminiscent of the suppression potential for transmitter release described at the squid giant synapse.[9,10] In some nerve terminals, we have found that large depolarizations that produce no inward current during the pulse may still lead to a small capacitance jump. These may well reflect the fact that there is still a large calcium tail current that might provide enough calcium to support release. It remains unclear whether all of the effect of voltage can be accounted for by the process of channel activation.

SLOW PHASES OF RELEASE

As mentioned above, the amplitude of the capacitance jump depends on the duration of the depolarizing pulse. Very brief pulses (1–5 ms) often fail to elicit any

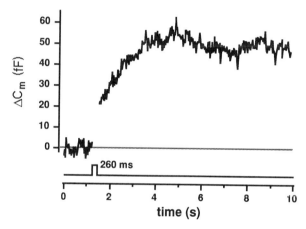

FIGURE 6. Illustration of a slow phase of capacitance increase (or release) in an isolated pituitary nerve ending. Immediately after the depolarization, a 20 fF increase was observed. In the following 2–3 seconds, an additional 30 fF of capacitance was added to the membrane.

ΔC_m response. Longer pulses, typically 10–100 ms, produce the characteristic jumps in the capacitance signal. As the pulse duration lengthens, a second and slower kinetic phase of capacitance increase appears (FIG. 6, and ref. 15). We have observed this same type of behavior in both chromaffin cells and the isolated nerve terminals. Thomas *et al.*[16] have observed a slow capacitance increase in melanotrophs isolated from the anterior pituitary. In this preparation, the ability to convert a cell's response from the rapid jump into the sustained slower increase by increasing the pulse duration was not explored. We would suspect that a similar behavior would be found when the cells are stimulated with longer pulses.

The interpretation of this slow phase is not simple. Does it reflect a slow step in excitation-secretion coupling that is now revealed? According to this hypothesis, a depletion of the releasable pool would be expected to slow the rate of release if reloading of the pool was both rate-limiting and now required for further exocytosis. Another possibility is that it might reflect exocytosis by a second pathway, perhaps bypassing the docked secretory granules and using different release machinery. Alternatively, the slow phase simply might reflect the relatively slow decay of the $[Ca^{2+}]_i$ transient. There are numerous pathways by which the Ca^{2+} brought in to the cell by the calcium current may be removed from the intracellular space. One that appears to play a major role in our fura-2 measurements occurs with approximately the same time-course as the diffusion of the dye into the cell from the pipette.

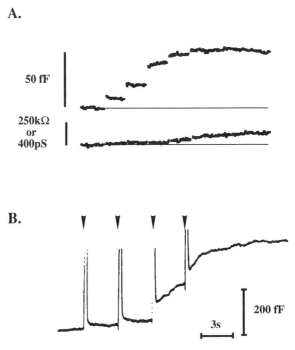

FIGURE 7. Examples of capacitance responses to multiple pulse protocols with isolated pituitary nerve endings (**A**) and chromaffin cells (**B**). In **A**, the terminal was depolarized for 45 ms to +30 mV every 750 ms. Note the clear fatigue of the capacitance response. In **B**, the chromaffin cell was depolarized to +20 mV for 200 ms every 3 seconds. The third and fourth pulses show not only facilitation but also a combined fast and slow response. The large transients are artifacts from the output filters in the lock-in amplifier. (**A** modified from Lim *et al.* [17]; **B** modified from Bookman and Schweizer. [15])

FACILITATION AND FATIGUE PHENOMENA

The basic capacitance responses described so far show the response of the system to a single depolarization. When such pulses are applied every 5–30 seconds, we presume that the cell has returned to the same initial condition (excluding the effects of rundown). In support of this idea is the fact that the amplitude of the capacitance jump remains approximately the same for many minutes during the recording. When we increased the pulse repetition rate to ~1 Hz, we observed both facilitation and fatigue of the capacitance response in the nerve terminals (FIG. 7A) and in chromaffin cells (FIG. 7B).

The response to the first pulse of a five-pulse series appears to be representative of the response of that particular cell to a depolarization of that amplitude and duration. Subsequent pulses, however, applied 0.75–3 s later, often produce a capacitance jump amplitude that is greater than the single pulse value. The third pulse can produce an even larger amount of facilitation of the capacitance response. In the example shown here from a chromaffin cell recording, the third pulse not only produced the largest fast capacitance response, but it also triggered a slow phase increase in the C signal that continued during the interpulse interval. Subsequent pulses have varying effects that depend on the cell or terminal. Many show an apparent fatigue of the secretory process, as judged by the fact that the capacitance response is diminished. Recovery from this fatigue is possible, because depolarizations applied after 1–2 minutes of rest can produce a robust response.[17] Furthermore, we believe that the fatigue cannot be ascribed to Ca channel inactivation, inasmuch as the time-course of recovery from inactivation is much faster than the recovery from secretory fatigue.[17] The proper interpretation of these data must await further investigation. Ca indicator measurements on chromaffin cells, however, show that there is a clear elevation in the resting level of $[Ca^{2+}]_i$ during these multiple pulse protocols.[18]

SUMMARY AND PROSPECTS

By adjusting the pattern of stimulation, it is possible to probe the excitation-secretion pathway of an excitable cell with an arbitrary stimulus. Such control over the input combined with the ability to measure simultaneously changes in intracellular $[Ca^{2+}]_i$ and increase in cell surface area in a single cell has already produced important new insights into the mechanisms underlying excitation-secretion coupling from an increasing number of laboratories.

Although this report has emphasized those features that we find in common in these two neuroendocrine tissues, it should be remembered that in these preparations not all cells are alike. We have not yet made an effort to distinguish cells on the basis of their secreted product. Given that the pattern of electrical activity underlying release in posterior pituitary is different in the oxytocin- and vasopressin-releasing neurons, it is possible that the release process differs in subtle ways that are now beyond our view. Similarly, the cells of the adrenal medulla are divided among those that release epinephrine and those that release norepinephrine. Future work will focus increasingly on the specializations that are necessary for each of these cell types to perform a unique physiological role.

ACKNOWLEDGMENT

We would like to thank our colleague, Dr. Theo Schäfer, for his unending encouragement of the chromaffin cell work.

REFERENCES

1. GILLESPIE, J. I. 1979. The effect of repetitive stimulation on the passive electrical properties of the presynaptic terminal of the squid giant synapse. J. Physiol. **206:** 293–306.

2. NEHER, E. & A. MARTY. 1982. Discrete changes of cell membrane capacitance observed under conditions of enhanced secretion in bovine adrenal chromaffin cells. Proc. Natl. Acad. Sci. USA **79:** 6712–6716.

3. DESOER, C. A. & E. S. KUH. 1969. Basic circuit theory. 1969. McGraw-Hill. New York.

4. BROWN, P. B., G. N. FRANZ & H. MORAFF. 1982. Electronics for the modern scientist. Elsevier. New York.

5. LINDAU, M. & E. NEHER. 1988. Patch-clamp techniques for time-resolved capacitance measurements in single cells. Pfluegers Archiv. **411:** 137–146.

6. JOSHI, C. & J. M. FERNANDEZ. 1988. Capacitance measurements: an analysis of the phase detector technique used to study exocytosis and endocytosis. Biophys. J. **53:** 885–892.

7. FIDLER, N. H. & J. M. FERNANDEZ. 1989. Phase tracking: an improved phase detection technique for cell membrane capacitance measurement. Biophys. J. **56**(6): 1153–1162.

8. LINDAU, M. & J. M. FERNANDEZ. 1986. IgE-mediated degranulation of mast cells does not require opening of ion channels. Nature **319:** 150–153.

9. LLINÁS, R., I. Z. STEINBERG & K. WALTON. 1981. Presynaptic calcium currents in squid giant synapse. Biophys. J. **33:** 289–322.

10. AUGUSTINE, G. J., M. P. CHARLTON & S. J. SMITH. 1985. Calcium entry and transmitter release at voltage-clamped nerve terminals of the squid. J. Physiol. **367:** 163–181.

11. SCHÄFER, T., U. O. KARLI, F. E. SCHWEIZER & M. M. BURGER. 1987. Docking of chromaffin granules—a necessary step in exocytosis? Biosci. Rep. **7:** 269–279.

12. PALADE, G. 1975. Intracellular aspects of the process of protein synthesis. Science. **189:** 347–358.

13. SCHWEIZER, F. E., T. SCHÄFER, C. TAPARELLI, M. GROB, U. KARLI, R. HEUMANN, H. THOENEN, R. J. BOOKMAN & M. M. BURGER. 1989. Inhibition of exocytosis by intracellularly applied antibodies against a chromaffin granule-binding protein. Nature **339:** 709–712.

14. PUSCH, M. & E. NEHER. 1988. Rates of diffusional exchange between small cells and a measuring patch pipette. Pfluegers Arch. **411:** 204–211.

15. BOOKMAN, R. J. & F. E. SCHWEIZER. 1988. Fast and slow phases in chromaffin cell exocytosis depend on Ca entry and Ca buffering. J. Gen. Physiol. **92:** 4a.

16. THOMAS, P., A. SUPRENANT & W. ALMERS. 1990. Cytosolic Ca^{2+}, exocytosis, and endocytosis in single melanotrophs of the rat pituitary. Neuron. **5:** 723–733.

17. LIM, N. H., M. NOWYCKY & R. J. BOOKMAN. 1990. Direct measurement of exocytosis and calcium currents in single isolated nerve terminals. Nature **344:** 449–451.

18. GOLDSMITH, B. & R. J. BOOKMAN. 1990. Imaging Ca^{2+} transients in single, voltage clamped bovine adrenal chromaffin cells. Biophys. J. **57:** 302.

The Calcium Signal for Transmitter Secretion from Presynaptic Nerve Terminals[a]

GEORGE J. AUGUSTINE,[b,d] E. M. ADLER,[c,d,e] AND
MILTON P. CHARLTON[c,d]

[b]Department of Neurobiology
Duke University Medical Center
Bryan Neuroscience Building
Durham, North Carolina 27710

[c]Department of Physiology
University of Toronto
Toronto, Ontario M5S 1A8 Canada

[d]Marine Biological Laboratory
Woods Hole, Massachusetts 02543

Although it has been known for more than 30 years that Ca ions trigger the exocytotic release of neurotransmitters,[1] it still is not clear how a rise in Ca concentration ($[Ca]_i$) within a presynaptic terminal is transduced into an increased probability of exocytosis.[2,3] One of the reasons that we do not know how Ca causes exocytosis is that we do not know how much Ca is needed for exocytosis. Clarification of this question will define the Ca binding properties of the receptor molecule that triggers exocytosis and provide an important clue to the identity of the receptor molecule.[4] This article addresses the calcium requirements for transmitter release by summarizing some recent insights into the magnitude and spatio-temporal dimensions of the presynaptic Ca signal that triggers transmitter release.

In experimental terms, there are two ways that this question can be approached. First, one could manipulate $[Ca]_i$ and ask how high it must be raised in order to mimic physiological rates of secretion.[5,6] Alternatively, one can ask how high $[Ca]_i$ rises during the secretion event. The latter approach, as applied to the unique 'giant' presynaptic terminal of squid,[7] will provide the theme for our article.

DIRECT MEASUREMENTS OF PRESYNAPTIC CALCIUM CHANGES DURING TRANSMITTER RELEASE

The most obvious way to ask how high $[Ca]_i$ gets during transmitter release is to use an intracellular Ca indicator to directly measure presynaptic $[Ca]_i$ during stimuli that trigger release. The fluorescent dye, fura-2,[8] is presently the indicator of choice for measuring the magnitude of the presynaptic $[Ca]_i$ changes associated with

[a]This work was supported by NIH Grant NS-21624 to G. J. Augustine and an MRC Grant to M. P. Charlton.
[e]Present address: Laboratory of Molecular Neurobiology, Massachusetts General Hospital East, 149 13th Street, Charlestown, MA 02129.

transmitter release. Applications of earlier, less precise Ca indicators have been summarized in reference 2. At the squid giant synapse, photomultiplier measurements of fura-2 fluorescence allow quantification of the presynaptic $[Ca]_i$ changes caused by action potentials. Such measurements reveal that a single presynaptic action potential raises $[Ca]_i$ by a surprisingly small amount, approximately 5 nM from a resting level of approximately 50–100 nM.[9]

One important consideration in evaluating such measurements is that they reflect a spatial average, so that spatial gradients of $[Ca]_i$ within the presynaptic terminal will not be detected. In particular, it is possible that $[Ca]_i$ changes in the vicinity of sites of secretion may be higher than those in the bulk cytoplasm, because the voltage-gated Ca channels that are the source of the $[Ca]_i$ signal are clustered in the vicinity of the active zones, the sites of secretion in these terminals.[10,11] In order to address this possibility, video-imaging methods have been used to make spatially resolved measurements of $[Ca]_i$ within small presynaptic compartments in the vicinity of the sites of exocytosis. Such measurements, however, still indicate nM changes in $[Ca]_i$ in response to a single presynaptic action potential.[12]

Two features of the time-course of the $[Ca]_i$ changes measured with video-imaging techniques suggest limitations even in these measurements of presynaptic $[Ca]_i$. First, the decay time of the measured $[Ca]_i$ changes do not coincide with those expected at the release sites: presynaptic $[Ca]_i$ changes evoked by action potentials decay over tens of seconds, even though transmitter release ends within a couple of milliseconds following an action potential.[7] Second, the pattern of Ca signals evoked by trains of action potentials is unexpected: $[Ca]_i$ gradually rises in a ramp-like fashion, so there are no changes with kinetic properties similar to an action potential.

Part of the solution to these two problems could be the limited time resolution (ca. 100 ms) of the video cameras used to make spatial maps of $[Ca]_i$ in these experiments. However, similar slow changes in $[Ca]_i$ are detected even when using faster detectors such as a photomultiplier or photodiode. A more likely explanation can be found in the limited spatial resolution of the imaging methods, which is on the order of a few micrometers in this tissue.[13] It is likely that the spatial compartmentalization of the presynaptic $[Ca]_i$ signal exceeds this limit, and thus the $[Ca]_i$ signal at the secretory sites still is underestimated by our imaging measurements.

Theoretical studies of the diffusion of Ca ions into presynaptic cytoplasm suggest that presynaptic Ca signals drop off steeply in the vicinity of open Ca channels.[14–17] FIGURE 1 is a cartoon that summarizes the expected changes in $[Ca]_i$ in two presynaptic compartments. The idea is that near an open Ca channel, $[Ca]_i$ should rapidly rise to high levels and then decline very rapidly when the channel closes. At some distance away from the channel, however, the change in $[Ca]_i$ will be much smaller and much slower because this signal is low-pass filtered by diffusion throughout the terminal. The video camera is likely to be measuring the $[Ca]_i$ away from the open channels, because most of the volume of the presynaptic terminal is far from any Ca channels. Thus, this measured signal will be relatively small and slow in comparison to the signal near the open Ca channels, which is presumably the signal that triggers release. Thus, the imaging probably is only revealing the proverbial tip of the iceberg. In fact, depending upon the distances and volumes involved, the actual value of $[Ca]_i$ changes at active zones could be orders of magnitudes higher than a few nM per action potential. So the problem we faced is how to selectively measure $[Ca]_i$ within the minute microenvironment of the active zones.

CALCIUM BUFFERS AS PROBES OF THE
PRESYNAPTIC CALCIUM SIGNAL

The only sensor that selectively detects $[Ca]_i$ at the release sites is the Ca receptor that triggers secretion. We therefore have used the secretory event as an assay to tell us something about the relative $[Ca]_i$ levels at the release site. Armed with this assay, we then microinjected Ca buffers to try to compete with this receptor and used the resultant changes in secretion, along with the known Ca binding properties of these buffers, to deduce the magnitude and time-course of the Ca signal for secretion.[18]

Examples of results obtained with this approach are shown in FIGURE 2. This FIGURE illustrates the differential effects of EGTA and BAPTA, two buffers with

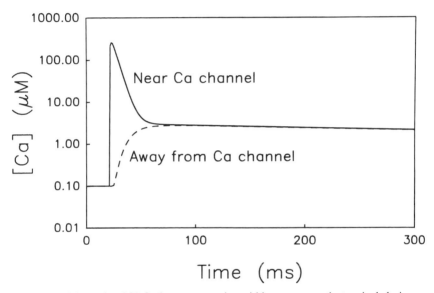

FIGURE 1. Schematic of $[Ca]_i$ changes occurring within a presynaptic terminal during an action potential. In the vicinity of the Ca channels opened by the action potential, $[Ca]_i$ will rise rapidly to high levels and decline rapidly after the channels close. Farther away from the Ca channels, the $[Ca]_i$ changes will be smaller and slower.

similar affinities for calcium. When injected into presynaptic terminals at concentrations estimated to be in excess of 10 mM, BAPTA produced a prompt and reversible reduction in action potential–evoked transmitter release, whereas EGTA had negligible effects (see also ref. 19). This shows that despite their similar affinities for Ca, BAPTA can successfully compete with the Ca receptor for Ca ions, whereas EGTA cannot.

This unexpected difference in buffer efficacy presumably is due to differences in the kinetics of Ca binding by the two buffers.[20] Previous voltage-clamp experiments at the squid giant synapse show that the minimal delay between Ca entry into the presynaptic terminal and initiation of postsynaptic electrical responses is on the order of a few hundred microseconds.[14,21] The Ca binding properties of these two Ca buffers during this brief time period is illustrated in FIGURE 3. Under conditions where the concentration of buffer is high relative to the magnitude of the presynaptic $[Ca]_i$ change, BAPTA should bind Ca within a fraction of a μs, whereas the time constant for Ca binding to EGTA is on the order of 400 times slower.[18] It therefore appears that EGTA is too slow to bind Ca before the Ca receptor does, so that release can proceed undiminished. The more rapid kinetics of BAPTA allow it to successfully compete with the receptor and attenuate transmitter release. This suggests that the Ca receptor must bind Ca very rapidly, in the order of tens of

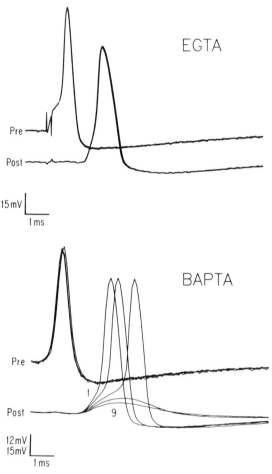

FIGURE 2. Differential effects of EGTA and BAPTA on transmitter release. Either EGTA (top) or BAPTA (bottom) were microinjected into squid presynaptic terminals to estimated concentrations in excess of 10 mM. Although EGTA had no effect on postsynaptic responses (Post) elicited by presynaptic action potentials (Pre), BAPTA produced a progressive reduction in synaptic transmission. Traces 1 and 9 in the BAPTA experiment indicate postsynaptic responses evoked after 1 and 9 had brief injections of BAPTA. (Adler *et al.*[18] With permission from the *Journal of Neuroscience*.)

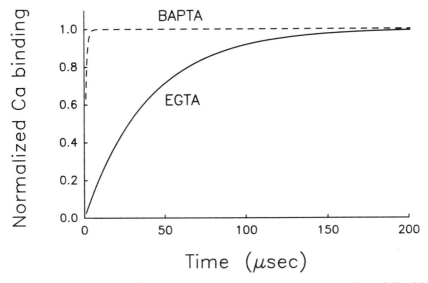

FIGURE 3. BAPTA and EGTA bind Ca at different rates. At concentrations of 50 mM, BAPTA will bind Ca with a time constant of less than 1 μs (dashed line), whereas EGTA will bind 400 times more slowly (solid line).

microseconds, because EGTA will start binding Ca at later times. Thus, it appears that the Ca binding step that triggers release is a relatively small fraction of the total, few hundred microsecond–long synaptic delay. Further, because Ca has a finite rate of diffusion, this also means that the Ca receptor responsible for triggering exocytosis must be within a few tens of nanometers of the open Ca channel.

This analysis also suggests that BAPTA binding to Ca may be so fast as to be at equilibrium during a BAPTA-buffered release event. Under such conditions, one can then chemically alter the Ca affinity of the BAPTA molecule and determine how changes in affinity alter the ability of BAPTA to attenuate transmitter release. We found that BAPTA derivitives with different affinities (K_ds) for Ca have different abilities to compete with the release receptor (FIG. 4). The most effective was dibromoBAPTA (K_d = 4.9 μM); dimethylBAPTA (K_d = 0.2 μM) and BAPTA (K_d = 0.5 μM) were next in potency, whereas dinitroBAPTA, with a K_d of approximately 30 mM, was much less effective.

A SIMPLE NUMERICAL MODEL FOR DIFFERENTIAL BUFFER EFFICACY

To translate this pattern of buffer efficacy into information regarding [Ca]$_i$ levels at the release site, we used a simple numerical model of Ca-buffer interactions. In this model the primary free parameter was the size of the Ca concentration change to which the buffers were responding. If the presynaptic concentration and K_d of a buffer are known, and the reaction between calcium and buffer reaches equilibrium during the transient rise in [Ca]$_i$ produced by an action potential, then the relative attenuation of the [Ca]$_i$ change produced by the buffer can be estimated from the following steady-state equations:

$$[Ca]_i = \frac{K_d[CaBuffer]}{[Buffer]} \tag{1}$$

$$[Ca_{total}] = [Ca]_i + [CaBuffer] \tag{2}$$

$$[Buffer_{total}] = [CaBuffer] + [Buffer], \tag{3}$$

in which $[Ca_{total}]$ is the level of $[Ca]_i$ produced by an action potential before injection of buffer; [CaBuffer] and $[Ca]_i$ are the fraction bound to buffer and remaining free,

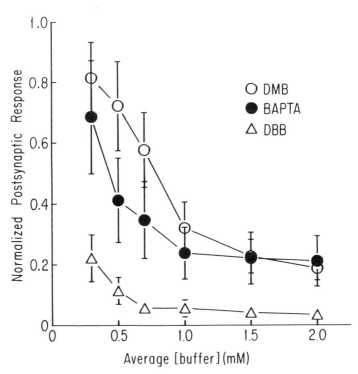

FIGURE 4. Relative efficacy of BAPTA derivatives in attenuating transmitter release. Release, measured as amplitude of postsynaptic response evoked by a presynaptic action potential, decreased with higher concentration of buffer within the presynaptic terminal. DMB = dimethylBAPTA and DBB = dibromoBAPTA. (Adler *et al.*[18] With permission from the *Journal of Neuroscience.*)

respectively; $[Buffer_{total}]$ is the total concentration of buffer injected into the terminal; and [Buffer] is the fraction remaining uncomplexed with Ca. The equations can be combined to determine $[Ca]_i$ (see refs. 22 and 23):

$$[Ca]_i = \frac{[([Ca^{total}] - K_d - [Buffer_{total}]) \pm [(K_d + [Buffer_{total}] - [Ca_{total}])^2 + 4K_d[Ca_{total}]]^{1/2}]}{2}. \tag{4}$$

This treatment assumes that the concentration of exogenous buffer is much higher than that of any endogenous buffer, so that the contribution of such a putative endogenous buffer under these conditions is negligible.

Equation 4 was used to predict the relative reduction in presynaptic $[Ca]_i$ produced by different concentrations of the various buffers. The results of this calculation are that the buffers should reduce transmitter release roughly in proportion to their K_D values, with buffers having lower K_Ds more effective in reducing transmitter release. These differences between the theory and experimental observations indicate that equation 4 is not sufficient to predict the ability of a buffer to reduce evoked transmitter release.

One limitation of the above calculation is that it does not account for buffer binding to calcium present in the resting nerve terminal (resting $[Ca]_i$) prior to nerve stimulation. With a resting $[Ca]_i$ of 50–100 nM,[9] the reduction in free buffer concentration for a buffer load of 300 μM to several millimolar is negligible if the chelation of resting $[Ca]_i$ is uncompensated and $[Ca]_i$ is allowed to drop to levels on the order of 10^{-9} M. Studies in other systems (see references in ref. 24), however, suggest that homeostatic mechanisms can maintain resting $[Ca]_i$ at normal levels in the presence of several mM exogenous calcium buffer.

If it is assumed that resting $[Ca]_i$ gravitates to a set point, with Ca from the extracellular fluid and intracellular stores replacing that which is chelated by the buffer, a certain fraction of the buffer will be bound to resting Ca and will therefore be unavailable to chelate the additional Ca added by an action potential, that is, $[Ca_{total}]$. The exact fraction of a given buffer load that is still available to chelate $[Ca_{total}]$ will depend on the buffer K_d and the resting $[Ca]_i$ set point. Under equilibrium conditions, free buffer concentrations will be predicted by the following equation:

$$[\text{Buffer}] = \frac{(K_d[\text{Buffer}_{total}])}{([Ca_{rest}] + K_d)}, \tag{5}$$

in which $[Ca_{rest}]$ is the set point for resting $[Ca]_i$. If a correction is made for the reduction of free buffer by resting Ca, and a term added to equation 4 so that $[Ca]$ during the transient cannot be buffered to levels below 5×10^{-8} M, predicted $[Ca]$ for the range of concentrations of the BAPTA-family buffers resembles the pattern of buffer efficacy in reducing transmitter release observed experimentally (FIG. 5A). The resemblance is apparent regardless of whether it is assumed that the relationship between $[Ca]_i$ and transmitter release is a linear function[14] or a power function.[21,25,26]

The exact form of the predicted relationship between buffer concentration and $[Ca]_i$ is strongly dependent on the specific values chosen for parameters, such as the exact size of the $[Ca]_i$ change produced by an action potential and the resting $[Ca]_i$ level. Therefore the predictions of the model can be used to estimate these values. In particular, if the peak $[Ca]_i$ change during an action potential is less than 100 μM, dimethylBAPTA is predicted to be more effective that dibromoBAPTA, which was not observed. Thus, our results are consistent with $[Ca]_i$ levels on the order of one-hundred micromolar in the vicinity of the release sites during an action potential.

One consideration ignored in the above calculations is the influence of endogenous buffers on presynaptic $[Ca]_i$ and the effect of injected buffers on $[Ca]_i$. Although relatively little is known about the properties of such a buffer, if its concentration and K_d are known, then equations 1–3 can also be used to evaluate the impact of this endogenous buffer on $[Ca]_i$. For the purposes of calculation, we assumed that the presynaptic terminal might have 1 mM of an endogenous buffer having a K_d of 1 μM. After including this endogenous buffer, the minimum [Ca_{total}] needed to replicate the observed order of buffer efficacy was 2 mM, with [Ca]$_i$ in this situation being 1.1 mM or greater after complexation by the endogenous buffer (FIG. 5B). Thus, any endogenous buffer present in the presynaptic terminal will raise the total amount of Ca needed to account for our experimental results.

The results of these simple calculations force us to conclude that the presynaptic Ca change caused by an action potential is on the order of one-hundred μM or higher, depending on the amount of endogenous buffer in the presynaptic terminal. Similar conclusions have been reached in other secretory cells. By using Ca-activated

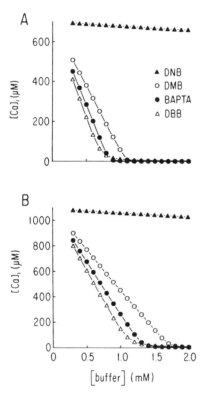

FIGURE 5. Numerical model of attenuation of the presynaptic Ca signal by different BAPTA derivitives. **A:** Reduction in [Ca]$_i$ predicted with [Ca_{total}] = 700 μM, [Ca_{rest}] = 100 nM. **B:** Reduction in [Ca]$_i$ predicted with [Ca_{total}] = 2 mM, [Ca_{rest}] = 100 nM, and the addition of 1 mM endogenous buffer with a K_d of 1 μM.

K channels as indicators of [Ca]$_i$ in hair cells, Roberts et al.[27] suggest that [Ca]$_i$ in the secretory region of these cells may reach 100 μM or even higher during depolarization. A similar use of the secretory response as an indicator of [Ca]$_i$ in adrenal chromaffin cells also suggests levels on the order of 10–100 μM during depolarization.[6] Thus, three different technical approaches applied to three different experimental systems all suggest that [Ca]$_i$ at secretory sites is fairly high during exocytosis, perhaps as high as several hundred μM. This indicates that the measurements of a few nM change in [Ca]$_i$ during a presynaptic action potential were indeed severe underestimates of the magnitude of the changes in the vicinity of the secretory sites and that steep spatial gradients of $[Ca]_i$ occur in the presynaptic terminal during an action potential.

HIGH PRESYNAPTIC CALCIUM LEVELS ARE PRODUCED BY DISCRETE DOMAINS OF CALCIUM ELEVATION

We will end our discussion of the presynaptic $[Ca]_i$ signal by considering how the presynaptic terminal is able to generate such a large change in Ca concentration. We believe that the answer lies in localized "domains" of elevated $[Ca]_i$ in the immediate vicinity of open Ca channels. The relevant calculations for such a situation (first performed as reported in refs. 28, 16, and 17) present two possible scenarios for generating tens or hundreds of μM Ca^{2+} at a release site.

One possibility, schematized in FIGURE 6A, is that $[Ca]_i$ can reach these concentrations within a single domain if the release site is only a few nanometers away from the open channel (FIG. 6B). This small separation is consistent with the spacing estimates derived from the lack of effect of EGTA, as described above.

An alternative possibility is that even if the release site is not so close to a single open Ca channel, high $[Ca]_i$ levels could result if many open Ca channels are clustered close together. This possibility is diagrammed in FIGURE 6C. In this situation, the resulting domains will overlap and produce a generalized rise in Ca_i throughout the active zone (FIG. 6D). The clustering of Ca channels illustrated in FIGURE 6C is consistent with video-imaging observations indicating the clustering of Ca channels at secretory sites[13] and also is consistent with freeze-fracture measurements of the spacing between large intramembranous particles in the presynaptic membrane.[10,29]

The key distinction between these two possibilities is whether or not the $[Ca]_i$ domains associated with open Ca channels overlap with each other. We have performed experiments designed to look for signs of domain overlap by again using transmitter release as an indicator of relative $[Ca]_i$ levels at the active zones. In these experiments the number of domains was increased by prolonging the duration of the presynaptic action potential, using pharmacological agents that block the voltage-gated K channels responsible for the repolarization phase of the action potential.[30] Such broadening increases the macroscopic Ca current by increasing the number of open Ca channels, which results in an increased number of domains being generated.

Interpretation of these experiments relies on the cooperative behavior of transmitter release[21,25,26] to yield information on the relative level of $[Ca]_i$ at the release sites. The assumption is that there is a nonlinear, cooperative relationship between the amount of Ca entering into a domain and the release that results (FIG. 7A). The best experimental support for this assumption comes from voltage-clamp experiments performed on the squid giant synapse.[26] In these experiments, presynaptic Ca influx was varied by changing the external Ca concentration, while repeatedly depolarizing the presynaptic terminal to a constant membrane potential to open a constant number of Ca channels (FIG. 7B).

Under these conditions the number of domains produced is constant, while the single channel Ca current, and thus the size of the $[Ca]_i$ signal within each domain, is reduced as $[Ca]_o$ is lowered. The resultant power-function relationship between the size of the presynaptic Ca current and amount of transmitter release can be interpreted as being due to changes in the size of the $[Ca]_i$ signal within each domain. These results therefore illustrate that the cooperative nature of transmitter release causes increases in $[Ca]_i$ within a domain to produce exponential increments in

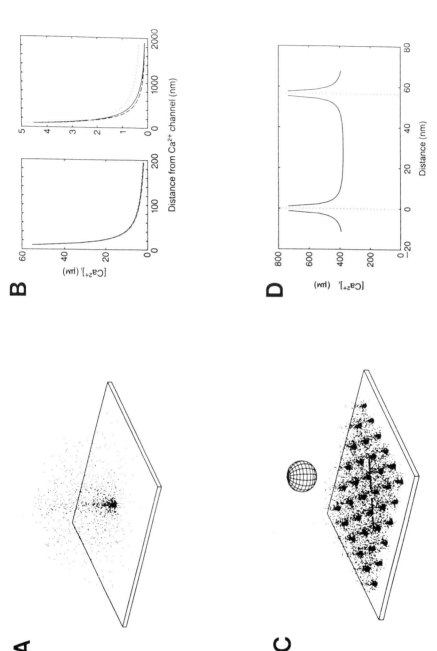

FIGURE 6. [Ca]$_i$ changes in the vicinity of open Ca channels. **A:** Diagram of predicted distribution of Ca ions (dots) diffusing away from a single open Ca channel. **B:** Dependence of the magnitude of [Ca]$_i$ changes on the distance away from a single open Ca channel, shown on two different scales. **C:** Diagram of predicted distribution of Ca ions diffusing within an array of many open Ca channels. The spacing between adjacent channels was set to be 40 nm, and a sphere comparable in dimensions to a synaptic vesicle is shown above the array. **D:** Distribution of [Ca]$_i$ changes along the transect shown by the line in C. (Smith & Augustine.[4] With permission from *Trends in Neuroscience*.)

transmitter release. Similar observations are made when the presynaptic Ca channels are opened with action potentials instead of voltage-clamp pulses.[25,31,32]

Based on such considerations, the cooperative triggering of transmitter release within single domains can be used to ask how $[Ca]_i$ within domains changes when the number of domains is increased by broadening the presynaptic action potential. If the domains do not overlap, then release will depend on the number of new domains produced and will increase in proportion to the increment in the magnitude of the macroscopic Ca current (FIG. 8A). Conversely, if domains overlap then release will increase more than the number of domains, because the additional overlap produced by recruitment of new domains will elevate $[Ca]_i$ within these domains and cause the cooperative relationship between $[Ca]_i$ and release to be expressed. In the extreme case of complete overlap between domains, then release will increase in proportion to the fourth power of the increment in macroscopic Ca current (FIG. 8B). Thus, the relationship between the increment in macroscopic Ca current and transmitter release provides a means of determining whether or not domains overlap.

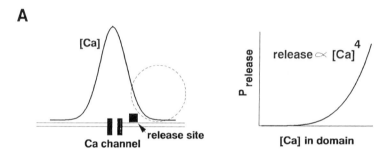

FIGURE 7A. Cooperative triggering of release within a single domain. Left: schematic diagram of distribution of $[Ca]_i$ changes (bold line) within a domain centered over a single Ca channel. Right: cooperative relationship between $[Ca]_i$ and probability that release will take place within the domain.

At the squid giant synapse, the K channel blockers, tetraethylammonium and 3,4-diaminopyridine, were used to increase the duration of the presynaptic action potential and thereby increase the number of domains generated by the action potential.[30] Broadening of the presynaptic action potential caused large increases in transmitter release, as assayed by an increase in the magnitude of the postsynaptic current evoked by a presynaptic action potential (FIG. 9A). At other synapses, K channel blockers also enhance transmitter release (*e.g.* ref. 33). A plot of the relationship between the duration of the action potential and the amplitude of the postsynaptic current yields a linear relationship, with a slope of approximately 6.3% change in release for a 1% increase in action potential duration (FIG. 9B).

In order to estimate the magnitude of the macroscopic Ca current flowing into the presynapse during these action potentials, a numerical simulation[30] was performed based on the Hodgkin and Huxley[34] mathematical model of an action potential and previous voltage-clamp measurements of the voltage-dependent gating of the Ca channels of the squid presynaptic terminal.[35,36] This kind of simulation, with no free parameters except for the duration of the presynaptic action potential, indicates that the magnitude of the macroscopic Ca current greatly increases as the

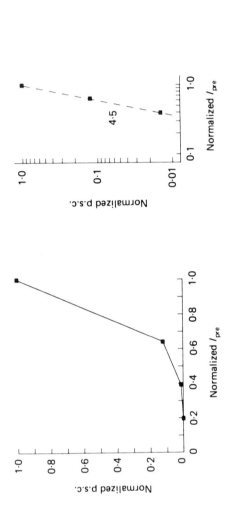

FIGURE 7B. Cooperative triggering of release within a single domain. Experimental evidence for cooperativity within domains. Left: varying presynaptic Ca current (I_{pre}) by altering external Ca concentration produces an exponential change in release, measured as postsynaptic current (p.s.c.). Right: on logarithmic coordinates, the data shown at the left can be described by a power function with an exponent of 4.5. (Augustine & Charlton.[26] With permission from the *Journal of Physiology (London)*.)

A If domains do not overlap

B If domains overlap

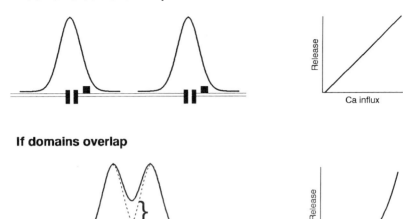

FIGURE 8. Predicted effects of increased number of domains depend upon whether or not domains overlap. **A:** If domains do not overlap, then increasing the number of domains will produce a linear rise in release. **B:** If domains overlap, then release will increase in a supralinear fashion, due to the increment in $[Ca]_i$ (bracket) at the release sites within the domains.

action potential broadens (FIG. 10A). The quantitative relationship between the duration of the action potential and the integral of the Ca current is a linear function, with an approximate slope of 7% change in Ca influx per 1% change in action potential duration (FIG. 10B).

Knowledge of the relationship between action potential duration and magnitude of the macroscopic Ca current (FIG. 10B) allows the relationship shown in FIGURE 9B to be expressed in terms of Ca influx rather than action-potential duration. Such a

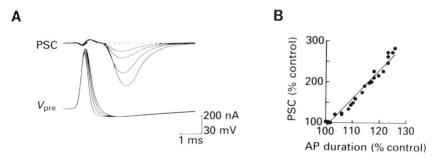

FIGURE 9. A: Broadening presynaptic action potentials (V_{pre}) by treatment with 3,4-diaminopyridine causes large increases in postsynaptic current responses (PSC) evoked by the action potentials. **B:** Linear relationship between presynaptic action potential (AP) duration and peak amplitude of PSCs. (Augustine.[30] With permission from the *Journal of Physiology (London).*)

A   **B**

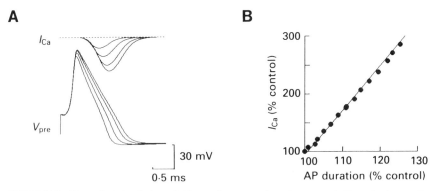

FIGURE 10. Numerical simulation of effects of presynaptic action potential broadening on Ca current. **A:** Increasing the duration of the simulated presynaptic action potential (V_{pre}) causes a large increase in the amplitude of the presynaptic Ca current (I_{Ca}). **B:** Predicted relationship between presynaptic action potential (AP) duration and presynaptic I_{Ca}. (Augustine.[30] With permission from the *Journal of Physiology (London)*.)

transformation reveals that transmitter release increases in direct proportion to the amount of Ca entry (FIG. 11), as has also been reported by Llinás *et al.*[37] This relationship is as predicted for the case where domains do not overlap (FIG. 8A). Thus, these results suggest that the high [Ca]$_i$ levels generated at active zones during action potentials are generated within single, nonoverlapping domains. Similar conclusions have been reached on the basis of different experiments performed at frog neuromuscular synapses.[38] Both sets of results suggest that the Ca receptor that triggers release must be very near (within a few nanometers) the voltage-gated Ca channel, because the [Ca]$_i$ signal cannot reach levels on the order of 100 μM at distances greater than a few nanometers away from the channel (*e.g.* FIG. 6B).

At odds with these conclusions are two suggestions of apparent domain overlap in presynaptic terminals. First, high local [Ca]$_i$ levels in active zones of hair cells

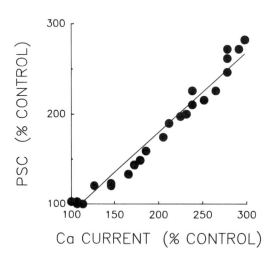

FIGURE 11. Combining the results shown in FIGS. 9B and 10B allows an estimate of the relationship between presynaptic Ca current and magnitude of postsynaptic current (PSC).

appear to be caused by domain overlap,[27] but the Ca channels in this cell appear to be packed in a very high density in comparison to the squid terminal.[10] Thus, Ca channels of hair cells, but perhaps not those of most presynaptic terminals, may be specially organized to produce overlap. Second, at voltage-clamped squid synapses the relationship between macroscopic Ca current and postsynaptic response has been reported to be a high-order, power function when the number of domains is increased by voltage-clamp depolarizations to different membrane potentials.[21,28] This suggests a high degree of spatial overlap of domains (as in FIG. 8B). The difference between these end results and those shown in FIGURE 11, however, is probably due to differences in the number of domains generated by these two kinds of stimuli: during an action potential, only about 10% of the Ca channels are opened,[10] whereas much larger numbers of channels were probably opened in the voltage-clamp experiments because they used depolarizations much longer-lasting than an action potential. Thus, at the squid synapse it seems that during an action potential the average distance between open Ca channels is sufficiently large to prevent overlap, but during voltage-clamp pulses this distance is decreased and allows overlap to occur.

Getting back to the question posed at the beginning of this article, it seems that the receptor to which Ca binds to trigger release experiences high $[Ca]_i$ levels, perhaps on the order of hundreds of μM, and binds Ca within a few tens of microseconds. Because of the concentrations and times involved, as well as the apparently nonoverlapping nature of the local $[Ca]_i$ domains within an active zone, this receptor must be located within a few tens of nanometers of the voltage-gated Ca channels of the active zone. The cooperative triggering of release within a single domain suggests the presence of multiple Ca binding sites on one or more molecules important in release, perhaps simply on the Ca receptor itself. These considerations should help molecular biologists to identify more plausible candidates for the Ca receptor that mediates release.

ACKNOWLEDGMENT

We thank Shelli Sedlak for typing this manuscript.

REFERENCES

1. KATZ, B. 1969. The Release of Neural Transmitter Substances. Liverpool University Press. Liverpool.
2. AUGUSTINE, G. J., M. P. CHARLTON & S. J. SMITH. 1987. Calcium action in synaptic transmitter release. Annu. Rev. Neurosci. **10:** 633–693.
3. KELLY, R. B. 1988. The cell biology of the nerve terminal. Neuron **1:** 431–438.
4. SMITH, S. J. & G. J. AUGUSTINE. 1988. Calcium ions, active zones and synaptic transmitter release. Trends Neurosci. **11:** 458–464.
5. DELANEY, K. R. & R. S. ZUCKER. 1990. Calcium released by photolysis of DM-nitrophen stimulates transmitter release at squid giant synapse. J. Physiol. (Lond.) **426:** 473–498.
6. AUGUSTINE, G. J. & E. NEHER. 1991. Calcium requirements for secretion in bovine chromaffin cells. J. Physiol. (Lond.) In press.
7. LLINÁS, R. R. 1982. Calcium in synaptic transmission. Sci. Am. **247:** 56–65.
8. GRYNKIEWICZ, G., M. POENIE & R. Y. TSIEN. 1985. A new generation of Ca^{2+} indicators with greatly improved fluorescence properties. J. Biol. Chem. **260:** 3440–3450.
9. ZIPSER, K., G. J. AUGUSTINE & J. DEITMER. 1991. Na/Ca exchange regulates presynaptic calcium levels. Biophys. J. **59:** 594a.

10. PUMPLIN, D. W., T. S. REESE & R. LLINÁS. 1981. Are the presynaptic membrane particles the calcium channels? Proc. Natl. Acad. Sci. USA **78:** 7210–7213.

11. SMITH, S. J., L. R. OSSES & G. J. AUGUSTINE. 1988. Fura-2 imaging of localized calcium accumulation within squid 'giant' presynaptic terminal. *In* Calcium and Ion Channel Modulation. A. D. Grinnell, D. Armstrong & M. B. Jackson, Eds.: 147–155. Plenum Press. New York.

12. SMITH, S. J., J. BUCHANAN, L. R. OSSES, M. P. CHARLTON & G. J. AUGUSTINE. 1991. Clustering of presynaptic calcium channels at active zones. In preparation.

13. AUGUSTINE, G. J., J. BUCHANAN, M. P. CHARLTON, L. R. OSSES & S. J. SMITH. 1989. Fingering the trigger for neurotransmitter secretion: Studies on the calcium channels of squid giant presynaptic terminals. *In* Secretion and Its Control G. S. Oxford & C. M. Armstrong, Eds.: 203–223. Rockefeller University Press. New York.

14. LLINÁS, R., I. Z. STEINBERG & K. WALTON. 1981. Relationship between presynaptic calcium current and postsynaptic potential in squid giant synapse. Biophys. J. **33:** 323–352.

15. ZUCKER, R. S. & N. STOCKBRIDGE. 1983. Presynaptic calcium diffusion and the time courses of transmitter release and synaptic faciliatation at squid giant synapse. J. Neurosci. **3:** 1263–1269.

16. SIMON, S. M. & R. R. LLINÁS. 1985. Compartmentalization of the submembrane calcium activity during calcium influx and its significance in transmitter release. Biophys. J. **48:** 485–498.

17. ZUCKER, R. S. & A. L. FOGELSON. 1986. Relationship between transmitter release and presynaptic calcium influx when calcium enters through discrete channels. Proc. Natl. Acad. Sci. USA **83:** 3032–3036.

18. ADLER, E. M., G. J. AUGUSTINE, S. N. DUFFY & M. P. CHARLTON. 1991. Alien intracellular calcium chelators attentuate neurotransmitter release at the squid giant synapse. J. Neurosci. **11:** 1496–1507.

19. ADAMS, D. J., K. TAKEDA & J. A. UMBACH. 1985. Inhibitors of calcium buffering depress evoked transmitter release at the squid giant synapse. J. Physiol. (Lond.) **369:** 145–159.

20. MARTY, A. & E. NEHER. 1985. Potassium channels in cultured bovine adrenal chromaffin cells. J. Physiol. (Lond.) **367:** 117–141.

21. AUGUSTINE, G. J., M. P. CHARLTON & S. J. SMITH. 1985. Calcium entry and transmitter release at voltage-clamped nerve terminals of squid. J. Physiol. (Lond.) **367:** 163–181.

22. ZUCKER, R. S. & R. A. STEINHARDT. 1978. Prevention of the cortical reaction in fertilized sea urchin eggs by injection of calcium-chelating ligands. Biochim. Biophys. Acta **541:** 459–466.

23. NACHSEN, D. A. & P. DRAPEAU. 1982. A buffering model for calcium-dependent neurotransmitter release. Biophys. J. **38:** 205–208.

24. TSIEN, R. Y., T. POZZAN & T. J. RINK. 1984. Measuring and manipulating cytosolic Ca^{2+} with trapped indicators. Trends Biochem. Sci. **9:** 263–266.

25. DODGE, F. A. & R. RAHAMIMOFF. 1967. Co-operative action of calcium ions in transmitter release at the neuromuscular junction. J. Physiol. (Lond.) **193:** 419–432.

26. AUGUSTINE, G. J. & M. P. CHARLTON. 1986. Calcium dependence of presynaptic calcium current and post-synaptic response at the giant squid synapse. J. Physiol. (Lond.) **381:** 619–640.

27. ROBERTS, W. M., R. A. JACOBS & A. J. HUDSPETH. 1990. Colocalization of ion channels involved in frequency selectivity and synaptic transmission at presynaptic active zones of hair cells. J. Neurosci. **10:** 3664–3684.

28. CHAD, J. E. & R. ECKERT. 1984. Calcium domains associated with individual channels can account for anomalous voltage relations of Ca-dependent responses. Biophys. J. **45:** 993–999.

29. HEUSER, J. E., T. S. REESE & D. M. D. LANDIS. 1974. Functional changes in frog neuromuscular junctions studied with freeze-fracture. J. Neurocytol. **3:** 109–131.

30. AUGUSTINE, G. J. 1990. Regulation of transmitter release at the squid giant synapse by presynaptic delayed rectifier potassium current. J. Physiol. (Lond.) **431:** 343–364.

31. LESTER, H. A. 1970. Transmitter release by presynaptic impulses in the squid stellate ganglion. Nature **227:** 493–496.

32. STANLEY, E. F. 1986. Decline in calcium cooperativity as the basis of facilitation at the squid giant synapse. J. Neurosci. **6:** 782–789.
33. LIN, J. W. & D. S. FABER. 1988. Synaptic transmission mediated by single club endings on the goldfish Mauthner cell. II. Plasticity of excitatory postsynaptic potentials. J. Neurosci. **8:** 1313–1325.
34. HODGKIN, A. L. & A. F. HUXLEY. 1952. A quantitative description of membrane current and its application to conduction and excitation in nerve. J. Physiol. (Lond.) **117:** 500–544.
35. LLINÁS, R., I. Z. STEINBERG & K. WALTON. 1981. Presynaptic calcium current in squid giant synapse. Biophys. J. **33:** 289–322.
36. AUGUSTINE, G. J., M. P. CHARLTON & S. J. SMITH. 1985. Calcium entry into voltage-clamped presynaptic terminals of squid. J. Physiol. (Lond.) **367:** 143–162.
37. LLINÁS, R., M. SUGIMORI & S. M. SIMON. 1982. Transmission by spike-like depolarizations in the squid synapse. Proc. Natl. Acad. Sci. USA **79:** 2415–2419.
38. YOSHIKAMI, D., Z. BAGABALDO & B. M. OLIVERA. 1989. The inhibitory effects of omega-contotoxins on Ca channels and synapses. Ann. N.Y. Acad. Sci. **560:** 230–248.

Mechanisms Involved in
Calcium-Dependent Exocytosis[a]

RONALD W. HOLZ, JAN SENYSHYN,
AND MARY A. BITTNER

Department of Pharmacology
M6322 Medical Science I
University of Michigan Medical School
Ann Arbor, Michigan 48109-0626

Although a great deal is known concerning the membrane events controlling Ca^{2+} influx and metabolism, the events triggered by Ca^{2+} that lead to exocytosis in neurons and other cells are poorly understood. The purpose of this article is to consider some of the processes that control exocytosis, with special emphasis on the bovine adrenal chromaffin cell as a model system. Chromaffin cells are excitable cells and, like sympathetic nerves, are derived from the neural crest. Although chromaffin cells do not contain long processes or nerve terminals, secretion from chromaffin cells is stimulated by Ca^{2+} influx and inhibited by the clostridial neurotoxins (see below), which block exocytosis from the nerve terminals of peripheral and central nervous system neurons. Thus, it is likely that the secretory pathway in chromaffin cells is similar to that in neurons. Chromaffin cell secretory vesicles (chromaffin granules) are large, dense core vesicles that contain proteins, peptides, ATP, and the catecholamines epinephrine and norepinephrine. Ca^{2+} influx is stimulated in bovine chromaffin cells by activation of the nicotinic receptor/channel complex and voltage-sensitive Ca^{2+} channels.

EXOCYTOSIS AND GTP-BINDING PROTEINS

Exocytosis is the last fusion event in the repeated sequence of vesicle budding and fusion that characterizes the passage of secretory proteins from the endoplasmic reticulum to the cell exterior (for review see ref. 1). Secretory vesicles leaving the *trans* golgi network are targeted to different locations. Some vesicles are targeted to lysosomes. Some go quickly to the plasma membrane where exocytosis occurs in a seemingly unregulated manner (constitutive secretion).[2] Other vesicles fuse with the plasma membrane in a highly regulated manner. In the neuron, regulated exocytosis can occur meters away from the cell body where synthesis of the secretory vesicle membrane and intravesicular proteins occurs. Secretory vesicles involved in synaptic transmission journey to the nerve terminal by way of a microtubule-based transport system. After fusion with the plasma membrane, vesicle membrane recycles by way of endocytosis. In the case of small synaptic vesicles that store nonprotein neurotransmitters (*e.g.,* acetylcholine), the recycled vesicles are reused locally for exocytosis.[3]

In endocrine cells and nerve terminals, the events leading to fusion of the

[a]This work was supported by NIH Grants RO1 DK27959 and PO1 HL18575. Part of the work presented was done when R. W. Holz was an Established Investigator of the American Heart Association.

secretory vesicle with the plasma membrane are highly regulated. In most cases a rise in cytosolic Ca^{2+} from 0.1 μM to micromolar or higher concentrations is the primary trigger for exocytosis. One of the major challenges in the study of the biochemistry of exocytosis is to distinguish those processes that are intimately involved in regulating exocytosis from the many processes activated by Ca^{2+}. Although there are many possibilities (e.g., protein phosphorylation, cytoskeletal changes, changes in lipid metabolism: see below), at this time we do not know the critical events activated by Ca^{2+}. An alternative approach is to consider whether regulated exocytosis in either endocrine cells or in nerve terminals has elements in common with the multiple fusion events occurring earlier in the biosynthetic pathway of secretory proteins.

The genetic analysis of protein secretion in yeast led to the identification and purification of SEC4p, which is necessary for fusion of post-Golgi vesicles with the plasma membrane,[4,5] and YPT1p, which is necessary for protein transfer from endoplasmic reticulum (ER) to Golgi.[6] Both SEC4p and YPT1p are 23 kDa, GTP-binding proteins homologous to the ras family of GTP-binding proteins. They share 45% homology with each other. GTP-binding proteins are involved in the transfer and fusion of vesicles formed from donor cisternae (ER or Golgi compartments) to subsequent cisternae in the eukaryotic biosynthetic pathway. A nonhydrolyzable analogue of GTP (GTPγS) prevents transfer of protein from ER to Golgi,[7] and between Golgi compartments,[8] and induces the accumulation of coated vesicles in the Golgi region[9] and the accumulation of tubular-vesicular membranes near the ER. It has been postulated that GTP binding to vesicular protein and subsequent GTP hydrolysis are required for proper targeting and transfer of budding vesicles.[10] An epitope in common with YPT1p is associated with mammalian Golgi.[6]

Do low molecular weight, GTP-binding proteins generally play an important role in targeting secretory vesicles or controlling fusion in regulated exocytosis? At this time the answer is unclear. Both chromaffin granules, the secretory vesicles in adrenal chromaffin cells,[2,11] and bovine brain synaptic vesicles[12,13] contain numerous GTP-binding proteins between 20 and 30 kDa. FIGURE 1A demonstrates the multitude of these proteins that are found on secretory vesicles. One can distinguish at least six proteins on bovine chromaffin granule membranes and on bovine brain synaptic vesicles. (These brain synaptic vesicles display active glutamate uptake.[14,15]) GTP-binding proteins from chromaffin granules and synaptic vesicles have identical mobilities in SDS-PAGE. A GTP-binding protein of approximately 45 kDa can also be detected that probably corresponds to either α_o or α_i, the pertussis toxin substrates for ADP-ribosylation that have been previously demonstrated on chromaffin granules.[16] A quantitative analysis of GTP-binding sites on chromaffin granules (FIG. 1B) indicates that there are approximately 60 GTP-binding sites per chromaffin granule, which accounts for approximately 5% of the total granule membrane protein (see FIG. 1B legend). Nonhydrolyzable guanine nucleotides have a number of effects on secretion in permeabilized secretory cells. GTPγS inhibits Ca^{2+}-dependent secretion from electropermeabilized bovine chromaffin cells when added together with Ca^{2+}[17] and from digitonin-permeabilized bovine chromaffin cells when a low concentration of GTPγS is incubated with permeabilized cells prior to stimulation with Ca^{2+} (FIG. 2). These effects are consistent with the effects of GTPγS to inhibit transfer and fusion of vesicles in earlier steps in the biosynthetic pathway of secretory proteins. The effects, however, depend upon cell type, method of plasma membrane permeabilization and experimental design. For example, nonhydrolyzable guanine nucleotides stimulate Ca^{2+}-dependent secretion in electropermeabilized chicken chromaffin cells[17] and in bovine chromaffin cells permeabilized by α-toxin.[18] Guanine nucleotides and Ca^{2+} are required for secretion from streptolysin-O- or digitonin-permeabilized mast cells in the presence of high concentrations of Cl^-.[19,20] When the

Cl⁻ concentration, however, is reduced[19] or when protein kinase C is activated,[20] either GTPγS or Ca^{2+} alone stimulates submaximal secretion. GTPγS also stimulates Ca^{2+}-independent secretion from digitonin-permeabilized bovine chromaffin cells,[21,22] and PC12 cells,[23] and from mast cells using whole cell recording with the patch clamp.[24-26] The multitude of effects of nonhydrolyzable guanine nucleotides on secretion is not surprising inasmuch as guanine nucleotides can activate a host of

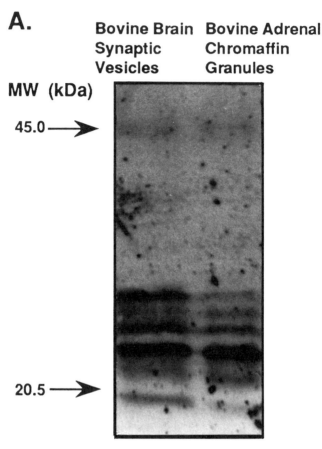

FIGURE 1A. GTP-binding proteins associated with bovine chromaffin granules and bovine brain glutamatergic synaptic vesicles. Chromaffin granules were purified from fresh bovine adrenal medulla. Adrenal glands were homogenized in 0.29 M sucrose, 10 mM Hepes (pH 7.1), 1 mM Na_2EDTA, 1 mM PMSF, and chromaffin granules purified using a discontinuous sucrose gradient according to Smith and Winkler,[73] except that the large granule fraction was layered over a 1.7 M sucrose solution. The gradient was centrifuged at $146,000 \times g_{ave} \times 70$ min in a Beckman 50.2 Ti rotor. The chromaffin granules were collected in the pellet, lysed in 10 mM Hepes (pH 7.1), and washed twice and stored at −70. Synaptic vesicles were purified from bovine brain according to the methods of Ueda and colleagues[14,15] with an additional gel filtration step using Sephacryl 1000. The vesicle fraction concentrated glutamate in an ATP-dependent manner. The molecular masses of the GTP-binding proteins are 20.1 kDa, 22.4 kDa, 23.0 kDa (dense band), 24.6 kDa, 26.5 kDa, 27.5 kDa, and 45 kDa.

B.

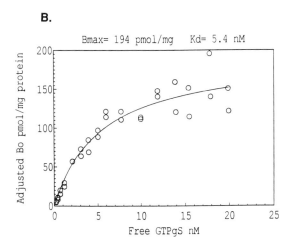

FIGURE 1B. Specific GTPγS binding to chromaffin granule membranes. Purified chromaffin granules (2 μg/mL) were incubated with various concentrations of nonradioactive GTPγS and 0.235 nM [³⁵S]GTPγS (0.23 μC$_i$/mL) for 90 min at 30°C. The suspension was passed through a nitrocellulose filter. The filter was washed extensively and the radioactivity determined.[74] The data were analyzed by a nonlinear, least squares algorithm. Assuming a chromaffin granule diameter of 2800 angstroms, 17 μL chromaffin granule volume/mg membrane protein and maximal binding of 194 pmoles/mg membrane protein, one calculates 78 GTPγS binding sites/chromaffin granule. A similar experiment using a different preparation of granules yielded 130 pmoles GTPγS binding/mg membrane protein and 52 GTPγS binding sites/chromaffin granule. Approximately 4–6% of the total chromaffin granule membrane protein is GTP-binding protein, assuming an average molecular mass of 30 kDa for GTP-binding proteins.

enzymes either directly or indirectly (*e.g.,* adenylate cyclase, phospholipase C, phospholipase A$_2$, protein kinase C) that could influence the secretory response. Thus, it is unclear which, if any, of the effects of guanine nucleotides on secretion requires GTP-binding proteins on secretory vesicles. Furthermore, it is possible that the GTP-binding proteins associated with secretory vesicles are not directly involved in secretion but with other functions of the vesicles related to biosynthesis of the membrane[27] or recycling after exocytosis.

THE ROLE OF ATP IN SECRETION: PRIMING OF SECRETION, PROTEIN PHOSPHORYLATION, AND MAINTENANCE OF POLYPHOSPHOINOSITIDES

Experiments with permeabilized chromaffin cells by Baker and Knight[28,29] conclusively demonstrated a role for ATP hydrolysis in the intracellular pathway for exocytosis. Synaptic transmission occurs within less than a millisecond after invasion of the terminal by the action potential and the opening of voltage-sensitive Ca^{2+} channels. Because this is insufficient time for a cascade of biochemical reactions,[30] the exocytotic machinary must be poised to respond rapidly to the rise in Ca^{2+}. In experiments with the patch clamp in which incorporation of the granule membrane into the plasma membrane is measured by increases in plasma-membrane capacitance, depolarization-induced secretion from chromaffin cells occurs within the time

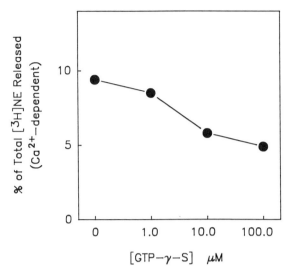

FIGURE 2. GTPγS inhibits secretion from digitonin-permeabilized chromaffin cells. [³H]nor-epinephrine-labeled chromaffin cells were permeabilized by incubation in KGEP [139 mM potassium glutamate, 5 mM EGTA, 20 mM PIPES (pH 6.6), 1 mM $MgCl_2$, and 5 mg/mL BSA] containing 2 mM MgATP, 20 μM digitonin, and various concentrations of GTPγS. After 4 min, the solution was replaced with digitonin-free KGEP without MgATP and GTPγS, and with and without 10 μM free Ca^{2+}. Ca^{2+}-dependent secretion was determined after 2 min. Secretion in the absence of Ca^{2+} was 1.6–2.4%. GTPγS at all concentrations released less than 1% of the catecholamine during the incubation with digitonin. There were 3 wells/group.

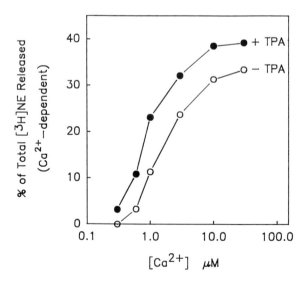

FIGURE 3. The phorbol es-ter TPA enhances secretion from digitonin-perme-abilized chromaffin cells. [³H]norepinephrine-labeled cells were incubated for 30 min in MEM with or with-out 20 nM TPA. The cells were permeabilized in KGEP containing 2 mM MgATP with indicated [Ca^{2+}]. Ca^{2+}-dependent se-cretion was determined af-ter 15 min. Secretion in the absence of Ca^{2+} was 3.4–3.6%. There were 3 wells/group.

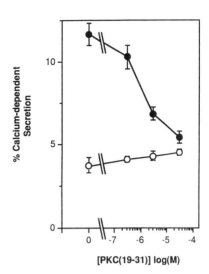

FIGURE 4. The protein kinase C inhibitor peptide PKC(19-31) inhibits Ca^{2+}-dependent secretion in TPA-treated but not in TPA-untreated chromaffin cells. [³H]norepinephrine-labeled cells were incubated for 15 min with (filled circles) or without (unfilled circles) 60 nM TPA in physiological salt solution. Cells were permeabilized for 6 min in Ca^{2+}-free potassium glutamate solution (KGEP) containing 20 μM digitonin in the presence or absence of increasing concentrations of PKC(19-31). The solution was replaced with KGEP with or without 1 μM Ca^{2+} in the continuing presence or absence of PKC(19-31). Ca^{2+}-dependent secretion was measured after 5 min. Release in the absence of Ca^{2+} was 3.1–4.4%. There were 3 wells/group.[42]

resolution of the experiments (several hundred milliseconds).[31] In experiments in which release of catecholamine is detected biochemically, the maximal rate of secretion occurs within the first 1–2 min and then slows[32]; secretion can be reproducibly detected within 10 seconds.[33] We found that the rapid initial rate of catecholamine secretion requires prior incubation with ATP.[32] Although the time scale of the experiments is orders of magnitude slower than the events following Ca^{2+} entry in the nerve terminal, the experiments nevertheless demonstrate that ATP acts before Ca^{2+} to prime the cell to respond to Ca^{2+}. A similar conclusion can be drawn from experiments with mast cells.[34]

ATP is required for protein phosphorylation, and there is abundant evidence that protein phosphorylation modulates exocytosis. In the squid giant synapse[35] and mammalian synaptosomes[36] Ca/calmodulin kinase II enhances secretion, perhaps by

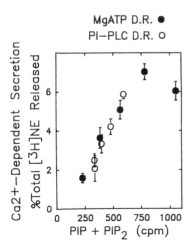

FIGURE 5. The relationship between the levels of the polyphosphoinositides and Ca^{2+}-dependent secretion in digitonin-permeabilized chromaffin cells. The polyphosphoinositides were varied in digitonin-permeabilized cells by varying the concentrations of MgATP or by varying the concentrations of a PtdIns-specific phospholipase C from *Bacillus thuringiensis*. [³H]Inositol-labeled cells were permeabilized for 8 min in Ca^{2+}-free potassium glutamate solution (KGEP) containing either various amounts of MgATP or 2 mM MgATP and various amounts of bacterial phospholipase C. The levels of [³H]inositol-labeled PtdIns, PtdInsP, and PtdInsP₂ were determined after an additional 3 min incubation in 10 μM Ca^{2+} in the continuing presence of MgATP. Bacterial phospholpase C was not present in the last incubation. Ca^{2+}-dependent secretion from [³H]norepinephrine-labeled cells was determined in parallel experiments at 6 min. For details see FIG. 5 in ref. 45.

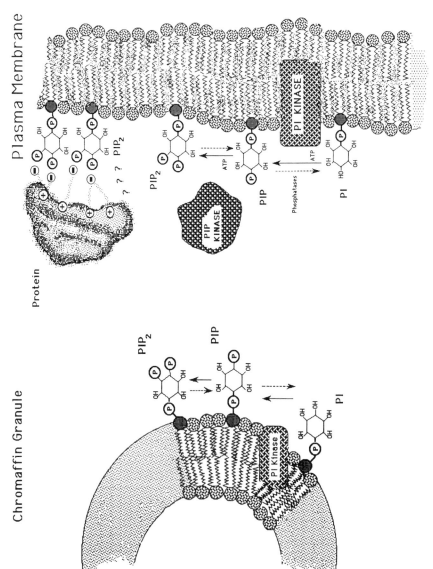

FIGURE 6

phosphorylation of synapsin I. In many secretory cells including chromaffin cells, activation of protein kinase C increases the ability of cells to respond to submicromolar and micromolar Ca^{2+}.[37-39] FIGURE 3 demonstrates effects of the protein kinase C activator TPA (12-O-tetradecanoylphorbol acetate) on the Ca^{2+} dose-response relation for secretion from permeabilized cells. Because cellular protein kinase C can be activated by Ca^{2+} in the absence of exogenous activators,[33,40] an important issue is whether protein kinase C is required for secretion and is responsible for the ATP dependency. We have recently addressed this issue in permeabilized chromaffin cells using a specific inhibitor of protein kinase C. The synthetic peptide PKC(19-31), which is derived from the pseudosubstrate sequence of protein kinase C, is a potent inhibitor of protein kinase C *in vitro*[41] and *in situ* within permeabilized cells.[42] Although it inhibited phorbol ester-induced secretion in the presence of Ca^{2+} almost completely, it had no effect on Ca^{2+}-dependent secretion in the absence of phorbol ester (FIG. 4). Thus, it is unlikely that the ATP-dependency for secretion reflects the necessary involvement of protein kinase C in the secretory pathway. Similarly, it is unlikely that calmodulin-dependent protein kinase or other calmodulin-dependent processes play a necessary role in secretion from permeabilized cells. Relatively high concentrations of the calmodulin antagonists trifluoperazine and calmidazolium have either partial effects in electropermeabilized chromaffin cells[29,43] or virtually no effects in digitonin-permeabilized chromaffin cells (Holz, unpublished observations). Furthermore, an anticalmodulin antibody (Holz, unpublished observations) and a calmodulin-binding peptide[42] have no effect on secretion from digitonin-permeabilized chromaffin cells. The ability of an anticalmodulin antibody to inhibit secretion when injected into intact cells[44] may reflect a role for calmodulin in the events leading to a rise in cytosolic Ca^{2+}.

These data led us to consider other reactions in which ATP may be involved. We found that the maintenance of the polyphosphoinositides by PI and PIP kinases occurred over the same MgATP concentration range as that necessary to maintain exocytosis.[45] We also found that in the presence of MgATP we could manipulate the levels of the polyphosphoinositides by a bacterial phospholipase C that hydrolyzed their precursor, phosphatidylinositol. The polyphosphoinositides declined because of the action of endogenous lipid phosphatases in the absence of continued synthesis. The relationship between Ca^{2+}-dependent secretion and the polyphosphoinositides was the same whether the lipids were manipulated by varying the MgATP concentration or by varying the concentration of the bacterial phospholipase C (FIGURES 5 and 6). The inhibitory effects of the exogenous phospholipase C could not be explained by the products of the bacterial phospholipase C reaction (IP_1 and diacylglycerol) or the loss of products from the endogenous phospholipase C (due to the loss of the polyphosphoinositide substrates). The simplest and most compelling interpretation is that the polyphosphoinositides are necessary in the secretory pathway. Thus, ATP

FIGURE 6. Polyphosphoinositide metabolism in chromaffin cells. The polyphosphoinositides are synthesized from phosphatidylinositol by PI and PIP kinases. In resting cells, PIP_2 phosphatase and PIP phosphatase are responsible for degrading the polyphosphoinositides. Phospholipase C activated by receptor-mediated mechanisms or by a rise in cytosolic Ca^{2+}[75] breaks down PIP_2 to IP_3 and diacylglycerol (not shown). Experiments in which the polyphosphoinositides are decreased by ATP or by hydrolysis of PI with a bacterial phospholipase C demonstrate a close correlation between the levels of the polyphosphoinositides and Ca^{2+}-dependent secretion.[45] Thus, reducing either substrate for PI kinase reduces the polyphosphoinositides and Ca^{2+}-dependent secretion. The requirement for the polyphosphoinositides in secretion could reflect the importance of a protein that binds to and is regulated by these lipids.

is important not only for modulation of secretion by protein kinases, but also for maintenance of the polyphosphoinositides.

Polyphosphoinositides are synthesized both on the plasma membrane[47] and on the chromaffin granule membrane[48-50] (FIG. 6). The binding of a protein to PIP_2 (and/or PIP) on either membrane may regulate its function in secretion. There are at least two proteins, myosin I and gelsolin, that bind to the polyphosphoinositides and to actin. Myosin I, which causes actin-dependent organelle movement, has recently been demonstrated to bind to PIP_2.[51] The ability of gelsolin to cause Ca^{2+}-dependent severing of f-actin is inhibited by polyphosphoinositides[52] (for review see [53]). Because chromaffin granules also interact with f-actin,[54-56] it is possible that the PIP_2 or PIP localizes these proteins to secretory sites and controls the interaction of chromaffin granules with the cortical cytoskeleton and the plasma membrane. In addition, calpactin I, which interacts with acidic phospholipids including the polyphosphoinositides,[57] aggregates and under some conditions allows fusion of chromaffin granules *in vitro*.[58,59] Indeed, recent reports suggest that calpactin is in intimate contact with chromaffin granules, and the plasma membrane in intact cells,[60] and can maintain secretion in digitonin-permeabilized chromaffin cells.[61,62]

CLOSTRIDIAL NEUROTOXINS DIRECTLY INHIBIT THE EXOCYTOTIC PATHWAY

Botulinum and tetanus neurotoxins (clostridial neurotoxins) block neurotransmitter release from various neurons and are thought to interact with critical sites in the exocytotic pathway.[63] Botulinum type D neurotoxin interacts with bovine tissues and inhibits secretion from both intact and electropermeabilized bovine chromaffin cells.[64] Extracellular application of botulinum types A, B, or E neurotoxin or tetanus neurotoxin has no effect on intact bovine chromaffin cells because of the absence of receptors on the plasma membrane. The introduction of these toxins, however, into cells through a patch-clamp electrode[65] or by incubation with digitonin- or streptolysin O (SL-O)-permeabilized cells[66-69] inhibits secretion. Experiments with permeabilized cells demonstrate that the light chain (50 kDa) of the dichain molecules (150 kDa) is responsible for the inhibition of secretion.[67,68,70] The ability of these classical inhibitors of synaptic transmission to inhibit exocytosis from chromaffin cells indicates that there are common elements in the secretory pathway in neurons and chromaffin cells. The toxins decrease the maximal extent of secretion and not the sensitivity to Ca^{2+}.[66,67] Interestingly, the toxins do not all act alike. Both tetanus toxin and botulinum B neurotoxins completely inhibit secretion, whereas botulinum A neurotoxin, even at high concentrations, inhibits secretion by no more than 70 percent. Thus, the toxins may interact with different sites in the secretory pathway. At the intact neuromuscular junction, the effects of tetanus and botulinum B neurotoxins can also be distinguished from those of botulinum A neurotoxin. Tetanus and botulinum B neurotoxins reduce evoked miniature end-plate potentials (MEPPS) and desynchronize those MEPPS that are observed.[71] Botulinum A neurotoxin also reduces evoked MEPPS but without desynchronizing the residual MEPPS. Key issues for future investigation are the sites of interaction of the light chains of these toxins within nerve terminals and chromaffin cells and the possibility that they may act through an unknown enzymatic activity. The ADP-ribosylating activity of neurotoxin preparations is likely to be caused by contaminating ADP-ribosyl transferase activity (C-3 toxin).[72]

ACKNOWLEDGMENTS

We are grateful to Dr. T. Ueda and Dr. J. Tabb (Mental Health Research Institute and the Department of Pharmacology, University of Michigan) for providing us with purified bovine brain synaptic vesicles. We thank Peter Wick (Department of Pharmacology, University of Michigan Medical School) for preparing FIGURE 6.

REFERENCES

1. BALCH, W. E. 1989. J. Biol. Chem. **264:** 16965–16968.
2. BURGESS, T. L. & R. B. KELLY. 1987. Annu. Rev. Cell Biol. **3:** 243–294.
3. TORRI-TARELLI, F., A. VILLA, F. VALTORTA, P. DE CAMILLI, P. GREENGARD & B. CECCARELLI. 1990. J. Cell Biol. **459:** 449–459.
4. NOVICK, P., C. FIELD & R. SCHEKMAN. 1980. Cell **21:** 205–215.
5. GOUD, B., A. SALMINEN, N. C. WALWORTH & P. J. NOVICK. 1988. Cell **53:** 753–768.
6. SEGEV, N., J. MULHOLLAND & D. BOTSTEIN. 1988. Cell **52:** 915–924.
7. BECKERS, C. J. & W. E. BALCH. 1989. J. Cell Biol. **108:** 1245–1256.
8. MELANCON, P., B. S. GLICK, V. MALHOTRA, P. J. WEIDMAN, T. SERAFINI, M. L. GLEASON, L. ORCI & J. E. ROTHMAN. 1987. Cell **51:** 1053–1062.
9. ROTHMAN, J. E. & L. ORCI. 1990. FASEB J. **4:** 1460–1468.
10. BOURNE, H. R. 1988. Cell **53:** 669–671.
11. BURGOYNE, R. D. & A. MORGAN. 1989. FEBS Lett. **245:** 122–126.
12. BIELINSKI, D. F., P. J. MORIN, B. F. DICKERY & R. E. FINE. 1989. J. Biol. Chem. **264:** 18363–18367.
13. MOLLARD, G. F. V., G. A. MIGNERY, M. BAUMERT, M. S. PERIN, R. J. HANSON, P. M. BURGER, R. JAHN & T. C. SUDHOF. 1990. Proc. Natl. Acad. Sci. USA **87:** 1988–1992.
14. KISH, P. E. & T. UEDA. 1986. Glutamate accumulation into synaptic vesicles. *In* Methods in Enzymology Biomembranes Part V. S. Fleischer & B. Fleischer, Eds.: **174:** 9–25. Academic Press. New York.
15. CARLSON, M. D., P. E. KISH & T. UEDA. 1989. J. Biol. Chem. **264:** 7369–7376.
16. TOUTANT, M., D. AUNIS, J. BOCKAERT, V. HOMBURGER & B. ROUOT. 1987. FEBS Lett. **215:** 339–344.
17. KNIGHT, D. E. & P. F. BAKER. 1985. FEBS Lett. **189:** 345–349.
18. BADER, M.-F., J.-M. SONTAG, D. THIERSE & D. AUNIS. 1989. J. Biol. Chem. **264:** 16426–16434.
19. CHURCHER, Y. & B. D. GOMPERTS. 1990. Cell Regul. **1:** 337–346.
20. KOOPMAN, W. R. & R. C. JACKSON. 1990. Biochem. J. **265:** 365–373.
21. BITTNER, M. A., R. W. HOLZ & R. R. NEUBIG. 1986. J. Biol. Chem. **261:** 10182–10188.
22. MORGAN, A. & R. D. BURGOYNE. 1990. Biochem. J. **269:** 521–526.
23. CARROLL, A. G., A. R. RHOADS & P. D. WAGNER. 1990. J. Neurochem. **55:** 930–936.
24. FERNANDEZ, J. M., E. NEHER & B. D. GOMPERTS. 1984. Nature **312:** 453–455.
25. ZIMMERBERG, J., M. CURRAN, F. S. COHEN & M. BRODWICK. 1987. Proc. Natl. Acad. Sci. USA **84:** 1585–1589.
26. BRECKENRIDGE, L. J. & W. ALMERS. 1987. Proc. Natl. Acad. Sci. USA **84:** 1945–1949.
27. TOOZE, S. A., U. WEISS & W. B. HUTTNER. 1990. Nature **347:** 207–208.
28. BAKER, P. F. & D. E. KNIGHT. 1978. Nature **276:** 620–622.
29. KNIGHT, D. E. & P. F. BAKER. 1982. J. Membr. Biol. **68:** 107–140.
30. ALMERS, W. 1990. Annu. Rev. Physiol. **52:** 607–624.
31. NEHER, E. & A. MARTY. 1982. Proc. Natl. Acad. Sci. USA **79:** 6712–6716.
32. HOLZ, R. W., M. A. BITTNER, S. C. PEPPERS, R. A. SENTER & D. A. EBERHARD. 1989. J. Biol. Chem. **264:** 5412–5419.
33. TERBUSH, D. R., M. A. BITTNER & R. W. HOLZ. 1988. J. Biol. Chem. **263:** 18873–18879.
34. HOWELL, T. W., I. M. KRAMER & B. D. GOMPERTS. 1989. Cellular Signal. **1:** 157–163.
35. LLINÁS, R., R. L. MCGUINNESS, C. S. LEONARD, M. SUGIMORI & P. GREENGARD. 1985. Proc. Natl. Acad. Sci. USA **82:** 3035–3039.

36. NICHOLS, R. A., T. S. SIHRA, A. J. CZERNIK, A. C. NAIRN & P. GREENGARD. 1990. Nature **343:** 647–651.
37. KNIGHT, D. E. & P. F. BAKER. 1983. FEBS Lett. **160:** 98–100.
38. POCOTTE, S. L., R. A. FRYE, R. A. SENTER, D. R. TERBUSH, S. A. LEE & R. W. HOLZ. 1985. Proc. Natl. Acad. Sci. USA **82:** 930–934.
39. BROCKLEHURST, K. W., K. MORITA & H. B. POLLARD. 1985. Biochem. J. **228:** 35–42.
40. TERBUSH, D. R. & R. W. HOLZ. 1986. J. Biol. Chem. **261:** 17099–17106.
41. HOUSE, C. & B. E. KEMP. 1987. Science **238:** 1726–1728.
42. TERBUSH, D. R. & R. W. HOLZ. 1990. J. Biol. Chem. **265:** 21179–21184.
43. KNIGHT, D. E., D. SUGDEN & P. F. BAKER. 1988. J. Membr. Biol. **104:** 21–34.
44. KENIGSBERG, R. L. & J. M. TRIFARO. 1985. Neurosci. **14:** 335–347.
45. EBERHARD, D. A., C. L. COOPER, M. G. LOW & R. W. HOLZ. 1990. Biochem. J. **268:** 15–25.
46. EDELMAN, A. M., D. K. BLUMENTHAL & E. G. KREBS. 1987. Annu. Rev. Biochem. **56:** 567–613.
47. BERRIDGE, M. J. 1987. Annu. Rev. Biochem. **56:** 159–193.
48. BUCKLEY, J. T., Y. A. LEFEBVRE & J. N. HAWTHORNE. 1971. Biochim. Biophys. Acta **239:** 517–519.
49. MULLER, T. W. & N. KIRSHNER. 1975. J. Neurochem. **24:** 1155–1161.
50. PHILLIPS, J. H. 1973. Biochem. J. **136:** 579–587.
51. ADAMS, R. J. & T. D. POLLARD. 1989. Nature **340:** 565–568.
52. JANMEY, P. A. & T. P. STOSSEL. 1989. J. Biol. Chem. **264:** 4825–4831.
53. YIN, H. L. 1987. Bioessays **7:** 176–179.
54. BURRIDGE, K. & J. A. PHILLIPS. 1975. Nature **254:** 526–529.
55. WILKINS, J. A. & S. LIN. 1981. Biochim. Biophys. Acta **642:** 55–66.
56. FOWLER, V. M. & H. B. POLLARD. 1982. Nature **295:** 336–339.
57. GLENNEY, J. 1986. J. Biol. Chem. **261:** 7247–7252.
58. DRUST, D. S. & C. E. CREUTZ. 1988. Nature **331:** 88–91.
59. GLENNEY, J. R. 1987. Bioessays **7:** 173–175.
60. NAKATA, T., K. SOBUE & N. HIROKAWA. 1990. J. Cell Biol. **110:** 13–25.
61. ALI, S. M., M. J. GEISOW & R. D. BURGOYNE. 1989. Nature **340:** 313–315.
62. ALI, S. M. & R. D. BURGOYNE. 1990. Cellular Signal. **2:** 265–276.
63. SIMPSON, L. L. 1986. Annu. Rev. Pharmacol. Toxicol. **26:** 427–453.
64. KNIGHT, D. E., D. A. TONGE & P. F. BAKER. 1985. Nature **317:** 719–721.
65. PENNER, R., E. NEHER & F. DREYER. 1986. Nature **324:** 76–78.
66. BITTNER, M. A. & R. W. HOLZ. 1988. J. Neurochem. **51:** 451–456.
67. BITTNER, M. A., B. R. DASGUPTA & R. W. HOLZ. 1989. J. Biol. Chem. **264:** 10354–10360.
68. AHNERT-HILGER, G., U. WELLER, M. E. DAUZENROTH, E. HABERMANN & M. GRATZL. 1989. FEBS Lett. **242:** 245–248.
69. STECHER, B., M. GRATZL & G. AHNERT-HILGER. 1989. FEBS Lett. **248:** 23–27.
70. BITTNER, M. A., W. H. HABIG & R. W. HOLZ. 1989. J. Neurochem. **53:** 966–968.
71. GANSEL, M., R. PENNER & F. DREYER. 1987. Pfluegers Arch. **409:** 533–539.
72. ADAM-VIZI, V., S. ROSENER, K. AKTORIES & D. E. KNIGHT. 1988. FEBS Lett. **238:** 277–280.
73. SMITH, A. D. & H. WINKLER. 1967. Biochem. J. **103:** 480–482.
74. STERNWEIS, P. C. & J. D. ROBISHAW. 1984. J. Biol. Chem. **259:** 13806–13813.
75. EBERHARD, D. A. & R. W. HOLZ. 1987. J. Neurochem. **49:** 1634–1643.

MPP$^+$ Enhances Potassium-Evoked Striatal Dopamine Release through a ω-Conotoxin-Insensitive, Tetrodotoxin- and Nimodipine-Sensitive Calcium-Dependent Mechanism

C. C. CHIUEH AND S.-J. HUANG

Laboratory of Cerebral Metabolism
National Institute of Mental Health
National Institutes of Health
Building 10, Room 2D-55
Bethesda, Maryland 20892

Presynaptic function of calcium ions in neural transmission and exocytoic secretion is well-documented.[1] Calcium ions can enter neuronal membrane through either voltage-regulated calcium channels, such as T-, N-, L-, and P-type channels, or through receptor-linked calcium channels. Previous studies indicate that calcium entry through the presynaptic N-type (ω-conotoxin GVIA-sensitive) rather than the L-type (1,4-dihydropyridine-sensitive) channels regulates transmitter release from nerve terminals.[2,3] Entry and cycling of extracellular calcium ions, however, through dihydropyridine-sensitive L-type voltage-regulated calcium channels, play a key role in mediating a sustained secretion of pituitary hormones, adrenal catecholamines, and neuropeptides.[4,5]

Similar to cardiac and vascular smooth muscles, the presence of highly specific dihydropyridine binding sites has been demonstrated in brain tissue.[6] The specific function mediated by these binding sites for L-type calcium antagonist is mostly unknown. Recently, clinical case reports have suggested the involvement of calcium channel blockers in regulating brain functions. For example, depression and parkinsonism have been observed in aged patients after receiving nondihydropyridine calcium channel blockers.[7] Available evidence suggests nimodipine, a CNS L-type calcium antagonist, is promising for treatment of mania, tardive dyskinesia, and also for retarding the progressive dementia seen in Alzheimer's disease.[8,9] Consequently, it is of interest to investigate the role of nimodipine-sensitive L-type calcium channels in mediating the release of endogenous dopamine from the caudate nucleus evoked by potassium depolarization and MPP$^+$ (1-methyl-4-phenylpyridine).

MPP$^+$ is one of the most potent dopamine- and serotonin-releasing agents[10] when it is infused through a microdialysis probe[11] (1 µL/min, CMA-20 Carnegie Medicin, Sweden) placed in the dorsolateral caudate nucleus of anesthetized rats. Additionally, intracranially administered MPP$^+$ is capable of inducing calcium uptake and overload leading to cell death.[12] In this *in vivo* intrastriatal dialysis study, potassium depolarization (30 nmol/min, for 5 min) potentiated dopamine release elicited by 50 pmol MPP$^+$ (TABLE 1). Potassium-evoked dopamine release was also enhanced by 5 nmol 4-aminopyridine.

Perfusion of the striatum with either tetrodotoxin (10 pmol/min) or calcium-free Ringer's solution containing EGTA (1 nmol/min) antagonized the enhanced potas-

TABLE I. Effects of MPP$^+$ and 4-Aminopyridine on Potassium-Induced Dopamine Release from the Caudate Nucleus *in Vivo*[a]

	Net Dopamine Efflux[b] (pmol)
KCl	0.10 ± 0.01
MPP$^+$	0.41 ± 0.06
4-AP	0.10 ± 0.03
KCl + MPP$^+$	1.97 ± 0.23
KCl + 4-AP	1.10 ± 0.24

[a]An intrastriatal microdialysis perfusion[11] was used to investigate the effects of KCl (150 nmol), MPP$^+$ (50 pmol), and 4-AP (5 nmol) on the release of endogenous dopamine from the nigrostrital dopaminergic terminals of anesthetized rats. Following a 60 min washout, drugs were added to Ringer's solution and perfused (1 μL/min for 5 min) through the microdialysis probe; dialysates were collected every 5 min and assayed for dopamine by HPLC procedure.[10] Resting efflux of dopamine was about 0.03 pmol/min. Results show mean and one SEM of drug-induced–increased dopamine release obtained from 4 animals.

[b]$p < 0.05$.

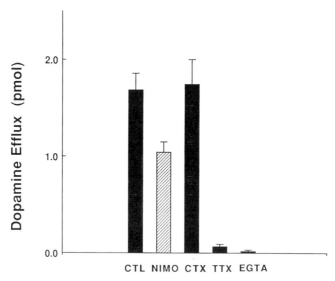

FIGURE 1. Effects of pretreatment with nimodipine (NIMO), ω-conotoxin GVIA (CTX), tetrodotoxin (TTX), and EGTA (calcium-free) on MPP$^+$-enhanced dopamine release evoked by potassium depolarization. Similar to the experimental procedure described in TABLE 1, enhanced dopamine release was evoked by infusing Ringer's solution containing 50 pmol MPP$^+$ and 150 nmol KCl through a microdialysis probe placed in the striatum of anesthetized rats. During the pretreatment studies, drugs (nimodipine, ω-cocotoxin GVIA, or tetrodotoxin, 10 pmol/μL/min each) were added to the Ringer's solution one hour prior to the infusion of MPP$^+$ and KCl. In the EGTA group, the striatum was perfused with calcium-free Ringer's solution containing EGTA (1 mmol/L) instead of the normal Ringer's solution with 2.3 mmol/L calcium ions. N = 3 to 7. Each column depicts the net dopamine efflux following a 5 min perfusion with MPP$^+$ and KCl.

sium-induced dopamine efflux in the presence of 50 picomoles MPP[+] (FIG. 1). This calcium-mediated dopamine release elicited by MPP[+] in the presence of potassium was modified by pretreating with nimodipine but not ω-conotoxin GVIA (FIG. 1). Nimodipine antagonism of dopamine release evoked by potassium and MPP[+] seems to be regulated by membrane potential[13]; this inhibitory effect increases to about 70% when voltage is clamped to near 0 mV *in vivo* by infusing 120 nmol/min potassium. Nimodipine also blocks increased dopamine efflux from a newly synthesized amine pool in mesolimbic nerve terminals of the nucleus accumbens following haloperidol (i.p.).[14]

In conclusion, picomoles MPP[+]–potentiated depolarization-induced brain dopamine release is a calcium-dependent exocytotic secretion. This observed potentiation of endogenous dopamine release elicited by MPP[+] is thought to be mediated by calcium entry through nimodipine-sensitive and ω-conotoxin-insensitive L-type calcium channels. These neuronal L-type calcium channels on dopamine nerve terminals are highly voltage-gated; their exocytotic function can be up-regulated by depolarization and down-regulated by tetrodotoxin. Therefore, these *in vivo* results suggest that calcium uptake through neuronal L-type voltage-sensitive calcium channels on dopaminergic nerve terminals mediates a sustained exocytotic release of "newly synthesized" brain dopamine in response to prolonged depolarization as evoked by potassium and/or MPP[+]. CNS therapeutic effects of nimodipine might be mainly due to its ability in antagonizing a sustained calcium-mediated efflux of brain dopamine evoked by prolonged depolarization as shown by this study.

ACKNOWLEDGMENTS

Nimodipine was kindly supplied by Dr. A. Scriabine of the Institute of Preclinical Pharmacology, Miles Inc. We thank Dr. E. Stanley for donating ω-conotoxin GVIA to this project.

REFERENCES

1. MILLER, R. J. 1987. Multiple calcium channels and neuronal function. Science **235:** 46–62.
2. HIRNING, L. D., A. P. FOX, E. W. MCCESKEY, B. M. OLIVERA, S. A. THAYER, R. J. MILLER & R. W. TSIEN. 1988. Dominent role of N-type Ca[+] channels in evoked release of norepinephrine from sympathetic neurons. Science **239:** 57–61.
3. HERDON, H. & S. R. NABORSKI. 1989. Investigation of the role of dihydropyridine and ω-conotoxin-sensitive calcium channels in mediating depolarization-evoked endogenous dopamine release from striatal slices. Naunyn-Schmiedeberg's Arch. Pharmakol. **340:** 36–40.
4. LADONA, M. G., D. AUNIS, L. GANDIA & A. G. GARCIA. 1987. Dihydropyridine modulation of chromaffin cell secretory response. J. Neurochem. **48:** 483–490.
5. SHANGOLD, G. A., S. N. MURPHY & R. J. MILLER. 1988. Gonadotropin-releasing hormone-induced Ca[2+] transients in single identified gonadotropes require both intracellular Ca[2+] mobilization and Ca[2+] influx. Proc. Natl. Acad. Sci. USA **85:** 6566–6570.
6. MORANGOS, P. J., J. PATE, C. MILLER & A. M. MARTINO. 1982. Specific calcium antagonist binding sites in brain. Life Sci. **31:** 1575–1585.
7. CHOUZA, C., A. SCARAMELLI, J. L. CAAMANO, O. DEMEDINA, R. ALJANATI & S. ROMERO. 1896. Parkinsonism, tardive dyskinesia, akathisia and depression induced by flunarizine. Lancet **1:** 1301–1304.
8. BRUNET, G., B. CERLICH, P. ROBERT, S. DUMAS, E. SOUETRE & G. DARCOURT. 1990. Open trial of a calcium antagonist, nimodipine, in acute mania. Clin. Neuropharmacol. **13:** 224–228.

9. TOLLEFSON, G. D. 1990. Short-term effects of the calcium channel blocker nimodipine (Bay-e-9736) in the management of primary degenerative dementia. Biol. Psychiatry **27:** 1133–1142.

10. MIYAKE, H. & C. C. CHIUEH. 1989. Effects of MPP$^+$ on the release of serotonin and 5-hydroxyindoleacetic acid from rat striatum *in vivo.* Eur. J. Pharmacol. **166:** 49–55.

11. UNGERSTEDT, U. 1984. Measurement of neurotransmitter release by intracranial dialysis. *In* Measurement of Neurotransmitter Release *in Vivo.* C. A. Marsden, Ed.: 81–105. John Wiley & Sons. Chicester, England.

12. SUN, C. J., J. N. JOHANNESSEN, W. P. GESSNER, I. NAMURA, W. SINGHANIYOM, A. BROSSI & C. C. CHIUEH. 1988. Neurotoxic damage to the nigrostriatal system in rats following intranigral administration of MPDP$^+$ and MPP$^+$. J. Neural Transm. **74:** 75–86.

13. CHIUEH, C. C., H. MIYAKE, S.-J. HUANG & M.-T. PENG. 1990. Role of extracellular calcium ion on 1-methyl-4-phenylpyridine (MPP$^+$) induced sustained exocytosis of endogenous striatal dopamine *in vivo.* Eur. J. Pharmacol. **183:** 1069–1070.

14. DENG, F.-C. & C. C. CHIUEH. 1990. Mediation of haloperidol-enhanced dopamine release but not homovanillic acid efflux from mesolimbic neurons by calcium entry through nimodipine-sensitive L-type voltage-regulated calcium channels. Proc. Am. College Neuropsychopharmacol. (Abstract).

Depolarization-Induced Presynaptic Calcium Accumulation May Occur by an N-Type Channel That Is Blocked by Flunarizine

STANLEY L. COHAN, MEI CHEN, DAVID REDMOND,
AND DAHLIA WILSON

Department of Neurology
3800 Reservoir Road, N.W.
Georgetown University
Washington, D.C. 20007

The cerebral synaptosome is an important potential *in vitro* model for study of the pathophysiology and pharmacology of stroke. Sustained depolarization resulting primarily from excessive extracellular potassium (K^+) accumulation is known to occur in stroke[1] and promotes excessive cystosolic calcium (Ca^{2+}) accumulation by way of voltage-regulated channels.[2] Much of this Ca^{2+} accumulation occurs presynaptically,[3] which may directly promote cell damage[4] in the presynaptic compartment but also may promote damage in the postsynaptic compartment through Ca^{2+}-dependent release of neurotoxic excitatory amino acids.[5] It is for these reasons that we have chosen to study the effect of sustained K^+-induced depolarization upon synaptosomal Ca^{2+} uptake as a model of stroke.

METHODS

Gerbil cerebral synaptosomes were prepared by homogenization and differential centrifugation in sucrose[6] and suspended in Hepes buffer (2 mg synaptosomal protein/mL) containing (in mM) NaCl, 125; KCl, 5; NaH_2PO_4, 1.2; $MgCl_2$, 1.2; $NaHCO_3$, 5; D-glucose, 6; $CaCl_2$, 0.02; and Hepes 25, adjusted to pH 7.4 with NaOH; 1.0 mL of this suspension was incubated with the fluorescent Ca^{2+}-ligand fura-2 AM for 40 minutes at 30°C, and the incubation was terminated by the addition of 9.0 mL ice-cold Hepes buffer. Fura-2–loaded synaptosomes (75–150 μg protein/mL) were incubated at 30°C for 1 minute or 45 minutes in 5 mM K^+ or 60 mM K^{+a} Hepes buffer containing 1 mM $CaCl_2$. Fluorescence was determined (Shimadzu UV 5000) at an emission wavelength of 510 nM (Slit 10 nM) and excitation wavelengths of 340 and 380 nM (Slit 10 nM). Calcium concentration was calculated by the method of Grynkiewicz *et al.*[7] with R_{max} obtained by addition of 2 μM ionomycin and R_{min} obtained by addition of 10 mM EGTA and Tris pH 8.2.

---

[a] In 60 mM K^+ buffer, NaCl decreased to 70 mM to maintain isosmolarity.

TABLE 1. Intrasynaptosomal Calcium Concentrations $[Ca]_{is}$ as Measured by Fura-2 after 1 or 45 Minute Incubation in 5 mM or 60 mM K^+ Hepes Buffer at 30°C

K$^+$ Concentration	Time of Incubation	
	1 Min	45 Min
5 mM	$192^a \pm 12$	$542^c \pm 34$
60 mM	$718^b \pm 57$	$1188^d \pm 122$

^{a}Calcium concentration in nmoles.
$^b[Ca]_{is}$ significantly greater in 60 mM K$^+$ than in 5 mM K at 1 minute; $p < .01$ (Student t test)
$^c[Ca]_{is}$ significantly greater in 5 mM K$^+$ at 45 min than at 1 min; $p < .01$.
$^d[Ca]_{is}$ significantly greater in 60 mM K$^+$ than in 5 mM K$^+$ at 45 min; $p < .005$.

RESULTS

TABLE 1 demonstrates that depolarization with 60 mM K$^+$ resulted in a significant rise in the intrasynaptosomal Ca^{2+} concentration $[Ca]_{is}$ and a continued rise in $[Ca]_{is}$ over 45 min in both 5 mM and 60 mM K$^+$. This increase in $[Ca]_{is}$ was unaffected by incubation in Na-free buffer containing choline (125 mM) or preincubation with the Na$^+$-channel blocker tetrodotoxin (TABLE 2). In Ca^{2+}-free buffer, $[Ca]_{is}$ did not increase following depolarization. Nickel, a T-type Ca^{2+}-channel blocker, had no effect on $[Ca]_{is}$, but cadmium, an L-type and N-type Ca^{2+}-channel blocker, did reduce depolarization-induced increases in $[Ca]_{is}$ after 1 and 45 minutes (TABLE 2). Nimodipine, a specific L-type Ca^{2+}-channel blocker, had no effect on depolarization-induced changes in $[Ca]_{is}$. Flunarizine preincubation significantly inhibited depolarization-induced increases in $[Ca]_{is}$.

These results suggest that depolarization-induced increases in presynaptic cytosolic Ca^{2+} concentrations arise primarily from influx of extracellular calcium, are not

TABLE 2. Intrasynaptosomal Calcium Concentration $[Ca]_{is}$ as Measured by Fura-2: Role of Na$^+$, Ca^{2+}, Flunarizine, and Voltage-Regulated Calcium Channel Blockers at 1 and 45 Minutes after Depolarization in 60 mM K$^+$ Buffer

Incubation time	5 mM K$^+$		60 mM K$^+$	
	1 min	45 min	1 min	45 min
Ca^{2+}-free buffer	164 ± 32	277 ± 44	$200^a \pm 40$	$283^b \pm 70$
1 mM Ca^{2+} buffer	172 ± 22	350 ± 85	852 ± 64	1246 ± 212
Na$^+$-free buffer (choline 125 mM)	213 ± 42	536 ± 62	732 ± 173	1346 ± 254
125 mM Na$^+$ buffer	198 ± 48	472 ± 81	764 ± 90	1217 ± 147
Tetrodotoxin 1 µM	172 ± 37	512 ± 47	648 ± 78	1112 ± 241
No tetrodotoxin	191 ± 22	448 ± 66	622 ± 82	1171 ± 181
Nickel 100 µM	242 ± 34	442 ± 112	862 ± 88	1225 ± 77
No nickel	211 ± 38	394 ± 90	814 ± 101	1162 ± 104
Cadmium 50 µM	150 ± 45	295 ± 72	$340^c \pm 68$	$532^b \pm 72$
No cadmium	212 ± 27	419 ± 166	752 ± 60	1136 ± 187
Nimodipine 1 µM	214 ± 40	669 ± 84	592 ± 67	1178 ± 131
No nimodipine	192 ± 34	567 ± 89	544 ± 63	1096 ± 162
Flunarizine 50 nM	222 ± 32	$312^c \pm 37$	$375^c \pm 62$	$350^a \pm 76$
No flunarizine	231 ± 41	490 ± 52	490 ± 52	1262 ± 144

$^a p < .001$ (Student t test).
$^b p < .005$.
$^c p < .01$.

Na^+ or Na^+-channel dependent, and may occur by way of a voltage-regulated Ca^{2+} channel similar to the N-type Ca^{2+} channel indentified in single channel recordings.[8] Flunarizine, which has protective effects after cerebral ischemia,[9-11] reduces depolarization-induced presynaptic Ca^{2+} accumulation, possibly in part by blocking Ca^{2+} influx through a channel similar, if not identical, to the N-type channel. This pharmacologic action of flunarizine may be one of its mechanisms of protection following cerebral ischemia.

REFERENCES

1. HOLLER, M., H. DIERKING, D. DENGLER, F. TEGTMEYER & T. PETERS. 1986. Effect of flunarizine on extracellular ion concentration in the rat brain under hypoxia and ischemia. *In* Acute Brain Ischemia. N. Battistine, R. Courbier, P. Fiorani, F. Plum & C. Fieschi, Eds.: 229–233. Raven Press. New York.
2. SIESJO, B. K. 1981. Cell damage in the brain: a speculative synthesis. J. Cereb. Blood Flow Metab. **1:** 155–185.
3. VAN REEMPTS, J. & M. BORGERS. 1985. Ischemic brain injury and cell calcium; morphologic and therapeutic aspects. Ann. Emerg. Med. **14:** 736–742.
4. HASS, W. K. 1981. Beyond cerebral blood flow, metabolism, and ischemic thresholds: An examination of the role of calcium in the initiation of cerebral infarction. *In* Cerebral Vascular Disease. J. S. Meyer, H. Lochner, M. Reivich, E. O. Ott & R. Aranibar, Eds. **3:** 3–17. Excepta Medica. Amsterdam.
5. BENVENISTE, H., J. DREGER, A. SCHOUSBOE & N. H. DIEMER. 1985. Elevation of the extracellular concentrations of glutamate and aspartate in rat hippocampus during transient cerebral ischemia monitored by intracerebral microdialysis. J. Neurochem. **40:** 189–201.
6. KOMULAINEN H. & S. C. BONDY. 1987. The estimation of free calcium within synaptosomes and mitochondria with Fura-2; comparison to quin-2. Neurochem. Int. **10:** 55–64.
7. GRYNKIEWICZ, G., M. POENIE & R. Y. TSIEN. 1985. A new generation of Ca^{2+} indicators with greatly improved fluorescence properties. J. Biol. Chem. **260:** 3440–3450.
8. FOX, A. P., M. C. NOWYCKY & R. W. TSIEN. 1987. Kinetic and pharmacologic properties distinguishing three types of calcium currents in chick sensory neurones. J. Physiol. (Lond.) **394:** 149–172.
9. COHAN, S. L., D. VON LUBITZ, D. REDMOND, S. SZATHMARY & J. A. WAXMAN. 1989. The effects of flunarizine on survival following prolonged cerebral ischemia in the gerbil. *In* Cerebral Ischemia and Calcium. A. Hartmann and W. Kuschinsky, Eds.: 483–493. Springer-Verlag. Berlin.
10. VAN REEMPTS, J., M. HASELDONCKY, B. VAN DEUVEN, L. WOUTERS & M. BORGERS. 1986. Structural damage of the ischemic brain involvement of calcium and effects of postischemic treatment with calcium entry blockers. Drug Dev. Res. **8:** 387–395.
11. DERYCK, M. J. VAN REEMPTS, M. BORGERS, A. WAUQUIER & P. A. J. JANSSEN. 1989. Photochemical stroke model: flunarizine prevents sensormotor deficits after neocortical infarcts in rats. Stroke **20:** 1383–1390.

Subsecond Kinetics of Inositol 1,4,5-Trisphosphate-Induced Calcium Release Reveal Rapid Potentiation and Subsequent Inactivation by Calcium

E. A. FINCH,[a,c,e] T. J. TURNER,[d] AND S. M. GOLDIN[b,c]

[a]Program in Neuroscience and
[b]Biological Chemistry Department
Harvard Medical School
Boston, Massachusetts 02115

[c]Cambridge NeuroScience Research
Cambridge, Massachusetts 02139

[d]Department of Physiology
Tufts University School of Medicine
Boston, Massachusetts 02111

The kinetics and modulation by extravesicular Ca^{2+} (Ca_e^{2+}) of inositol 1,4,5-trisphosphate (IP3)-induced $^{45}Ca^{2+}$ release from synaptosome-derived microsomal vesicles were studied using a superfusion system affording 50 ms time resolution and the precise control of agonist and ionic concentrations.[1-4] We were thus able to examine the magnitude and time-course of $^{45}Ca^{2+}$ efflux in response to step changes in buffers of known IP3 and free Ca^{2+} concentrations.

Vesicles were loaded with $^{45}Ca^{2+}$ in an ATP-dependent manner, then washed with a buffer containing 100 nM free Ca^{2+} and 5 mM $MgCl_2$. Introduction of IP3 at various Ca_e^{2+} concentrations evoked a transient release of $^{45}Ca^{2+}$, which reached its maximum rate within 140 ms and decayed over the next second. The IP3-stimulated release was blocked by heparin (100 µg/mL), which has been shown to inhibit the binding of IP3 to its receptor.

The IP3 concentration dependence of the maximum rate of IP3-induced $^{45}Ca^{2+}$ release indicated that the [IP3] and $^{45}Ca^{2+}$ release rate are related in a normal hyperbolic manner over the range of 30 nM–10 µM (EC_{50} = 240 nM, n_H = 1.0).

Ca^{2+} modulated both the time-course and magnitude of IP3-induced $^{45}Ca^{2+}$ release. Superfusion with 1 µM IP3 at a range of free Ca^{2+} concentrations (100 nM–10 µM) demonstrated that elevation of Ca_e^{2+} markedly potentiated the maximum rate of IP3-induced $^{45}Ca^{2+}$ release in a manner suggesting that Ca^{2+} is a coagonist for the release mechanism (EC_{50} = 660 nM, n_H = 1.0) (FIG. 1). The IP3-induced $^{45}Ca^{2+}$ release rate, plotted as a function of Ca_e^{2+} concentration extrapolated to zero at or below 60 nm Ca_e^{2+}. Superfusion with IP3 at higher free Ca^{2+} concentrations resulted in a diminished maximum rate of $^{45}Ca^{2+}$ release, suggesting a second, inhibitory effect of Ca^{2+}, which was examined further. Elevation of Ca_e^{2+} prior to IP3 exposure resulted in a reversible [Ca_e^{2+}]- and time-dependent inactivation of $^{45}Ca^{2+}$ release (IC_{50} = 620 nM) (FIG. 2).

[e]Address for correspondence: Cambridge NeuroScience Research, Inc., One Kendall Square, Building 700, Cambridge, MA 02139.

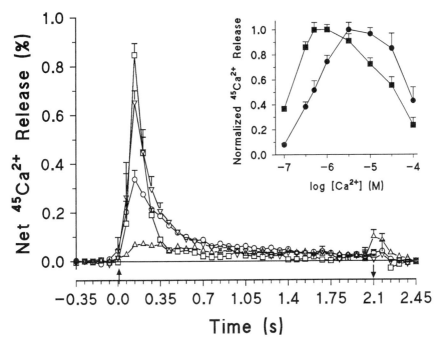

FIGURE 1. Dependence of IP3-induced $^{45}Ca^{2+}$ efflux on Ca_e^{2+} concentration. The 3500 ms superfusion protocol consisted of a 750 ms superfusion with wash buffer, 2000 ms of superfusion with stimulation buffer, and another 750 ms of wash. The upward arrow indicates switch to stimulation buffer (time = 0), and the downward arrow indicates switch back to wash buffer. Wash buffer contained (in mM) 20 MOPS, 100 KCl, 10 NaCl, 1 EGTA, 5 $MgCl_2$, pH 7.2 (free $[Ca^{2+}] \simeq 100$ nM). Stimulation buffer contained (in mM) 20 MOPS, 100 KCl, 10 NaCl, 1 EGTA, pH 7.2, and was supplemented with $CaCl_2$ to the desired free Ca^{2+} concentration, with or without IP3. $[Ca_e^{2+}]$ was determined using a Ca^{2+}-selective electrode. Each point on the x-axis represents $^{45}Ca^{2+}$ in a single superfusate fraction and corresponds to a 70 ms bin of $^{45}Ca^{2+}$ efflux. $^{45}Ca^{2+}$ release in these and subsequent experiments is expressed as the percent of the total $^{45}Ca^{2+}$, accumulated by the vesicles, that is released in each fraction, and thus is a measure of the average rate of $^{45}Ca^{2+}$ efflux during that 70 ms period. In all experiments, the [IP3] in the stimulation buffer was 1 μM. The range of $[Ca_e^{2+}]$ in different experiments was 100 nM–100 μM. Net IP3 induced $^{45}Ca^{2+}$ efflux at 100 nM ($\triangle$), 300 nM ($\bigcirc$), 1 μM ($\triangledown$), and 10 μM ($\square$) Ca_e^{2+}. Inset: Biphasic Ca_e^{2+} dependence of the maximum rate ($\bullet$) and cumulative amount ($\blacksquare$) of $^{45}Ca^{2+}$ efflux over a 2-s superfusion period at various Ca_e^{2+} concentrations (100 nM–100 μM). The data are normalized to the maximum value obtained for each of these measures. The data are from a series of experiments, a subset of which was used to generate the main figure. Data are the means $\pm$ SD for three to five separate experiments at each $[Ca_e^{2+}]$. Error bars are not shown when smaller than the symbol. (Finch *et al.*[4] With permission from *Science.* Copyright 1988 by the AAAS.)

The Ca_e^{2+}-dependent potentiation of maximal IP3-induced $^{45}Ca^{2+}$ release was more rapid (≤ 140 ms) than the Ca_e^{2+}-dependent inhibition ($\tau = 580$ ms at 10 μM Ca^{2+}). Our rapid kinetic measurements thus argue that, at constant IP3 levels, rapid elevation of cytosolic Ca^{2+} would initially potentiate and subsequently inactivate Ca^{2+} release *in vivo*.

The Ca_e^{2+}- and time-dependent control of the neuronal IP3 receptor is similar to that described for the structurally homologous[5,6] ryanodine-sensitive Ca^{2+} release channels associated with sarcoplasmic reticulum, which exhibit both Ca^{2+}-induced Ca^{2+} release and Ca^{2+}-dependent inactivation of Ca^{2+} release.[7,8] Sequential positive and negative feedback regulation of IP3-induced Ca^{2+} release by Ca^{2+} may play a role in the generation of cytosolic Ca^{2+} transients in a manner analogous to transients mediated by Ca^{2+}-induced Ca^{2+} release from sarcoplasmic reticulum,[7,8] and could

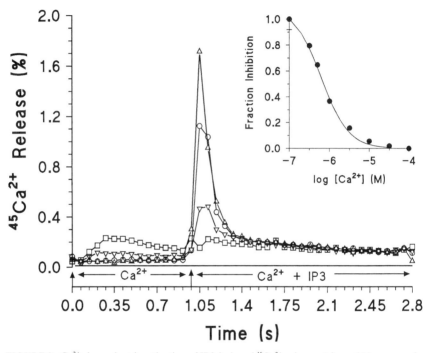

FIGURE 2. Ca_e^{2+}-dependent inactivation of IP3-induced $^{45}Ca^{2+}$ release. After a 350 ms superfusion with wash buffer (not shown), vesicles were exposed at time = 0 to a 1-s conditioning pulse of stimulation buffer containing 100 nM ($\triangle$), 300 nM ($\bigcirc$), 1 μM ($\triangledown$), and 10 μM ($\square$) Ca_e^{2+}. Subsequently (second vertical arrow) a standard 2-s test pulse of stimulation buffer containing 1 μM IP3 and 10 μM Ca^{2+} was delivered. Inset: Semi-log plot of $[Ca_e^{2+}]$-dependent inactivation of net IP3-induced $^{45}Ca^{2+}$ release. The data represent cumulative $^{45}Ca^{2+}$ release from a series of experiments, a subset of which was used to generate the main figure ($n = 2$ or 3 for each $[Ca_e^{2+}]$). Error bars are not shown when smaller than the symbol. (Finch *et al.*[4] With permission from *Science*. Copyright 1988 by the AAAS.)

help explain regulation of IP3-induced Ca^{2+} oscillations by Ca^{2+}.[9–12] If Ca^{2+} entry across the plasma membrane triggers IP3-induced Ca^{2+} release,[13-15] then Ca^{2+} release from these stores may contribute substantially to increased cytosolic Ca^{2+} levels in response to Ca^{2+} entry through voltage-gated Ca^{2+} channels. In nerve terminals, the rapid modulation of IP3-induced Ca^{2+} release by Ca^{2+} may be relevant to modulation of neurotransmitter release.

REFERENCES

1. PEARCE, L. B., R. D. CALHOON, P. R. BURNS, A. VINCENT & S. M. GOLDIN. 1988. Biochemistry **27:** 4396.
2. TURNER, T. J., L. B. PEARCE & S. M. GOLDIN. 1989. Anal. Biochem. **178:** 8.
3. TURNER, T. J. & S. M. GOLDIN. 1989. Biochemistry **28:** 586.
4. FINCH, E. A., T. J. TURNER & S. M. GOLDIN. 1991. Science **252:** 443.
5. FURUICHI, T. *et al.* 1989. Nature **342:** 32.
6. MIGNERY, G. A., T. C. SUDHOF, K. TAKEI & P. DE CAMILLI. 1989. Nature **342:** 92.
7. FABIATO, A. 1985. J. Gen. Physiol. **85:** 247.
8. MEISSNER, G., E. DARLING & J. EVELETH. 1986. Biochemistry **25:** 236.
9. JACOB, R., J. E. MERRITT, T. J. HALLAM & T. J. RINK. 1988. Nature **335:** 40.
10. WAKUI, M., B. V. L. POTTER & O. H. PETERSON. 1989. Nature **339:** 317.
11. BERRIDGE, M. J. & A. GALIONE. 1988. FASEB J. **2:** 3074.
12. RINK, T. J. & R. JACOB. 1989. Trends Neurosci. **12:** 43.
13. FABIATO, A. 1985. J. Gen. Physiol. **85:** 291.
14. NABAUER, M., G. CALLEWAERT, L. CLEEMANN & M. MORAD. 1989. Science **244:** 800.
15. LEBLANC, N. & J. R. HUME. 1990. Science **248:** 372.

The Effect of Low-Energy Combined AC and DC Magnetic Fields on Articular Cartilage Metabolism

D. A. GRANDE, F. P. MAGEE,[a,c] A. M. WEINSTEIN,
AND B. R. McLEOD[b]

North Shore University Hospital
350 Community Drive
Manhasset, New York 11030

[a]*Research and Development*
IatroMed, Inc.
2850 S. 36th Street
Phoenix, Arizona 85040

[b]*Department of Electrical Engineering*
Montana State University
Bozeman, Montana 59717

It has long been recognized that magnetic fields can influence cells in biologic systems. Magnetic field influence on ion transport across cell membranes is one of the possible mechanisms that has received recent attention. Liboff *et al.*[1] proposed the cyclotron resonance theory to describe the influence of magnetic fields on ion transport. The theory uses the Lorentz force equations to define magnetic field conditions that will enhance ion transport across cell membranes. The objective of this experiment is to expose resting bovine articular cartilage to magnetic fields that satisfy the Liboff hypothesis and evaluate the effect on metabolism.

MATERIAL AND METHODS

Explant Preparation

Full-thickness articular cartilage specimens were harvested from young adult bovine knee joints under aseptic conditions within six h of death. A sterile 4 mm trephine was used to create circular samples 1.5–2.0 mm thick, which were placed in a 60 mm petri dish (10/dish). Each petri dish contained exactly 2 mL of a previously defined low-serum medium known to maintain steady state viability of cartilage in organ culture for over three weeks.[2] Cartilage samples were allowed to equilibrate 48 h *in vitro* prior to initiation of the experiments.

Chondrocyte Isolation and Culture

Fresh articular cartilage was harvested sterilely and placed in a spinner flask with medium containing collagenase, hyaluronidase and DNase for 10–18 h to isolate free

---

[c]To whom correspondence should be addressed.

chondrocytes. Cells were then washed, counted, plated, and placed into monolayer culture using standard culture techniques.

Tissue Processing

Following these treatment periods, samples were washed five times with phosphate-buffered saline and then in 95% ethanol for three days with complete changes of ethanol every day until the ethanol reached background levels of radioactivity, (< 100 cpm) as assayed by scintillation counting. The cartilage explants were then frozen, lyophilized, weighed, solubilized by papain digestion, suspended in Aquasol-2, and counted in a liquid scintillation counter.

Magnetic Field Conditions

Chondrocyte cultures were placed between a pair of vertically oriented copper wire coils. This provided an arrangement that could produce uniform magnetic fields surrounding the cultures. In the cultures to be exposed, the coils were connected in parallel to a function generator. The control unstimulated cultures were handled identically with the exception that no power was applied to the coils. The magnetic fields were monitored using a flux gate magnetometer. According to the Liboff theory, to specifically stimulate one ion species transport requires the application of a static magnetic field combined in parallel with an alternating magnetic field.

The ratio of these two fields is adjusted according to the following equation:

$$f_A = \tfrac{1}{2}\pi \times B_S \times q/m,$$

where f_A = frequency of alternating field, B_S = magnitude of static field, and q/m = charge to mass ratio of ion to be stimulated.

In these experiments, the equation was solved for K^+, the f_A = 16 hz, B_S = 40.8 μT; Ca^{2+}, the f_A = 16 hz, B_S = 20.9; Mg^{2+}, the f_A = 16 hz, B_S = 12.7; and the Ca^{45} f_A = 14.3 hz, B_S = 20.0. The amplitude of the alternating fields was 40 μT p-p. To determine the flux of labeled calcium (Ca^{45}) across chondrocyte cell membranes, confluent chondrocyte cultures in tissue culture plates were prepared. The fields were set to stimulate Ca^{45}. At t = 0, medium containing Ca^{45} was added to replicate dishes with samples of cartilage. Samples were harvested at .5, 1, 3, and 24 h after field exposure and processed as described. DNA content was measured using flourescent binding of the dye Hoechst 33258. Data is expressed as CPM/μg DNA. Additionally, the effect of the potassium, calcium, and magnesium signals on cartilage metabolism was determined using the above-described explant system. Cultures were exposed for 24, 48, and 72 hours. Tritiated thymidine and sulfate incorporation was measured.

RESULTS

Calcium Ion

Thymidine and sulfate incorporation both reached significant ($p < .05$) increases over control samples by 48 hours. Both labels were nonsignificant at the 24-h time point. By 72 h, the 48 h increase in radiolabel incorporation had decreased to a nonsignificant value compared to controls (FIG. 1A).

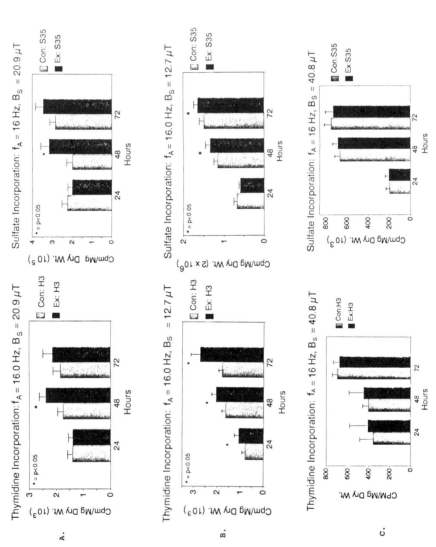

FIGURE 1, A, B, and C. Graphic representations of $[S^{35}]$- and $[H^3]$thymidine uptake in chondrocytes stimulated with magnetic fields tuned for Ca, Mg, and K ions compared to unstimulated controls.

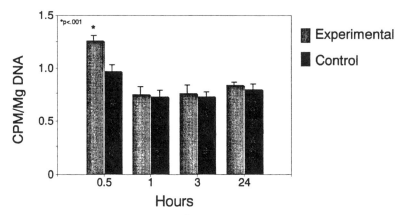

FIGURE 2. Graphic representation of Ca^{45} uptake of cells exposed to magnetic fields compared to unstimulated controls.

Magnesium Ion

Thymidine incorporation was increased significantly ($p < .05$) at all time points compared to controls. Sulfate incorporation did not reach a significant increase until 48 hr, but continued through 72 hours (FIG. 1B).

Potassium Ion

There were no significant differences at all time points for both radiolabels. Thymidine showed a high degree of variability at 24 and 48 h with an apparent trend toward increasing, but this effect was gone by 72 hours. Sulfate incorporation was nonsignificant in comparison with controls (FIG. 1C).

Ca^{45} Uptake

There was a significant increase in radioactive calcium uptake at 30 min of exposure that became insignificant at 1, 3, and 24 hours (FIG. 2). It can be stated in summary that low-energy combined AC and DC magnetic fields have the ability to stimulate the metabolism of resting articular cartilage, and that this increase in metabolic activity is associated with an increase in calcium ion uptake by the cells.

REFERENCES

1. LIBOFF, A. R., S. D. SMITH & B. R. McLEOD. 1987. *In* Mechanistic Approaches to Interactions of Electric and Electromagnetic Fields with Living Systems. M. Blank & E. Findl, Eds.: 109–132. Plenum Press. New York.
2. OSBORN, K. D., S. B. TRIPPEL & H. J. MANKIN. 1989. Growth Factor Stimulation of Adult Articular Cartilage. J. Orthop. Res. **7**: 35–42.

Developmental Changes in the Pharmacology of Ca^{2+}-Dependent Neurotransmitter Release

D. B. GRAY, N. MANTHAY, AND G. PILAR

Department of Physiology and Neurobiology
University of Connecticut
Storrs, Connecticut 06269

The intact synaptic terminals of ciliary ganglion neurons in the smooth muscle of the vascular choroid coat and the striated muscle of the iris of the chick eye have been used to characterize the onset of Ca^{2+}-dependent ACh release. We have previously shown that release of [³H]ACh during high-K^+ challenge from these mature posthatching terminals is not sensitive to dihydropyridine (DHP) but is irreversibly inhibited by ω-conotoxin.[1,2] The choroid terminals also contain somatostatin, which is released and acts to inhibit ACh release by blocking DHP-insensitive (N-type?) Ca^{2+} channels.[2] In this report we have examined embryonic St 40 ciliary ganglion terminals in both iris and choroid with respect to their Ca^{2+} channel pharmacology and ACh release characteristics. [³H]ACh release from whole irises and stereotypic wedges of the innervated choroid of the chick was measured as described previously.[2,3]

Although ACh release from embryonic terminals in both iris and choroid is Ca^{2+}-dependent and can be evoked with K^+, the pharmacological characteristics are quite different from release in posthatching terminals. In FIGURE 1, the sensitivity of

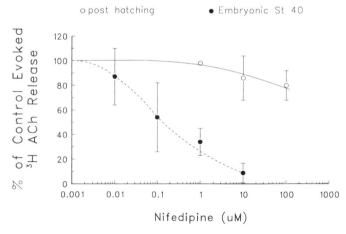

FIGURE 1. Dose-response relationship of nifedipine on K^+-evoked ACh release from isolated choroid terminals. Values are shown as percent of control [³H]ACh release evoked by 55 mM K^+ for 3 min. Open circles represent release from posthatching (0–5 days) choroids; filled circles represent release from embryonic St 40 choroids. All values with the exception of one posthatching point (at 1 μM) are averages of at least 4 experiments; bars indicate standard error.

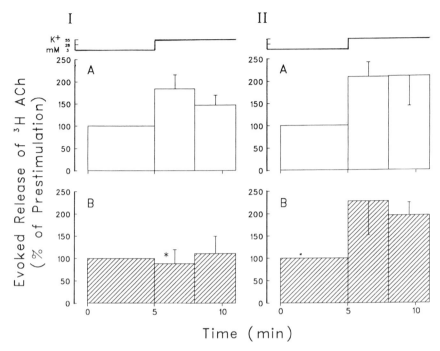

FIGURE 2. Effect of somatostatin on K^+-evoked [^{3}H]ACh release in embryonic St 40 choroids and irises. Values are normalized to 100% of the last prestimulation release. Potassium concentration in the Tyrode's incubation solution is indicated at the top of the FIGURE. IA represents control ACh release (clear bars) from choroids, and IB, release in the presence of 100 nM somatostatin (shaded bars). Values in II A + B are from embryonic irises. All values are means of at least 5 experiments with standard errors. * = significantly different from control stimulation at $p < 0.05$.

evoked ACh release in embryonic choroid preparations to nifedipine is compared to that of posthatching tissues. Although ACh release in older choroids is only fractionally sensitive to nifedipine even at concentrations approaching millimolar levels, St 40 terminals display an ID_{50} for nifedipine on evoked ACh release of approximately 10^{-6} M. In this portion of the concentration range, variance in release values were reproducibly high from experiment to experiment.

This developmental change in sensitivity to a DHP antagonist is mirrored by the fact that the DHP agonist, Bay K 8644, enhances embryonic ACh release but not at posthatching in these preparations (data not shown). In addition, ω-conotoxin, which irreversibly inhibits 100% of K^+-evoked ACh release in posthatching terminals, blocks only approximately 50% of release in embryonic terminals.

FIGURE 2 shows the effect of exogenous somatostatin on ACh release in both embryonic iris and choroid. As in posthatching terminals, somatostatin abolishes evoked release in the choroid but not in the iris. Thus, ciliary ganglion terminals at St 40 are already distinguished in terms of the presence of somatostatin receptors coupled to neuromodulation of ACh release in a fashion similar to that of mature terminals after hatching. Inasmuch as studies have implicated Ca^{2+} channels as the site of somatostatin's action, these results suggest that activation of somatostatin receptors can inhibit more than one type of voltage-dependent Ca^{2+} channel in this preparation.

REFERENCES

1. GRAY, D. B., G. R. PILAR & M. J. FORD. 1989. Opiate and peptide inhibition of transmitter release in parasympathetic nerve terminals. J. Neurosci. **9:** 1683–1692.
2. GRAY, D. B., D. ZELAZNY, N. MANTHAY & G. R. PILAR. 1990. Endogenous modulation of ACh release by somatostatin and the differential roles of calcium channels. J. Neurosci. **10:** 2687–2699.
3. VACA, K. & G. R. PILAR. 1979. Mechanisms controlling choline transport and acetylcholine synthesis in motor nerve terminals during electrical stimulation. J. Gen. Physiol. **73:** 605–628.

Reduced Ca Currents in Frog Nerve Terminals at High Pressure[a]

Y. GROSSMAN, J. S. COLTON, AND S. C. GILMAN

Department of Physiology
Faculty of Health Sciences
Ben-Gurion University of the Negev
Beer-Sheva 84105, Israel
and
Diving Biomedical Technology
Naval Medical Research Institute
Bethesda, Maryland 20889-5055

Exposure to high pressure (HP) causes suppression of synaptic transmission in individual synapses.[1] This suppression is due to a decrease in presynaptic transmitter release.[2] Indirect evidence suggests that HP primarily affects Ca^{2+} influx (I_{Ca}) in nerve terminals.[3] We examined the effect of HP on such I_{Ca}, using a "loose" patch-clamp technique, in an isolated cutaneous pectoris nerve-muscle preparation of the frog (*Rana pipiens*).[4] When the electrode (3–5 M ohms) was inserted under the perineurial sheath proximal to the nerve terminals, the local circuit currents flowing between the terminals and the parent axons could be recorded.[4] The preparation was placed in a pressure chamber and was perfused constantly with oxygenated physiological solution of the following composition (mM): NaCl,116; KCl,2; $CaCl_2$,1.8; Tris buffer,5; pH 7.4, at 18°C. Tubocurarine (5 mg/L) was added to block muscle contraction. Compression up to 6.9 MPa was accomplished with helium. The normal response was composed of a fast large inward current of sodium (I_{Na}) at the nodes, followed by a small inward current that reflects the outward potassium current (I_K) at the repolarizing terminals[4] (FIG. 1A). Blocking I_K by tetraethylammonium (TEA, 10 mM) disclosed a Ca-dependent outward current that was comprised of fast (I_{Ca_F}) and slow (I_{Ca_S}) components (FIG. 1B). Both phases, which reflect inward I_{Ca} at the terminals, were blocked by 10 μM Cd^{2+} and 1–5 μM omega-conotoxin, and only I_{Ca_S} was diminished by nifedipine and nitrendipine (15–25 μM). HP suppressed the maximal I_{Ca} by 87 ± 10% (mean ± SD, n = 13) and concomitantly reduced the action potential I_{Na} by 29 ± 11% in a pressure-dependent manner (FIG. 1C–E). I_{Ca_S} was more resistant to HP effect and could be partially restored by increased $[Ca^{2+}]_0$ (FIG. 1F–H). The data indicate that HP decreases the maximal I_{Ca} through L-type, voltage-gated Ca^{2+} channels[5] in vertebrate nerve terminals, and more so, in the N-type. It is not clear, however, whether this is a direct effect of HP on Ca^{2+} channels, because HP also reduced to some extent the amplitude of action potential invading the motor nerve terminals.

[a]This work was supported by NMRDC Work Unit M0099.01c-1010 and ONR Grant N00014-91-J-1908 to Y. Grossman. Y. Grossman is a National Research Council-NMRI Research Associate.

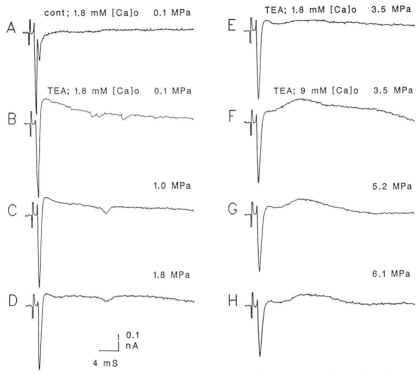

FIGURE 1. Nerve terminal currents and high pressure. All current records are from the same site. Holding potential was zero with respect to ground. A, control at normal pressure (0.1 MPa); B, TEA blocks all potassium currents and discloses a large calcium current; C–E, pressure-dependent reduction of calcium current; F, increased $[Ca^{2+}]_0$ may oppose pressure effect on the current amplitude; G-H, with increased pressure, the calcium current is further suppressed. Note that the node-sodium current (fast inward current) is also decreased in a pressure-dependent manner.

REFERENCES

1. GROSSMAN, Y. & J. J. KENDIG. 1988. J. Neurophysiol. **60:** 1497–1512.
2. ASHFORD, M. L. J., A. G. MACDONALD & K. T. WANN. 1982. J. Physiol. (Lond.) **333:** 531–543.
3. GROSSMAN, Y. & J. J. KENDIG. 1990. J. Physiol. (Lond.) **420:** 355–364.
4. MALLART, A. 1984. Pfluegers Arch. **400:** 8–13.
5. TSIEN, R. W., D. LIPSCOMBE, D. V. MADISON, K. R. BLEY & A. P. FOX. 1988. Trends Neurosci. **11:** 431–438.

Drug Actions and Regulation at Voltage-Dependent Neuronal Ca^{2+} Channels (VDCCs)[a]

M. H. HAWTHORN, J. FERRANTE, Y. W. KWON,
A. RUTLEDGE, E. LUCHOWSKI, AND D. J. TRIGGLE

Department of Biochemical Pharmacology
School of Pharmacy
State University of New York at Buffalo
Buffalo, New York 14260

It is now apparent that VDCCs are subject to homologous and heterologous regulatory influences.[1] Although the mechanisms of regulation are as yet unclear, calcium itself may play an important role. To investigate this further we examined the effects of chronic depolarization on VDCCs. Chick retinal neuronal cells were grown for four days in the presence of elevated K$^+$ concentrations (12–73 mM). This produced a concentration-dependent reduction in VDCC density as assessed by [^{3}H]PN200-110 binding (FIG. 1) without a change in K_d and was prevented by the

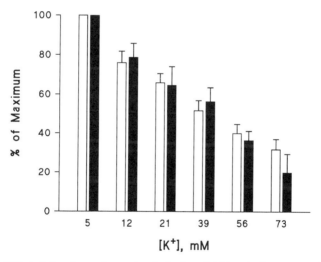

FIGURE 1. Effect of chronic membrane depolarization of chick retinal neurons on [^{3}H]PN200-110 binding density (open columns) and ^{45}Ca^{2+} uptake (filled columns). Cells were incubated for four days in the presence of the indicated concentration of potassium. Results are expressed as a percentage of the control values (*i.e.* in 5 mM K$^+$).

[a]This work was supported by Grants from the NIAAA (AA08182) to M. H. Hawthorn and NIH (HL 16003) to D. J. Triggle.

VDCC antagonist D600. The reduction in VDCC density was initially observed at 4 h and continued for six days. Chronic depolarization resulted in a reduction in K^+-stimulated $^{45}Ca^{2+}$ uptake, which correlated well with the VDCC down-regulation (FIG. 1). A down-regulation of VDCCs was also produced by the calcium ionophore A23187, further illustrating the importance of $^{45}Ca^{2+}$ in the regulatory mechanism. It is interesting to note that neither chronic depolarization nor A23187 had any effect on VDCC density in rat neonatal ventricular myocytes, although these cells express functional L-type channels.

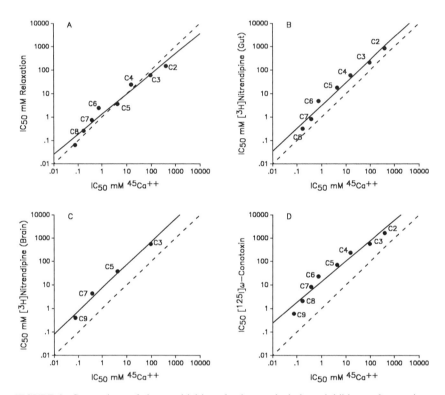

FIGURE 2. Comparison of the sensitivities of primary alcohols as inhibitors of potassium-contracted ileal smooth muscle (A), binding of [^{3}H]nitrendipine to smooth muscle membranes (B), and binding of [^{3}H]nitrendipine and [^{125}I]omega-conotoxin in neuronal membranes (C and D) to synaptosomal $^{45}Ca^{2+}$ uptake.

Ca^{2+} also appears to play a central role in VDCC regulation caused by ethanol. Although ethanol inhibits K^+-stimulated $^{45}Ca^{2+}$ into neuronal tissue,[2] it is unclear which of the VDCC subtypes (L, N, T, or P) are affected. As higher alcohols have been suggested to show channel selectivity, we compared the effects of a homologous series of primary alcohols on potassium-stimulated $^{45}Ca^{2+}$ uptake into synaptosomes, [^{3}H]nitrendipine and [^{125}I]omega-conotoxin binding to neuronal membranes to their actions on K^+-contracted ileal longitudinal smooth muscle, a process dependent on Ca^{2+} entry through L-type calcium channels.[3] FIGURE 2 shows the similar sensitivity of the alcohols as relaxants of smooth muscle, inhibitors of calcium entry into neurons, and inhibitors of [^{3}H]nitrendipine binding. In neuronal tissue, however, the alcohols were 5–30 times more potent at inhibiting $^{45}Ca^{2+}$ uptake than displacing [^{3}H]Nitrendipine and [^{125}I]omega-conotoxin binding, suggesting an action on a channel type other than L or N.

Chronic exposure to ethanol results in an up-regulation of VDCCs in response to the acute inhibition[4] of Ca^{2+} entry. The recent observation that ethanol also inhibits Ca^{2+} entry through the NMDA-linked calcium channel[5] suggests that VDCC inhibition may not be solely responsible for this up-regulation. To investigate this observation, rats were treated with either 10 mg/kg CGS-19755 or 2 mg/kg MK801 in saline every 12 h for 7 days, and the density of L-type calcium channels in the striatum, cortex, hippocampus, and heart were determined using [^{3}H]PN200-110. With the exception of the hippocampus in which a 36% reduction in density was observed after CGS-19775 treatment, chronic inhibition of the NMDA-linked channel had no effect on the density of voltage-dependent calcium channels. The inability of NMDA antagonists to up-regulate the voltage-dependent channel suggests that although the acute effects of ethanol may be mediated in part by inhibition of the NMDA receptor, its chronic effects on the voltage-dependent calcium channel are not.

REFERENCES

1. FERRANTE, J. & D. J. TRIGGLE. 1990. Pharmacol. Rev. **42:** 29–44.
2. STOKES, J. A. & R. A. HARRIS. 1982. Mol. Pharmacol. **22:** 99–104.
3. ROSENBERGER, L. B., M. K. TICKU & D. J. TRIGGLE. 1979. Can. J. Physiol. Pharmacol. **57:** 333–342.
4. DOLIN, S. & H. J. LITTLE. 1989. J. Pharmacol. Exp. Ther. **250:** 985–991.
5. LOVINGER, D. M., G. WHITE & F. F. WEIGHT. 1990. Science **243:** 1721–1724.

Stimulus-Induced Nuclear Ca^{2+} Signals in Fura-2–Loaded Amphibian Neurons

A. HERNÁNDEZ-CRUZ, F. SALA,[a] AND J. A. CONNOR

Department of Neurosciences
Roche Institute of Molecular Biology
Nutley, New Jersey 07110
and
[a]*Departamento de Neuroquímica*
Universidad de Alicante
San Juan Alicante, Spain

Several recent examples support the notion that Ca^{2+} signaling often involves heterogeneity in intracellular [Ca^{2+}] regulation. The spatial distribution and kinetic properties of Ca^{2+} influx pathways, cytosolic calcium buffering, and Ca^{2+} release from intracellular Ca^{2+} stores are thought to be the key factors in local shaping of neuronal Ca^{2+} signals.[1]

A recent Ca^{2+} imaging study with confocal microscopy in the soma of bullfrog sympathetic neurons[2] demonstrated that following electrical stimulation, the expected inward spread of Ca^{2+} in the bulk of the cytosol governed by radial diffusion theory[3] coexisted with an unexpected local amplification of the Ca^{2+} signal in the nucleus. This phenomenon could be relevant to the proposed role of changes of intranuclear [Ca^{2+}] in the tranduction pathway linking neuronal excitation to long-term modifications of nerve cell function and structure.[4]

The need for more accurate estimates of the Ca^{2+} levels involved prompted us to conduct ratio-imaging experiments in fura-2–loaded neurons.[5] To ascertain whether this finding was common to other neuronal types, we also examined neurons from the dorsal root ganglion and expanded our study to two unrelated amphibian species, clawed frog (*Xenopus laevis*) and salamander (*Ambystoma tigrinum*).

Fura-2–imaging experiments (time resolution ~400 ms) in amphibian neurons showed that (1) depolarization-induced Ca^{2+} influx through the plasma membrane or

---

FIGURE 1. Caffeine-induced release of intracellular Ca^{2+}. **A:** a through i: Series of consecutive ratio images (600 ms interval) taken before and during the rising phase of the caffeine response of a fura-2 AM loaded DRG salamader neuron. The gray scale ranges from 0 to 1 μM. Data are more often displayed with a pseudo-color scale to provide quantitative information. A 1.5 s pulse of 10 mM caffeine was applied near the lower left edge of the cell following the acquisition of frame a. The nucleus position is shown in B as region no. 3. Caffeine initiates a wave of Ca^{2+} release that quickly engulfs the whole cell. Notice the delayed, passive penetration of Ca^{2+} into the nucleus (b) and the subsequent nucleus-cytoplasm gradient at the peak of the response (d and e, nucleus response). Scale in b was expanded 1.5-fold to emphasize perinuclear gradients. **B:** Ca^{2+} transients monitored at the three cell locations indicated in the diagram. Cells were enzymatically isolated[2] and loaded with indicator dye either by 15 min incubation in 2 μM fura-2 AM or by pressure injection with a micropipette containing 4 mM ionic fura-2. Fast application with a puffer pipette of either isotonic KCl or caffeine (10 mM) was used to trigger transmembrane Ca^{2+} influx or intracellular Ca^{2+} release, respectively. When required, CCCP and rotenone were also applied by pressure from a broken-tip micropipette. The ratio imaging apparatus is described elsewhere.[5]

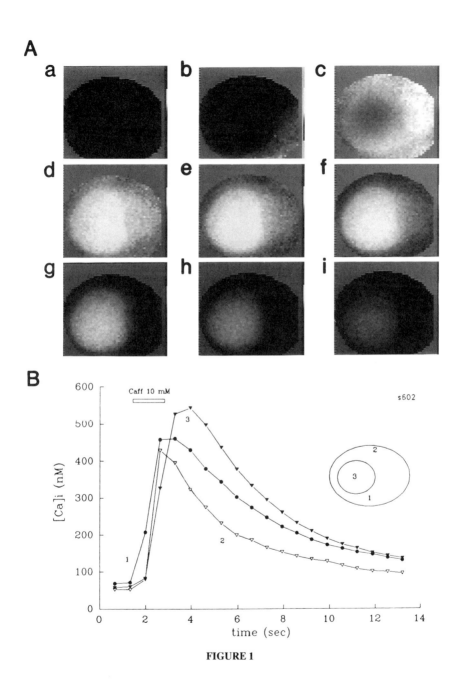

FIGURE 1

release from intracellular stores by caffeine produces conspicuous, transient intracellular [Ca²⁺] gradients (FIGURES 1A and 2A); (2) initially, Ca²⁺ spreads into the nucleus at a slower rate than in the rest of the cytosol, suggesting that the nuclear envelope presents a significant barrier to passive Ca²⁺ diffusion (FIGURES 1b and 2b); (3) nuclear [Ca²⁺] then can temporarily rise above levels expected from passive diffusion, generating a nuclear/cytoplasm gradient of several hundred nanomolar, which dissipates slowly after the cessation of the stimulus (called the nucleus response hereafter; see FIGURES 1 d–i and 2 c–h); (4) nuclear responses could be

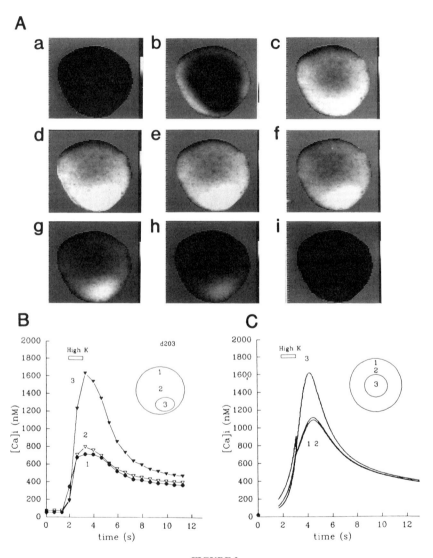

FIGURE 2

seen both in ester-loaded– and fura-2–injected cells, suggesting that nucleus/cytosol Ca^{2+} gradients do not result from dye internalization artifacts. These results provided the physiological constraints needed to evaluate a theoretical model of subcellular Ca^{2+} dynamics in these cells (see below).

Bullfrog and clawed frog sympathetic neurons showed striking differences in their response to caffeine. Unlike bullfrog cells, which consistently gave large Ca^{2+} responses that could be repeated several times (provided a few minutes were allowed for the cell to recover), *Xenopus* neurons gave either no response or a single small response. When the caffeine pulse was applied within a few minutes of a prior 10 s K^+-depolarization, however, a Ca^{2+} release similar to that of nonstimulated bullfrog cells could be recorded (not shown). This suggests that caffeine-sensitive Ca^{2+} stores in *Xenopus* sympathetic neurons are relatively abundant, but "leakier" than their bullfrog counterparts.

Nuclear signals elicited by caffeine or membrane depolarization require relatively strong cytosolic transients to develop. Small cytoplasmic Ca^{2+} increases in response to short pulses of caffeine or high K^+ failed to produce a conspicuous

---

FIGURE 2. Changes in $[Ca^{2+}]$ distribution following a brief membrane depolarization with a pulse of high K^+. Experimental results and theoretical modeling. **A:** a through h: Consecutive ratio images (600 ms interval) taken before (a) and during the rising phase of the response to a pulse of high K^+; i is the last ratio image of the series, about 7 s after the peak. Gray scale ranges from 0 to 2.3 µM; scale in b was expanded 1.5-fold. **B:** $[Ca^{2+}]_i$ transients monitored at the cell positions indicated in the diagram. Notice the 800 nM nucleus-cytoplasm gradient at the peak of the response. Clawed frog DRG neuron loaded with fura-2 AM. **C:** Simulation of depolarization-induced Ca^{2+} transients with a theoretical model. Calculated transients obtained from the positions indicated in the diagram, with a modified radial diffusion model,[3] which includes a central nucleus region 8 µm in diameter, whose most external shell (nuclear envelope) has a diffusion coefficient of 1/20 of the rest of shells. Within the cytoplasm and in the nuclear envelope we also included a Ca-induced Ca-release mechanism (CICR), defined by the equation

$$\Delta Ca/\Delta t = Rm \cdot m \cdot h,$$

where Rm is the maximal release, and m and h are Hodgkin-Huxley–type variables that describe the "gating" of the CICR mechanism. Rate constants αm and αh are $[Ca^{2+}]$-dependent:

$$\alpha m = \alpha m(max) \cdot [Ca/Ca + K_{dm}]^{nm}$$

and

$$\alpha h = \alpha h(max) \cdot [Ca/Ca + K_{dh}]^{nh},$$

where $\alpha m(max)$ and $\alpha h(max)$ are the maximal rates, K_{dm} and K_{dh} are affinity constants, and n_m and n_h are integers representing the stoichiometry of the reaction. Initial values for m and h were calculated for $[Ca]$ initial = 100 nM as follows:

$$m_0 = \alpha m([Ca]_{init})/\alpha m([Ca]_{init} = \beta m,$$

and

$$h_0 = \beta h/\beta h + \alpha h([Ca]_{init}).$$

A calcium removal mechanism, described by
$$\Delta Ca/\Delta t = -Rm \cdot m_0 \cdot h_0$$

was included to keep the system at steady state in the absence of stimulus. K^+ depolarization was assumed to elicit 40 pA Ca currents. (Full details to be published elsewhere).

nucleus response. Consistent differences between cell types and species were evident. Dorsal root ganglia (DRG) neurons from all three species examined showed nucleus responses under appropriate conditions of intracellular Ca^{2+} loading. About 70% of bullfrog sympathetic neurons, however, and virtually all of clawed frog sympathetic neurons examined lacked nuclear responses, in spite of large depolarization-induced changes in cytosolic $[Ca^{2+}]$. This suggests that some cells lack the mechanism necessary to generate nucleus responses.

Amphibian neurons are capable of maintaining long-lasting nucleus/cytosol Ca^{2+} gradients as well. For instance, cell injury during fura-2 injection, causing sustained entry of calcium, gives rise to nucleus responses lasting for several minutes. The collapse of the mitochondrial proton gradient by superfusion with 20 μM carbonyl cyanide m-chlorophenyl hydrazone (CCCP) and the subsequent massive release of mitochondrial Ca^{2+} gives rise within 10 minutes to maintained nucleus cytoplasmic gradients in excess of 3 μM (not shown). *Rotenone* (100 μM) produced similar effects, but with a slower time-course.

To simulate the depolarization-induced nucleus response, our radial diffusion model of a spherical neuron[3] was modified to include a central nucleus region whose most external shell (nuclear envelope) behaves as a weak diffusional barrier. A Ca-induced Ca-release mechanism, distributed throughout the cytoplasm and at the nuclear envelope (CICR) and "gated" by Hodgkin-Huxley type kinetics, was also included (see FIG. 2C). This new model confirmed our earlier conclusion[2] that nuclear responses could not be produced without the additional Ca^{2+} provided by the intracellular release mechanism. The diffusional barrier at the "nuclear envelope" proved to be essential to generate sustained nucleus/cytoplasmic gradients.

REFERENCES

1. MILLER, R. J. 1988. TINS **11:** 415–419.
2. HERNÁNDEZ-CRUZ, A., F. SALA & P. R. ADAMS. 1990. Science **247:** 858–862.
3. SALA, F. & A. HERNÁNDEZ-CRUZ. 1990. Biophys. J. **57:** 313–324.
4. MORGAN, J. I. & T. CURRAN. 1989. TINS **12:** 459–462.
5. CONNOR, J. A. 1986. Proc. Natl. Acad. Sci. USA **83:** 6179–6183.

The Effect of ω-Conotoxin GVIA on Field Potentials in the Hippocampus and Nucleus Accumbens *in Vitro*

A. L. HORNE AND J. A. KEMP

Merck Sharp & Dohme Research Laboratories
Terlings Park
Harlow, United Kingdom CM20 2QR

The use of isolated preparations in the study of synaptic transmission has facilitated our understanding of many of the important physiological mechanisms involved. The versatility of such preparations and their obvious application to medium change and ion-substitution experiments has allowed detailed investigations into the role of calcium in central synapses. In this study, we have used slices of rat brain to study the effects of the calcium channel blocker ω-conotoxin (ω-CgTx) on evoked synaptic potentials in the hippocampus and nucleus accumbens.

In the hippocampus, electrical stimulation of the stratum radiatum activated Schaffer collateral and commissural fibers that formed excitatory synaptic connections onto CA1 pyramidal cells.[1] This activity is curtailed by inhibitory interneurons that are also synaptically activated following the electrical stimulus. Recording extracellularly in the stratum radiatum, where the excitatory synapses were formed, the evoked excitatory postsynaptic potential EPSPs resulted in the production of a negative (downward) wave (FIG. 1A). In the cell body layer these EPSPs summated

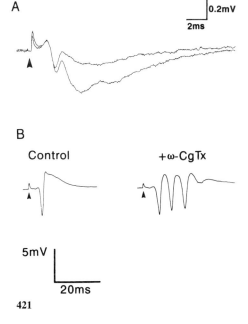

FIGURE 1. Effect of ω-CgTx on field potentials in the hippocampus. **A:** Superimposed field potentials recorded in the stratum radiatum before and after application of 100 nM ω-CgTx (10 min). Each trace is an average of four successive sweeps. The presynaptic (early) component is largely unaffected, whereas the postsynaptic (later) component is reduced in amplitude and gradient following exposure to the toxin. There was a gradual recovery from these effects. **B:** Population spikes, recorded in the cell-body layer, were also inhibited transiently by ω-CgTx, and multiple population spikes were irreversibly produced. This suggests that a more powerful block of inhibitory synapses was produced. In all figures the stimulus artifacts have been replaced with an arrow.

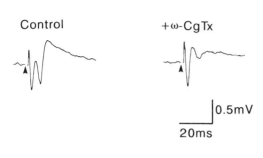

Control   +ω-CgTx

|0.5mV
20ms

FIGURE 2. Effect of ω-CgTx on field potentials in the nucleus accumbens. Stimulation of the dorsal regions of the nucleus accumbens evoked field potentials similar to those of the CA1 cell-body layer of the hippocampus. The first negative (downward) deflection was probably the result of action potentials in the presynaptic elements, whereas the second negative wave was the result of synaptic activation of the nucleus accumbens cells. ω-CgTx selectively reduced the postsynaptic component of the field. This effect was not reversed by either increasing the stimulus strength or by a period of washout of up to two hours.

to produce action potentials. If recordings were made in the cell body layer, these action potentials produced large negative going population spikes (FIG. 1B). The recurrent inhibition limited the firing of these cells so that normally only one population spike was produced. Population spikes were also recorded from slices of nucleus accumbens (FIG. 2). The afferent fibers were stimulated by focal stimulation within the accumbens tissue.[2]

Application of 100 nM ω-CgTx for 10 min reduced the rate of rise of hippocampal EPSPs recorded in the stratum radiatum (FIG. 1A) by a mean (±SEM) value of 44.2 ± 13.3% (n = 4). ω-CgTx also reduced the amplitude of the population spike in the nucleus accumbens (FIG. 2) by 75.6 ± 5.5% (n = 5). As ω-CgTx has been shown to be an antagonist of N-type calcium channels,[3] these results indicate that N-channels are involved in the calcium entry into the presynaptic terminals of these synapses.[4,5]

As expected, when recording in the CA1 cell body layer, ω-CgTx produced a reduction in the population spike amplitude of 31.2 ± 4.2% (n = 7). Multiple population spikes, however, were produced in each slice (FIG. 1B), and spontaneous discharges also occurred in four slices following exposure to the toxin. This indicates that inhibition was reduced to a greater extent than excitation. This was confirmed using intracellular recordings. Furthermore, both the reduction in the population spike amplitude and the reduction in the rate of rise of the EPSP, produced by ω-CgTx in the hippocampus, could be reversed by increasing the stimulus strength. The effects of ω-CgTx in the nucleus accumbens, or on the hippocampal EPSP, could not be reversed by this procedure.

These results suggest that the release of the excitatory transmitter in the CA1 may be less susceptible to ω-CgTx compared to either the release of the inhibitory transmitter in this region or the release of the excitatory transmitter in the nucleus accumbens.

REFERENCES

1. ANDERSEN, P., T. V. P. BLISS & K. K. SKREDE. 1971. Unit analysis of hippocampal population spikes. Exp. Brain Res. **13:** 208–221.
2. HORNE, A. L., G. N. WOODRUFF & J. A. KEMP. 1990. Synaptic potentials mediated by

excitatory amino acid receptors in the nucleus accumbens of the rat, *in-vitro.* Neuropharmacology **29:** 917–921.

3. Fox, A. P., M. C. Nowycky & R. W. Tsien. 1987. Kinetic and pharmacological properties distinguishing three types of calcium currents in chick sensory neurones. J. Physiol. (Lond.) **394:** 149–172.

4. Krishtal, O. A., A. V. Petrov, S. V. Smirnov & M. C. Nowycky. 1989. Hippocampal synaptic plasticity induced by excitatory amino acids includes changes in sensitivity to the calcium channel blocker ω-conotoxin. Neurosci. Lett. **102:** 197–204.

5. Dutar, P., O. Rascol & Y. Lamour. 1989. ω-Conotoxin GVIA blocks synaptic transmission in the CA1 field of the hippocampus. Eur. J. Pharmacol. **174:** 261–266.

Calcium Currents in Presynaptic Varicosities of Embryonic Motoneurons[a]

SUSAN C. HULSIZER, STEPHEN D. MERINEY,
AND ALAN D. GRINNELL

Jerry Lewis Neuromuscular Research Center
UCLA School of Medicine
Los Angeles, California 90024

The presynaptic calcium currents that regulate transmitter release have been difficult to study directly. With the notable exception of the squid giant synapse,[1,2] few presynaptic structures have been shown to be amenable to a direct voltage clamp study of calcium fluxes. We have chosen to study the varicose enlargements that motoneurons elaborate on muscle cells *in vitro.* Within two days of plating embryonic nerve and muscle cells from the African clawed frog (*Xenopus laevis*), motoneurons send out neurites that usually contact nearby muscle cells. Within minutes of this contact, quanta of acetylcholine are released both spontaneously[3] and in response to nerve stimulation.[4] In addition, these functional synaptic varicosities have been shown to contain ultrastructural specializations reminiscent of mature presynaptic nerve terminals.[5] In this study, we have begun a characterization of the calcium currents in neurite varicosities, with the expectation that we will be able to determine which currents are tightly coupled to transmitter release.

Embryonic nerve and muscle cells (ST 19-22) were dissected, dissociated, and plated on clean glass coverslips, and cocultured for two to four days in a standard medium with 1% fetal calf serum.[6] The varicosities are very small (2–8 μm in

---

FIGURE 1. The typical current-voltage relationship (**A**) of calcium currents recorded from neurite varicosities (arrows in **B**; M = muscle cell). **C:** The family of currents plotted in **A** were activated from a holding potential of −60 mV with step potentials (135 ms duration) to −50 through 100 in 10 mV increments. Before patch-clamp recordings were made, the cells were gradually equilibrated from their growth medium to an external solution (125 mM NaCl, 2 mM KCl, 2 mM $CaCl_2$, 1 mM $MgCl_2$, 20 mM Hepes, pH 7.8, with NaOH). This solution kept the cells in good health while the patch pipette seal (> 10 GΩ) was made. Patch pipettes were fabricated from Corning 7052 glass, coated with Sylgard, and fire-polished such that the pipette resistance was 2–5 MΩ. For traditional whole-cell recording, the pipette was filled with 108 mM CsCl, 1.8 mM $MgCl_2$, 4.5 mM EGTA, 36 mM Hepes, 0.9 mM $CaCl_2$, pH 7.2, with CsOH. For nystatin-induced access, the tip of a filament-containing pipette was filled with 43 mM $CsCl_2$, 60 mM Cs_2SO_4, 5 mM $MgCl_2$, and 10 mM Hepes. The shank and shaft of the pipette were filled with the same solution plus up to 1500 μg/mL nystatin. The nystatin usually required 2–15 minutes to diffuse to the tip of the pipette and provide complete access to the varicosity interior. After electrical access was established, the bath was changed to a solution of either 81 mM $BaCl_2$, 18 mM TEA-Cl, 1.8 μM TTX, 9 mM Hepes, 18 mM glucose, pH 7.4, with TEA-OH or one that consisted of 25 mM $CaCl_2$, 110 mM TEA-Cl, 2 μM TTX, 20 mM NaCl, 10 mM Hepes, pH 7.4, with TEA-OH. Calcium currents were evoked by 90–135 ms depolarizations to −50 through +100 mV in 10 mV increments from a holding potential of either −40, −60, or −80 mV.

[a]This work was supported by Grants from the NSF and the NIH.

424

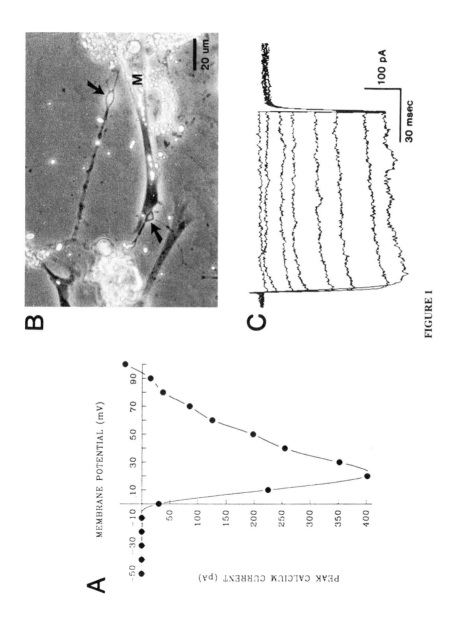

FIGURE 1

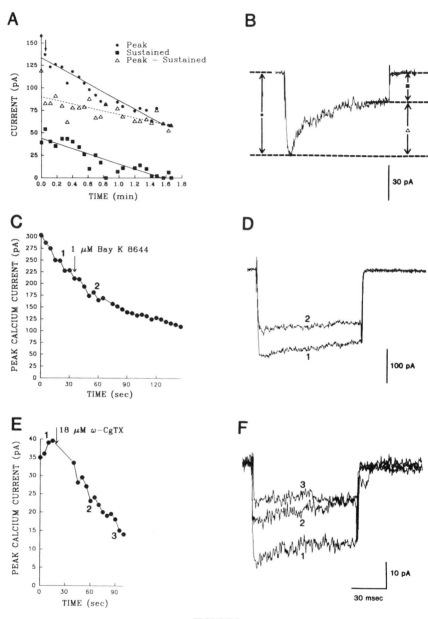

FIGURE 2

diameter) and have highly distensible membranes. In most cases, and especially when it was deemed necessary to maintain good voltage control, the neurites extending on either side of the varicosity were cut with a glass pipette.[7] Whole-cell patch-clamp recordings were made with either traditional methods of access to the varicosity interior (added suction), or nystatin-induced perforation of the cell-attached patch of membrane.[8] To isolate calcium currents, the bath was changed to a solution that blocked sodium and potassium channels and enhanced the observation of flux through calcium channels (see FIG. 1).

FIGURE 1 shows a typical varicosity and a representative family of currents with the plot of the current-voltage relationship. In all varicosities studied, only high-voltage activated currents were encountered. In most varicosities, both rapidly and noninactivating components of the current were evident during a 100 ms pulse. In all cases, the noninactivating component was more sensitive to washout (see FIGURES 2A and B). The pharmacologic sensitivity of the currents was examined to further characterize them and to compare their sensitivity with known sensitivities of transmitter release. Mature neuromuscular transmission has been shown to be very sensitive to omega-conotoxin (ω-CgTX) and relatively insensitive to dihydropyridines. FIGURES 2C and D demonstrate that these calcium currents are not sensitive to the dihydropyridine agonist Bay K 8644. FIGURES 2E and F show that the currents are sensitive to ω-CgTX (GVIA) and that the rapidly inactivating current component appears to be completely blocked. All of the current was rapidly and completely blocked by 400 μM cadmium (not shown).

On average, the current density in varicosities was 135 pA/pF with 81 mM Ba^{2+} as the charge carrier and 35 pA/pF with 25 mM Ca^{2+} as the charge carrier (varicosity capacitance ranged from 0.45 to 7.7 pF). Previously O'Dowd *et al.*[9] have shown that the soma has a Ca^{2+} current density of 55 pA/pF with 10 mM Ca^{2+} as the charge carrier. Therefore, 2–4-day-old neurite varicosities appear to have a lower current density than the somata. It is possible that further maturation will increase varicosity calcium current density.

There are several lines of evidence that suggest that two types of calcium current are present in embryonic neurite varicosities: (1) there is a variable amount of inactivation of the composite calcium current in different varicosities; (2) the noninactivating component of the calcium current washes out faster than the rapidly inactivating component; and (3) ω-CgTX blockade is not complete, with the rapidly inactivating component more sensitive than the noninactivating component. The noninactivating component has many of the characteristics of the L-type calcium

---

FIGURE 2. **A:** The noninactivating current washes out at a greater rate than the rapidly inactivating current. Calcium current is evoked once every five seconds from a holding potential of −60 mV with a 90 ms step to 30 mV. **B:** The current measured at the peak (filled circles; solid line) is compared with the sustained current measured at the end of the depolarization pulse (filled squares; solid line). The rapidly inactivating component of the current (open triangles; dashed line) is derived by subtracting the sustained current from the peak current. The small arrow in **A** indicated the point at which the current record in **B** is taken. **C:** In a varicosity that showed some calcium current run-down, Bay K 8644 was not able to increase the calcium current or lengthen the time-course of the tail current decay. The currents are evoked as in **A,** and 1 μM Bay K 8644 is added as indicated by the arrow. **D:** The numbers 1 and 2 indicate the times at which sample records are displayed. **E:** ω-CgTX blocks the varicosity calcium current in a nystatin-induced whole-cell recording. The currents are evoked as in **A,** and 18 μM ω-CgTX (GVIA) is added as indicated by the arrow. **F:** The gradual block of the current is displayed by sample records 1–3 with their positions indicated on the graph (**E**).

current described in dorsal root ganglia (DRG) cells,[10] except that it does not appear
to be sensitive to Bay K 8644. This lack of effect cannot be attributed to an excessively
hyperpolarized holding potential, inasmuch as Bay K 8644 can strongly affect
calcium currents in *Xenopus* motoneuron somata at this potential (-60 mV; not
shown). The rapidly inactivating component of the varicosity calcium currents is
similar to the N-type current described in DRG cells.[10]

The calcium currents described in this report are all from varicosities that were
either in contact with, or near, nerve-muscle contacts. We look forward to comparing
these observations to currents encountered in isolated neuronal cultures. It is
anticipated that nerve-muscle contact will induce the expression of synapse-specific
properties of the varicosity, which may include the type or quantity of calcium
channels. In addition, we look forward to recording the postsynaptic end-plate
potentials associated with activation of varicosity calcium currents in an attempt to
determine which current type(s) are most closely coupled to transmitter release.

REFERENCES

1. LLINÁS, R. I., I. Z. STEINBERG & K. WALTON. 1981. Presynaptic calcium currents in squid giant synapse. Biophys. J. **33**: 289–322.
2. AUGUSTINE, G. J., M. P. CHARLTON & S. J. SMITH. 1985. Calcium entry into voltage-clamped presynaptic terminals of squid. J. Physiol. (Lond.) **367**: 143–162.
3. CHOW, I. & M-M. POO. 1985. Release of acetylcholine from embryonic neurons upon contact with muscle cell. J. Neurosci. **5**: 1076–1082.
4. KIDOKORO, Y. & E. YEH. 1982. Initial synaptic transmission at the growth cone in *Xenopus* nerve-muscle cultures. Proc. Natl. Acad. Sci. USA **79**: 6727–6731.
5. WELDON, P. R. & M. W. COHEN. 1979. Development of synaptic ultrastructure at neuromuscular contacts in an amphibian cell culture system. J. Neurocytol. **8**: 239–259.
6. CHOW, I. & M-M. POO. 1984. Formation of electrical coupling between embryonic *Xenopus* muscle cells in culture. J. Physiol. (Lond.) **346**: 181–194.
7. KIDOKORO, Y., O. SAND & B. CHEN. 1986. Membrane electrical properties at various regions of embryonic neurons in *Xenopus* cultures. Soc. Neurosci. (Abstr.) **12**: 545.
8. HORN, R. & A. MARTY. 1988. Muscarinic activation of ionic currents measured by a new whole cell recording method. J. Gen. Physiol. **92**: 145–159.
9. O'DOWD, D. K., A. B. RIBERA & N. C. SPITZER. 1988. Development of voltage-dependent calcium, sodium, and potassium currents in *Xenopus* spinal neurons. J. Neurosci. **8**: 792–805.
10. FOX, A. P., M. C. NOWYCKY & R. W. TSIEN. 1987. Kinetic and pharmacological properties distinguishing three types of calcium currents in chick sensory neurons. J. Physiol. (Lond.) **394**: 149–172.

Ionizing Radiation and Calcium Channels

S. B. KANDASAMY

Behavioral Sciences Department
Armed Forces Radiobiology Research Institute
Bethesda, Maryland 20889-5145

INTRODUCTION

Ionizing radiation alters many neuronal systems that are regulated by calcium ions. Because ionizing radiation reduces voltage-sensitive (VS) calcium uptake in rat brain synaptosomes, experiments were conducted to elucidate the mechanisms of reduced calcium uptake. This paper reviews the work being done in this laboratory.[1-5]

METHODS

A crude, synaptosomal fraction preparation from the brains of male Sprague-Dawley rats and gamma irradiation from a ^{60}Co source at a dose rate of 10 Gy/min were used as described by Mullin *et al.*[6] KCl-stimulated $^{45}Ca^{2+}$ uptake into rat brain synaptosomes was measured as described by Leslie *et al.*[7] [^{3}H]nimodipine binding assays were based on the methods reported by Skattebol and Triggle.[8]

RESULTS

The fastest and highest rate of VS calcium uptake occurred at 3 s with 65 mM KCl. Irradiation (3 Gy and 10 Gy/min) reduced calcium uptake at all incubation times (3, 10, 30, and 60 s) and KCl concentrations (15–65 mM). Irradiation (1–30 Gy) reduced 65 mM KCl-stimulated calcium uptake after 3 s (FIG. 1). Enhancement of 15 mM KCl-stimulated calcium uptake by Bay K 8644 was reduced by irradiation. Nimodipine binding to dihydropyridine (DHP) L-type calcium channel receptors was not altered following irradiation. Prostaglandin $F_2\alpha$ ($PGF_2\alpha$), inositol 1,4,5-trisphosphate (IP3), phorbol esters (PE), Bay K 8644, and interleukin 1α (IL-1α) alone did not reverse the decrease in calcium influx caused by irradiation, but in combination they did reverse it. For example, pretreatment with 1 nM to 100 nM of PE and 1 nM of IP3, 1 nM of Bay K 8644, 10 nM $PGF_2\alpha$, or 20-hr pretreatment with 2,000 units of IL-1α significantly reversed decreases in calcium uptake induced by irradiation (TABLE 1).

DISCUSSION

Ionizing radiation significantly reduced KCl-stimulated, VS calcium uptake in rat brain synaptosomes. The inhibitory effect of irradiation on the VS calcium channels

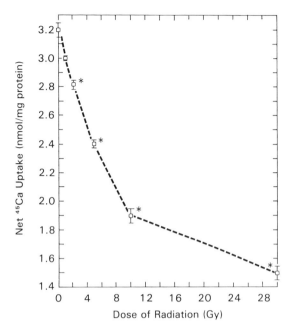

FIGURE 1. Effect of gamma irradiation on 65 mM KCl-stimulated calcium uptake by rat whole-brain synaptosomes, measured during 3-s periods. Points and bars represent mean ±SEM values from three separate experiments, each using triplicate samples. *Significantly different from control value: $p < 0.05$.

was not mediated by DHP receptors because irradiation did not alter nimodipine binding to DHP L-type calcium channel receptors.

If pretreatment with IP3, PE, or $PGF_2\alpha$ reversed the radiation-induced reduction in calcium influx, it would indicate that the formation of IP3, diacylglycerol, and $PGF_2\alpha$ is necessary for calcium influx and that radiation interferes with their

TABLE 1. Effect of PE in Combination with IP3, Bay K 8644, $PGF_2\alpha$, or 2,000 Units of IL-1α on Calcium Uptake (nmol/mg protein) in Irradiated (3 Gy and 10 Gy/min gamma rays) and Nonirradiated Rat Whole-Brain Synaptosomes

Concentration of Drug	Concentration of PE (nM)[a]			
	0	1	10	100
1 nM IP3				
Irradiated	1.9 ± 0.05	3.2 ± 0.05[b]	4.1 ± 0.15[b]	4.6 ± 0.10[b]
Nonirradiated	2.6 ± 0.05	3.6 ± 0.10[c]	4.3 ± 0.10[c]	4.8 ± 0.05[c]
1 nM Bay K 8644				
Irradiated	2.2 ± 0.10	3.3 ± 0.10[b]	4.0 ± 0.15[b]	4.4 ± 0.15[b]
Nonirradiated	2.8 ± 0.10	3.5 ± 0.10[c]	3.9 ± 0.10[c]	4.6 ± 0.10[c]
10 nM $PGF_2\alpha$				
Irradiated	2.0 ± 0.10	3.0 ± 0.10[b]	3.8 ± 0.15[b]	4.7 ± 0.10[b]
Nonirradiated	2.7 ± 0.10	3.5 ± 0.10[c]	3.9 ± 0.10[c]	4.8 ± 0.15[c]
2,000 units IL-1α				
Irradiated	1.8 ± 0.15	3.3 ± 0.10[b]	4.2 ± 0.15[b]	4.5 ± 0.10[b]
Nonirradiated	2.4 ± 0.10	3.5 ± 0.05[c]	4.2 ± 0.05[c]	4.6 ± 0.10[c]

[a]Values are mean ± SEM of three separate experiments, each using triplicate samples.
[b]Significantly different from irradiated 0 PE values: $p < 0.05$.
[c]Significantly different from nonirradiated 0 PE values: $p < 0.05$.

formation. So, IP3, PE, Bay K 8644, $PGF_2\alpha$, and IL-1α were tested to determine if they could reverse the radiation-induced decrease in calcium influx. None of the compounds alone reversed the decrease in calcium uptake induced by irradiation, but in combination they did reverse it, suggesting that ionizing radiation might affect protein kinase C activity, which is linked to the opening and closing of ion channels[9] and the mobilization of calcium. These experiments demonstrate that the stimulation of protein kinase C by PE together with the mobilization/influx of calcium by calcium ionophores is necessary to attenuate radiation-induced decreases in calcium influx. Currently, we are comparing protein kinase C activity and G protein receptor binding of irradiated and nonirradiated synaptosomes to determine whether decreases in calcium uptake induced by irradiation are due to impairment of protein kinase C, alterations in G protein receptors, or both.

REFERENCES

1. KANDASAMY, S. B. & W. A. HUNT. 1988. Effect of ionizing radiation on calcium channels in rat brain synaptosomes. Soc. Neurosci. (Abstr.) **54:** 13.
2. KANDASAMY, S. B., W. A. HUNT & A. DUBOIS. 1989. Effect of ionizing radiation on calcium channels in rat ileum myenteric plexus synaptosomes. Soc. Neurosci. (Abstr.) **147:** 19.
3. KANDASAMY, S. B., T. C. HOWERTON & W. A. HUNT. 1991. Reductions in calcium uptake induced in rat brain synaptosomes by ionizing radiation. Radiat. Res. **125:** 158–162.
4. KANDASAMY, S. B. & W. A. HUNT. 1990. Arachidonic acid and prostaglandins enhance potassium-stimulated calcium influx into rat brain synaptosomes. Neuropharmacol. **29:** 825–829.
5. KANDASAMY, S. B. & W. A. HUNT. 1990. Role of protein kinase C in radiation-induced decreased calcium-uptake in rat brain synaptosomes. The Toxicologist. (Abstr.) 422.
6. MULLIN, M. J., W. A. HUNT & R. A. HARRIS. 1986. Ionizing radiation alters the properties of sodium channels in rat brain synaptosomes. J. Neurochem. **47:** 489–495.
7. LESLIE, S. W., M. B. FRIEDMAN, R. E. WILCOX & S. Y. ELROD. 1980. Acute and chronic effects of barbiturates on depolarization-induced calcium influx into rat synaptosomes. Brain Res. **185:** 409–417.
8. SKATTEBOL, A. & D. J. TRIGGLE. 1987. Regional distribution of calcium channel ligand (1,4-dihydropyridine) binding sites and $^{45}Ca^{2+}$ uptake processes in rat brain. Biochem. Pharmacol. **36:** 4163–4166.
9. MARX, J. L. 1987. Polyphosphoinositide research updated. Science **235:** 974–976.

Diazepam Enhances Ca²⁺ Levels in Rat Brain Synaptosomes

JOSEPH V. MARTIN, DON R. KEIR, AND HSIN-YI LEE

Biology Department
Rutgers University
Camden, New Jersey 08102

A variety of neurophysiological evidence now indicates stimulatory effects of benzo-diazepines (BZ),[1] in addition to the well-known inhibitory effects mediated through a chloride channel in the BZ/γ-aminobutyric acid$_A$ ($GABA_A$) receptor complex.[2] Several studies have shown effects of BZ on fluxes of Ca^{2+} to presynaptic preparations, including synaptosomes.[3,4] Using $^{45}Ca^{2+}$ as a tracer, low μM doses of BZ were found to increase the uptake of radioactivity to depolarized synaptosomes,[3] whereas much higher (100 μM) doses of BZ inhibited depolarization-induced $^{45}Ca^{2+}$ uptake.[4] The present study measured total unbound cytoplasmic Ca^{2+} by the method of Grynkiewicz and co-workers[5] in synaptosomes exposed to a wide range of doses of the BZ, diazepam.

If synaptosomes are maintained in a physiological buffered saline including Na^+, excess cytoplasmic Na^+ accumulates.[6] Elevated intrasynaptosomal Na^+ causes the Na^+/Ca^{2+} exchanger to act in a reversed mode, taking up extracellular Ca^{2+}. When synaptosomes are maintained in a buffer that includes choline Cl in place of NaCl, the effects of a reversed Na^+/Ca^{2+} exchanger are minimized.[6] Therefore, in order to evaluate the effects of a reversed Na^+/Ca^{2+} exchanger, synaptosomes were maintained in buffered salt solution with NaCl (Na^+ BSS) or a similar solution in which NaCl was replaced by isomolar choline Cl (choline BSS).

Synaptosomes were prepared from rat brain and were suspended in either Na^+ BSS or choline BSS. The synaptosomal suspension was then incubated with the acetoxymethyl ester of fura-2 (fura-2/AM) at a concentration of 10 μM for 45 min at 37°C. The solution was diluted fivefold and incubated 15 min at 37°C to allow regeneration of the free fura-2 by endogenous esterases within the synaptosomes. The synaptosomes were then washed twice by centrifugation at 3,200 $\times$ *g* for 10 min and resuspension in the appropriate BSS. Synaptosomes (2 mL) loaded with dye were then equilibrated with vehicle (10 μL ethanol) or with 1–100 μM diazepam for 45 min at 0–4°C. Fluorescence was measured at 500 nm for excitation at 340 and 385 nanometers. Synaptosomes were depolarized with a solution containing KCl and $CaCl_2$ (final concentrations = 45 mM KCl and 1.2 mM $CaCl_2$). Fluorescence measurements were then taken for 2 min (depolarized condition). The minimal dye response in the presence of very low Ca^{2+} (R_{MIN})[5] was measured in parallel incubates in 0.5% sodium dodecylsulfate (SDS) in 4 mM ethyleneglycolbis-(β-aminoethyl ether) N,N'-tetraacetic acid (EGTA). Measures of background fluorescence were made on synaptosomes without dye. R_{max} was measured at 3 min after addition of 5 μM of the nonquenching Ca^{2+} ionophore 4-Br A23187, and the concentration of Ca^{2+} was calculated.[7]

Nondepolarized synaptosomes incubated in Na^+ BSS (FIG. 1) contained 54% more free Ca^{2+} than synaptosomes maintained in choline BSS (FIG. 2). Depolarization caused a proportionately smaller increase of 32% in levels of synaptoplasmic Ca^{2+} in choline BSS (FIG. 2) compared to a 155% increase in the presence of Na^+

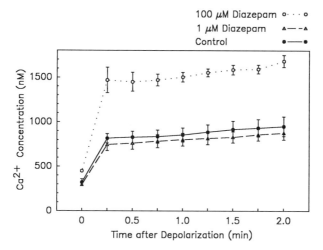

FIGURE 1. Effect of 0, 1, or 100 μM diazepam on the depolarization-induced increase in Ca^{2+} in synaptosomes in Na^+ BSS. Measurements of Ca^{2+} levels at time 0 were made in nondepolarized synaptosomes loaded with the fluorescent dye fura-2 in Na^+ BSS (136 mM NaCl, 5.6 mM KCl, 1.3 mM $MgCl_2$, 11 mM glucose, 20 mM Tris HCl, pH 7.4). Following this initial measurement, 0.1 mL of a depolarizing solution was added to bring the final concentration of KCl to 45 mM and $CaCl_2$ to 1.2 mM. Fluorescence measurements were then taken for 2 min. Results are presented as mean ± standard error of the mean (SEM) for 6 replicates at each point.

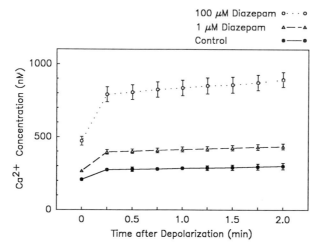

FIGURE 2. Effect of 0, 1, or 100 μM diazepam on the depolarization-induced increase in Ca^{2+} in synaptosomes in choline BSS without Na^+. Measurements of Ca^{2+} levels at time 0 were made in nondepolarized synaptosomes loaded with the fluorescent dye fura-2 in choline BSS (136 mM choline Cl, 5.6 mM KCl, 1.3 mM $MgCl_2$, 11 mM glucose, 20 mM Tris HCl, pH 7.4). Following this initial measurement, 0.1 mL of a depolarizing solution was added to bring the final concentration of KCl to 45 mM and $CaCl_2$ to 1.2 mM. Fluorescence measurements were then taken for 2 min. Results are presented as mean ± standard error of the mean (SEM) for 6 replicates at each point.

(FIG. 1). Against this lowered background level of Ca^{2+}, the effect of diazepam was more readily apparent in choline BSS than in Na^+ BSS. Both types of synaptosomal incubates showed dramatic increases in Ca^{2+} in response to 100 μM diazepam under depolarizing conditions. In synaptosomes maintained in choline BSS, significant increases in Ca^{2+} were also found for doses of diazepam as low as 1 μM in both depolarizing and nondepolarizing conditions. Analysis of variance also indicated a significant interaction of drug treatment group by time after depolarization ($p < 10^{-6}$).

In contrast to earlier studies using $^{45}Ca^{2+}$ as a tracer,[3,4] the present studies measured total free synaptoplasmic Ca^{2+} under conditions designed to minimize the contribution of a reversed Na^+/Ca^{2+} exchanger. In the present studies both low and high micromolar doses of Ca^{2+} had similar qualitative effects: to increase synaptoplasmic Ca^{2+}. Also in contrast to the earlier studies, when a solution lacking Na^+ (choline BSS) was used, effects of BZ were seen in nondepolarized synaptosomes. In choline BSS, the effects of depolarization and BZ action in enhancing Ca^{2+} levels were synergistic.

REFERENCES

1. POLC, P. 1988. Prog. Neurobiol. (Oxf.) **31:** 349–423.
2. STEPHENSON, F. A. 1988. Biochem. J. **249:** 21–32.
3. MENDELSON, W. B., P. SKOLNICK, J. V. MARTIN, M. D. LUU, R. WAGNER & S. M. PAUL. 1984. Eur. J. Pharmacol. **104:** 181–183.
4. LESLIE, S. W., L. J. CHANDLER, A. Y. CHWEH & E. A. SWINYARD. 1986. Eur. J. Pharmacol. **126:** 129–134.
5. GRYNKIEWICZ, G., M. POENIE & R. Y. TSIEN. 1985. J. Biol. Chem. **260:** 3440–3450.
6. SUSZKIW, J. B., M. M. MURAWSKY & M. SHI. 1989. J. Neurochem. **52:** 1260–1269.
7. DEBER, C. M., J. TOM-KUN, E. MACK & S. GRINSTEIN. 1985. Anal. Biochem. **146:** 349.

Evidence for Subtypes of the ω-Conotoxin GVIA Receptor

Identification of the Properties Intrinsic to the High-Affinity Receptor

MAUREEN W. McENERY, ADELE M. SNOWMAN,
AND SOLOMON H. SNYDER

Department of Neuroscience
The Johns Hopkins University School of Medicine
Baltimore, Maryland 21205

The neuropeptide toxin ω-conotoxin GVIA (CTX)[1] present in the venom of the predatory cone snail *Conus geographus* has been shown to inhibit the voltage-gated calcium channel (VGCC) present in both rat hippocampus and rat sympathetic neurons.[2] The inhibitory action of CTX on VGCC has been extended to other peripheral nerve terminals[3] and brain synaptosomal preparations from many species.[4] As the CTX peptide is believed to have evolved to target a structurally related set of receptor molecules,[5] apparent differences in affinity for the toxin may reflect subunit heterogeneity within a family of receptors as has been demonstrated in the case of the acetylcholine receptor.[6] As shown in TABLE 1, a [125I]CTX binding site can be identified in the brain of several species as well as in rat retina, spinal cord, pituitary, and in *Torpedo* electroplax membranes. Scatchard analysis of these sites indicate that [125I]CTX interacts with endogenous receptors that can be pharmacologically distinguished from each other. The [125I]CTX receptor in rat and human brain is of similiar affinity (7 and 15 pM, respectively) and is present in similiar amounts (2.3 and 1.3 pmol/mg, respectively). By contrast, the [125I]CTX receptor in frog brain possesses a much lower affinity (K_d value of 78.8 pM) and is present in much greater quantity (B_{max} of 377 pmol/mg). The [125I]CTX binding site in rat retina and spinal cord is similar to the brain site in affinity (K_d values of 16 and 21 pM, respectively), but is present in low abundance (0.03 and 0.06 pmol/mg, respectively). These

TABLE 1. Summary of Properties That Distinguish between Central (C) and Peripheral (P)-Type Receptors for [125I]ω Conotoxin GVIA

Tissues (C- or P-type)	K_d (pM)	B_{max} (pmol/mg)	Molecular weight (kDa) of HSA-[125I]CTX cross-linked receptor
Rat brain synaptosomes (C)	7	2.3	230
Human frontal cortex (C)	15	1.3	230, 210
Chicken brain (C)	56	1.5	230
Frog brain (P)	965	78.8	56
Torpedo electroplax (P)	3000	377.0	71, 68.5, 55, 51, 47
Rat retina (P)	16	0.03	65, 56
Rat spinal cord (P)	21	0.1	50
Rat olfactory bulb (C)	37	0.06	230, 38
Rat pituitary (P)	190	2.13	56, 50

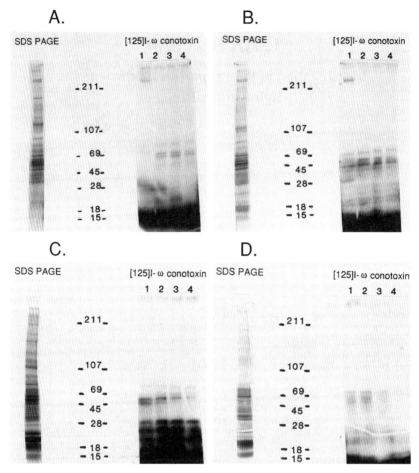

FIGURE 1. Identification of the [^{125}I]ω-Conotoxin GVIA ([^{125}I]CTX) binding sites in central and peripheral neurons by photoaffinity labeling with HSA-[^{125}I]CTX. Membrane samples from several tissues: (**A**) rat brain synaptosomes, (**B**) rat olfactory bulb, (**C**) rat pituitary gland, and (**D**) rat retina were labeled with N-hydroxysuccinimidyl-4-azidobenzoate (HSA)–derivatized [^{125}I]CTX according to the method of Glossmann and Striessnig[7] in the presence of increasing concentrations of unlabeled CTX; lane 1: no additional cold, lane 2: 0.5 nM, lane 3: 50 nM, and lane 4: 1000 nM. The total amount of [^{125}I]CTX receptor present in the photo-crosslinking experiments was normalized to 16 fmol of [^{125}I]CTX receptor/lane. After a 40-min incubation of the membranes in the dark with HSA-[^{125}I]CTX, the samples were irradiated for 40 min with ultraviolet light. The reaction was quenched by the addition of Laemmli sample buffer and resolved on a 7–15% discontinuous gradient gel. The positions of the molecular weight standards (kDa) are as indicated.

findings regarding peripheral neurons are in contrast to the results of [^{125}I]CTX binding in pituitary that has a K_d of 190 pM and a B_{max} of 2.13 pmol/mg. The molecular properties of the endogenous [^{125}I]CTX receptors were further examined by cross-linking with [^{125}I]CTX derivatized with a photoactivatible cross-linker.[7] The results of these experiments are shown in FIGURE 1 and summarized in TABLE 1. In rat brain synaptosomes (panel A) and rat olfactory bulb (panel B) HSA-[^{125}I]CTX identifies a 230 kDa protein. The binding of HSA-[^{125}I]CTX is inhibited by the addition of <0.5 nM unlabeled CTX. This apparent high-affinity 230 kDa protein can be regarded as the central type (C-type) CTX receptor. As presented in TABLE 1, a protein with similiar apparent molecular weight is identified in both chick and human brain (human brain also has a 210 kDa protein). In peripheral neurons such as rat pituitary (FIG. 1, panel C) and rat retina (panel D), the HSA-[^{125}I]CTX labeling pattern is very different: 50, 56, and 65 kDa proteins are identified, and this labeling is inhibited by concentrations of cold CTX in the range of 50–1000 nM. These low molecular weight HSA-[^{125}I]CTX binding proteins (a putative peripheral (P)-type) are also present in frog brain and *Torpedo*.[8]

[NOTE ADDED IN PROOF: We have purified the C-type CTX receptor from rat forebrain to homogeneity retaining the molecular properties of the membrane-bound receptor as defined above. CTX receptor from rat forebrain membranes were solubilized with CHAPS, then further purified by negative chromatography on heparin-sepharose, arginine sepharose, and zinc/metal chelate chromatography. The CTX receptor was then chromatographed on hydroxylapatite and wheat germ agglutinin-sepharose. The 230 kDa band specifically photolabeled by HSA-[^{125}I]CTX copurifies with the active receptor. In addition to the 230 kDa CTX binding protein, four additional proteins with apparent molecular weights of 140, 110, 70, and 60 are observed in the purified preparation. These bands appear to be integral components of the receptor. The subunit composition of the C-type CTX receptor closely resembles the α_1, α_2, and β subunit structure of the 1,4-dihydropyridine-sensitive L-calcium channel receptor.[9]]

REFERENCES

1. OLIVERA, B. M., W. R. GRAY, R. ZEIKUS, J. M. McINTOSH, J. VARG, J. RIVIER, V. DE SANTOS & L. J. CRUZ. 1985. Science **230:** 1338–1343.
2. McCLESKY, E. W., A. P. FOX, D. H. FELDMAN, L. J. CRUZ, B. M. OLIVERA, R. W. TSIEN & D. YOSHIKAMI. 1987. Proc. Natl. Acad. Sci. USA **84:** 4327–4331.
3. LUNDY, P. M. & R. FREW. 1988. Eur. J. Pharmacol. **156:** 325–330.
4. SUSZKIW, J. B., M. M. MURAWSKY & R. C. FORTNER. 1987. Biochem. Biophys. Res. Commun. **145:** 1283–1286.
5. OLIVERA, B. M., J. RIVIER, C. CLARK, C. A. RAMILO, G. P. CORPUS, F. C. ABOGADIE, E. E. MENA, S. R. WOODWARD, D. R. HILLYARD & L. J. CRUZ. 1990. Science **249:** 257–263.
6. LUETJE, C. W., K. WADA, S. ROGERS, S. N. ABRAMSON, K. TSUJI, S. HEINEMANN & J. PATRICK. 1990. J. Neurochem. **55:** 632–640.
7. GLOSSMANN, H. & J. STRIESSNIG. 1988. ISI Atlas Sci. Pharmacol. **2:** 202–210.
8. HORNE, W., R. R. DELAY & R. W. TSIEN. 1990. Neurosci. (Abstr.) **16:** 957.
9. TAKAHASHI, M. SEAGAR, M. JONES, B. REBER & W. A. CATTERALL. 1987. Proc. Natl. Acad. Sci. USA **84:** 5478–5482.

5-HT, MDMA (Ecstasy), and Nimodipine Effects on ^{45}Ca-Uptake into Rat Brain Synaptosomes

W. K. PARK AND E. C. AZMITIA

Department of Biology
New York University
100 Washington Square East
New York, New York 10003

Ca^{2+} entry into cells is one of the initial steps in cell death.[1-4] MDMA-induced neuropathology of cultured serotonergic neurons is linked to 5-HT release and attenuated by nimodipine.[5] Rat brain synaptosomes were used as an *in vitro* system to measure $^{45}Ca^{2+}$ entry. To test the possible mechanism of MDMA-induced stimulation of Ca entry and the role of the 5-HT system on regulating brain Ca^{2+} channels, we modified an *in vitro* microassay system[6] for use with 96-well plates (NUNC, Denmark).

SUBJECT AND METHOD

Whole rat brain, except cerebellum, synaptosomal preparations were used to measure Ca^{2+} entry into synaptosomes. After preincubation at 30°C for 15 min, tissue was added to start uptake. All drugs were tested in resting (4.5 mM K^+) and stimulating (68.5 mM K^+) media at 30°C for 1 second. In addition, the synaptosomes were pretreated with ethyleneglycol tetraacetate (EGTA; 12 mM) in the preincubation step to test the possible dependency of Ca^{2+} entry on endogeneous Ca^{2+} level with or without caffeine treatment. Furthermore, the effect of MDMA on ^{45}Ca entry was tested both with and without pretreatment with fluoxetine (10^{-7}M), a selective 5-HT uptake blocker.

RESULTS

MDMA (10^{-5}M), 5-HT (10^{-6}M), and nimodipine (10^{-9}M) significantly stimulated ^{45}Ca entry in both basal and high K^+ media. Nimodipine with MDMA enhanced ^{45}Ca uptake even further than either alone (FIG. 1). MDMA-induced $^{45}Ca^{2+}$ entry was completely blocked by fluoxetine pretreatment (FIG. 2). In EGTA-pretreated synaptosomes no K^+-stimulated ^{45}Ca entry was observed. MDMA and 5-HT both significantly stimulated ^{45}Ca entry as in the control condition, however. Caffeine (10^{-5}M), a nucleotide phosphodiesterase inhibitor, stimulated ^{45}Ca uptake under depolarizing condition after preincubation with EGTA (not shown).

CONCLUSION AND DISCUSSION

A microassay system was developed to measure the uptake of $^{45}Ca^{2+}$ into adult rat brain synatosomes under basal and K^+-stimulated conditions. Approximately a 50%

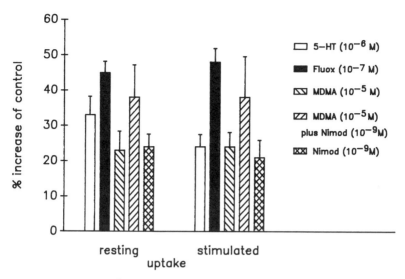

FIGURE 1. Stimulation of ^{45}Ca uptake into rat brain synaptosomes by 5-HT (10^{-6}M), MDMA (10^{-5}M), fluoxetine (10^{-7}M), nimodipine (10^{-9}M), and MDMA with nimodipine. Data shown are expressed as percentage increase of control value in resting (4.5 m MK$^+$) and stimulating (68.5 m MK$^+$) buffer (mean ± SE; quadruplicates, n = 5–8).

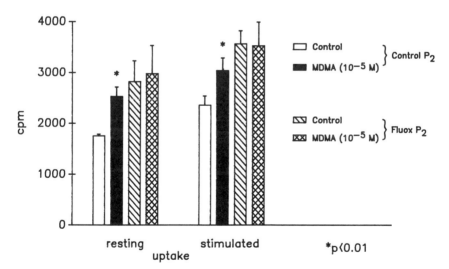

FIGURE 2. Fluoxetine inhibits MDMA-induced increase in ^{45}Ca uptake. MDMA effect on ^{45}Ca entry in fluoxetine-pretreated synaptosomes was compared to control synaptosomes in resting and stimulating buffers. From control synaptosomes in resting condition, MDMA (10^{-5}M) caused 44% increase in ^{45}Ca uptake, whereas in fluoxetine (10^{-7}M, final concn)-pretreated synaptosomes, MDMA increased only 5.6%. Under stimulating conditions, MDMA stimulated ^{45}Ca uptake 29% with control synaptosomes, whereas in fluoxetine-treated synaptosomes, MDMA effect was negligible (1% decrease) (quadruplicates, n = 3). * p < .01 with respect to appropriate control.

increase was seen in the K^+-stimulated conditions. The basal and K^+-stimulated uptake of $^{45}Ca^{2+}$ was increased by exposure to MDMA, a potent drug of abuse that produces neuropathology of serotonergic neurons. Interestingly, a stimulation was also seen with 5-HT and fluoxetine. It is known that MDMA releases 5-HT (Gu and Azmitia, submitted) and binds to the 5-HT transporter,[7] which also binds fluoxetine, a potent 5-HT reuptake blocker. It is suggested that Ca^{2+} influx may be altered by drugs that act on the 5-HT transporter. It is interesting to note that verapamil, a Ca^{2+} channel antagonist has been shown to block [^{3}H]5-HT uptake into synaptosomes. Thus, 5-HT and Ca^{2+} may use a similar mechanism for uptake into the synaptosomes. Furthermore, the brain synaptosomal Ca^{2+} channels must be phosphorylated by endogenous Ca^{2+} or through cyclic-AMP–mediated phosphorylation. MDMA and 5-HT–induced stimulation of $^{45}Ca^{2+}$ entry appears to be independent of endogenous Ca^{2+} levels. Finally, the Ca^{2+} L-type channel blocker (nimodipine) increased Ca^{2+} accumulation in the synaptosome either by stimulating uptake or by inhibiting release.

REFERENCES

1. SHANNE, F. A. X., A. B. KANE, E. E. YOUNG & J. L. FARBER. 1979. Science **206:** 700–702.
2. HAYDON, P. G., D. P. MCCOBB & S. B. KATER. 1984. Science **262:** 561–564.
3. DREYER, E. B., P. K. KAISER, J. T. OFFERMANN & S. A. LIPTON. 1990. Science **248:** 364–367.
4. CHOI, D. W. 1985. Neurosci Lett. **58:** 293–297.
5. AZMITIA, E. C., R. B. MURPHY & P. M. WHITAKER-AZMITIA. 1990. Brain Res. **510:** 97–103.
6. SKATTEBOL, A. & D. J. TRIGGLE. 1987. Biochem. Pharmacol. **36:** 4163–4166.
7. POBLETE, J. C., P. M. WHITAKER-AZMITIA & E. C. AZMITIA. 1989. Soc. Neurosci. (Abstr.) **15:** 418.

Relationship between Membrane Depolarization and Intracellular Free Calcium in Individual Nerve Terminals from the Neurohypophysis

EDWARD L. STUENKEL

Department of Physiology
University of Michigan
Ann Arbor, Michigan 48109-0622

The release of transmitter/hormone from nerve terminals is dependent on depolarization-induced changes in intraterminal free $[Ca^{2+}]$, yet anatomical limitations of vertebrate nerve endings have largely precluded direct monitoring of such changes at single axon endings. As a result the quantitative relationship of the change in $[Ca^{2+}]_i$ to exocytosis in vertebrate endings remains virtually uncharacterized. Using axon terminals isolated from the neurohypophysis of the rat, changes in $[Ca^{2+}]_i$ in individual endings in response to depolarizing stimuli were directly quantitated by dual wavelength microspectrofluorometry of cytoplasmic fura-2. The mean basal $[Ca^{2+}]_i$ was 66 ± 4 nM (n = 212, $\pm$SEM), a value similar to most excitable and nonexcitable cells. Membrane depolarization evoked by elevation of extracellular $[K^+]$ resulted in a rapid, dose-dependent increase in $[Ca^{2+}]_i$ that was not present in medium lacking extracellular Ca^{2+} (no added Ca^{2+} plus 1 mM EGTA) and was greatly reduced by the inorganic Ca^{2+} channel blockers Cd^{2+} and La^{3+}. Application of the dihydropyridine nicardipine dose dependently reduced the rise in $[Ca^{2+}]_i$ evoked by 50 mM K^+ (93% block at 10 µM) as did desmethoxyverapamil (D888). These results suggest that the evoked rise in $[Ca^{2+}]$ is mediated by an L-type Ca^{2+} channel under these depolarizing conditions. Recovery of basal $[Ca^{2+}]_i$ on removal of elevated K^+ showed an initial rapid decline followed by a slower phase.

Initial studies have found the change in $[Ca^{2+}]_i$ in single nerve endings, in response to given K^+-induced depolarizations, to closely correlate to vasopressin release monitored from populations of isolated endings.[1] The close correlation suggests that Ca^{2+} influx by way of the L-type Ca^{2+} channel is associated with release under these depolarizing conditions. A strengthening of this conclusion was provided by the close relationship between dihydropyridine block of secretion (IC_{50} = 4 µM)[1] with the observed block of Ca^{2+} influx and rise in $[Ca^{2+}]_i$ (approx. IC_{50} = 2 µM). Furthermore, there is a close relationship between the kinetics of a change in $[Ca^{2+}]_i$ and that of vasopressin release in the present study when challenged with a 30-s pulse of 50 mM $^+$ [arginine vasopressin release graciously performed by Dr. J. J. Nordmann]. For depolarizations longer than 30 sec, however, $[Ca^{2+}]_i$ remained elevated, although release rapidly declined. Thus, the phasic nature of the vasopressin secretory response is not limited by inactivation of Ca^{2+} entry.

Vasopressin release from the neurohypophysis has been reported to be directly influenced at the level of the nerve endings by a variety of bioactive peptides. These include dynorphin[2] and cholecystokinin,[3] which are believed to be autoregulatory, and by the peptide hormone relaxin.[4] None of these peptides were found to affect either the basal $[Ca^{2+}]_i$ value or to alter the change in $[Ca^{2+}]_i$ evoked by either 25 mM or 50 mM extracellular K^+. By contrast, the opioid receptor agonist, U50488 (a selective kappa agonist), did significantly reduce the evoked rise in $[Ca^{2+}]_i$ to K^+ depolarization without affecting the basal value.

REFERENCES

1. CAZALIS, M., G. DAYANITHI & J. J. NORDMANN. 1987. Hormone release from isolated nerve endings of the rat neurohypophysis. J. Physiol. (Lond.) **390:** 55–70.
2. ZHAO, B. G., C. CHAPMAN & R. J. BICKNELL. 1988. Functional kappa-opioid receptors on oxytocin and vasopressin nerve terminals isolated from the rat neurohypophysis. Brain Res. **462:** 62–66.
3. BONDY, C. A., R. T. JENSEN, L. S. BRADY & H. GAINER. 1989. Cholecystokinin evokes secretion of oxytocin and vasopressin from rat neural lobe independent of external calcium. Proc. Natl. Acad. Sci. USA **86:** 5198–5201.
4. DAYANITHI, G., M. CAZALIS & J. J. NORDMANN. 1987. Relaxin affects the release of oxytocin and vasopressin from the neurohypophysis. Nature **325:** 813–816.

Suppression Cloning of a cDNA Fragment for a Candidate Presynaptic Calcium Channel

J. A. UMBACH AND C. B. GUNDERSEN

Department of Pharmacology and Jerry Lewis Neuromuscular Research Center
University of California at Los Angeles School of Medicine
Los Angeles, California 90024-1735

When *Xenopus* oocytes are injected with mRNA from the neurons that innervate the electric organ of *Torpedo,* they express an ω-conotoxin (CgTx)-sensitive, dihydropyridine (DHP)-resistant calcium (Ca) channel.[1] Sucrose-gradient fractionation of this mRNA reveals that transcripts exceeding 7 kb in mass are sufficient to induce the expression of these Ca channels in oocytes. We have attempted unsuccessfully to isolate the cDNA for this channel through expression cloning. To circumvent problems in obtaining full-length cDNAs (a prerequisite for expression cloning), we have been using a complementary, "suppression cloning" strategy. This approach relies on the observation[2] that antisense RNAs that block the 5' coding region of the corresponding mRNAs can completely inhibit the expression of that mRNA in oocytes. Thus, we constructed in Bluescript, a randomly primed cDNA library from fractionated *Torpedo* mRNA (7 kb and larger), and sought cDNA clones whose RNA transcripts would selectively block the expression of CgTx-sensitive, DHP-resistant Ca channels in oocytes coinjected with the native *Torpedo* mRNA. Using this protocol, we isolated a 1.55 kb cDNA that yields RNA transcripts with the following properties (see FIG. 1): (1) T3 RNA transcripts virtually completely suppress the expression of CgTx-sensitive, DHP-resistant Ca channels in oocytes; RNA transcribed in the opposite, T7, direction does not affect Ca channel expression; (2) neither the T3, nor the T7, transcripts appreciably alter the expression of potassium (K$^+$) channels or kainate receptors that are coexpressed in oocytes injected with this *Torpedo* mRNA. These results were confirmed using more than 20 oocytes for each RNA preparation. The directional specificity (T3 vs T7) of this RNA-mediated suppression of Ca channels, plus the fact that K$^+$ channels and kainate receptors are spared, is presumptive evidence that the 1.55 kb cDNA encodes part of the CgTx-sensitive, DHP-resistant Ca channel. Two additional lines of evidence support this contention. First, high stringency Northern analysis with the 1.55 kb cDNA as a probe reveals a single mRNA species of about 8 kb in *Torpedo* electric lobe mRNA (see FIG. 2). This mass of RNA is consistent with our earlier fractionation data indicating that mRNA exceeding a size of 7 kb is sufficient to induce expression of the CgTx-sensitive Ca channels in oocytes. Moreover, this mRNA species is detected only in preparations of RNA from *Torpedo* nervous tissue, and not in RNA from liver, muscle, or electric organ. This distribution is compatible with what one would expect of the mRNA for a presynaptic Ca channel. On the basis of these results, we conclude that the 1.55 kb clone is likely to encode a portion of the CgTx-sensitive, DHP-resistant Ca channel. Efforts are underway to isolate the full-length clone.

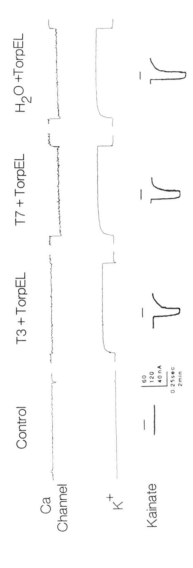

FIGURE 1. Effect of T3 and T7 RNA transcripts on ion channel expression in *Xenopus* oocytes coinjected with *Torpedo* electric lobe mRNA. Records depict voltage-clamp currents through Ca channels, K channels, and kainate-gated channels in uninjected, control oocytes or in oocytes injected with *Torpedo* electric lobe (TorpEL) mRNA (40–50 ng) with or without 10 ng either of T3 or T7 transcripts synthesized from the 1.55 kb clone. Each column displays records from one oocyte. Ca channel currents for each oocyte were evoked by a voltage step to +10 mV from a holding potential of −60 mV in a 40 mM Ba, 10 mM tetraethylammonium (TEA) Ringer[1] in the presence or absence of 10 μM CgTx and were subtracted to reveal the CgTx-sensitive component of inward current. K channel currents represent the TEA-sensitive component (10 mM TEA) of outward current elicited by depolarizing to 0 mV from a holding potential of −60 mV. Kainate-triggered currents were recorded at −60 mV by applying kainate (1 mM) for the time indicated by the bar above the record. All results were obtained from the same-donor oocytes 7 days after injection of mRNA/RNA. These particular control oocytes have little or no endogenous K or Ca current and exhibit no response to kainate. Oocytes injected with TorpEL lobe mRNA give sustained Ca (Ba) and K current activity and a robust response to kainate. These responses are affected little, if at all, by coinjection of T7 transcripts. Coinjection of T3 transcripts, however, almost completely abolishes the Ca channel current while leaving K and kainate responses intact. Note the difference in scale for the different currents.

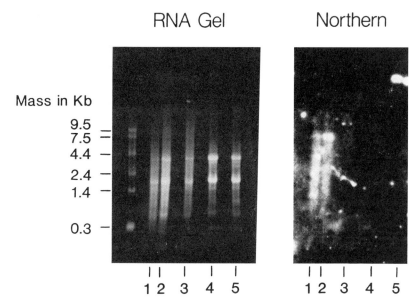

FIGURE 2. *Torpedo* RNA gel and corresponding Northern probed with 1.55 kb cDNA. RNA gel: reproduction of an ethidium bromide–stained formaldehyde-agarose gel. Lanes were loaded with 2–3 micrograms of poly(A)$^+$RNA or with 2 micrograms of the BRL (Bethesda Research Labs, Gaithersburg, MD) RNA ladder. Corresponding masses are indicated. Northern: using capillary transfer, the RNA was blotted onto MSI (Micron Separations, Inc., Westboro, MA) Nitroplus 2000, fixed, and prehybridized prior to hybridization for 24 h at 45°C (in 50% formamide, 10% dextran sulfate, 5X SSPE, 0.5% SDS, 5X Denhardt's, 0.01% yeast tRNA, and ^{32}P-labeled probe). The 1.55 kb probe was gel-purified, oligolabeled (Pharmacia, Piscataway, NJ), and denatured prior to hybridization. The blot was washed using the ABN (American Bionetics, Hayward, CA) Omniblot and final, high-stringency conditions of 0.1% SDS, 0.1X SSPE at 65°C. Lane identification: 1 and 2, electric lobe; 3, electric organ; 4, liver; 5, muscle.

REFERENCES

1. UMBACH, J. A. & C. B. GUNDERSEN. 1987. Proc. Natl. Acad. Sci. USA **86:** 5464–5468.
2. MELTON, D. A. 1985. Proc. Natl. Acad. Sci. USA **82:** 144–148.

Calcium- and Barium-Activated Acetylcholine Synthesis and Release from Isolated Nerve Terminals

Do Divalent Cations Alter Membrane Potential?

THOMAS W. VICKROY

Departments of Physiological Sciences and Neuroscience
University of Florida College of Veterinary Medicine
Box J-144 J. Hillis Miller Health Center
Gainesville, Florida 32610-0144

Ionized calcium (Ca^{2+}) is perhaps the single most universally recognized molecular species associated with exocytosis in secretory cells. For CNS neurons, investigations in isolated tissues have proven invaluable in delineating the mechanistic and regulatory events associated with Ca^{2+}-dependent neurotransmitter release. Among the different tissue preparations that have been used widely, few have offered the promise and frustrations encountered with isolated nerve-ending preparations (synaptosomes). Synaptosomes offer a convenient preparation that is readily amenable to most neurochemical and pharmacological analyses; however, the lack of an exocytotic response to quasiphysiological stimuli, particularly short depolarizing electrical pulses, is viewed as a significant shortcoming. Several release-promoting chemical stimuli have been used successfully with synaptosomes (notably, elevated extracellular potassium), but are often considered nonphysiological in view of basic mechanistic differences from naturally occurring neurotransmitter release *in vivo.* Recently, a novel method has been reported in which chemically induced synaptosomal neurotransmitter release displays properties that are more typical of release *in vivo.* This procedure, which uses low millimolar amounts of Ca^{2+} to initiate release from synaptosomes that are prepared in a Ca^{2+}-free medium (containing micromolar amounts of EGTA), is unusual in that release is strongly inhibited by tetrodotoxin (TTX) as well as drugs that stimulate presynaptic autoreceptors.[1] The former observation is particularly curious as it implies that brief exposure to Ca^{2+} promotes membrane depolarization and voltage-gated sodium influx into EGTA-pretreated synaptosomes. In this report, studies are described for EGTA-pretreated hippocampal cholinergic synaptosomes in which Ca^{2+} and Ba^{2+} promote neurochemical changes that are consistent with plasmalemmal membrane depolarization.

METHODS

All studies were carried out in hippocampal P_2 fractions from male albino Sprague-Dawley rats as described in legends for FIGURES 1 and 2 and as previously reported.[2] A Student's *t* test was used for statistical comparisons with p < 0.05 as the minimum acceptable level for differences.

RESULTS AND DISCUSSION

Preliminary studies have revealed that Ca^{2+}, Ba^{2+}, and strontium (Sr^{2+}) all elicit a saturable yet reversible secretagogue effect in EGTA-pretreated hippocampal synaptosomes. As shown in FIGURE 1, brief infusion of low millimolar amounts of Ca^{2+} or Ba^{2+} promotes a substantial and rapid stimulation of [³H]ACh efflux. Although the maximal effect for Ba^{2+} is approximately 2.5-fold greater than that of Ca^{2+} (and Sr^{2+}) (not shown), all three cations display nearly equivalent potencies ($K_m = 0.3 - 0.5$ mM, data not shown). The different maximal secretagogue effects of Ca^{2+} and Ba^{2+} are eliminated in the presence of 30 mM KCl (FIG. 2), which, in conjunction with

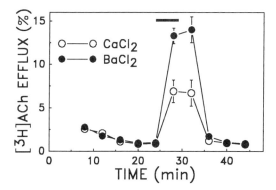

FIGURE 1. Stimulated [³H]acetylcholine release from EGTA-pretreated rat hippocampal synaptosomes by brief exposure to Calcium or barium chloride. Crude synaptosomal fractions were isolated from tissue homogenates in 0.32 M sucrose and resuspended in a solution containing (in mM) NaCl (137), KCl (4.7), $MgCl_2$ (1.0), ethylene glycol bis(beta-aminoethyl ether)-N,N'-tetraacetic acid (EGTA, 0.05), glucose (10), NaH_2PO_4 (1.25), $NaHCO_3$ (25) and eserine hemisulfate (0.1) that was saturated with a 95:5 mixture of O_2/CO_2 (pH 7.4 at 37°C). Following a 10 min incubation under O_2/CO_2 atmosphere, 100 nM choline chloride [methyl-³H]- was added to the homogenate and incubated for an additional 15 min. [³H]Choline-labeled homogenates were subsequently transferred to Whatman GF/B filter paper in chambers (maintained at 37°C) and superfused with warm oxygenated buffer. Superfusate fractions (4 min) and final tissue extract were assayed for [³H]ACh content by a paired choline kinase-ion extraction method. Data points represent the fractional efflux of [³H]ACh (percent efflux/4 min) before, during, and after a 5 min infusion (solid bar at top) of EGTA-free buffer containing 1 mM $CaCl_2$ (open circles) or 0.5 mM $BaCl_2$ (filled circles). Net [³H]ACh efflux (area of peak above baseline) was 10.8% and 25.1% for calcium and barium, respectively.

other data (manuscript submitted), is consistent with the hypothesis that the greater secretagogue efficacy of Ba^{2+} under these conditions derives from blockade of plasmalemmal potassium channels. As shown in FIGURE 2, synaptosomal pretreatment with TTX, an inhibitor of voltage-activated sodium channels, markedly attenuates both Ca^{2+}- and Ba^{2+}-induced [³H]ACh efflux. Blockade by TTX clearly differentiates Ca^{2+}-evoked exocytosis from potassium-induced [³H]ACh release and is similar to release evoked by electrical stimulation of hippocampal slices as noted above. Because a similar result has been reported for Ca^{2+}-evoked [³H]dopamine release from striatal tissue,[1] it appears that TTX sensitivity is the rule rather than the exception for divalent cation-evoked neurotransmitter release from EGTA-

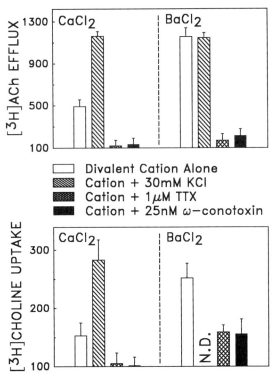

FIGURE 2. Comparative profiles for divalent cation-stimulated [³H]acetylcholine release and [³H]choline uptake by EGTA-pretreated synaptosomes. [³H]ACH release (top panel) was measured as described under FIG. 1. Additions or changes in the composition of superfusion buffer were carried out 10 min prior to infusion of Ca^{2+} (1 mM)- or Ba^{2+} (0.5 mM)-containing solutions. For experiments involving estimation of [³H]choline uptake (bottom panel), synaptosomes were first exposed to buffer containing Ca^{2+} or Ba^{2+} (with or without indicated drugs), then re-collected and assayed in fresh EGTA-containing buffer (no $CaCl_2$, $BaCl_2$, or drugs) with approximately 50 μg tissue protein and 50 nM [³H]choline for 3 min at 37°C. Uptake was terminated with 1 mL of ice-cold stop buffer (assay buffer containing 5 μM hemicholinium-3) followed by rapid vacuum filtration through Whatman GF/B filters and two 2 mL rinses with stop buffer. Filters were extracted and radioactivity quantified by liquid scintillation counting. Uptake values represent the net difference between triplicate samples incubated without (total uptake) or with 5 μM hemicholinium-3 (nonspecific uptake). All results were normalized with respect to protein content and are expressed as percent of control (arithmetic mean + SEM).

pretreated synaptosomes. Furthermore, a participatory role for N-type plasmalemmal Ca^{2+} channels is supported by the inhibitory effect of ω-conotoxin (FIG. 2) and the absence of effect by the dihydropyridine Ca^{2+} channel antagonist nifedipine (data not shown). Whereas these data support the concept that divalent cations promote membrane depolarization and activation of voltage-gated plasmalemmal sodium channels in EGTA-treated synaptosomes, the novelty of this observation led us to seek additional support for this finding. It is well-recognized that sodium-dependent, carrier-mediated uptake of numerous small molecules is highly dependent upon the transmembrane potential of synaptosomes and is strongly regulated by neuronal activity immediately preceding assay of the uptake process. For choline, the biosynthetic precursor of ACh, sodium-dependent uptake is activated by prior depolarization of tissues *in vitro*.[3] In view of this, we have used [^{3}H]choline uptake as a secondary indicator for the effects of divalent cations on membrane potential in EGTA-pretreated synaptosomes. The investigation revealed almost identical results to those obtained from [^{3}H]ACh release studies. Pretreatment with Ca^{2+} or Ba^{2+} significantly enhanced the rate of [^{3}H]choline uptake when subsequently assayed in the absence of either divalent cation. Uptake was stimulated to a greater degree by Ba^{2+} than Ca^{2+} and was substantially blocked by TTX or ω-conotoxin (FIGURE 2). Therefore, using two separate neurobiochemical indices of synaptosomal membrane potential ([^{3}H]ACh release and high-affinity [^{3}H]choline uptake), it appears that brief exposure to physiological amounts of Ca^{2+} or Ba^{2+} promotes TTX-sensitive membrane depolarization in EGTA-pretreated synaptosomes. Although these results are internally consistent, the underlying mechanism(s) responsible for these observations are as yet unclear and require further investigation.

REFERENCES

1. BOWYER, J. F. & N. WEINER. 1987. Modulation of the Ca^{++}-evoked release of [^{3}H]dopamine from striatal synaptosomes by dopamine (D_2) agonists and antagonists. J. Pharmacol. Exp. Ther. **241:** 27–33.
2. VICKROY, T. W. 1991. Neurobiochemical evidence for calcium-stimulated depolarization of EGTA-pretreated hippocampal synaptosomes. Brain Res. **540:** 335–339.
3. BARKER, L. A. 1976. Modulation of synaptosomal high affinity choline transport. Life Sci. **18:** 725–732.

Properties and Modification of Recombinant Human Synexin (Annexin VII)

A. LEE BURNS, KARIN MAGENDZO,
MEERA SRIVASTAVA,[a] EDUARDO ROJAS,
CONSTANCE CULTRARO, MILTON DE LA FUENTE,
JUDY HELDMAN, CLAUDIO PARRA,
AND HARVEY B. POLLARD

Laboratory of Cell Biology and Genetics
National Institute of Diabetes and Digestive and Kidney Diseases
Building 8, Room 403
National Institutes of Health
Bethesda, Maryland 20892

[a]Cardiorenal Division
Food and Drug Administration
Bethesda, Maryland 20892

Exocytotic secretion is a general process by which different granule contents of various cell types are released to the exterior of the cell. Although the exact mechanism of this event in cell to cell communication remains obscure, it is generally agreed that the granule and cytoplasmic membranes must fuse. In 1978, this laboratory isolated synexin, a protein that aggregates chromaffin granules in the presence of calcium and fuses these aggregates upon the addition of arachidonic acid.[1-5] Electron microscopy of cells, stimulated to secrete, revealed structures similiar to those seen with synexin-fused granules.[4] In addition, synexin could directly fuse chromaffin granule ghosts and liposomes. Thus, synexin appears to possess many of the activities of a protein involved in mediating secretion.

More recently, however, synexin was also shown to be able to insert into the membrane bilayer and transport calcium ions across artificial membranes *in vitro*.[6-8] The voltage-sensitive synexin channels were highly selective for calcium and were blocked by lanthanum or phenothiazine drugs (trifluoperazine and promethazine). It is interesting that these drugs also block both secretion from stimulated intact cells and synexin-induced aggregation of granules. The synexin channels appear to be another type of calcium channel, inasmuch as dihydropyridine and cadmium did not inhibit the synexin channels.

Concurrently with the biophysical analysis of synexin, molecular biological experiments to identify human synexin clones were successful. Sequencing of bovine and human tryptic peptides[9] and of human cDNAs[7] revealed that synexin belongs to the annexin gene family.[10] All annexins have a conserved C-terminal tetrad repeat (except for the octad repeat of calelectrin), that may be the region responsible for the common annexin activity of binding in a calcium-dependent manner to phospholipids. On the other hand, annexins generally have unique N-termini, with synexin having the longest and most hydrophobic. Although some other annexins besides

450

synexin can aggregate chromaffin granules and form calcium channels, the actual *in vivo* functions of the various annexins remain to be elucidated.

Following the identification of the human synexin cDNA, several expression plasmids were constructed for the synthesis and modification of synexin in *E. coli.*[11] The clones in the pTrc99A vector[10] included the full-length synexin (pTrcFLS), synexin with the cassette exon (pTrcCES),[12] synexin with the four repeats (pTrcR4S), and an N-terminal endonexin II/C-terminal synexin chimera (pTrcEIIS). Synexins from the above constructs were immunoreactive with antisynexin antisera on Western blots. In addition, the synexins from pTrcEIIS and pTrcCES also reacted with antiendonexin II antisera (gift of Dr. Harry Haigler) and antisera specific to the peptide predicted by the cassette exon in the N-terminus of synexin, respectively. Because the full-length synexin (FLS) was the easiest to isolate, this recombinant protein was used for most experiments involving granule aggregation and calcium channels. The aggregation of chromaffin granule by FLS was dependent on calcium with a $K_{1/2}$ value of approximately 200 µM. In addition, artificial phosphatidylserine (PS) liposomes could be aggragated and fused with this preparation of synexin. Finally, recombinant synexin formed channels in PS bilayers in a similar manner as human lung synexin. Experiments are continuing with the other constructs as well as site-directed mutants.

REFERENCES

1. CREUTZ, C. E., C. J. PAZOLES & H. B. POLLARD. 1978. J. Biol. Chem. **253:** 2858–2866.
2. CREUTZ, C. E., C. J. PAZOLES & H. B. POLLARD. 1979. J. Biol. Chem. **254:** 553–558.
3. CREUTZ, C. E. 1981. J. Cell Biol. **91:** 247–256.
4. CREUTZ, C. E., J. H. SCOTT, C. J. PAZOLES & H. B. POLLARD. 1982. J. Cell Biochem. **18:** 87–97.
5. HONG, K., N. DUZGUNES & D. PAPAHADJOPOULOS. 1981. J. Biol. Chem. **256:** 3641–3644.
6. POLLARD, H. B. & E. ROJAS. 1988. Proc. Natl. Acad. Sci. USA **85:** 2974–2978.
7. BURNS, A. L., K. MAGENDZO, A. SHIRVAN, M. SRIVASTAVA, E. ROJAS, M. R. ALIJANI & H. B. POLLARD. 1989. Proc. Natl. Acad. Sci. USA **86:** 3798–3802.
8. POLLARD, H. B., A. L. BURNS & E. ROJAS. 1990. J. Membr. Biol. **117:** 101–112.
9. POLLARD, H. B., A. L. BURNS & E. ROJAS. 1988. J. Exp. Biol. **139:** 267–286.
10. DEDMAN, J. R. & M. J. CRUMPTON. 1990. Nature **345:** 212.
11. BURNS, A. L., K. MAGENDZO, M. SRIVASTAVA, E. ROJAS, C. PARRA, M. DE LA FUENTE, C. CULTRARO, A. SHIRVAN, T. VOGEL, J. HELDMAN, H. CAOHUY, D. TOMBACCINI & H. B. POLLARD. 1990. Biochem. Soc. Trans. **18:** 1128–1131.
12. MAGENDZO, K., A. SHIRVAN, C. CULTRARO, M. SRIVASTAVA, H. B. POLLARD & A. L. BURNS. 1991. J. Biol. Chem. **266:** 3228–3232.

Calcium-Dependent and Calcium-Independent Enhancement of Transmitter Release at the Crayfish Neuromuscular Junction Studied with Fura-2 Imaging

K. R. DELANEY AND D. W. TANK

AT&T Bell Laboratories
Murray Hill, New Jersey 07974

Although a wealth of experimental evidence exists linking increases in cytoplasmic calcium concentrations to enhancement of evoked transmitter release, quantitative studies that measure and compare the magnitude and temporal characteristics of "residual calcium" to synaptic facilitation are lacking. We have used fluorescent imaging of fura-2 in the intact functioning crayfish neuromuscular junction to address quantitatively the relationship between presynaptic calcium activity and facilitation of action potential–evoked release.

The much-studied neuromuscular junction of the crayfish claw opener muscle is an example of a highly facilitating, nondepressing, tonic synapse. We have further developed this preparation to permit simultaneous measurement of basal calcium concentrations in the presynaptic boutons that release transmitter while recording the postsynaptic responses in a muscle fiber.[1] We have made quantitative comparisons between the decay of calcium accumulations following tetanic stimulation and the decay of tetanically induced facilitation of transmission.

We have concentrated on two of the longer phases of frequency-dependent synaptic enhancement: augmentation, which typically decays with a time-constant of 5–7 seconds, and posttetanic potentiation (PTP), which decays with a time constant that is on the order of a few minutes, depending upon the rate and duration of the tetanus.[2] Starting about 1 s after short tetani, (up to a few hundred action potentials delivered at less than about 30 Hz), augmentation is present, and synaptic enhancement decays with a single exponential time-constant. The calcium accumulation in the presynaptic terminals decays with an identical time-course, indicating a linear correspondence between the residuum of calcium left by the tetanic stimulation and augmentation of release (FIG. 1).This linear relationship appears to persist even with 10-fold or more facilitation of the excitatory junction potential. The persistence of a linear relationship between residual calcium with high levels of facilitation would not be compatible with traditional "power-law" models[3] in which the residual calcium sums directly with calcium influx during the action potential.

With longer stimulation (several thousand action potentials at 20 Hz or greater), a second, longer-lasting phase of facilitation, termed PTP, is produced in addition to augmentation. Thus synaptic enhancement decays with two exponentials. Our measurements demonstrate that calcium accumulation also decays with these same two exponentials. Thus the two time-constants for the decay of calcium accumulations are reflected by two time-constants for the slow decay of synaptic facilitation following prolonged tetanic stimulation (FIG. 2).

Addition of exogenous calcium buffer prolongs the buildup of facilitation during tetanic stimulation and prolongs the decay of synaptic enhancement after the offset of an action potential train. In our experiments we use ethylenediamine acetate (EDTA) because its binding kinetics are slow enough that it does not block evoked release even when present at what we estimate to be low millimolar concentrations. The buffer-induced decrease in both the rate of rise and rate of decay of synaptic enhancement is exactly matched by the decrease in the rate of rise of calcium accumulations during tetanic stimulation and the decrease in the rate of recovery of calcium after stimulation. This suggests a causal relationship between the residual calcium and enhancement.

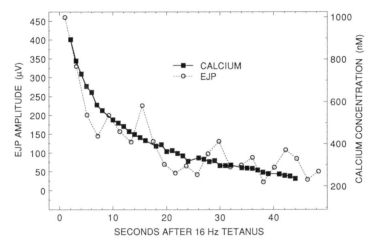

FIGURE 1. Decay of augmentation and calcium accumulations after short low-frequency tetanus. Calcium in crayfish claw opener exciter nerve terminals calculated every 1.1 s following the offset of 2 min of 16 Hz facilitation. Time-course of synaptic enhancement following tetanus tested at 0.5 Hz. Results are from a single trial. EDTA iontophoretically injected into the axon to an estimated 1 mM along with fura-2 (about 100 μM). Addition of exogenous buffer increased time-constant for both decay of calcium and synaptic facilitation from 6 to 13 s calculated from data greater than 2 s after the offset of 16 Hz stimulation. Calcium and junction potentials scaled to values at pretetanus and about 3 s after tetanus. EJP = excitatory junction potential.

We have also used imaging of calcium in presynaptic terminals to examine whether the facilitatory effects of serotonin[4] at this synapse involve increased basal cytoplasmic calcium concentrations or increased voltage-dependent, action potential–mediated calcium influx.[5] We found little or no increase in the steady-state calcium concentration in presynaptic terminals during a 5-min application of micromolar concentrations of serotonin. An increase of about 50 nM was seen in axonal regions of several preparations, which was reversed quickly after washout whereas enhanced transmitter release persisted for an hour or more. The level of calcium accumulation during 30-s long trains of action potentials was not increased by serotonin. Doubling the extracellular calcium concentration from 50% of normal to 100% of normal

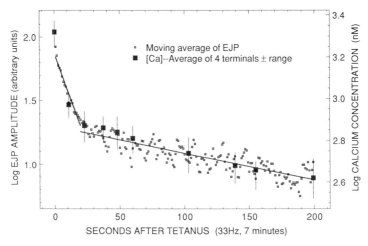

FIGURE 2. Stimulation at 33 Hz for 7 min produces an additional long-time constant for the decay of synaptic facilitation corresponding to PTP, which is accompanied by a second slow component of the decay of residual calcium. Solid line is least squared fit to EJP data, illustrating fit by two exponential decay rates. Calcium and EJP scaled to values before tetanic stimulation and approximately 11 s after offset of stimulus. Note semilog coordinates. Adapted from data of Delaney et al.[1].

produced about the same facilitation (4-fold) as serotonin with a clearly detectable 30% increase in accumulation. Broadening the presynaptic action potential with 2–5 mM tetraethylammonium had an even greater effect on calcium accumulations for the same amount of facilitation, indicating that it is unlikely that serotonin acts by broadening the presynaptic action potential. We favor the suggestion that serotonin acts to increase the efficacy of the release apparatus so that normal calcium concentrations result in enhanced transmitter release.

REFERENCES

1. DELANEY, K. R., R. S. ZUCKER & D. W. TANK. 1989. Calcium in motor nerve terminals associated with posttetanic potentiation. J. Neurosci. **9(10):** 3558–3567.
2. MAGLEBY, K. 1987. Short-term changes in synaptic efficacy. *In* Synaptic Function. G. M. Edelman, W. E. Gall & W. Maxwell Cowan, Eds. John Wiley & Sons. New York.
3. KATZ, B. & R. MILEDI. 1968. The role of calcium in neuromuscular facilitation. J. Physiol. (Lond.) **196:** 75–86.
4. DIXON, D. & H. L. ATWOOD. 1985. Crayfish motor nerve terminal's response to serotonin examined by intracellular microelectrode. J. Neurobiol. **16:** 409–432.
5. DELANEY, K. R., D. W. TANK & R. S. ZUCKER. Presynaptic calcium and serotonin-mediated enhancement of transmitter release at crayfish neuromuscular junction. J. Neurosci. **11**(9). In press.

G-Protein Modulation of [^{3}H]Serotonin Release through the L-Type Calcium Channel[a]

V. C. GANDHI AND D. J. JONES

Departments of Anesthesiology and Pharmacology
The University of Texas Health Science Center
San Antonio, Texas 78284-7838

Recent studies using the 1,4 dihydropyridine (DHP) agonist Bay K 8644 have demonstrated coupling of L-type voltage-dependent calcium channels (VDCC) to neurotransmitter release in neuronal tissue.[1-3] In our studies this was demonstrated in spinal cord synaptosomes as enhancement of K$^+$-stimulated [^{3}H]serotonin ([^{3}H]5HT) release by Bay K 8644 with inhibition of the response by DHP antagonists such as nimodipine and nitrendipine. In agreement with other studies, submaximal depolarization (15 mM K$^+$) of neuronal preparations was required to demonstrate the role of the L-type VDCC in modulating transmitter release. In order to explore second messenger systems that might couple the L-type VDCC to neurotransmitter release, the role of protein kinase C (PKC) in modulating neurotransmitter release under similar depolarizing conditions was investigated in the present studies. In addition, the role of G proteins was investigated as a possible mechanism of linking the DHP receptor directly to the L-type VDCC or indirectly to phospholipase C, the activation of which would lead to PIP$_2$ hydrolysis and the formation of products known to stimulate PKC. The results, in general, point to both direct and indirect coupling of G proteins to the L-type VDCC and to PKC.

K$^+$-stimulated release of [^{3}H]5HT in spinal cord synaptosomes was measured according to Stauderman and Jones.[4] The spinal cord synaptosomes (P$_2$ fraction) were superfused with either 3 mM (basal) or 15–60 mM K$^+$ (depolarizing) buffers with agents added 20 min prior to K$^+$ depolarization. Synaptosomes were treated with cholera toxin (CTX, preactivated with 20 mM DTT at 37°C for 10 min) at 10 μg/7 mg protein for 20 min prior to initiation of superfusion. Pertussis toxin (PTX) was pretreated with 1 mM ATP and 10 mM DTT at 37°C for 10 min prior to addition to synaptosomes. Synaptosomes were exposed to PTX (25 μg/7 mg protein) for 20 min at 37°C prior to initiation of superfusion.

The results demonstrated that similar depolarizing conditions are required for either Bay K 8644 or PKC activators to enhance K$^+$-stimulated release. As in our previous studies[3] where Bay K 8644 enhanced K$^+$-stimulated release only at 15 mM K$^+$, phorbol myristate acetate (PMA) and 1,2-oleoylacetylglycerol (OAG), activators of PKC, enhanced K$^+$-stimulated release only at 15 mM K$^+$ (FIG. 1). Enhanced release in the presence of Bay K 8644 or PMA was concentration-dependent, and the effects of both agents were blocked by the 1,4 DHP antagonist nimodipine (NIM) (FIG. 2). Enhanced release of [^{3}H]5HT induced by Bay K 8644 and PMA were also antagonized by the PKC inhibitors polymyxin B(PMX-B) and staurosporine (TABLE 1).

NaF, a known activator of G proteins produced a concentration-dependent

[a]This work was supported by the National Science Foundation (BNS 88–20008).

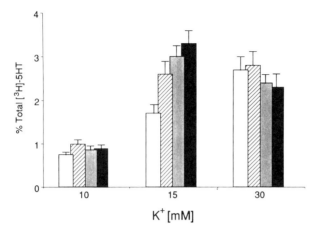

FIGURE 1. Effects of Bay K 8644, PMA, and OAG on depolarization-induced [³H]5HT release at various K⁺ concentrations. (□) control; (▨) Bay K 8644 (1 μM); (▦) PMA (0.2 μM); (■) OAG (50 μM).

enhancement of 15 mM K⁺-evoked [³H]5HT release, which was inhibited by both NIM and PMX-B (data not shown). These results suggested that a G protein may be involved in the enhanced release of [³H]5HT noted in the presence of either Bay K 8644 or activators of PKC. The sensitivity of G proteins to ADP-ribosylation by CTX and PTX has been used to differentiate the roles of G proteins in various cellular processes. Our results show that CTX pretreatment of synaptosomes, while not significantly altering K⁺-stimulated release (av. $1.77 \pm 0.13\%$ vs $1.83 \pm 0.10\%$), blocked the enhancement of [³H]5HT release by Bay K 8644 without altering PMA-enhanced release (FIG. 3). PTX pretreatment of spinal cord synaptosomes also did not alter basal release. This pretreatment, however, blocked PMA-enhanced release without altering the effects of Bay K 8644.

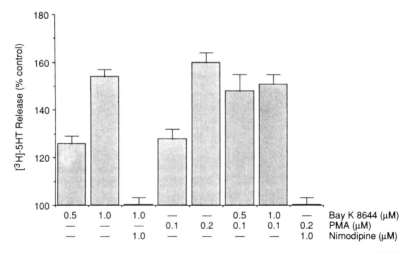

FIGURE 2. PMA- and Bay K 8644–induced enhancement of 15 mM K⁺-evoked [³H]5HT release and their attenuation by nimodipine.

TABLE 1. Inhibition of PMA and Bay K 8644–Enhanced K[+]-Evoked [^{3}H] 5HT Release by PKC Inhibitors Polymyxin B (PMX-B) or Staurosporine[a]

	Percent control + SEM
PMA (02. μM)	149 ± 4
PMA (0.2 μM) + PMX-B (1 μM)	123 ± 9[b]
(2 μM)	115 ± 4[c]
(6.6 μM)	92 ± 6
PMA (0.2 μM) + staurosporine (50 nM)	102 ± 3
Bay K 8644 (1 μM)	150 ± 5
Bay K 8644 (1 μM) + PMX-B (1 μM)	133 ± 9[b]
(2 μM)	123 ± 5[c]
(6.6 μM)	96 ± 3
Bay K 8644 (1 μM) + staurosporine (50 nM)	100 ± 3

[a]PMX-B at 6.6 μM decreased 15 mM K[+]-evoked [^{3}H]5HT release by 18%.
[b]$p < 0.02$ vs. agent in the absence of PMX-B.
[c]$p < 0.001$ vs. agent in the absence of PMX-B.

The present results indicate that depolarization of synaptosomes with 15 mM K[+] "sensitizes" the L-type VDCC for subsequent stimulation of [^{3}H]5HT release by either DHP agonists or activators of PKC. The fact that the enhancement of release by either Bay K 8644 or PMA is blocked by DHP antagonists and PKC inhibitors and vice versa suggests that Ca^{2+} influx and subsequent release of [^{3}H]5HT may involve a common process. These results suggest that in the presence of 15 mM K[+], Bay K 8644 activates phospholipase C to form diacylglycerol (DAG), which subsequently stimu-

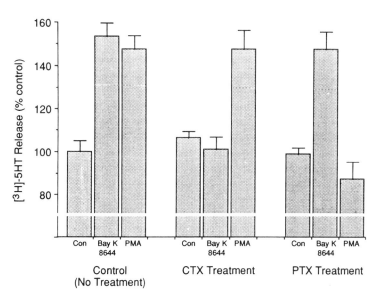

FIGURE 3. Cholera toxin (CTX)- and pertussis toxin (PTX)-induced alterations in PMA (0.2 μM)—and Bay K 8644 (1 μM)—enhanced release of [^{3}H]5HT in spinal cord synaptosomes. Synaptosomes were exposed to CTX (10 μg/7 mg protein) or PTX (25 μg/7 mg protein) for 20 or 30 min, respectively, prior to initiation of perfusion.

lates PKC. Thus in the presence of 15 mM K^+ and activation of either the DHP receptor or PKC, PKC-dependent phosphorylation of the L-type VDCC leads to channel opening, Ca^{2+} influx, and neurotransmitter release. This mechanism agrees with the work of Armstrong and Eckert[5] who demonstrated that phosphorylation of the L-type channel was required for opening of the channel and Ca^{2+} influx. Phosphorylation-independent activation of the L-type VDCC by DHP agonists may also play a role in modulating transmitter release.

Previously, Brown and Birnbaumer[6] indicated that gating of ion channels by G proteins appears to require the membranes "being brought into a voltage responsive state" before the modulatory effects of these proteins are observed. Our results point to this possibility and the involvement of a G protein in spinal cord synaptosomes, because both Bay K 8644 and PMA require membrane depolarization to produce enhancement of [³H]5HT release. Thus it is possible that G protein–dependent gating of the L-type VDCC occurs when Bay K 8644 binds to its receptor and/or with activation of phospholipase C to form DAG and hence stimulation of PKC.

Differential sensitivity of Bay K 8644- versus PMA-mediated enhancement of K^+-stimulated release was demonstrated by pretreatment of synaptosomes with either CTX or PTX. CTX interferes with the action of a G protein by maintaining it in an activated state where it cannot be further activated by agonists. Our results demonstrate that following CTX treatment, the G protein is not available to gate the L-type VDCC in the presence of Bay K 8644, and channel opening and enhanced release do not occur. The effects of PKC stimulation with PMA, however, are not altered by CTX pretreatment. The effects of PMA are, however, blocked by PTX exposure, whereas the Bay K 8644 effects are not. These results suggest that both CTX-sensitive and PTX-sensitive G proteins mediate gating of the L-type VDCC. These effects possibly occur through both direct and indirect means by way of the DHP receptor on the channel and/or the second messenger PKC, respectively. When the G protein effects are isolated as with pretreatment of synaptosomes with CTX or PTX, the relative contribution of each can be measured. Studies are currently in progress to determine which G proteins are involved in modulating L-type VDCC function.

REFERENCES

1. MIDDLEMISS, D. N. & M. SPEDDING. 1985. Nature **314:** 94.
2. WOODWARD, J. J. & S. W. LESLIE. 1986. Brain Res. **370:** 397.
3. GANDHI, V. C. & D. J. JONES. 1990. Eur. J. Pharmacol. **187:** 271.
4. STAUDERMAN, K. A. & D. J. JONES. 1986. Eur. J. Pharmacol. **120:** 107.
5. ARMSTRONG, D. & R. ECKERT. 1987. Proc. Natl. Acad. Sci. USA **84:** 2518.
6. BROWN, A. M. & L. BIRNBAUMER. 1988. Am. J. Physiol. **254:** H401.

Modulation by Voltage of Calcium Channels and Adrenal Catecholamine Release

BENITO GARRIDO, FRANCISCO ABAD,
AND ANTONIO G. GARCÍA

Departamento de Farmacología
Facultad de Medicina
Universidad Autonoma de Madrid
Arzobispo Morcillo, 4
28029 Madrid, Spain

INTRODUCTION

Radioligand-binding studies,[1] and measurements of $^{45}Ca^{2+}$ fluxes,[1] Ca_i^{2+} transients,[2] and Ca^{2+} currents[3] suggest that adrenal medulla chromaffin cells contain various subtypes of voltage-dependent Ca^{2+} channels. The questions are, Which channels contribute to the regulation of the physiological acetylcholine-evoked catecholamine release from such cells? and How do these channels contribute? Because various voltage protocols affect differently the kinetics of T, L, and N channels,[4] it seems logical to presume that those protocols could also influence differently the rates of $^{45}Ca^{2+}$ uptake and secretion in chromaffin cells. This approach, together with the judicious use of drugs that act on specific channel subtypes could provide clues on the participation of each channel type in the regulation of the secretory process. We present here recent data on the effects of voltage changes on catecholamine release from cat and ox adrenals perfused at high rates with oxygenated Krebs-Tris solutions at 37°C.

INACTIVATION BY VOLTAGE PREPULSES OF $^{45}CA^{2+}$ UPTAKE AND SECRETION IN CAT ADRENALS

Experimental conditions were selected so that adrenal medullary chromaffin cells were depolarized for different time periods and with various K^+ concentrations in the absence of Ca^{2+}, prior to the application of 0.5 mM Ca^{2+} for 10 s in the presence of 118 mM K^+ to test the rate of secretion (the "Ca^{2+} pulse"). Prepulses of 30 s with increasing $[K^+]$ produced gradual inactivation of secretion (FIG. 1A). Using prepulses of 118 mM K^+, the inactivation of secretion was shown to be time-dependent (FIG. 1B). Inactivation of $^{45}Ca^{2+}$ uptake into adrenal medullary tissues by depolarizing prepulses (118 mM K^+) paralleled inactivation of secretion. This, together with the fact that Cd^{2+} blocked secretion completely and inactivation was seen equally using Ca^{2+} or Ba^{2+} as secretagogues, suggests that inactivation by voltage of a certain class of Ca^{2+} channel is responsible for the blockade of secretion. Inasmuch as isradipine (an L-type Ca^{2+} channel blocker) enhanced the rate of

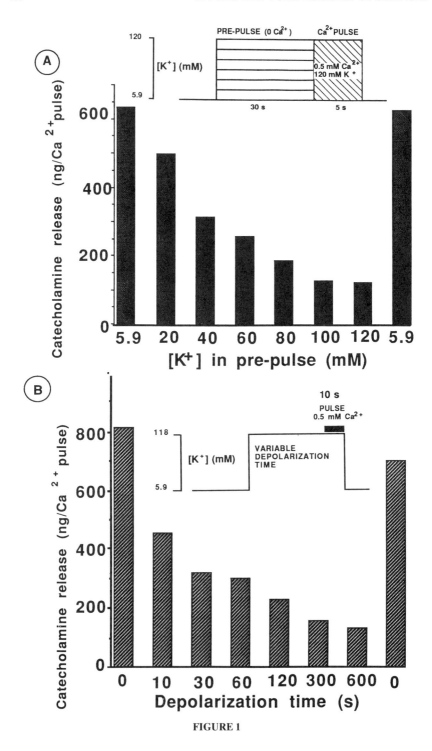

FIGURE 1

inactivation, and Bay K 8644 (an L-type Ca^{2+} channel activator) prevented it,[5] it seems that the channel might belong to the L subtype.

FACILITATION BY VOLTAGE PREPULSES OF CATECHOLAMINE RELEASE IN BOVINE ADRENALS

Opposite to the cat, catecholamine release evoked by Ca^{2+} pulses from bovine adrenals was increased about 35% using depolarizing prepulses (FIG. 2A). This facilitated release was further enhanced in the presence of Bay K 8644. Nisoldipine (an L-type Ca^{2+} channel blocker) inhibited the facilitated component of the secretory response (FIG. 2B) and reduced by 50% the "standard" component of secretion. Nisoldipine, however, was unable to block completely the secretory response, either with or without prepulse. The facilitated component of secretion could be associated to a facilitated Ca^{2+} current seen in chromaffin cells when strong prepulses to positive potentials were applied prior to test pulses.[6] This facilitated current is highly sensitive to Bay K 8644 and nisoldipine, and has been suggested to be due to recruitment of L-type Ca^{2+} channels different from those carrying the standard current.[3]

The sensitivity to Bay K 8644 and nisoldipine of the facilitated component of secretion strengthens the view that L-type Ca^{2+} channels are controlling this component of the overall secretory response. Partial blockade of secretion by nisoldipine, however, suggests that a significant portion of the secretory response is regulated by dihydropyridine-resistant Ca^{2+} channels, probably those carrying the so-called standard Ca^{2+} current.[3] Contrary to a previous view,[7] this secretory component does not seem to inactivate in a voltage-dependent manner.

CONCLUSIONS

Cat adrenal chromaffin cells contain most likely L-type Ca^{2+} channels that are inactivated in a voltage-dependent manner; they play major roles in controlling catecholamine release. Bovine adrenal chromaffin cells probably have Ca^{2+} channels that do not seem to suffer voltage-inactivation. In fact, Ca_i^{2+}- but not voltage-mediated inactivation of those channels has been previously shown by measuring fast divalent cation fluxes[8] or Ca^{2+} currents.[9] The diversity of Ca^{2+} channels controlling

---

FIGURE 1. A: Inactivation by different K^+ concentrations of catecholamine release in cat adrenal glands. In this experiment the gland was perfused with a Krebs-Tris solution containing 5.9 mM K^+ and 2.5 mM Ca^{2+} for 10 min (5.9 K^+/2.5 Ca^{2+}); then, it was changed to a Ca^{2+}-free solution (5.9 K^+/0 Ca^{2+}) for 2 min. Later, it was perfused for 30 s with a depolarizing solution containing 0 Ca^{2+} and different K^+ concentrations (prepulse), and the catecholamine release was evoked by switching this solution to another containing 120 K^+/0.5 Ca^{2+} (test Ca^{2+}-pulse) for 5 s. B: Time-dependence of catecholamine release inactivation by voltage in cat adrenal glands. Glands were perfused as above with the following differences: the basal perfusing solution was a 5.9 K^+/0 Ca^{2+} solution, the prepulse solution was 118 K^+/0 Ca^{2+} applied for variable periods of time, and the test Ca^{2+}-pulse solution was 118 K^+/0.5 Ca^{2+} for 10 s. Catecholamine release in each Ca^{2+}-pulse was estimated fluorometrically and expressed as ng/pulse. Data are from a typical experiment out of 6 (A) and 3 (B).

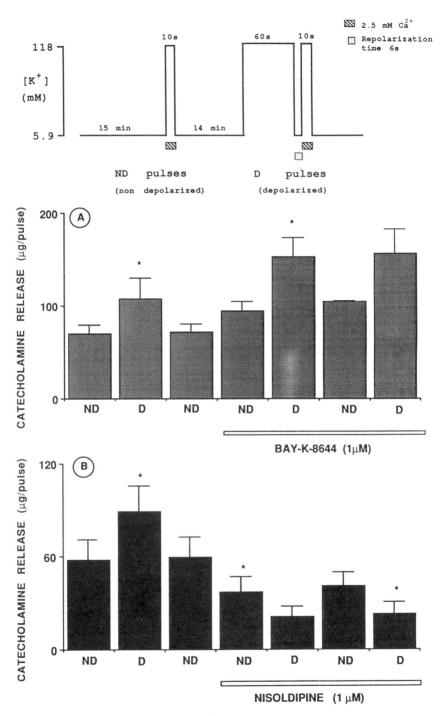

FIGURE 2

FIGURE 2. Facilitation by voltage of catecholamine release in bovine adrenal glands. This experiment has two parts taking place in the same gland. First, glands were perfused with a Krebs-Tris-0 Ca^{2+} solution containing 5.9 mM K^+ (5.9 K^+/0 Ca^{2+}), and every 15 min a catecholamine release was evoked by switching to another solution containing 118 K^+/2.5 Ca^{2+} for 10 s (test Ca^{2+}-pulse). Test Ca^{2+}-pulses were alternatively applied without prepulses (nondepolarized, ND) or preceded by prepulses of 30 s duration with 118 K^+/0 Ca^{2+} (depolarized, D). The second part of the experiment was similar to the first one, but in the presence of Bay K 8644 (10^{-6} M, **A**) or nisoldipine (10^{-6} M, **B**). Data are means ± SE of 5 (**A**) and 5 (**B**) glands. They are expressed as μg total catecholamine secreted per pulse. *p < 0.01 with respect to control ND.

secretion in cat and bovine adrenal glands might reflect different regulatory mechanisms of the catecholamine secretory responses in two animal species that may react differently in stressful situations.[10]

REFERENCES

1. BALLESTA, J. J., M. PALMERO, M. J. HIDALGO, L. M. GUTIERREZ, J. A. REIG, S. VINIEGRA & A. G. GARCÍA. 1989. J. Neurochem. **53:** 1050–1056.
2. ROSARIO, L. M., B. SORIA, G. FEUERSTEIN & H. B. POLLARD. 1989. Neurosci. **29:** 735–747.
3. ARTALEJO, C. R., M. DAHMER, R. L. PERLMAN & A. P. FOX. 1990. Biophys. J. **57:** 23a.
4. TSIEN, R. W., D. LIPSCOMBE, D. V. MADISON, K. R. BLEY & A. P. FOX. 1988. TINS **11:** 431–438.
5. GARRIDO, B., M. G. LÓPEZ, M. A. MORO, R. DE PASCUAL & A. G. GARCÍA. 1990. J. Physiol. (Lond.) **428:** 615–637.
6. FENWICK, E. M., A. MARTI & E. NEHER. 1982. J. Physiol. (Lond.) **331:** 599–635.
7. BAKER, P. F. & T. J. RINK. 1975. J. Physiol. (Lond.) **253:** 593–620.
8. ARTALEJO, C. R., A. G. GARCÍA & D. AUNIS. 1987. J. Biol. Chem. **262:** 915–926.
9. HIRNING, L. D., C. R. ARTALEJO, M. DAHMER, R. L. PERLMAN & A. P. FOX. 1989. Biophys. J. **55:** 593a.
10. GANDÍA, L., P. MICHELENA, R. DE PASCUAL, M. G. LÓPEZ & A. G. GARCÍA. 1990. NeuroReport. **1:** 119–122.

Long-Term Monitoring of Depolarization-Induced Exocytosis from Adrenal Medullary Chromaffin Cells and Pancreatic Islet B Cells Using "Perforated Patch Recording"[a]

KEVIN D. GILLIS,[b,d] RAYMUND Y. K. PUN,[c] AND
STANLEY MISLER[b,d]

[b]*Departments of Medicine (Jewish Hospital),
Cell Biology and Physiology, and Electrical Engineering
Washington University
St. Louis, Missouri 63110*
[c]*Department of Physiology and Biophysics
University of Cincinnati
Cincinnati, Ohio 45267*

Like neurons, many endocrine cells use Ca^{2+} entry through voltage-dependent Ca^{2+} channels as the major link between stimulus-induced depolarization and vesicular secretion.[1] The study of the dynamics of depolarization-secretion coupling in neurons has one distinct advantage over that in endocrine cells: neurons make synaptic contacts; endocrine cells do not. For neurons, the postsynaptic membrane provides an exquisitely sensitive, instantaneous bioassay for locally released neurotransmitter. By contrast, methods for monitoring stimulation-induced hormone release from single endocrine cells using immunochemistry (*e.g.* the reverse hemolytic plaque assay)[2] or the formation of artificial "synapses" (*e.g.* co-culturing of secretory cells with target cells)[3] are still crude, slow, or uncertain.

Ideally, the combination of whole-cell patch-clamp electrophysiology (WCR) with phase detector techniques permits detection of membrane capacitance changes of several femtofarads (fF) (or the equivalent of a single 250 nm diameter secretory granule) against a background cell capacitance of 5–10 pF.[4] This should provide a sensitive, instantaneous assay for the actual process of secretion. In practice, however, evoked secretion rapidly declines in WCR due to the rapid dialysis of soluble cytoplasmic contents, the "rundown" of Ca^{2+} currents, and the loss of endogenous intracellular Ca^{2+} buffering. Recently, a novel "perforated patch" variant of whole cell recording (PPR), which uses antifungal pore-formers, such as nystatin, to permeabilize plasma membrane and to gain electrical access to the cytoplasm, has been shown to greatly reduce these problems.[5–7] By combining PPR with phase detection techniques we have demonstrated stable depolarization-induced increases in membrane capacitance for up to two hours in single bovine adrenal chromaffin cells and rat pancreatic islet B cells. The results with chromaffin cells are in print.[8]

[a]This work was supported by NIH Grant DK37380 and an AHA Established Investigator Grant to S. Misler.
[d]Address for correspondence: Renal Division, Yalem 713, The Jewish Hospital of St. Louis, 216 S. Kingshighway Boulevard, St. Louis, Missouri 63110.

RESULTS AND DISCUSSION

Ca²⁺ and Voltage Dependence of Depolarization-Induced Capacitance Changes in Adrenal Chromaffin Cells and B Cells

With PPR, performed at room temperature, single chromaffin and B cells often display Ca_o^{2+}-dependent increases in C_m following one or more pulses of membrane depolarization, which activate Ca^{2+} currents (see FIG. 1 for sample results with

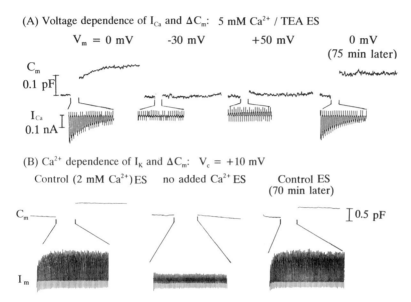

FIGURE 1. Voltage and calcium dependence of depolarization-induced capacitance changes as well as long-term maintenance of depolarization-induced capacitance changes in bovine adrenal chromaffin cells during perforated patch recording. (**A**) Trains of depolarization to 0 mV, which evoke sizable Ca^{2+} currents (I_{Ca}), evoke membrane capacitance increases (ΔC_m), whereas trains of depolarizations to -30 mV and $+50$ mV, which evoked little or no I_{Ca}, similarly produced little ΔC_m. Note that the amplitudes of I_{Ca} and ΔC_m at 0 mV are maintained even after 70 minutes. The pipette solution contained in mM: 28 Cs_2SO_4; 64 CsCl; 12 NaCl; 0.5 EGTA; 1 $MgCl_2$; and 20 tetraethylammonium⁺ Hepes at pH 7.3. The bath solution (ES) contained (in mM): 140 NaCl; 5.5 KCl; 5 $CaCl_2$; 1 Mg Cl_2; 5 glucose; and 20 Na⁺ Hepes, at pH 7.35. (**B**) Trains of depolarization separated by a 70-minute interval produced similar ΔC_ms and similar staircases of outward K⁺ currents. Because I_K is predominantly Ca^{2+}-activated in that it is mostly blocked by reduction in $[Ca^{2+}]_o$, the maintenance of the I_K build-up during a long train suggests the maintenance of endogenous Ca^{2+} buffering. The relative intactness of Ca_i^{2+} buffering is underscored by the ability of cells undergoing PPR to maintain stable resting C_ms and depolarization-induced increments in C_m even with 0.1 mM free Ca^{2+} in the pipette. The pipette solution was the same as in **A**, except that the Cs salts were replaced by equimolar concentrations of KCl and K_2SO_4. The bath solution was the same as in **A**. General methods: An experiment was initiated once the access resistance (R_a) of the perforated patch, achieved with nystatin, reached <30 MΩ. ΔC_m was monitored by applying to a patch clamp amplifier a 10 mV peak-to-peak amplitude, 500 Hz sinusoid stimulus about $V_h = -70$ mV, and feeding the output current to a lock-in amplifier set to a phase angle sensitive to ΔC_m (least sensitive to a change in series resistance).

chromaffin cells). Increases in C_m in response to either single pulses or trains of pulses show a very similar bell-shaped dependence on clamping voltage (V_c) as does peak inward Ca^{2+} current (I_{Ca}); both have thresholds about -20 mV and maximal values maximal between $+10$ and $+20$ mV. Both ΔC_m and I_{Ca} are blocked by the addition of 50 μM Cd^{2+} to the extracellular solution. Cells with similar peak I_{Ca}s displayed a wide variety of amplitudes of evoked C_m response. In a given cell, however, similar depolarization regimes evoked similar I_{Ca}s and ΔC_ms over 1–2 hours after adequate patch perforation.

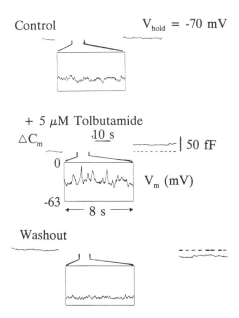

FIGURE 2. Secretogogue-induced electrical activity produces transient increases in C_m. Example: tolbutamide induces action potentials and ΔC_m in single pancreatic islet B cell. Top panel: 40 seconds of exposure, in a low (0.8 mM) glucose ES, at a membrane potential (V_m) of about -50 mV resulted in a negligible ΔC_m. Middle panel: 40-second exposure to depolarization caused by 5 μM tolbutamide resulted in a 25 fF increase in C_m. Bottom panel: prolonged exposure to resting levels of V_m, seen after the washout of tolbutamide, resulted in a net decrease in C_m, presumably due to background endocytosis.

*Capacitance Changes Resulting from Secretogogue Induced Depolarization in
Pancreatic B Cells*

Perhaps the most general use of stable capacitance monitoring in secretory cells will be to examine the effect of different patterns of electrical activity on exocytosis. Changes in C_m (measured by continuous phase detection in the voltage-clamp mode) should be seen immediately after short periods of electrical activity (measured during intermittent current clamp recording). In preliminary experiments, unstimulated rat B cells, with membrane potentials of -55 to -60 mV, show no detectable increments in C_m over several minutes. The same cells exposed to 40 s of depolarization to -30 mV, however, provoked by the addition of 5 μM tolbutamide, a known blocker of background ATP-sensitive K^+ channels, increase their C_m by 25–30 fF, roughly corresponding to the release of 15–20 granules (FIG. 2). Because glucose is the most critical physiological secretogogue, future experiments of this type shall focus on determining which patterns of glucose-induced depolarization and electrical activity optimize insulin granule exocytosis. Correlation of capacitance data with *in situ* evidence of insulin secretion (*e.g.* cell surface staining for insulin or chroma-granin) will be needed.

SUMMARY

(1) Membrane capacitance measurements using perforated patch recording offer the possibility of studying the process of depolarization-secretion coupling (DSC) in single endocrine cells with unprecedented time resolution and stability. (2) Early results with catecholamine-secreting adrenal chromaffin cells and insulin-secreting pancreatic B cells support longstanding ideas that the Ca^{2+}-dependent processes underlying DSC are fundamentally similar to those of nerve terminals. (3) Future experiments using these approaches should prove useful in sorting out those effects of humoral substances that have a predominant effect on excitability and Ca^{2+} entry from those that affect the secretory process itself.

ACKNOWLEDGMENTS

We thank Richard Bookman for stimulating discussions and our late colleague Lee Falke for participation in pilot experiments. We dedicate this work to the memories of John R. Segal and Bruno Ceccarelli.

REFERENCES

1. OZAWA, S. & O. SAND. 1986. Physiol. Rev. **66:** 887–952.
2. SMITH, P. F., E. H. LUGUE & J. D. NEILL. 1986. Methods Enzymol. **124:** 443–465.
3. CHEEK, T. R., T. R. JACKSON, A. J. O'SULLIVAN, R. B. MORETON, M. J. BERRIDGE & R. D. BURGOYNE. 1989. J. Cell Biol. **109:** 1219–1228.
4. NEHER, E. & A. MARTY. 1982. Proc. Natl. Acad. Sci. USA **79:** 6712–6716.
5. HORN, R. & A. MARTY. 1988. J. Gen. Physiol. **92:** 145–159.
6. KORN, S. J. & R. HORN. 1989. J. Gen. Physiol. **94:** 789–812.
7. FALKE, L., K. GILLIS, D. PRESSEL & S. MISLER. 1989. FEBS Lett. **251:** 167–172.
8. GILLIS, K., R. PUN & S. MISLER. 1991. Pfluegers Arch. (Eur. J. Physiol.) **418:** 611–613.

Signal Transmission at the Photoreceptor Synapse

Role of Calcium Ions and Protons

JOCHEN KLEINSCHMIDT

Department of Ophthalmology
New York University Medical Center
550 First Avenue
New York, New York 10016

Vertebrate photoreceptors respond to changes in incident light with slow and graded changes in membrane potential. In the dark, photoreceptors are depolarized ($V_m \approx -40$ mV), and they release their neurotransmitter continuously at a maximal rate. In the light, photoreceptors hyperpolarize by up to 30 mV, and transmitter release is reduced. Presynaptic potential changes as small as 10–100 μV can be transmitted reliably to second-order neurons.[1] These signals are transmitted at presynaptic active zones that contain many synaptic vesicles a well as a characteristic organelle, the synaptic ribbon. Most of our knowledge on the role of calcium in synaptic transmission derives from the study of a few model synapses such as the vertebrate neuromuscular junction and the squid giant synapse. These synapses are optimized for speed and reliability of transmission. By contrast, little is known about the operating characteristics of photoreceptor ribbon synapses. It is likely, however, that these slow, tonic synapses operate by rules different from the rules holding for fast, phasic synapses. Two unique characteristics of photoreceptor ribbon synapses are described below: an inversion of the sign of signal transfer at low external calcium,[2] and a high sensitivity of synaptic transmission to small changes in external pH.[3]

Normal synaptic transmission from rods and cones to horizontal cells (HC) in the superfused isolated salamander retina persists when the medium is "Ca-free" (no Ca salts added; 5–10 μM trace Ca) or when external free Ca (Ca_o) is buffered to ≥ 25 μM (2.5 mM Hedta and 2.5 mM nitrilotriacetic acid (NTA)). Transmission fails rapidly and completely, however, when Ca_o is buffered to ≤ 1 μM. When Ca_o is buffered to 5–10 μM, cone input to HC is abolished, whereas rod input persists but inverts its sign (see FIG. 1). Rods under these conditions produce purely hyperpolarizing light responses. Hyperpolarizing light responses of HC at 1 mM Ca_o and depolarizing light responses at 5–10 μM Ca_o are fully blocked by 1 mM kynurenate or 10 μM 6,7-dinitroquinoxaline-2,3-dione (DNQX), indicating that both types of response are mediated by activation of kainate-type glutamate receptors on HC. Depolarizing light responses at low Ca_o have also been observed in purely cone-driven HC in goldfish[4] and turtle[5] retina. Under normal conditions, transmitter release from photoreceptor terminals is thought to be modulated by tonic Ca entry through voltage-gated Ca channels. At 5–10 μM Ca_o, little Ca influx should be present. Hence, HC light responses in this range of Ca_o appear to reflect a mode of sign-inverting signal transfer from photoreceptors to HC, with a mechanism that differs from that of normal Ca_o-dependent vesicular transmitter release.

Synaptic transmission from both rods and cones to HC in the salamander retina is also blocked when extracellular pH (buffered with 20–40 mM Hepes) is lowered from 7.8 to 7.2. HC hyperpolarize by as much as 45 mV in response to this treatment, and their light-evoked responses are virtually abolished (see FIG. 2). The relationship between HC dark resting potential and pH_o is very steep and can be fitted with a Hill equation with an exponent of n = 4 and inflection point at pH 7.64 (for Ca_o = 1 mM). The sensitivity of HC to glutamate, the putative photoreceptor transmitter, is unaffected by this treatment, and rod and cone photoresponses are affected only weakly. Bipolar, amacrine, and ganglion cell light responses, however, are also blocked at pH 7.2. Hence, it appears that lowering pH_o blocks photoreceptor

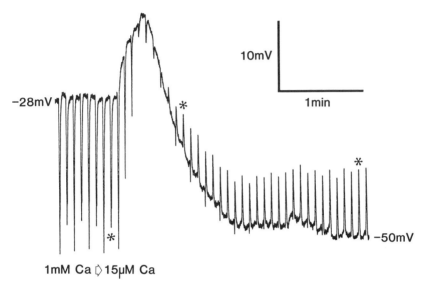

FIGURE 1. Sign inversion of intracellularly recorded light responses of horizontal cells in the isolated, superfused salamander retina at low external Ca concentration. At the time indicated by the arrow, the normal superfusate (1 mM Ca) was switched to a superfusate in which free Ca was buffered to approximately 15 µM (3 mM Hedta, 0.75 mM total Ca, 3.8 mM total Mg, pH 7.8). The retina was stimulated with alternating red (660 nm) and green (555 nm) full-field flashes of 100 ms duration, separated by 5 seconds. Irradiances of red and green flashes were matched to give equal rod responses. Irradiance at 555 nm: 288 photons/$\mu m^{-2} \cdot s^{-1}$; irradiance at 660 nm: 8960 photons/$\mu m^{-2} \cdot s^{-1}$. Selected responses to green flashes are marked with asterisks.

transmitter release. Normal synaptic transmission can be restored at pH 7.2 by treatments that greatly depolarize rods and cones and increase their photoresponses (*e.g.,* lowering Ca_o from 1 to 0.1 mM or adding 0.1 mM 3-isobutyl-1-methyl-xanthine (IBMX) at 1 mM Ca_o). Further, Ca/Sr spikes, induced in rods at pH 7.8 by adding 12 mM TEA and 7 mM Sr to the medium, are blocked at pH 7.2. These results can be explained by a direct effect of pH_o on voltage-gated Ca channels mediating normal transmitter release from photoreceptor terminals. pH titration of specific external sites on these channels may alter their surface potential and consequently the voltage dependence of gating of these channels. Because photoreceptor synaptic transmis-

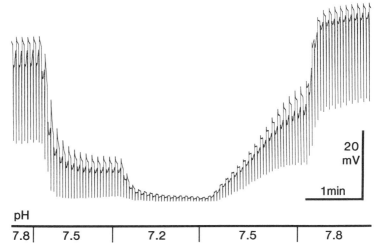

pH

| 7.8 | 7.5 | 7.2 | 7.5 | 7.8 |

FIGURE 2. pH dependence of dark resting potential and light-evoked responses of sala-mander horizontal cells. pH buffered with 20 mM Hepes at 1 mM Ca; alternating red (660 nm) and green (555 nm) 100 ms full-field flashes, separated by 3 seconds. Irradiances of red and green flashes were matched to give equal cone responses (both flashes 10^4 photons/$\mu m^{-2} \cdot s^{-1}$). Responses to green and to red light can be distinguished by the small rod-driven tails found only in green responses.

sion is extremely sensitive to pH_o changes in the physiological range, it is possible that variation in pH_o caused by retinal activity[6] modulates signal transmission at this synapse.

REFERENCES

1. HAGINS, W. A., R. D. PENN & S. YOSHIKAMI. 1970. Biophys. J. **10:** 380–412.
2. KLEINSCHMIDT, J. 1990. Invest. Ophthalmol. Vis. Sci. **31**(Suppl.): 388.
3. KLEINSCHMIDT, J. 1990. Soc. Neurosci. (Abstr.) **16:** 465.
4. ROWE, J. S. 1987. Neurosci. Res. (Suppl.) **6:** s147–s164.
5. NORMANN, R. A., I. PERLMAN & P. J. ANDERTON. 1988. Brain Res. **443:** 95–100.
6. YAMAMOTO, F. & R. H. STEINBERG. 1989. Soc. Neurosci. (Abstr.) **15:** 206.

Immunoelectron Microscopy of the Calcium-Binding Protein Synexin in Isolated Adrenal Chromaffin Granules and Chromaffin Cells

GEMMA A. J. KUIJPERS, GEORGE LEE,
AND HARVEY B. POLLARD

Laboratory of Cell Biology and Genetics
National Institute of Diabetes and Digestive and Kidney Diseases
National Institutes of Health
Bethesda, Maryland 20892

The protein synexin, annexin VII, was originally found in the adrenal medulla and has been shown to cause aggregation and support fusion of adrenal medullary chromaffin granules in a Ca^{2+}-dependent manner.[1] The exocytotic fusion of chromaffin granules with the plasma membrane of the chromaffin cell is triggered by a rise in the concentration of cytosolic Ca^{2+} upon cell activation. We have suggested that synexin may therefore play a role in the exocytotic fusion process.[2] In order to obtain ultrastructural information on synexin, we performed immunoelectron microscopy on frozen ultrathin sections of both isolated chromaffin granules and chromaffin cells.

METHODS

Chromaffin granules were isolated from bovine adrenal medulla, and synexin was isolated from bovine lung.[3] Granules were incubated in the presence or absence of synexin (24 μg/mg granule protein) and Ca^{2+} (1 mM), which induces maximal granule aggregation in 0.3 M sucrose/40 mM MES buffer (pH 6.0). Granules were pelleted, washed twice in buffer without synexin, and fixed with 2% glutaraldehyde/2% paraformaldehyde in 0.1 M phosphate buffer (GA/PFA) for 30 minutes.

Chromaffin cells were isolated and cultured for 3–5 days, and washed and incubated in Krebs solution with or without 20 μM nicotine.[4] Cells were fixed 90 s after onset of stimulation with GA/PFA for 30 minutes. Fixed granule or cell pellets were prepared for cryoultramicrotomy according to the method of Tokuyasu.[5] Sections (ca. 100 nm) were indirectly immunolabeled with a mouse monoclonal antibody against synexin (10E7) and 10 nm gold-labeled goat antimouse IgG, and embedded in methylcellulose.

RESULTS AND CONCLUSIONS

Cryosections of chromaffin granules labeled with synexin antibody are shown in FIGURE 1. In sections of control granules, only few gold particles are visible (FIG. 1a),

471

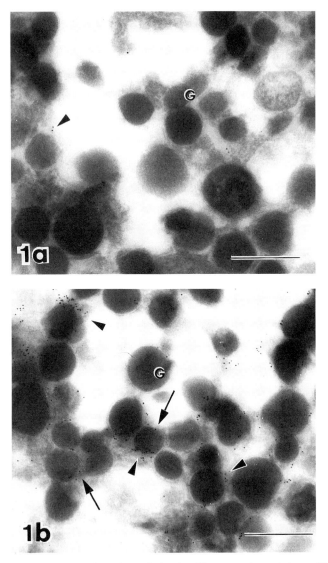

FIGURE 1. Immunogold labeling of synexin in ultrathin cryosections of chromaffin granules incubated in the absence (**a**) or presence (**b**) of synexin and Ca^{2+}. G = granule. Note granule aggregates (arrows) and abundant gold label (arrowheads) in **b.** Bar = 0.5 μm.

whereas sections of granules aggregated with synexin and Ca^{2+} show extensive gold label (FIG. 1b), indicating that the label observed is largely specific. In sections of chromaffin cells, gold label is present in the cell region rich in granule structures, the cytosol including Golgi and endoplasmic reticulum, and the nucleus (FIG. 2). The label is most prominent in the granule-rich cell areas (9 particles/μm^2). Upon stimulation, which induces a 5–10% release of total cell catecholamines, the label is decreased especially in the granule-rich areas.

We conclude that synexin in the chromaffin cell is localized throughout the cell but mainly around the granules, and that the increase in intracellular Ca^{2+} upon cell activation induces a decrease of the amount of immunoreactive synexin molecules, which is possibly related to a mobilization of synexin for membrane fusion.

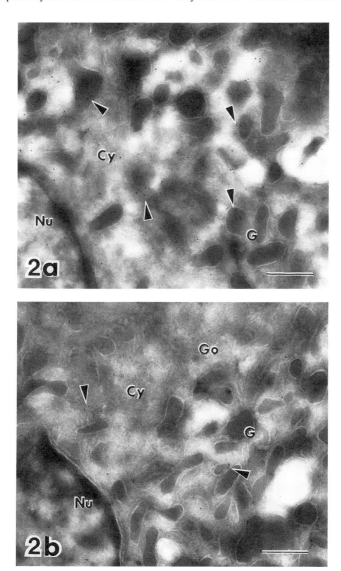

FIGURE 2. Immunogold labeling of synexin in resting (**a**) and nicotine-stimulated (**b**) chromaffin cell. Gold particles (arrowheads) are observed over granules (G), cytosol (Cy), and nucleus (Nu). Go = Golgi. In stimulated cell, density of label is reduced. Bar = 0.5 μm.

REFERENCES

1. CREUTZ, C. E., C. J. PAZOLES & H. B. POLLARD. 1978. J. Biol. Chem. **253**(8): 2858–2866.
2. POLLARD, H. B., A. L. BURNS & E. ROJAS. 1990. J. Membr. Biol. **117:** 101–112.
3. POLLARD, H. B., A. L. BURNS, E. ROJAS, D. D. SCHLAEPFER, H. HAIGLER & K. BROCKLE-
   HURST. 1989. *In* Methods in Cell Biology. A. M. Tartakoff, Ed. Vol. **31:** 207–227.
   Academic Press, Inc. New York.
4. KUIJPERS, G. A. J., L. M. ROSARIO & R. L. ORNBERG. 1989. J. Biol. Chem. **264**(2): 698–705.
5. TOKUYASU, K. T. 1980. Histochem. J. **12:** 381–403.

Calcium Dynamics in the Presynaptic Terminal of Barnacle Photoreceptors

NECHAMA LASSER-ROSS,[a] JOSEPH C. CALLAWAY,[b]
ANN E. STUART,[b] AND WILLIAM N. ROSS[a]

[a] Department of Physiology
Basic Sciences Building
New York Medical College
Valhalla, New York 10595
[b] Department of Physiology
University of North Carolina
Chapel Hill, North Carolina 27514

In the barnacle, *Balanus nubilus,* each of the four medial photoreceptors enters the supraesophageal ganglion at the commissure, bifurcates, and terminates in a spray of 1 to 4 μm diameter processes. Electron-microscopic reconstructions show that contacts with second-order I cells occur in this terminal region.[1] Previous electrophysiological experiments[2] and optical recordings using Arsenazo III[3] have shown that there is a voltage-dependent calcium conductance largely confined to the terminal region. For these experiments we followed the calcium changes in this region with high spatial and temporal resolution using the fluorescent calcium indicator fura-2 together with a cooled CCD camera. The dye was injected with a microelectrode inserted near the bifurcation. The same electrode was used to stimulate the cell and to record membrane potential using a switched current clamp. Time-course measurements were made every 25 ms using excitation at a single wavelength (380 nm). Steady state calcium levels at different membrane potentials were estimated by the ratio method.[4]

Depolarizing pulses (1 to 6 s) produced voltage-dependent calcium entry that was largely confined to the last 50 μm of the terminal regions (FIG. 1). In this region calcium entry began with the onset of the pulse, reached a steady level that was maintained for the duration of the pulse, and began to decline immediately at the end of the pulse. With increasing distance from the terminal, the rise-time of the calcium change was slower, and the peak calcium level was lower. Further, the decline in calcium level began at increasingly later times after the end of the pulse. These different time-courses suggest that calcium was entering through noninactivating calcium channels in the terminal region and diffusing out of this region into the much larger axon branches. Computer simulations incorporating these assumptions qualitatively reproduced the measured curves. Further evidence for removal by diffusion comes from the fact that we were not able to alter the time-course by blocking Na/Ca exchange or altering the $[Ca]_o$ or peak $[Ca]_i$.

A clear threshold for calcium entry was detected at about -60 mV. Approximately the same threshold for postsynaptic responses was reported by Hayashi, Moore, and Stuart.[5] Near this threshold, maintained depolarizations, which correspond to sustained postsynaptic responses, produced mean increases in $[Ca]_i$ of a few hundred nM (assuming the Ca:fura $K_d = 760$ nM and a viscosity correction of 0.3). In the fine processes in this part of the cell, diffusional equilibrium in the radial direction would be expected to occur rapidly compared to the time-course of the graded receptor potential or the time-course of the postsynaptic response. Therefore, these optical measurements of [Ca]$_i$ (which average over the volume of the terminal) should reflect the mean level of [Ca]$_i$ under the membrane.

In phasic synapses it is believed that peak [Ca]$_i$ at the release site is much higher than the mean [Ca]$_i$ in the cell inasmuch as the short synaptic delay requires that the release site be very close to the calcium channels. In this tonic synapse, however, this requirement is not necessary. In addition, the increased calcium levels during sustained release are constantly maintained instead of instantly declining following the action potential. Under these conditions the mean calcium levels we measured may be close to the values at the release site.

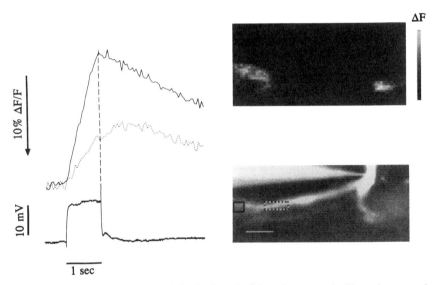

FIGURE 1. Time-course and spatial distribution of calcium changes evoked by an intraaxonal pulse. The left panel shows that in the terminal region (black box, solid trace), the transient begins to recover immediately at the end of the pulse. Away from the terminal (dotted box and trace), calcium continues to rise at this time. The grey scale image shows the location of fluorescence changes at the end of the pulse (dotted line). Calcium increases are largely confined to the terminal. Scale bar is 50 μm.

REFERENCES

1. SCHNAPP, B. J. & A. E. STUART. 1983. J. Neurosci. **3:** 1100–1115.
2. ROSS, W. N. & A. E. STUART. 1978. J. Physiol. (Lond.) **274:** 173–191.
3. STOCKBRIDGE, N. L. & W. N. ROSS. 1984. Nature **309:** 266–268.
4. GRYNKIEWICZ, G., M. POENIE & R. Y. TSIEN. 1985. J. Biol. Chem. **260:** 3440–3450.
5. HAYASHI, J., J. W. MOORE & A. E. STUART. 1985. J. Physiol. (Lond.) **368:** 179–195.

A Barium-Dependent Chromaffin Granule Aggregating Protein from Bovine Adrenal Medulla and Other Tissues

GEORGE LEE, MILTON DE LA FUENTE,
AND HARVEY B. POLLARD

Laboratory of Cell Biology and Genetics
National Institute of Diabetes and Digestive and Kidney Diseases
National Institutes of Health
Bethesda, Maryland 20892

Exocytosis is a process of secretion in which the membranes of the secretory granules or vesicles fuse with a region of the plasma membrane, with subsequent release of the contents of the granules to the outside of the cell.[1] In chromaffin cells, the secretion of catecholamines occurs after the fusion of chromaffin granule membranes with the plasma membrane. In addition to this process of simple exocytosis, compound exocytosis also occurs where the membranes of intact secretory granules fuse with those membranes of expended granules, still fused to the plasma membrane.[2] Furthermore, the secretory response in these cells depends on the influx of Ca^{2+} following exposure to a secretagogue such as nicotine, or depolarizing concentrations of KCl.[3,4] The exact mechanism of Ca^{2+} action is not known, but we have proposed that synexin, a Ca^{2+}-binding protein, from adrenal medulla and other tissues, might be a possible intracellular mediator of the Ca^{2+}-dependent membrane fusion process during exocytosis.[5,6]

Ba^{2+}, however, is also a potent secretagogue and needs no Ca^{2+} to promote secretion.[7] Indeed, recent evidence indicated that Ca^{2+} and Ba^{2+} can promote secretion by separate and coincident kinetic processes.[8] Thus, because synexin is selective only for Ca^{2+}, some other protein like synexin could be necessary to support Ba^{2+}-induced secretion. We therefore searched for a cellular protein that would promote Ba^{2+}-dependent contact and fusion, analogous to that found previously for synexin and Ca^{2+}. Recently we detected the presence of such a protein in bovine adrenal medulla, trachea, and lung and have termed it G-36. The isolation procedure included EGTA extraction, ammonium sulfate fractionation, ion exchange column chromatography, and gel filtration. G-36 caused isolated chromaffin granules to aggregate in the presence of Ba^{2+}, with a $K_{1/2}$ for Ba^{2+} of ca. 200 μM. We measured this aggregating activity in terms of increase in the absorbance at 540 nM of chromaffin granule suspensions mixed with active fractions (FIG. 1). We found the active species to be soluble, nondialyzable, trypsin-sensitive, and quite heat labile. For example, when heated to 60°C for 5 min, greater than 50% of aggregating activity was lost. It has an apparent molecular weight of 36,000 when subjected to SDS gel electrophoresis or gel filtration.

Amino acid analysis of G-36 indicated that the protein contains about equal amounts of hydrophobic and hydrophilic amino acids (approximately 70% of the total amino acids) and lysine and arginine (15%). Fluorescence studies showed that G-36 has no tryptophan. G-36 also caused chromaffin granules to aggregate, not only in the presence of Ba^{2+}, but also in the presence of Ca^{2+} or Sr^{2+}. G-36, however, was inactive in Mg^{2+} or EGTA. We also investigated the interaction of G-36 with phospholipids by incubating G-36 with large, thin-walled phosphatidylserine vesicles for 10 min in the presence of Ba^{2+}, Ca^{2+}, Mg^{2+}, or EGTA. We then centrifuged the solution to pellet the vesicles and analyzed the fractions by separating them on SDS-PAGE and staining with Coomassie blue. G-36 was found to be associated with phospholipid only in the presence of Ba^{2+} and Ca^{2+}, but not in the presence of Mg^{2+} or EGTA. We next tested this protein directly for fusion ability on large unilamellar liposomes. We found that this protein enhances aggregation and fusion of liposomes in the presence of Ba^{2+}. By contrast, synexin has no fusion activity in the presence of Ba^{2+}.

In summary, we have isolated a Ba^{2+}-sensitive protein from bovine tissues that causes chromaffin granules to aggregate and phospholipid liposomes to fuse. We

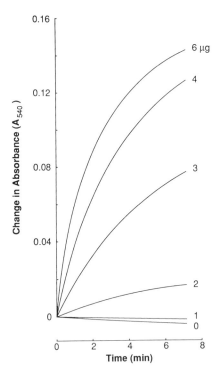

FIGURE 1. Time-course of turbidity changes in a chromaffin granule suspension induced by various amounts of G-36 in the presence of Ba^{2+}.

suggested that this protein is a possible candidate of the sought-after Ba^{2+}-dependent fusion protein in chromaffin cells, and that a number of properties of this protein are consistent with those that we might anticipate from kinetic studies of secreting cells.

REFERENCES

1. PALADE, G. 1975. Science 189: 347–358.
2. POLLARD, H. B., C. E. CREUTZ, V. FOWLER, J. SCOTT & C. J. PAZOLES. 1982. Cold Spring Harbor Symp. Quant. Biol. 46: 819–834.

3. ROSARIO, L. M., B. SORIA, G. FEUERSTEIN & H. B. POLLARD. 1989. Neurosci. **29:** 735–747.
4. CENA, V., A. STUTZIN & E. ROJAS. 1989. J. Membr. Biol. **112:** 101–112.
5. POLLARD, H. B., A. L. BURNS & E. ROJAS. 1988. J. Exp. Biol. **139:** 267–286.
6. POLLARD, H. B., A. L. BURNS & E. ROJAS. 1990. J. Membr. Biol. **117:** 101–112.
7. DOUGLAS, W. W. & P. P. RUBIN. 1964. Nature **203:** 305–307.
8. HELDMAN, E., M. LEVINE, L. RAVEH & H. B. POLLARD. 1989. J. Biol. Chem. **264:** 7914–7920.

Possible Role for Neurosecretory Granule Channel That Resembles Gap Junctions

JOSÉ R. LEMOS, CHEOL J. LEE,[a] KAREN A. OCORR,[b]

GOVINDAN DAYANITHI,[c] AND JEAN J. NORDMANN[c]

Worcester Foundation for Experimental Biology
Shrewsbury, Massachusetts 01545

The anatomy of the neurohypophysis and biochemical separation techniques[1] made possible the reconstitution of ionic channel proteins from neurosecretory granules (NSG), in order to analyze their possible roles in depolarization-secretion coupling. Our evidence indicates that these NSG membranes contain at least two ionic channels, the smaller one being more selective for anions.[2] In symmetrical 150 mM KCl, the larger amplitude channel has a linear slope conductance of 130 pS. In asymmetrical salt gradients the reversal potentials indicate that this channel appears to be permeable to most cations, but with Ca^{2+} and Ba^{2+} permeating better than K^+, Na^+, or Cs^+.

The gating kinetics for this channel are much more complicated than for the anion channel.[3] For example, the cation channel can open to more than one conductance level at a variety of pipet potentials. If an I-V curve is constructed in such asymmetrical solutions, all conductances reverse at the same potential. As many as four different conductance levels have been observed in a single patch, with openings occurring between any and all levels.[3] Furthermore, its gating shows little voltage dependence at pH 7.4, although lowering the pH greatly decreased the open probability of the channel.

In order to study the mechanism underlying depolarization-secretion coupling, nerve terminals isolated from the rat neurohypophysis were permeabilized with digitonin, and vasopressin (AVP) release was evoked by 10 μM Ca^{2+}.[4] Both C-10 and bis C-10 compounds inhibited this evoked release in a dose-dependent (1–10 μM) manner. At a concentration of 10 μM, C-10 also significantly inhibited the gating of the NSG cation channel.

This cation channel is bimodally regulated by Ca^{2+}. It opens only in the presence of greater than 30 nM free Ca^{2+}, with maximal effects at about 5 μM, where the channel is almost always open.[3] Surprisingly, its gating is inhibited at concentrations above 10 μM. The relationship between the amount of AVP released from digitonin-permeabilized neurohypophysial nerve terminals in response to different concentrations of internal Ca^{2+} also shows a similar biphasic dependence on increasing concentrations of the second messenger.

Alcohols were applied to the internal face of patches containing the Ca^{2+}-activated NSG cation channel. Ethanol (EtOH) did not affect channel openings even at a concentration of 50 mM. By contrast, much lower concentrations of heptanol and octanol (OcOH) significantly reduce the larger conductance channel openings. Digitonin-permeabilized nerve terminals were incubated with different concentrations (0.01–5 mM) of OcOH or 50 mM EtOH. Upon evoking vasopressin release with

---

[a] Present address: University of Wisconsin, Madison, WI.

[b] Present address: University of Michigan, Ann Arbor, MI.

[c] Present address: Centre de Neurochimie, Strasbourg, France.

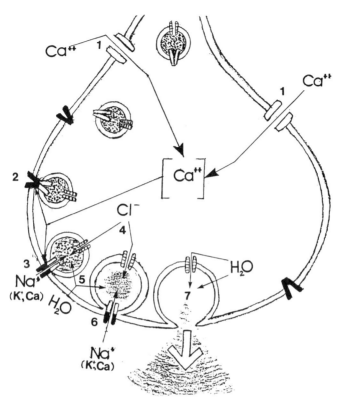

FIGURE 1. Model of depolarization-secretion coupling showing hypothesized role(s) of NSG channels and calcium. It is postulated that channels in both plasma and NSG membranes, when apposed, could form a fusion pore analogous to a gap junction–like connection between the inside of the NSG and the extracellular milieu. Representational drawing of neurohypophysial nerve terminal. Neurosecretory granules are dense-core vesicles entering from axon (at top). (1) Calcium (Ca^{++}) enters through two types of channels and elevates its intracellular levels [Ca^{++}]. (2) It is probable that in nerve terminals the interaction between the NSG cation channel (clear) and a similar channel in plasma membrane (dark) would have to precede Ca^{++} entry. In this context the plasma membrane hemichannel would act as a "docking protein" localizing release to specific sites on the plasma membrane. (3) Ca^{++} entry would lead to the opening of the two channels, and, when apposed, they could form a gap junction–like fusion pore. When the fusion pore is open, extracellular cations would move into the NSG down their concentration and/or electrical gradients. The primary cation would be sodium (Na^+), although Ca^{++} and potassium (K^+) could also enter. (4) As positive charges accumulated inside the NSG, anions, such as chloride (Cl^-), could also flow in through the NSG anion channel (striped). (5) This osmotic increase would force water (H_2O) to enter the NSG and cause them to swell. This swelling could tend to drive the NSG and plasma membranes closer, especially with the channel anchoring them together, and promote adhesion. (6) Osmotic swelling may not be enough, or even necessary, to cause fusion, however, and fusogenic proteins or lipids might be required. (7) The entry of ions would, in any case, disrupt the matrix inside the vesicle and lead to subsequent expulsion (large white arrow) of the contents of the NSG: the neuropeptides oxytocin and vasopressin.

10 μM Ca^{2+}, OcOH showed a dose-dependent inhibition of secretion, whereas EtOH had no significant effect.

Taken together, our data suggest that these NSG ion channels could be directly involved in the molecular mechanism underlying release. Because the cation NSG channel shows similarities to gap junctions,[5] this Ca^{2+}-activated channel could be the analogous "fusion pore" for nerve cells[6] reported[7] to occur during mast cell exocytosis. In the case of gap junctions the two hemichannels or connexons are coupled together in their gating when the two bilayers are apposed. An analogous situation could exist for exocytosis where the NSG bilayer has to come into close apposition with the plasma membrane of the terminal (see FIG. 1). More work is, of course, necessary to determine if this is indeed the mechanism for depolarization-secretion coupling.

REFERENCES

1. NORDMANN, J. J., F. LOUIS & S. J. MORRIS. 1979. Neurosci. **4:** 1367–1375.
2. LEMOS, J. R. & J. J. NORDMANN. 1986. J. Exp. Biol. **124:** 53–72.
3. LEMOS, J. R., K. A. OCORR & J. J. NORDMANN. 1989. Soc. Gen. Physiol. Ser. **44:** 333–347.
4. NORDMANN, J. J., G. DAYANITHI & J. R. LEMOS. 1987. Biosci. Rep. **7:** 411–425.
5. SPRAY, D. C. & M. V. L. BENNET. 1985. Ann. Rev. Physiol. **47:** 281–303.
6. RAHAMIMOFF, R., S. A. DERIEMER, B. SAKMANN, H. STADLER & N. YAKIR. 1988. Proc. Natl. Acad. Sci USA **85:** 5310–5314.
7. BRECKENRIDGE, L. J. & W. ALMERS. 1987. Nature **328:** 814–817.

Tissue-Regulated Alternative Splicing of Synexin mRNA

K. MAGENDZO, A. SHIRVAN, H. B. POLLARD,
AND A. L. BURNS

Laboratory of Cell Biology and Genetics
National Institute of Diabetes and Digestive and Kidney Diseases
National Institutes of Health
Bethesda, Maryland 20892

Synexin (annexin VII) is a cytosolic calcium-dependent membrane binding protein that aggregates chromaffin granules, promotes membrane fusion, and forms voltage-dependent calcium channels in artificial and natural membranes.[1] Recent sequencing of human cDNA has revealed that synexin belongs to the annexin gene family,[2] members of which are thought to be involved in such diverse processes as inflammation, blood coagulation, and cellular transformation. In fact, their precise physiological roles remain unresolved.[3]

The sequence of several different synexin cDNA and genomic clones has shown that synexin is encoded by a complex transcriptional unit involving alternative splicing of a cassette exon and alternate polyadenylation signals.[4] The selection of alternate poly(A) signals gives rise to two synexin mRNAs differing in the length of their 3' noncoding regions. Northern analysis of human RNA from fibroblast and liver showed the presence of two bands (2.0 and 2.4 kb) when hybridized to a cDNA fragment of the coding region of synexin, but only the 2.4 kb band hybridized to a probe made from the longer 3' end (FIG. 1). On the other hand, the alternative splicing predicts two isoforms of synexin differing in the N-terminal domain. The inclusion of the cassette exon may be important for the structure of the N terminus,

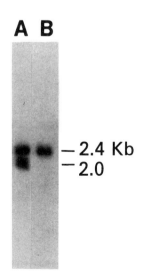

FIGURE 1. Northern blot analysis of human synexin mRNA. Five μg of human fibroblast mRNA hybridized with (A) a cDNA probe (PstI-SspI fragment) derived from the coding region of the synexin clone and (B) a PCR fragment obtained from the longer 3' end.

A B

— 2.4 Kb
— 2.0

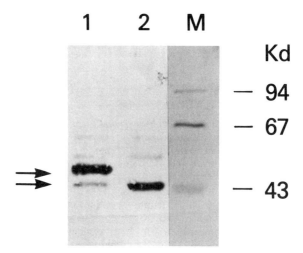

FIGURE 2. Western blot analysis of synexin isotypes. Lane 1: 5 μg of synexin from human skeletal muscle (partially purified to the second ammonium sulfate precipitation). Lane 2: 10 μg of synexin from human lung (purified through ultragel column). M: molecular weight markers. Arrows indicate the two synexin isotypes. The blots were incubated with goat polyclonal antibodies raised against bovine synexin, and the immunoreactive proteins were detected with streptavidin-biotinylated rabbit antigoat horseradish peroxidase.

because it results in the introduction of three acidic residues to an otherwise almost uncharged domain.[2]

Polymerase chain reaction analysis of synexin mRNA from various fetal and adult tissues of human and monkey revealed that the alternative splicing event is tissue-regulated. Synexin mRNA containing the cassette exon is prevalent in brain, heart, and skeletal muscle, whereas synexin mRNA lacking this exon is more abundant in other tissues (liver, lung, kidney, spleen, fibroblast cells, and placenta). This is supported by Western blot analysis showing that muscle synexin is larger than synexin from lung (FIG. 2). The difference in size is consistent with the molecular masses predicted from the proteins encoded by the alternatively spliced synexin mRNAs. Furthermore, specific antibodies raised against a synthetic peptide derived from the sequence of the cassette exon reacted only with the larger synexin isoform.

We anticipate that comparison of synexin from human muscle or brain with the smaller synexin isoform in lung will shed light on the functional significance of the tissue-regulated alternative processing of synexin mRNA. In addition, these studies may illuminate the question of possible subcellular localization and also may yield insight to the molecular basis of calcium-dependent binding to phospholipids, membrane fusion, and channel properties.

REFERENCES

1. POLLARD, H. B., A. L. BURNS & E. ROJAS. 1990. J. Membr. Biol. **117:** 101–112.
2. BURNS, A. L., K. MAGENDZO, A. SHIRVAN, M. SRIVASTAVA, E. ROJAS, M. R. ALIJANI & H. B. POLLARD. 1989. Proc. Natl. Acad. Sci. USA **86:** 3798–3802.
3. BURGOYNE, R. D. & M. D. GEISOW. 1989. Cell Calcium **10:** 1–10.
4. MAGENDZO, K., A. SHIRVAN, C. CULTRARO, M. SRIVASTAVA, H. B. POLLARD & A. L. BURNS. 1991. J. Biol. Chem. **266:** 3228–3232.

Tetrodotoxin-Sensitive Ciguatoxin Effects on Quantal Release, Synaptic Vesicle Depletion, and Calcium Mobilization[a]

JORDI MOLGO, JOAN X. COMELLA,[b] TAKESHI
SHIMAHARA, AND ANNE M. LEGRAND[c]

Laboratoire de Neurobiologie Cellulaire et Moléculaire
Centre National de la Recherche Scientifique
91198 Gif sur Yvette CEDEX, France

Ciguatoxin (CTX) is one of the main toxins responsible for a complex human food poisoning known as ciguatera.[1] Extracted from the moray eel *Gymnothorax javanicus,* CTX, which has a molecular formula of $C_{60}H_{86}O_{19}$, was recently disclosed to be a polyether having a brevetoxin-like structure.[2] Recent evidence indicates that CTX could result from oxidative modification of the toxins produced by the dinoflagellate *Gambierdiscus toxicus* during their transmission to fish through the marine food chain.[3]

CTX has been shown to affect selectively sodium channels inducing membrane depolarization and spontaneous action potentials in neuroblastoma cells,[4] myelinated axons,[5] and frog skeletal muscle fibers.[6] In addition, CTX (1.5–2.5 nM) increased the spontaneous quantal release of acetylcholine, measured electrophysiologically as an increase in miniature end-plate potential (MEPP) frequency (FIG. 1A, inset), at frog neuromuscular junctions independently of extracellular Ca^{2+}.[6] Tetrodotoxin (TTX) (0.5–1 μM), which by itself has no action on MEPP frequency, prevented CTX (2.5 nM) effects on neurotransmitter release (FIG. 1A). TTX inhibition of CTX action could be reversed by continuous washing with CTX-free and TTX-free solution (FIG. 1A). These results revealed that TTX was more easily reversible than CTX, prior action of TTX did not affect subsequent action of CTX, or vice versa, and CTX action depends upon Na^+ entry into motor terminals.

In order to determine whether CTX affected intracellular Ca^{2+} levels, experiments were performed in cultured mouse neuroblastoma × rat glioma NG108-15 hybrid cells, bathed with a nominally Ca^{2+}-free medium supplemented with 1 mM EGTA, using the fluorescent Ca^{2+} indicator fura-2[7] and an Olimpus OSP-3 system. As shown in FIG. 1B, addition of 1 μM TTX and subsequent addition of 2.5 nM CTX did not modify cytoplasmic Ca^{2+} concentration. By contrast, CTX increased about 2.5 times cytosolic basal Ca^{2+} levels when tested in the absence of TTX (FIG. 1C). Whether CTX-induced Ca^{2+} mobilization is mediated by second messengers remains to be determined.

In view that quantal transmitter release was exhausted irreversibly within 3–4 h of CTX (2.5 nM) action, an ultrastructural study was performed to assess eventual

[a]This research was supported, in part, by Direction des Recherches Etudes et Techniques and, in part, by the French Polynesian Government.

[b]Permanent address: Universitat de Barcelona, Estudi General de Lleida, Faculty of Medicine, Anselm Clave 22, E-25007 Lleida, Spain.
[c]Permanent address: Institut Territorial de Recherche Médicale Louis Malardé, Papeete, Tahiti, Polynésie Française.

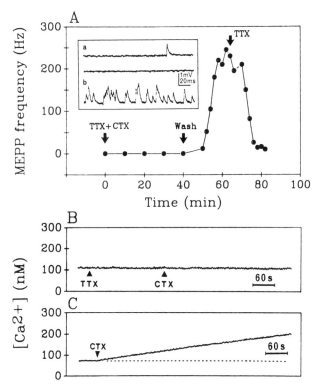

FIGURE 1. A: Failure of CTX (2.5 nM) to enhance the rate of occurrence of MEPPs when TTX (1 μM) was present in the bathing solution, the increase in MEPP frequency caused by washing with a TTX-free and CTX-free solution, and the ability of TTX to reverse the effect of CTX. Arrows indicate changes in bathing solutions. The inset shows MEPPs recorded at a single neuromuscular junction of a frog cutaneous pectoris muscle bathed in standard Ringer's solution before (a) and after (b) 20 min of CTX action. Temperature 20°C. **B** and **C:** Fluorometrical recordings from single neuronal hybrid cells (NG108-15) showing that prior treatment with TTX (1 μM) and subsequent addition of CTX (2.5 nM), in the continuous presence of TTX, had no effect on cytosolic Ca^{2+} concentration (**B**), whereas in the absence of TTX, CTX caused an increase in cytosolic Ca^{2+} concentration (**C**). Recordings in **B** and **C** were made on different cells. In **B** and **C**, the extracellular medium contained no added Ca^{2+} and 1 mM EGTA. Triangles indicate the changes in perfusing solutions. Temperature 37°C.

FIGURE 2. Effects of CTX and TTX on the ultrastructure of frog neuromuscular junctions. Panel **a** and **b:** electron micrographs of cross-sectioned terminals treated for 3 h with 2.5 nM CTX, in a nominally Ca^{2+}-free solution with 1 mM EGTA, in the presence of 1 μM TTX (**a**) or in its absence (**b**). Notice the normal appearance of the terminal, the mitochondria, and the complement of synaptic vesicles in **a,** whereas in **b,** the terminal is swollen, practically devoid of synaptic vesicles, and the mitochondria exhibit signs of internal disruption. Arrows in **b** show a few coated vesicles. Panel **c:** portion of a transversally sectioned terminal showing coated structures in relation to the prejunctional membrane. Scale marker in **b** is 0.5 μm, and in **c,** 0.1 μm.

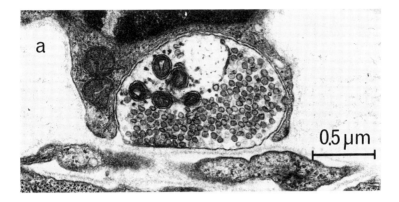

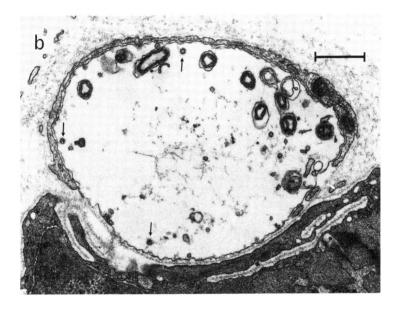

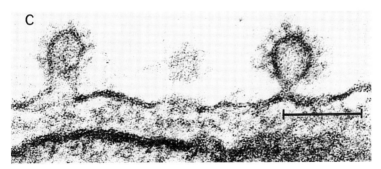

FIGURE 2

changes caused by the toxin at the subcellular level of motor nerve terminals. As depicted in FIGURE 2a, 2.5 nM CTX applied for 3 h in the presence of 1 μM TTX caused no evident alterations in the typical components of the nerve endings. When the same concentration of CTX was applied for 3 h in the absence of TTX, however, a marked reduction in the number of synaptic vesicles per nerve terminal cross-section was observed (FIG. 2b). Depletion of vesicles was accompanied by the enlargement of the presynaptic membrane coupled to the swelling of the terminal. In addition, an increase in the number of coated vesicles and pits was observed (FIG. 2c). Coated structures were usually associated either with elements of the endoplasmic reticulum or with cisternae-like double membranes. These results suggest that CTX impairs the recycling process that is believed, under normal conditions, to conserve the synaptic vesicle population during quantal release.

In conclusion, CTX effects on quantal release, synaptic vesicle depletion, and Ca^{2+} mobilization were completely prevented by TTX, indicating that such effects are mediated by Na^+ influx through TTX-sensitive channels. In addition, it is suggested that CTX blocks synaptic vesicle recycling and mobilizes Ca^{2+} from intracellular stores in an Na^+-dependent way.

REFERENCES

1. HOKAMA, Y. & J. T. MIYAHARA. 1986. J. Toxicol. Toxin Rev. **5:** 25–53.
2. LEGRAND, A. M., M. FUKUI, P. CRUCHET, Y. ISHIBASHI & T. YASUMOTO. 1990. Proceedings of the 3rd International Conference on ciguatera. In press.
3. MURATA, M., A. M. LEGRAND, Y. ISHIBASHI, M. FUKUI & T. YASUMOTO. 1990. J. Am. Chem. Soc. **112:** 4380–4386.
4. BIDART, J. N., H. P. M. VIJVERBERG, C. FRELIN, E. CHUNGUE, A. M. LEGRAND, R. BAGNIS & M. LAZDUNSKI. 1984. J. Biol. Chem. **259:** 8353–8357.
5. BENOIT, E., A. M. LEGRAND & J. M. DUBOIS. 1986. Toxicon **24:** 357–364.
6. MOLGO, J., J. X. COMELLA & A. M. LEGRAND. 1990. Br. J. Pharmacol. **99:** 695–700.
7. GRYNKIEWICZ, G., M. POENIE & R. Y. TSIEN. 1985. J. Biol. Chem. **260:** 3440–3450.

Effect of Antibodies on Calcium Channels[a]

H. J. PHILLIPS, G. G. WILSON, S. BALDWIN,[b]
R. NORMAN,[c] AND D. WRAY

Pharmacology Department
Worsley Medical and Dental Building
The University of Leeds
Leeds LS2 9JT, United Kingdom

[b]*Biochemistry Department*
Royal Free Hospital School of Medicine
London NW3 2PF, United Kingdom

[c]*Department of Medicine*
Leicester Royal Infirmary
Leicester LE2 7LX, United Kingdom

In this work, we have used antibodies against the L-type calcium channel in order to investigate structure/function relationships of this channel. Two antibodies were used: a monoclonal antibody raised against the α_2 subunit of the calcium channel and a polyclonal antibody raised against a peptide corresponding to a known region of the α_1 subunit of the channel.

MONOCLONAL ANTIBODY AGAINST THE α_2 SUBUNIT

The α_2 calcium channel subunit purified from rabbit skeletal muscle t tubules was used to raise monoclonal antibody[1] in order to study a possible role of the α_2 subunit in channel function. The ion channel pore is thought to be contained within the α_1 subunit,[2] but the role of the α_2 subunit is not clear.

The monoclonal antibody was applied to differentiated neuroblastoma × glioma hybrid cells (NG 108 15) for 24 hours at 37°C. Whole-cell patch-clamp recordings were then made from these cells at 22–24°C using 10 mM barium as charge carrier in the presence of 25 mM tetraethylammonium and 2.5 μM tetrodotoxin in the bath, and 140 mM cesium in the patch pipette. Currents were recorded in response to 200 ms depolarizing command potentials at 0.1 Hz from a holding potential of −80 mV.

Currents in these cells have transient and sustained components corresponding to T- and L-type currents.

The antibody reduced significantly the sustained (L-type) currents (FIG. 1). This indicates that the α_2 subunit may have a modulating role in channel function. Because the antibody was incubated with the cells for 24 hours, however, the effect could equally be explained by channel down-regulation by antibody-induced channel internalization. To test this, the antibody was applied for up to 10–15 minutes. Under these circumstances, the antibody had no significant effect on L-type currents, suggesting that down-regulation was the mechanism of the above effect. Inasmuch as the antibody was raised against the α_2 subunit, these results suggest that either the α_2 subunit is tightly bound to the rest of the channel so that the whole channel is

[a]This work was supported by the Medical Research Council and Wellcome Trust.

down-regulated, or alternatively only the α_2 subunit is down-regulated with loss of channel function indicating an important role of the α_2 subunit in channel function. The antibody did not significantly affect transient currents evoked by small depolarizing steps (T-type currents), as might be expected because the antibody was raised against the L-type channel subunit. Thus the region probed by this antibody must be antigenically (and structurally) different between L- and T-type channels, or perhaps the α_2 subunit is not a structural component present in the T-type channel.

PEPTIDE-SPECIFIC ANTIBODY AGAINST THE α_1 SUBUNIT

For the α_1 subunit of the L-type channel, the amino acid sequence is known,[2-4] but the molecular regions of the protein concerned with channel function are not understood. We have studied the possible role of a putative extracellular sequence in channel function by using a polyclonal antibody raised against a specific channel sequence as a probe.

Antibody was raised against a synthetic peptide corresponding to residues 143–158 of the α_1 subunit of rabbit skeletal muscle L-type channel. This sequence is predicted to be located in the extracellular loop region between the membrane-spanning regions S3 and S4 of the first domain. The antibody was applied to NG 108 cells for 24 hours, and electrophysiological recordings made as above. The antibody caused significant reductions in peak current over a range of test potentials (FIG. 2). More specifically, there were reductions for small test potential steps where only transient (T-type) currents were activated. Reductions in sustained currents (L-type)

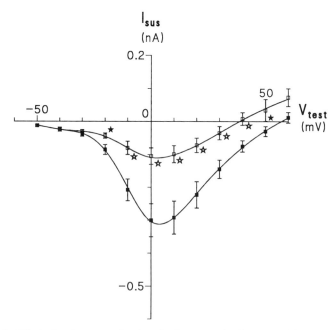

FIGURE 1. Effect of anti-α_2 monoclonal antibody on sustained currents. The I-V curves were obtained for NG 108 15 cells from a holding potential of −80 mV. Mean and SE of the mean are shown from 17 control cells (■) and 16 antibody-treated cells (□). Significant differences between control and test (Student's t test) ★ $p < 0.05$; ☆ $p < 0.005$.

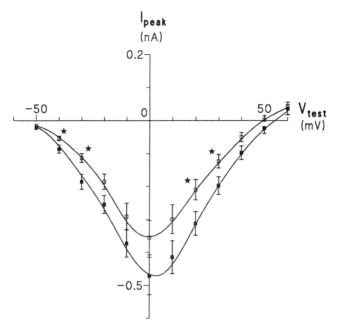

FIGURE 2. Effect of peptide-specific antibody on peak currents. The I-V curves were obtained as in FIG. 1 for 25 control cells (■) and 25 antibody-treated cells (□). Significant differences between control and test ★ $p < 0.05$.

also occurred, but these were not statistically significant, possibly because of large experimental scatter.

The experiments confirm the extracellular location of this amino acid sequence between segments S3 and S4, inasmuch as extracellular application produced functional effects.

The results appear to suggest that this extracellular region may play an important role in channel function; however, further experiments with short-term application of the antibody are required in order to distinguish whether functional block rather than down-regulation occurs.

It is interesting that this antibody raised against the L-type channel seems to have an effect on a low threshold T-type channel, suggesting that there may be a region of antigenic similarity and hence structural similarity between the α_1 subunit of these two channel types at least in the region probed by the antibody. Other regions (and/or subunits) may be different between T- and L-type channels, as indicated by our results with the anti-α_2 monoclonal antibody discussed above.

REFERENCES

1. NORMAN, R. I., A. J. BURGESS & T. M. HARRISON. 1989. Ann. N.Y. Acad. Sci. **560:** 258–268.
2. TANABE, T., H. TAKESHIMA, A. MIKAMI, V. FLOCKERZI, H. TAKAHAHSHI, K. KANGAWA, M. KOJIMA, H. MATSUO, T. HIROSE & S. NUMA. 1987. Nature **328:** 313–318.
3. MIKAMI, A., K. IMOTO, T. TANABE, T. NIIDOME, Y. MORI, H. TAKESHIMA, S. NARUMIYA & S. NUMA. 1989. Nature **340:** 230–233.
4. BIEL, M., P. RUTH, E. BOSSE, R. HULLIN, W. STUHMER, V. FLOCKERZI & F. HOFMANN. 1990. FEBS Lett. **269:** 409–412.

Frequency Facilitation Is Not Caused by Residual Ionized Calcium at the Frog Neuromuscular Junction

RICHARD ROBITAILLE AND MILTON P. CHARLTON

Department of Physiology
University of Toronto
Toronto, Canada, M5S 1A8

The most popular hypothesis used to explain frequency facilitation is the residual Ca^{2+} hypothesis. It proposes that facilitated release occurs when Ca^{2+} ions entering the nerve terminal add with the residual free Ca^{2+} from the previous synaptic activity.[1-3] We tested this hypothesis by increasing the intracellular Ca^{2+} buffering capacity of the frog neuromuscular junction (NMJ) by incorporation of the cell-permeant form of the mobile Ca^{2+} chelator 5,5'dimethyl-1,2-bis (2-aminophenoxy) ethane-*N,N,N,'N'*-tetraacetic acid (DMBAPTA-AM).[4] Mathematical models predict that mobile intracellular buffers should reduce the accumulation of free Ca^{2+} and increase its rate of diffusion from the release sites.[5] Thus, the amount of facilitation should be reduced and its rate of decay increased in the presence of the mobile intracellular Ca^{2+} chelator.

Experiments were performed on neuromuscular junctions of frog (*Rana pipiens*) cutaneous pectoris muscles at 19°C in low Ca^{2+}-high Mg^{2+} physiological solution (in mM: 120 NaCl; 2.0 KCl; 1 NaHCO$_3$; 0.5 CaCl$_2$; 3.6 MgCl$_2$; 5 Hepes; pH adjusted to 7.2). Synaptic transmission was recorded intracellularly in the muscle fiber using glass microelectrodes. DMBAPTA-AM was used at concentrations of 10 to 50 μM dissolved in low Ca^{2+}-high Mg^{2+} frog solution containing dimethyl sulfoxide at a final concentration of 1% v/v. Control solutions also contained 1% DMSO.

Loading the frog NMJ with the Ca^{2+} chelator caused a 50% reduction in transmitter release (FIG. 1A). This effect was presynaptic in origin because the amplitude of the miniature end-plate potentials (MEPP) was not affected (FIG. 1B). The Ca^{2+} chelator, however, induced a small increase in MEPP frequency (about 20%). Identical effects on transmitter release were obtained using BAPTA-AM. An increase of Ca^{2+} chelator concentration also induced a reduction in frequency facilitation by 73% ± 13% (FIG. 2A). This result is in agreement with the predictions of the mathematical models[4] and the residual Ca^{2+} hypothesis.[1-3] The increase in the buffering capacity of the nerve terminal, however, also caused a decrease in the rate of decay of facilitation as revealed by an increase in the time-constant (τ) from 30 ms in control to 65 ms in the presence of the buffer (FIG. 2B). This increase in τ does not agree with the predictions from the residual Ca^{2+} hypothesis and the mathematical models. It is predicted that a mobile buffer should increase the diffusion of Ca^{2+} away from the release sites because the diffusion rate of the buffer complexed with Ca^{2+}

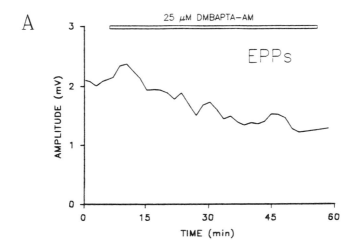

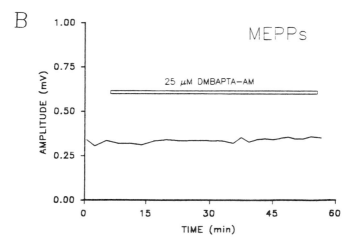

FIGURE 1. Effects of DMBAPTA-AM on transmitter release. **A:** Effects of exogenous Ca^{2+} buffer on EPP amplitude and (**B**) on MEPP amplitude for the same junction. DMBAPTA-AM (10 μM), applied during the period indicated by the bars, caused a reduction of 45% of EPP amplitude without affecting MEPP amplitude. This indicates that DMBAPTA-AM worked presynaptically and reduced the amount of transmitter released.

$(2 \times 10^{-6} \ cm^2/s)^{6,7}$ is greater then the diffusion rate of Ca^{2+} in cytoplasm. We therefore conclude that the residual free ionized Ca^{2+} is not directly the cause of frequency facilitation and that other mechanisms must be considered. These mechanisms must be characterized by a strong Ca^{2+} dependency because facilitation was greatly reduced in presence of the Ca^{2+} buffer.

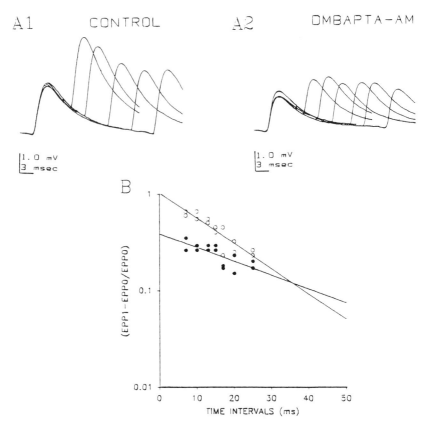

FIGURE 2. Effects of DMBAPTA-AM on the rate of decay of frequency facilitation. Conditioning EPPs were followed by a test EPP at different time intervals (between 7 and 25 ms) before (**A1**) and after (**A2**) the application of DMBAPTA-AM. Facilitation is defined by the ratio $EPP_1\text{-}EPP_0/EPP_0$. **B** illustrates the semilogarithmic plot of the facilitation ratios as a function of the testing time intervals before (open circles) and after (closed circles) loading with DM-BAPTA-AM (25 μM). Both the amount of facilitation and the rate of decay of facilitation were reduced.

REFERENCES

1. KATZ, B. & R. MILEDI. 1968. J. Physiol. (Lond.) **195:** 481–492.
2. MILEDI, R. & R. THIES. 1971. J. Physiol. (Lond.) **212:** 245–257.
3. ZUCKER, R. S. 1989. Annu. Rev. Neurosci. **12:** 13–31.
4. TSIEN, R. Y. 1980. Biochemistry **19:** 2396–2404.
5. DUFFY, S. N., J. L. WINSLOW & M. P. CHARLTON. 1989. Soc. Neurosc. (Abstr.) **19:** 475.
6. ADLER, E. M., S. N. DUFFY, G. J. AUGUSTINE & M. P. CHARLTON 1990. J. Neurosci. **11:** 1496–1507.
7. STRAUTMAN, A. F., R. J. CORK & K. R. ROBINSON. 1990. J. Neurosci. **10:** 3564–3575.

Presynaptic Inhibition Mediated by GABA$_B$ Receptors in Rat Striatal Brain Slices

G. R. SEABROOK,[a] M. L. EVANS, W. HOWSON,
C. D. BENHAM, AND M. G. LACEY

SmithKline Beecham Pharmaceuticals
The Frythe, Welwyn, Herts
AL6 9AR United Kingdom

The mechanism by which GABA$_B$ receptors depress synaptic transmission is not fully understood; baclofen modulates both neuronal calcium currents[1] and potassium currents.[2] Clarification of the role of GABA$_B$ receptors in presynaptic inhibition has been hampered by the lack of effective agonists and antagonists for these receptors. This study examines the comparative physiological effects of a novel GABA$_B$ agonist, 3-aminopropyl-methyl-phosphinic acid (SK&F 97541), in relation to these known actions of baclofen.

Excitatory postsynaptic potentials (EPSPs) were recorded from neurons in sagittal slices of rat dorsal striatum.[3] Recordings were also made from neurons in coronal slices of rat substantia nigra compacta.[2] Fifty-nine percent of these neurons fired spontaneously (2.3 ± 0.36 Hz); thus for drug quantification they were hyperpolarized beyond the threshold for firing (mean -56.6 ± 0.5 mV). Whole-cell calcium currents were recorded from rat dorsal root ganglion neurons in the presence of (in mM) BaCl$_2$ (10), TEA$_{external}$ (135), or CsCl (130) and tetrodotoxin (1 μM).

Baclofen and SK&F 97541 reversibly reduced the amplitude of EPSPs in rat striatum (FIG. 1). The half maximally effective concentrations (EC$_{50}$s) determined from single-site logistic fits to the data (fitted curves) were 92 nM (SK&F 97541) and 1.25 μM (baclofen); both drugs exhibited a maximal depression of 92 percent. The depression of EPSP amplitudes occurred without any observed postsynaptic effects. Baclofen and SK&F 97541 reversibly hyperpolarized neurons in substantia nigra compacta by up to 25 mV; this was accompanied by a fall in input resistance. The EC$_{50}$s were 0.15 μM for SK&F 97541 and 3.6 μM for baclofen. Both drugs exhibited a mean maximal hyperpolarization of 21 mV. The peak amplitude of whole-cell calcium currents recorded from cultured rat dorsal root ganglion neurons was reversibly reduced by baclofen and SK&F 97541. Ten μM SK&F 97541 was approximately equipotent to 100 μM baclofen, producing a mean depression of 26 ± 7% and 22 ± 2%, respectively (SE of 3 cells).

In conclusion, both baclofen and SK&F 97541 depress synaptic transmission in the dorsal striatum, hyperpolarize neurons in substantia nigra compacta, and decrease whole-cell calcium currents in neurons of dorsal root ganglia. Thus, the precise mechanism of presynaptic inhibition, whether by virtue of a presynaptic hyperpolarization or by a decrease in nerve terminal calcium conductance (or both),

---

[a]Address for correspondence: Department Pharmacology, Merck Sharp & Dohme Research Laboratories, Neuroscience Research Centre, Terling's Park, Eastwick Road, Harlow, Essex CM20 2QR, UK.

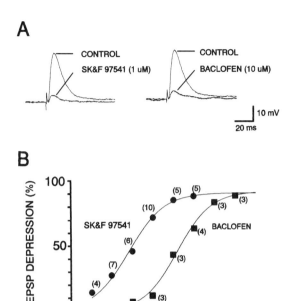

FIGURE 1. Striatal EPSPs recorded in the presence of 30 μM bicuculline methiodide were reversibly depressed by $GABA_B$ agonists in a concentration-dependent manner. **A:** Averaged (n = 10) records of EPSP from a single striatal neuron showing depression by SK&F 97541 (1 μM) and baclofen (10 μM). **B:** Dose-response curves constructed with data pooled from a number of cells as indicated in parentheses, ± SE. The calculated EC_{50} values and mean maximal inhibition were 0.092 μM and 92% for SK&F 97541 (circles), and 1.25 μM and 92% for baclofen (squares).

remains unclear. However, it is apparent, that SK&F 97541 is at least tenfold more potent than baclofen at $GABA_B$ receptors in neuronal tissue.

REFERENCES

1. SCOTT, R. H. & A. C. DOLPHIN. 1987. Nature **330:** 760–772.
2. LACEY, M. G., N. B. MERCURI & R. A. NORTH. 1988. J. Physiol. (Lond.) **401:** 437–453.
3. SEABROOK, G. R., W. HOWSON & M. G. LACEY. 1990. Electrophysiological characterization of potent agonists and antagonists at pre- and post-synaptic $GABA_B$ receptors in rat brain slices. Br. J. Pharmacol. **101:** 949–957.

A Comparison of the Subsecond Kinetics of Radiolabeled and Endogenous Glutamate Release from Rat Brain Synaptosomes

TIMOTHY J. TURNER AND KATHLEEN DUNLAP

Department of Physiology
Tufts University School of Medicine
Boston, Massachusetts 02111

Much of our knowledge of the mechanisms that underlie neurotransmitter release has come from studies of acetylcholine secretion at the vertebrate nerve-muscle junction. Although this body of work has provided us with a firm foundation on which to build an understanding of interneuronal synaptic transmission, it is becoming increasingly clear that many synapses in the central nervous system are characterized by properties different from those governing synaptic transmission in motor neurons, where release is thought to occur within one millisecond. Transmission of information between central or autonomic neurons and their targets often is complex. As a general rule, peptides are responsible for slower, modulatory effects, whereas classical transmitters control fast synaptic transmission. It remains to be determined, however, whether such differences reflect the time-course of the postsynaptic response, presynaptic release, or both, such that the pre- and postsynaptic mechanisms of neurotransmission are temporally coupled. Our aim has been to measure neurotransmitter release directly, on a time-scale approaching that on which synaptic events take place. In this report, we examined the kinetics of release of glutamate, an excitatory amino acid neurotransmitter in mammalian brain, from rat cortex synaptosomes, a preparation enriched in "pinched-off" nerve terminals. Glutamate release was measured by two techniques, by preloading synaptosomes with radiolabeled tracer ([^{3}H]glutamate), and by biochemical assay of endogenous glutamate, in order to assess whether measuring efflux of tritium is an accurate reflection of endogenous glutamate release.

The experiments were conducted using a device designed to measure release of transmitters on a subsecond time-scale.[1] The heart of the apparatus is a valve assembly in which three pressurized fluid reservoirs are connected to a central chamber fitted with three radially arranged solenoid valves. The superfusion chamber accommodates a filter "sandwich," the central layer of which contains the synaptosomes. This filter was layered between two others that protect the cells against shearing and turbulence. A 1 μm Millipore RA filter was placed beneath the filter sandwich to capture any debris that might have dislodged during superfusion. The routing of solutions from the pressurized reservoirs through the central chamber was controlled by an Apple IIe computer linked to the solenoid valves through an external relay device. This provided a simple, accurate means by which to rapidly switch between the different solutions during a single experimental run. The "dead volume" of the central chamber is small (ca. 30 μL) compared to the superfusion flow rate (1.5 mL/s), insuring a complete and rapid exchange of solutions. Control experiments have determined that solution exchange occurs with a time-constant of about 60 milliseconds. The synaptosomes were stimulated by superfusion with saline solutions containing an elevated potassium concentration. The superfusate flows through the central chamber and, after leaving the valve assembly, is collected in vials (15×45 mm) juxtaposed on the outer circumference of a circular platform, rotating on a phonographic turntable. At the speed at which these experiments were performed (16 r.p.m.), 50 fractions were collected in 3.6 s; that is, each fraction represents ~ 70 ms of release time.

When preloaded synaptosomes were superfused with solutions containing elevated KCl content (substituted symmetrically for NaCl), the rate of radioisotope efflux increased in proportion to the potassium concentration. The rate of release at [KCl] > 15 mM was maximally enhanced by adding millimolar concentrations of calcium. The calcium-dependent release (defined as the difference between release in the presence and absence of added calcium) is multiphasic; there is a fast component that lasts ≤ 200 ms accompanied by a slower component that lasts ~ 10 seconds. Note that Ca-dependent release continues well after the stimulating buffer is washed out of the chamber. Ca-independent release is probably mediated by reversal of the electrogenic, Na^+- and K^+-dependent glutamate transporter responsible for reuptake of released transmitter, inasmuch as Ca-independent release is largely eliminated by the glutamate uptake blocker β-3-hydroxyaspartate (not shown).

One of the major limitations of using radiolabeled transmitters to measure their release is the problem of incorporating the isotope uniformly in all releasable pools of transmitter. When glutaminergic nerve terminals are exposed to radiolabeled glutamate, specific, high-affinity transport pathways concentrate the isotope within the cytoplasm. A distinct, low-affinity, ATP-dependent, transport mechanism transports the labeled glutamate into secretory vesicles. The vesicles, however, are already laden with unlabeled endogenous transmitter. Thus, the specific activity of the transmitter stored in synaptic vesicles will be diluted, leading to an underestimate of release from these pools. Release of endogenous glutamate is not complicated by considerations of isotope penetration into various compartments. We adopted a biochemical approach to this problem, similar to that used by Nicholls et al.[2] to measure release of endogenous glutamate "on-line" using a fluorimetric assay employing glutamate dehydrogenase. The relatively small amounts of synaptosomal protein, however, combined with the rapid time-scales employed required a more sensitive cycling assay,[3] which could be performed "off-line" on samples collected using the superfusion device. For this enzymatic assay, glutamate is oxidized to α-ketoglutarate by glutamate dehydrogenase, which is cycled back to glutamate by glutamate-oxaloacetate transaminase (see diagram). The rate of NAD^+ formation is proportional to the glutamate concentration, and thus the signal is amplified linearly with cycling times up to 16 hours. The NAD^+ is converted quantitatively to a

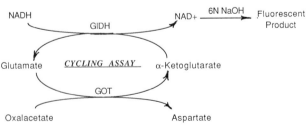

DIAGRAM 1.

A

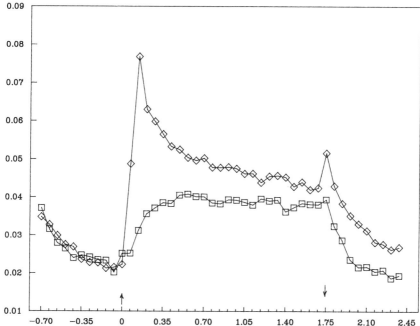

FIGURE 1. The subsecond time-course of synaptosomal release of radiolabeled (**A**) and endogenous (**B**) glutamate. **A:** Synaptosomes (50 μg/100 μL) were incubated with 5 μCi [³H]glutamate (46 Ci/mMol) at room temperature for 10 minutes, then applied to a filter sandwich and transferred to the superfusion device. The filter sandwich was washed with saline for 10 seconds, and efflux was measured in the same saline by collecting 15 fractions, 70 ms each. At time = 0, the superfusion solution was switched (indicated by "up" arrow) to a saline with 60 mM KCl, substituted on a equimolar basis for NaCl, either with (diamonds) or without (squares) 1.2 mM CaCl₂ added, and continued for 1.50 seconds, when the superfusion solution was switched back ("down" arrow) to the original saline. Results were calculated as a ratio of radioactivity in each fraction to the total radioactivity in all fractions plus radioactivity remaining on the filter at the end of the experiment. The results are plotted as [³H]glutamate release (% of total per fraction) versus time in seconds. **B:** Synaptosomes were treated as above, except the radiolabeling was omitted. Portions of each fraction were then transferred to 12 × 75 mm polystyrene tubes and reacted overnight in cycling assay mix. NAD⁺ formed was developed into a fluorescent product in 6 N NaOH and read in a Perkin-Elmer fluorimeter. Values were then obtained from a standard curve constructed with known amounts of added glutamate between 1 and 20 pmoles. The 20 pmole standard was at least 5 times greater than the uncorrected zero point and at least 20 times greater than the enzyme blank value. The results are plotted as pmoles of glutamate released versus time in seconds. Each data point is the average of three experiments performed on consecutive days.

fluorescent product in 6N NaOH, which is read in a fluorimeter (λ_{ex} = 365 nm, λ_{em} = 460 nm).

Synaptosomes were superfused with a solution containing 60 mM KCl +/− 1.2 mM Ca+2, and the fractions from each run were analyzed for glutamate content using the cycling assay. The kinetics of endogenous release were similar to those for the isotope (FIG. 1). The maximum release rate was 11.8 pmol/70 ms fraction; the comparable release rate observed with [³H]glutamate was 0.05% of total. The predicted synaptosomal content of glutamate (10 pmol per 100 µg/0.05%) is 200 nmole/mg. This predicted value is well above the reported values of synaptosomal glutamate content of 20–50 nmol/mg. Thus, the peak Ca-dependent release rates determined in isotope measurements probably underestimate release when calculated as a percent of total. This is consistent with a dilution of the specific activity of vesicular glutamate. Another difference is that Ca-independent release is below the level of detection of the assay, consistent with an overestimate of the Ca-independent component by isotope release measurements.

B

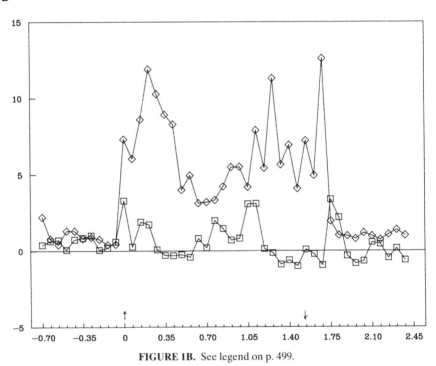

FIGURE 1B. See legend on p. 499.

We have developed methods to measure neurotransmitter release on a subsecond time-scale approaching that on which neurotransmission is thought to occur. We are arriving at a position to apply these methods to measuring release from intact cultured neurons, a system in which we hope to be able to evoke release using more relevant stimuli, such as field depolarization. This, coupled with parallel electrophysiological studies of neurotransmission between synaptically paired neurons, will provide a direct measure of the contribution of presynaptic release kinetics to the postsynaptic response.

REFERENCES

1. TURNER, T. J. & S. M. GOLDIN. 1989. Biochemistry **28:** 586–593.
2. NICHOLLS, D. G. 1989. J. Neurochem. **52:** 331–341.
3. LOWERY, O. H. & J. V. PASSONNEAU. 1972. *In* A Flexible System of Enzymatic Analysis.
    143. Academic Press. Orlando, FL.

Effect of Calcium on Presynaptic Inhibition in the Isolated Spinal Cord of Newborn Rats

ZHU LI-XIA AND CAO CHANG-QING

Department of Physiology
Institute of Acupuncture
Academy of Traditional Chinese Medicine
Beijing 100700, China

It was reported that presynaptic inhibition is due to a decrease in influx of calcium into the nerve terminal.[1] In this paper, the effect of calcium on presynaptic inhibition was further investigated by using Ca^{2+} agonist Bay K 8644 and Ca^{2+} antagonist nimodipine[2] in isolated spinal cord.

The spinal cords with four dorsal roots (L3–L6) were isolated from 6–12-day-old rats and superfused with artificial cerebrospinal fluid (CSF) containing 2.4 mM $CaCl_2$. Dorsal root potentials (DRP) were recorded with a suction electrode and induced by supramaximal stimulation of an adjacent dorsal root. The amplitude and the course of the fifth component (V wave) of DRP, which represents primary afferent depolarization, were measured. All drugs were bath-applied.

Bay K 8644 10^{-4}M markedly enhanced the V waves. Forty minutes after the application of Bay K 8644, the amplitude of V waves was increased to $136.7 \pm 11.7\%$ of the control ($p < 0.01$, n = 17), and the course was prolonged to $106.4 \pm 2.1\%$ ($p < 0.05$, n = 17). The vehicle (ethyl alcohol), however, did not show significant change. The enhancement was extremely long-lasting. In the majority of cases it

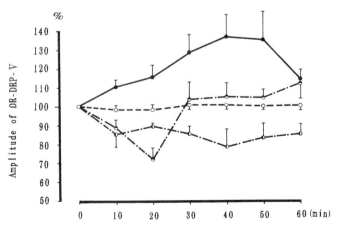

FIGURE 1. Bath application of Bay K 8644 (10^{-4}M) (●—●) could enhance the DR-DRP-V (n = 17, $p < 0.01$), whereas the vehicle did not show significant change (○—○, n = 6). The enhancement induced by Bay K 8644 could be reversed by bicuculline (10^{-4}M) (◓---◓, n = 6) or naloxone (10^{-4}M) (◐---◐, n = 6) ($p < 0.01$).

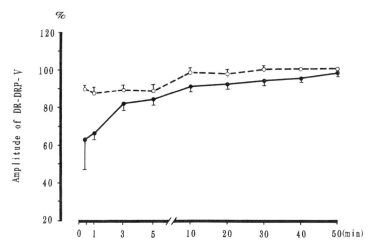

FIGURE 2. Bath application of nimodipine (10^{-4}M) (●—●) could significantly depress the DR-DRP-V (n = 10, p < 0.01), whereas the vehicle (○—○) slightly depresses. The difference between the two groups is significant (p < 0.01).

lasted up to 60 minutes, and in three cases it lasted up to about 180 minutes. When Bay K 8644 was applied together with bicuculline (10^{-4}M) or naloxone (10^{-4}M), the V waves were depressed rather than enhanced (FIG. 1). It means that the enhancement of V waves produced by Bay K 8644 could be reversed by bicuculline and naloxone (n = 6, p < 0.001).

In a further experiment, depolarization of dorsal root ganglion neurons recorded intracellularly could also be induced by bath applications of Bay K 8644, with a decrease in amplitude and prolongation of duration of the action potentials.

The new calcium antagonist nimodipine (10^{-4}M) produced marked depression on the V waves by 33.6 ± 6.1% (n = 10, p < 0.05), whereas the vehicle slightly reduced the V waves (FIG. 2). The difference between the two groups is of significance (p < 0.01).

In 13 preparations superfused with CSF containing 0.1 mM $CaCl_2$ and 2.3 mM $MgCl_2$, the V waves were totally abolished in 5 and depressed by 84–98% in the other eight.

These results indicate that the presence of calcium ions is an essential requirement for presynaptic inhibition. Calcium agonist Bay K 8644 can enhance DRP resulting from primary afferent depolarization through increasing the release of GABA and endogenous opioid peptides. Nimodipine can markedly depress the V wave by blocking the entry of calcium into the nerve terminals related to DRP.

REFERENCES

1. KANDEL, E. R. & J. H. SCHWARTZ, Eds. 1981. Principles of Neural Science. Elsevier/North-Holland.
2. BETZ, E. 1985. Nimodipine Pharmacological and Clinical Properties. Stuttgart Schattauer Verlag.

Index of Contributors

505